MEDICAL ASSISTING TEST PREP

Comprehensive Study Guide and Workbook for CMA(AAMA), 2025-2026

Published by

MERLINO EDUCATION

ISBN-13: 978-1-962766-01-2

Photo credits: Amanda Merlino, Desmond Merlino, Jeff Merlino, Starrisa Nordstrom, Ashley Capone, TJ Wilson, Rose Matthews, Frank Butler.

Stock photos via Shutterstock. Cover by Rocky McCahan.

Special Thanks: Every school and student who has used any of my guides, everyone who has supported me in my endeavors, my family, friends, Rocky McCahan, Tim Ferriss.

PUBLISHER'S DISCLAIMER

The material presented in this study guide is for informational purposes only. Any information regarding Medications, CPR, First Aid, and medical treatments should be researched by the reader to obtain the most up-to-date requirements, as these subjects are ever-changing.

"CMA" is a registered trademark of the American Association of Medical Assistants(AAMA). This study guide and the contents therein are not endorsed by the AAMA.

MERLINO EDUCATION

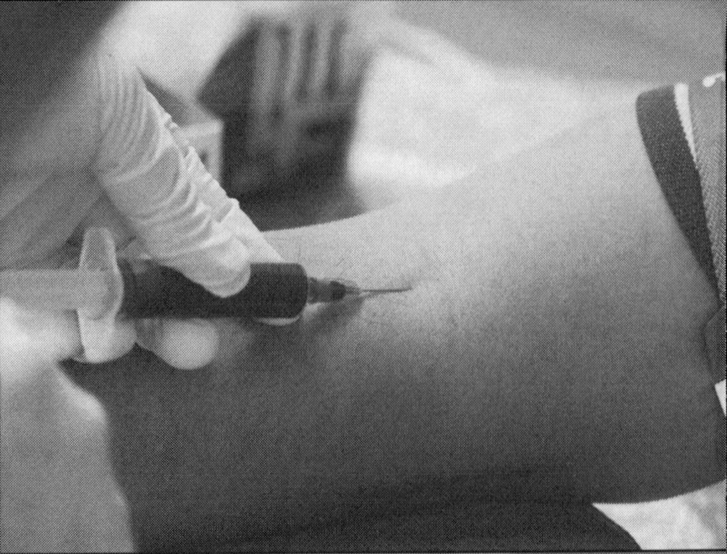

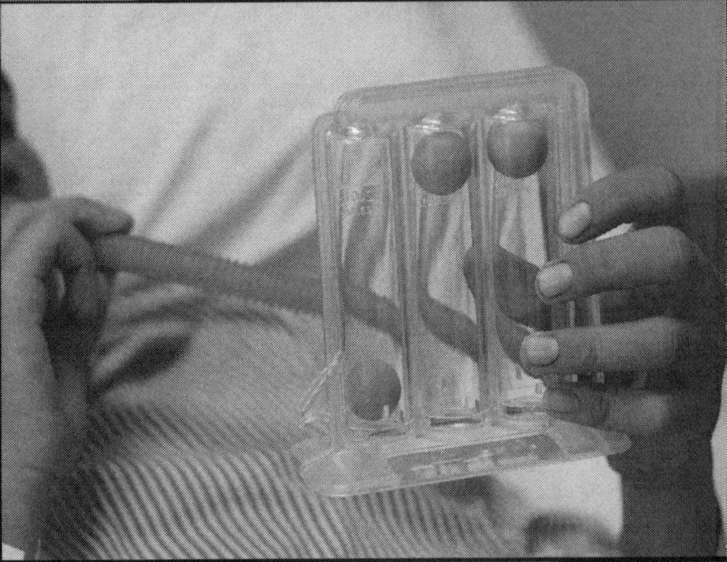

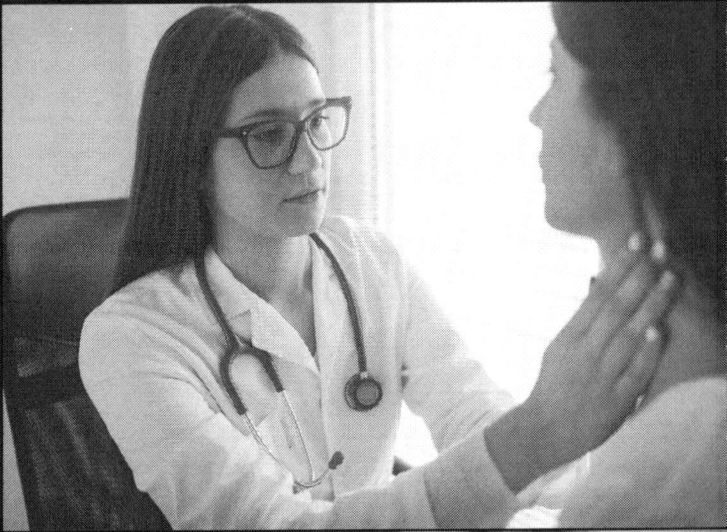

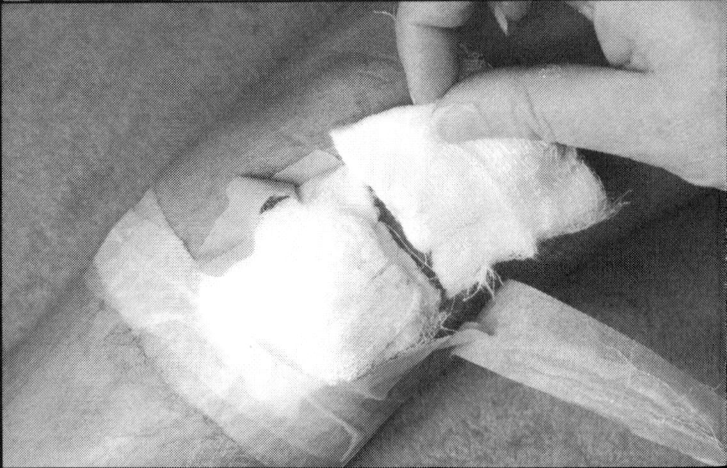

About the CMA(AAMA) Test

The Certified Medical Assistant Certification Exam is administered by the Certifying Board of the American Association of Medical Assistants. This exam is designed to test to competencies of those seeking to obtain certification in the field of Medical Assisting.

The CMA Exam, administered by the AAMA, is offered to students who are eligible to test via completion of a CAAHEP-accredited or ABHES-accredited medical assisting program. The student may take the exam up to 30 days before completion of education. A graduate of a postsecondary medical assisting program may also be eligible to test. Candidates may test up three times. If a candidate does not pass an attempt, they may reschedule the exam immediately and test again at the earliest opportunity.

The exam consists of three main sections: General, Administrative, and Clinical.

General consists of the following subcategories: Psychology, Communication, Professionalism, Medical Law/Regulatory Guidelines, Medical Ethics, Risk Management, Quality Assurance, and Safety, and Medical Terminology.

Administrative consists of the following subcategories: Medical Reception, Patient Navigator/Advocate, Medical Business Practices, Establish Patient Medical Record, Scheduling Appointments, and Practice Finances.

Clinical consists of the following subcategories: Anatomy and Physiology, Infection Control, Patient Intake and Documentation of Care, Patient Preparation and Assisting the Provider, Nutrition, Collecting and Processing Specimens, Diagnostic Testing, Pharmacology, and Emergency Management/Basic First Aid.

Each test consists of 200 questions, all multiple choice, and is split into four segments of 40 minutes each, for a total of 160 minutes of potential testing time. Short breaks are offered after each 40 minute segment.

How To Use This Study Guide

This study guide is designed to not just TELL information, but to help you LEARN information. This is achieved in many different ways, including standard study guides, assignments, and practice exams.

To get the complete, most effective and efficient experience from this study guide, I recommend the following:

Before starting, figure out the area you need to study the most: Clinical Workflow, Medical Terminology, Safety and Infection Control, Procedures/Examinations, Anatomy and Physiology, Pathology, Pharmacology, Legal and Ethical Issues, Communication, and Billing, Coding, Insurance, and Scheduling. A common study routine I've helped many students implement is the following(you can change the subjects as you see fit, depending on how comfortable you are with each), with an average of six weeks of study time before the exam:

What subjects do you need to study most? Write them down below and include the amount of time to study each!

Week 1: ____________________

Week 2: ____________________

Week 3: ____________________

Week 4: ____________________

Week 5: ____________________

Week 1: Study Subject 1 for five hours, and Subject 2 for five hours.
Week 2: Study Subjects 1 and 2 for two hours combined, Subject 3 for four hours, and Subject 4 for four hours.
Week 3: Study Subjects 1, 2, 3, and 4 for two hours combined, Subject 5 for four hours, and Subject 6 for four hours.
Week 4: Study Subjects 1, 2, 3, 4, 5, and 6 for two hours combined, Subject 7 for four hours, and Subject 8 for four hours.
Week 5: Study Subjects 1, 2, 3, 4, 5, 6, 7, and 8 for two hours combined, Subject 9 for four hours, and Subject 10 for four hours.
Week 6: Study every subject an equal amount of time, one hour per subject.

I've found that this way of studying is great for long-term memory growth in these subjects, as there is a consistent review of information every week.

While studying, be sure to finish the assignments and practice tests in the book. These are great for assessing your knowledge on the subjects you will have just covered, and help you figure out what you still need to study, and what you've learned.

I do have other products available that are by no means required, but they may be extremely beneficial in your studying efforts! Please check them out below and see if they can help you be even more prepared!

CMA Test Prep App

I have created a brand new smart phone app that is a fantastic compliment to this study guide! The free version of the app contains 180 free practice test questions, while upgrading to premium grants access to a complete content review, 2000+ practice test questions, 1600+ flash cards, and a matching assignment feature! Just search for "**CMA Test Prep**" on the Apple App Store or Google Play Store, or scan the QR code below for your device!

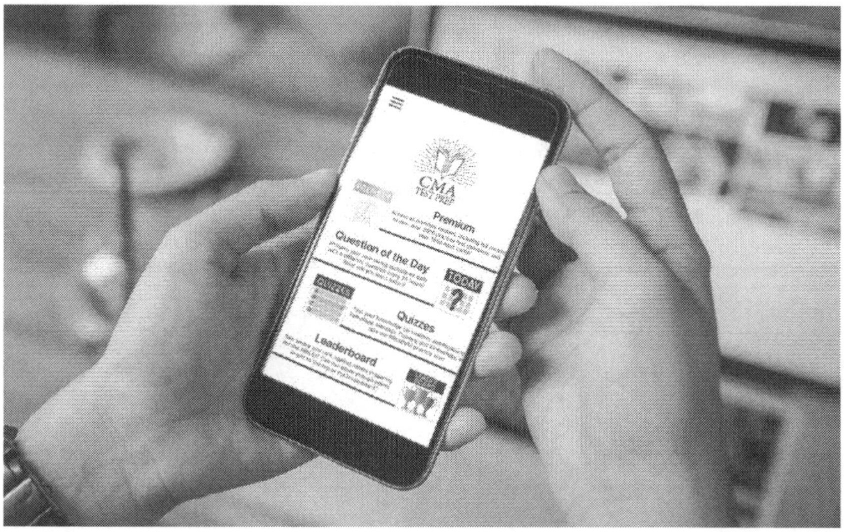

iPhone

Android

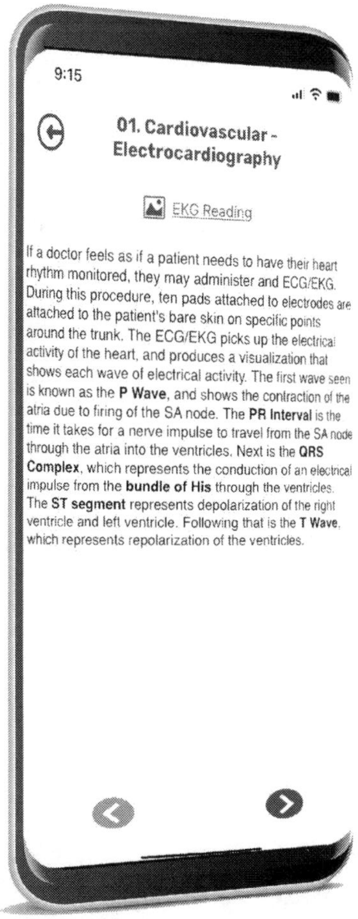

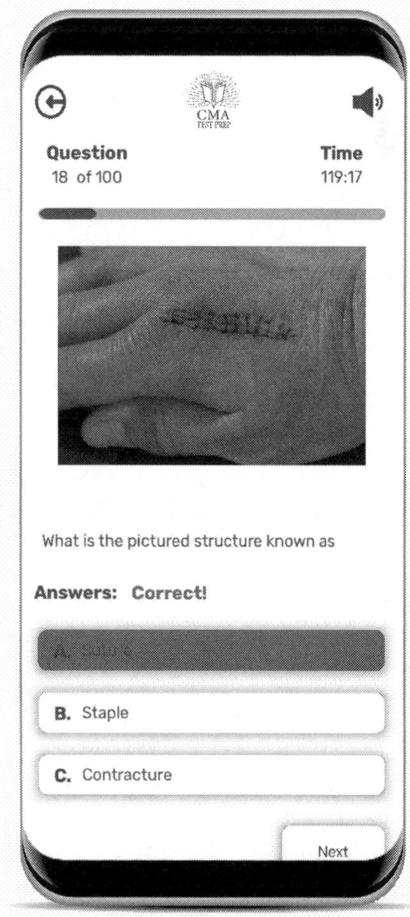

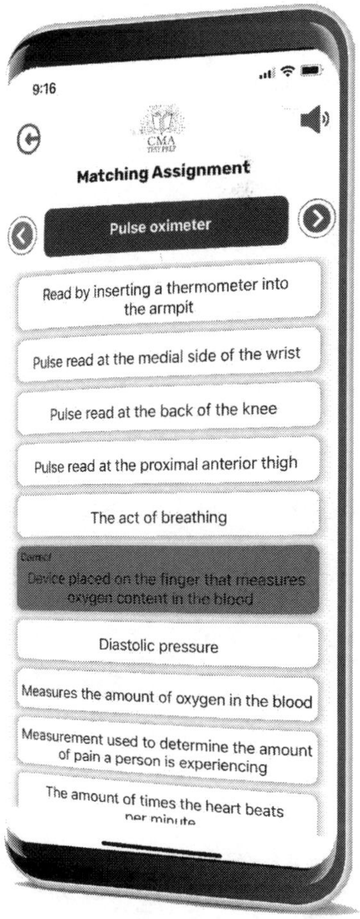

Study Skills

1. Do not do all of your studying the night before or day of the test. Study consistently, up to several times per week. Cramming is good for short-term learning, but does not help with long-term learning. The more you study, the more likely you are to retain the information.

2. Use all of your class and home work as study material. The information in these assignments is information that may be seen on the exam.

3. Take many short breaks as you study. Memory retention is higher at the beginning and end of study sessions than it is in the middle. This is called the Serial Position Effect. Study for no longer than ten minutes, then take a short break, and resume studying for another ten minutes.

4. Focus on one subject at a time while studying. You don't want to confuse yourself by mixing information.

5. Study the subject you have the most difficulty with more than the subjects you are comfortable with. Studying what you aren't weak in doesn't help. If you need work on a specific subject, focus the majority of your time learning that information, even if it means taking away study time from other areas. You're better off being 80% proficient in every subject than 100% in four subjects and only 50% in the last. Not studying this information could prevent you from passing the exam.

6. While studying, take notes on important information, especially if it's information you don't recognize or remember. Use this information to study with.

7. Assign yourself tests, reports, assignments, and projects to complete. You are more likely to remember information if you write a report on it than if you just read the information.

8. Teach information you are studying to another person. If you are responsible for someone learning something, you have to know and understand the material, and be able to put that information into the simplest terms possible, so someone else can understand it. This will only help you. Trust me, from personal experience, this works extremely well.

9. Understand the material you are studying. Do not just try to memorize certain answers you think may be on the test. Certain "key words" might not be on the test. Learn everything about a subject, and you'll never get any question on that subject wrong.

Test-Taking Tips

1. Go to the restroom before taking the exam. Using the restroom beforehand ensures that you are 100% focused on the exam, and not on your bladder.

2. Read the entire question slowly and carefully. Never make assumptions about what a question is asking. Assuming you know what a question is asking may lead you to missing key words in the question that tell you exactly what the question is asking. Read every single word in every single question, multiple times if necessary.

3. Understand what the question is asking before you try answering it.

4. Identify key words in each question. Key words are words that tell you exactly what the question is asking. Identify these words easily by reading question aloud to yourself. The words you find yourself emphasizing while reading aloud are likely the key words.

Here is an example. Read this question aloud:
Q. Which of the following statements is true regarding erythrocyte sedimentation rate?

In this question, there are two key words, which are telling you exactly what the question is asking. Which words did you find yourself putting emphasis on? Most likely, you read the question like this: "Which of the following statements is TRUE regarding ERYTHROCYTE SEDIMENTATION RATE?" These are the key words.

5. Do not change your answers, unless you misread the question. Changing your answers puts doubt into your mind, and leads to more changing of answers. The answer you put first is usually correct. Do not change your answers!

6. Match key words in the answers with key words in the questions. Sometimes it's as simple as matching terms, if you've exhausted all other avenues.

7. Eliminate answers you know aren't correct and justify the reason they aren't correct. If you can eliminate one answer from each question, that brings your odds of getting that question right up to 33%. If you can eliminate two answers that can't be right, that brings it up to 50%. Then it's just a coin flip!

Here's an example. Read the question, and the answers:
Q. Of the following, which is not contagious?
A. Athlete's foot
B. Herpes simplex
C. Influenza
D. Osgood-Schlatter Disease

Have you ever heard of Osgood-Schlatter Disease? Even if you haven't, you can still get this question right by eliminating the other answers. Athlete's foot is caused by a fungus, and is contagious. That leaves us with three possible answers(33% chance). Herpes simplex is caused by a virus, and is contagious. That leaves us with two possible answers(50% chance). So even if you're guessing at this point, it's only a 50/50 chance you get it right! Influenza is caused by a virus, and is contagious. This process of elimination just gave us the answer, D. Osgood-Schlatter Disease.

8. Read the entire question before looking at the answers. Again, never make assumptions about what the question is asking.

9. Come up with the answer in your head before looking at the answers. If the same answer you come up with is in the list of answers, that's most likely the right answer.

10. Read every answer given to make sure you are picking the most correct answer. Some questions have multiple right answers, and you need to make sure you're picking the most correct answer.

11. Make sure you are properly hydrated before the test. Studies have been done on the effects of proper hydration on those taking tests. People who are properly hydrated tend to score higher than those who are not.

12. Exercise for twenty minutes before the exam. Exercise has also been shown to increase test scores.

Reducing Test Anxiety

1. Study consistently. If you understand the material, you won't be as stressed out about the test. There are ways you can study without this book or your class notes as well. An example, whenever you take a bite of food, think about every structure the food passes through in the digestive tract and what each of the organs do. Another example, whenever you are massaging someone, tell yourself everything about every muscle you work on, like origin, insertion, and action.

2. Keep a positive attitude while preparing for the test and during the test. If you think you're going to fail, you will not be as motivated to study, you won't adhere to your test-taking techniques, you'll become stressed out during the exam much more easily, and you'll be more likely to fail.

3. Try to stay relaxed. Utilize deep breathing techniques to calm down if you start feeling nervous or stressed. You will have two hours to finish the exam. You can afford one or two minutes to calm yourself down if you need to.

4. Exercise consistently up until the day of the test to reduce anxiety. Exercise has been shown to significantly reduce stress, and also helps with memory retention. Try utilizing flash cards while riding an exercise bike.

5. Take your time on the test. If you find yourself rushing, slow down. Again, you have two hours to finish the exam. Do not rush through it. You may miss important information in the exam and answer questions incorrectly because of this.

I hated every minute of training, but I said "Don't quit. Suffer now and live the rest of your life as a champion."

- Muhammad Ali

Clinical Workflow

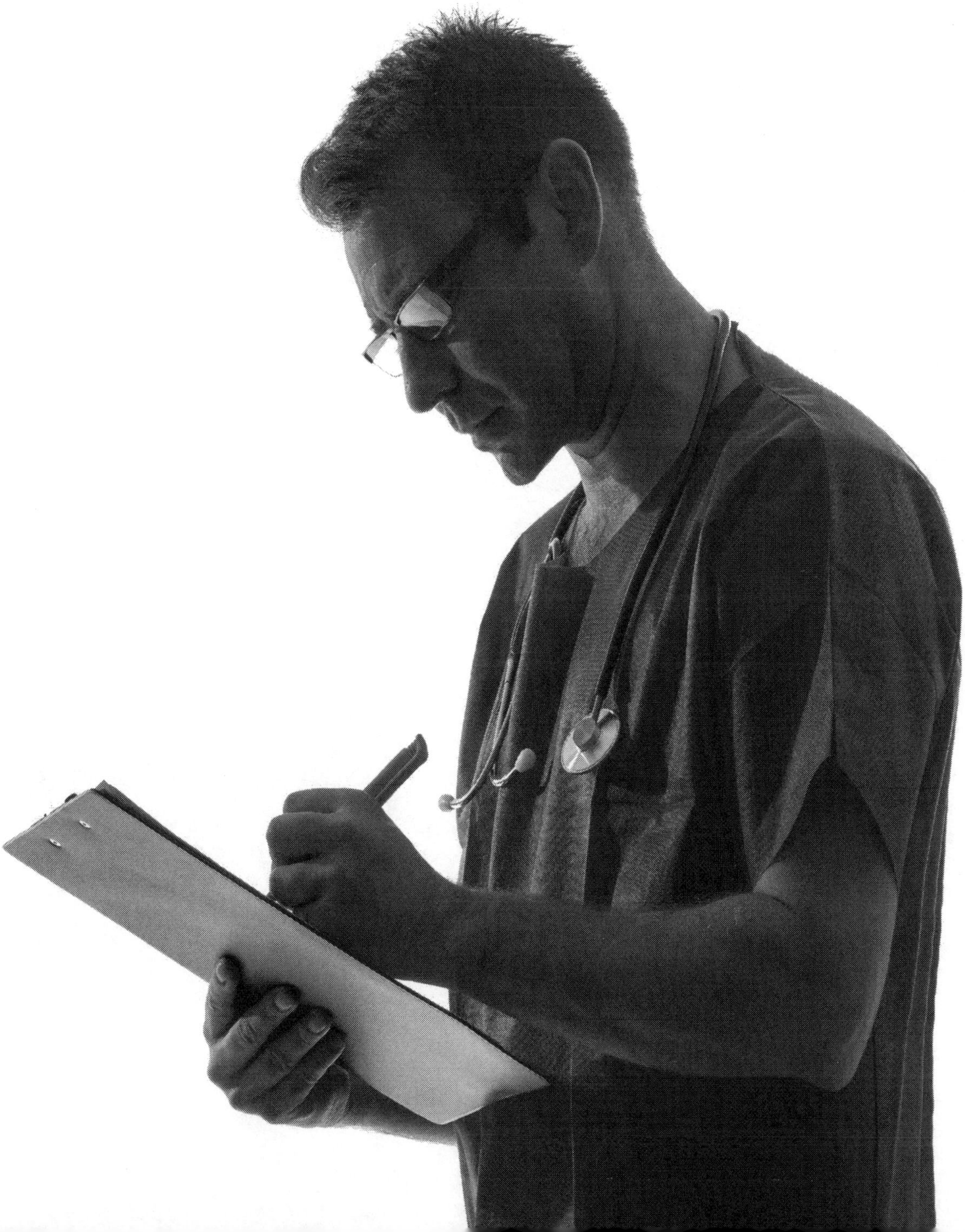

Vital Signs

Vital signs are the indication of the body's ability to maintain homeostasis. Primary vital signs include temperature, blood pressure, pulse, height, weight, oxygen saturation, and respiration.

Blood Pressure

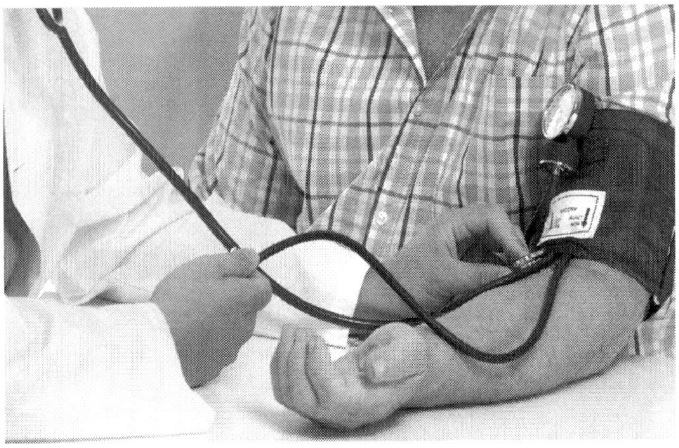

Blood pressure is the pressure felt in arteries as blood passes through them. Blood pressure is determined by the pressure exerted by the heart during ventricular contraction. Blood pressure is most commonly read using a **sphygmomanometer**. During a blood pressure reading, the sphygmomanometer cuff is wrapped around a person's arm and inflated at a pressure greater than systolic pressure, usually 180mmHg. A valve is then opened, and the pressure in the cuff is gradually decreased, until it reaches the same pressure as the systolic pressure. This produces sounds that can be heard using a **stethoscope** placed on the anterior elbow. The bell of the stethoscope picks up the sound of blood flowing through the arteries. If sound is unable to be heard at the antecubital fossa, the brachial artery may be used.

In a blood pressure reading, two numbers are given: **systolic pressure** and **diastolic pressure**. Systolic pressure measures the amount of pressure in the arteries as blood passes through them. This is caused by the left ventricle contracting, sending blood throughout the body. The diastolic pressure measures the amount of pressure in the arteries when there is not blood passing through them. This is caused by relaxation of the left ventricle between heart beats.

A normal blood pressure is read as systolic pressure over diastolic pressure. According to the American Heart Association, blood pressure is listed as: normal(below 120/below 80), elevated(120-129/less than 80), high blood pressure stage 1(130-139/80-89), high blood pressure stage 2(140+/90+), and hypertensive crisis(180+/120+).

Normal blood pressure ranges:
Infant: 60-95/50-65
1-5 years: 80-100/50-70
6-10 years: 80-120/50-80
11-15 years: 95-135/58-88
Adult: 90-120/60-80

Height, Weight, and BMI

Body Mass Index is a measurement of **body fat**, and is based on the **height and weight** of an adult. Adult weight should fall into a specified range based on their height. BMI can help determine if a person is too light, an average weight, overweight, or obese. However, BMI does not take into account the contributing weight due to muscle loss as a person ages, or muscle mass due to a person having a more athletic build. BMI can be measured using a BMI machine that sends an electric signal through the body. This electric signal moves slowly through fat, and the amount of electricity passing from one side of the body to the other helps determine fat percentage.

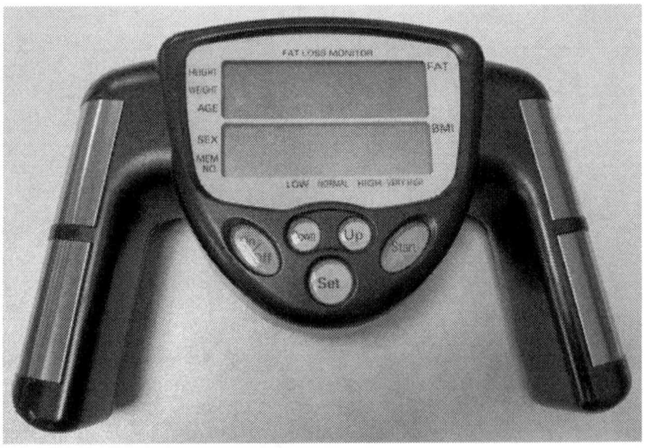

Pulse

A person's pulse is used to determine **heart rhythm** and **heart rate**. Heart rhythm refers to the regularity of the heart beat, the contractions of the atria and ventricles that pump blood through the heart and throughout the body. Heart rate refers to the **amount of times the heart beats per minute**. A pulse may be read manually by placing the index and middle fingers on the pulse point being tested. Certain pulse points, such as the apical pulse, are read with use of a stethoscope.

Pulse can be read at numerous different locations on the body.

- **Radial pulse** is read at the lateral side of the wrist, and is the most common site to read a pulse.
- **Ulnar pulse** is read at the medial side of the wrist.
- **Brachial pulse** is read at the medial side of the arm, and is commonly used to determine the pulse of infants.
- **Apical pulse** is read at the apex of the heart, and requires the use of a stethoscope.
- **Carotid pulse** is read at the neck, and is used to determine pulse in adults.
- **Femoral pulse** is read at the proximal anterior thigh, and is used to determine pulse in adults.
- **Popliteal pulse** is read at the back of the knee, or the popliteal region.
- **Dorsalis pedis** pulse is read on the dorsal surface of the foot.

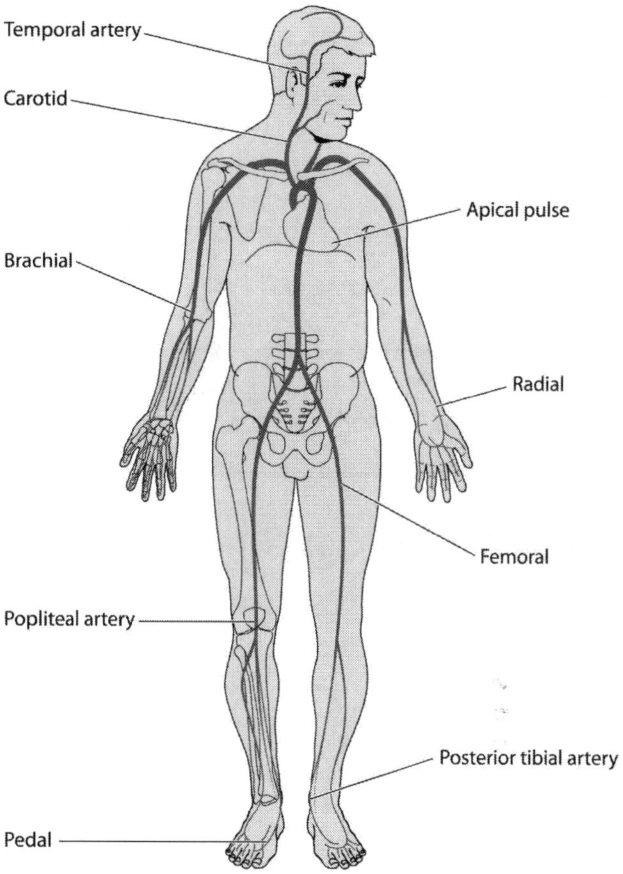

Normal pulse ranges:
Infant: 80-160 beats per minute
1-5 years: 75-130 beats per minute
6-10 years: 70-115 beats per minute
11-15 years: 55-110 beats per minute
Adult: 60-100 beats per minute

Body Temperature

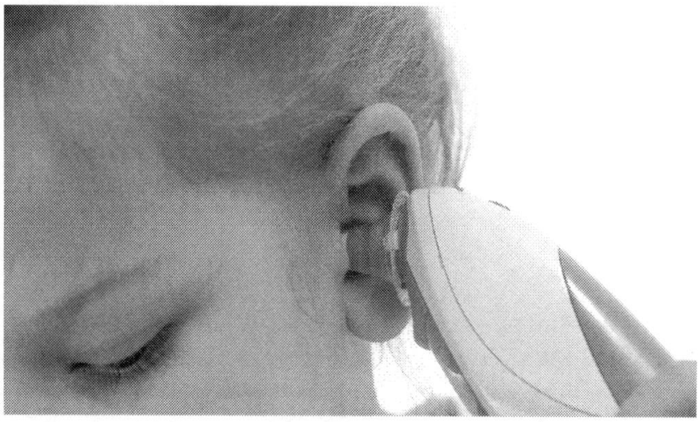

Temperature may be measured in several different areas, utilizing a thermometer. An elevated body temperature is often indicative of some sort of systemic infection, such as influenza. The type of thermometer used is dependent on the location of the temperature measurement. **Oral** or **sublingual** temperature is measured by inserting the thermometer **under the tongue**(sublingual) or **in the cheek**(buccal). Sublingual is the preferred oral measurement. Baseline temperature for an oral or sublingual temperature is 98.6 degrees Fahrenheit. An **axillary** temperature is measured by inserting the thermometer into the **armpit.** Baseline temperature is one degree less than oral/sublingual temperature. **Rectal** temperature is measured by inserting the thermometer into the **rectum.** Rectal temperature is considered the best way to measure core temperature. Baseline temperature is one degree higher than oral/sublingual temperature. **Aural** temperature is measured by reading the temperature of the **tympanic membrane** inside the ear.

Normal temperature ranges:
Infant: 96-100
1-5 years: 98-100
6-10 years: 97-99.5
11-15 years: 97.5-100.5
Adult: 97.5-100.5

Pulse Oximetry

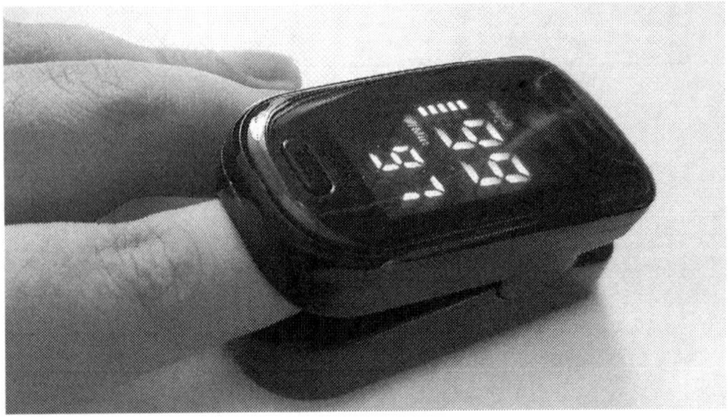

Pulse oximetry is used to measure the amount of **oxygen in the blood**. Pulse oximetry is measured with use of a **pulse oximeter**, a small device that is placed on a finger. Pulse oximeters work by passing light through the finger. The light read by the pulse oximeter provides information on the amount of oxygen in the blood. The amount of oxygen measured is known as the oxygen saturation level, which is the amount of oxygen currently being carried by the body compared to how much oxygen the body is capable of carrying.

Respiration

Respiration refers to the act of **breathing**. Respiration is measured by observing **breathing pattern**, **breathing rate**, and the **depth of breath**. Breathing pattern can be used to determine if there are abnormalities in breathing, such as apnea. Breathing rate refers to the amount of breaths a person takes during a one minute span. Depth of breath, also known as tidal volume, refers to the amount of air a person is able to take in during inspiration and expel during expiration. Inspiration is inhalation of oxygen into the body, and expiration is exhalation of carbon dioxide and other waste products.

Normal respiration rate:
Infant: 25-40 breaths per minute
1-5 years: 20-30 breaths per minute
6-10 years: 18-25 breaths per minute
11-15 years: 16-25 breaths per minute
Adult: 12-20 breaths per minute

Pain Scale

Pain levels may be utilized to determine exactly how painful an area or condition is. A **pain scale** is usually based on numerical value, ranging from **1-5 or 1-10**. The higher the number a patient states, the more pain they are experiencing. For example, if a patient were to state that their back pain was at a 6 out of 10, then the pain they are feeling is present and noticeable, but probably does not affect their ability to perform every day actions.

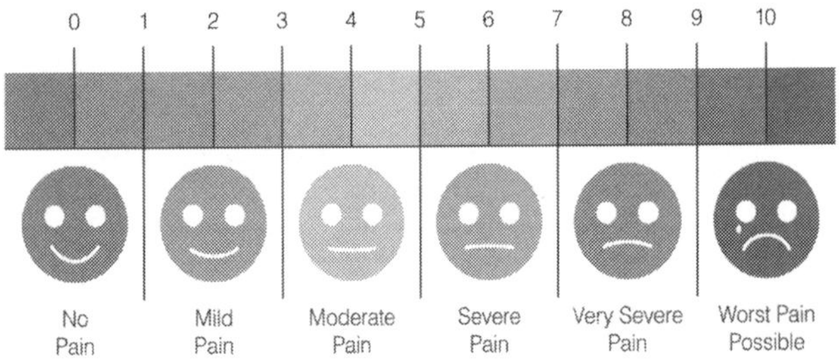

Some questions to consider when dealing with pain: Is this pain acute and localized in one specific area, such as sprained ankles? Is the pain widespread and more chronic, such as with Multiple Sclerosis? Does the pain come and go, or is it persistent? What does the pain feel like? How long has the pain been present?

Varying levels of chronic pain may require the patient to be prescribed certain types of pain medication. Patients with lower levels of pain may be prescribed non-opioid pain relievers such as acetaminophen, and adjuvants such as non-steroidal anti-inflammatory drugs. Moderate levels of pain may see the patient prescribed a weaker form of opioid such as oxycodone, in conjunction with acetaminophen and a non-steroidal anti-inflammatory drug. Severe pain typically sees the patient prescribed a stronger form of opioid such as morphine, along with acetaminophen and non-steroidal anti-inflammatory drugs. The goal for severe pain is to eliminate the pain altogether, while moderate and mild pain is treated by lessening the pain and preventing the pain from becoming worse for the patient.

Pediatric Exam

A **pediatric exam** is a physical examination of a **child**. This examination is performed to ensure the child is growing at a normal rate, both in height and weight, and developmentally. Each age has certain milestones that are likely for a child to have met, and each are examined and tested.

A **growth chart** is used to measure the **physical growth** of a child. Growth encompasses height, weight, and head circumference. These measurements are compared to the general population, and this gives an overall view of the child's growth rate compared to the majority of other children.

Interviewing Techniques

Obtaining accurate and concise information from the patient is an important step in successful treatment. If the information being requested of the patient is asked in a way the patient isn't open to, the patient may become defensive and uncooperative in providing sufficient answers. The prime way to influence a patient to become cooperative is by utilizing motivational interviewing techniques. The four processes of motivation interviewing are engaging, focusing, evoking, and planning. All four of these processes help an interviewer utilize the OARS technique effectively.

Engaging helps the interviewer build a **strong rapport** with the patient. The goal of engaging is to help the patient become comfortable with the interviewer, and to feel as if their needs are being heard and understood. These allow the patient to feel a sense of safety in the environment and with the person they are interacting with.

Focusing is the interviewer **determining a proper direction** or goal if one isn't established at the beginning of the interview. Some patients may take longer to open up to the interviewer about their goals and any changes they are hoping to make.

Evoking is used to help a patient identify **why** they are hoping to achieve **specific goals**. Is the goal they are hoping to reach for their own interest or betterment, or for someone else? What are the motivating factors for wanting to achieve this goal? What behaviors are needed, or need to change, to reach this goal? These can help define the reasons for the goal, and help the patient take necessary steps and stay motivated towards reaching their goal.

Planning involves **developing a commitment** from the patient to change behaviors to help achieve their stated goal. This step can involve establishing specific steps the patient can take that lead toward the goal being reached. Not only can these steps be from the patient, but they can involve the patient building a supportive culture around themselves to help keep them motivated and on track.

An effective motivational interviewing technique is utilizing **OARS**: open questioning, affirming, reflecting, and summarizing.

An **open-ended question** is a question used when asking for **feedback** from patients. Often, open-ended questions are meant to extract more detail or information. It allows the answer to be more open and abstract. This varies from a **close-ended question**, a question used when asking for a **yes-or-no response** only. These questions are used to extract important pieces of information in a short amount of time. When time is a factor, close-ended questions are primarily used to gather the important information without sacrificing too much time.

Affirming is **acknowledging a patient's behaviors**, and help the patient feel as if they are being understood and empathized with. Affirming positive behaviors can help the patient maintain positive changes leading towards desired outcomes, helping to improve the patient's confidence.

Reflecting helps the interviewer engage with the patient by ensuring the patient is being heard. The interviewer should utilize **active listening techniques**. After a patient makes a statement, the statement should be closely considered by the interviewer to determine if there was any miscommunication, if the patient actually meant to say something else and simply used the wrong terms, or if the interviewer has a different definition of what the patient has said. Reflecting on the statement with the patient, and restating what the patient has said, can help to clarify information the patient is providing. The statement may also be rephrased to help come to a better understanding, and/or paraphrased if the original statement was long and can be distilled down into a shorter statement with the same meaning.

Summarizing is an extension of reflecting. Summarizing is a useful tool to ensure there is no miscommunication, as the interviewer will summarize the patient's statement with their own leading statement such as, "If I understand correctly", or "I'm going to repeat back what I understand, please let me know if anything is incorrect." Summarizing the information helps assure the patient that they have been heard, understood, and that the interviewer is open to clarification from the patient. Summarizing also gives the interviewer an opportunity to transition to a new topic or question if no further clarification is needed on the statement.

Documentation of Care

Medical records are required to be documented, not only to protect the practice, but to protect the patient.

Subjective Data

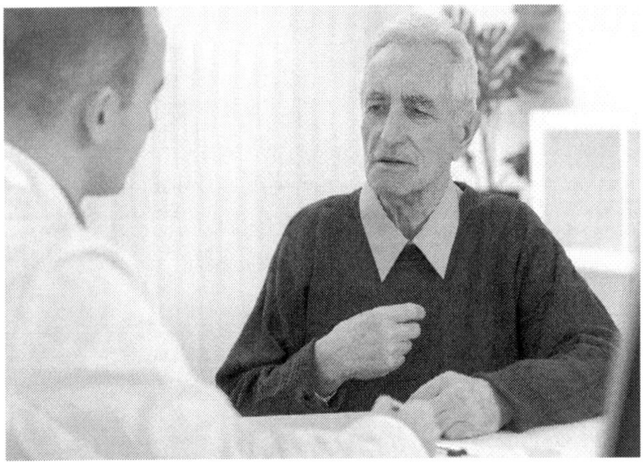

Subjective data is any information the **patient provides about themselves.** This information is typically not able to be measured, and is left up to the patient's interpretation. Documentation of subjective information should include the following information:

The **chief complaint**, which is the primary reason a patient has come in for treatment. There may be associated complaints, but the chief complaint is the primary reason for the visit.

Present illnesses the patient may be experiencing. These can give an indication of why a person may be experiencing the chief complaint, or the chief complaint may be causing the present illness.

Review of systems involves asking questions regarding specific **body systems and organs.** This can help determine if any specific structures or body systems are contributing to the patient's chief complaint.

Past medical history should be established to determine any patterns of the development of the chief complaint, to determine proper course of treatment based on prior health history, and to determine if the chief complaint is acute or chronic in nature.

Medications and allergies should be documented. Medications may play a role in a patient's chief complaint, and should be considered to rule out complications. A patient may have allergies, and be allergic to specific forms of medication or materials used in a medical environment, and these allergies should be documented to make efforts to avoid the allergen.

Family history should be established to determine in there is any likelihood that a chief complaint or illness is genetic, or if the patient has an increased chance of developing a specific disease or condition.

Social and occupational history should be documented to give insights into the person's daily life, what kind of activities they are performing each day, and if any of these activities can contribute to the development of a disease or condition. These activities may affect the person physically or mentally.

Objective Data

Objective data is any data that can actually be **physically measured.** This information is not up to opinion, but is factual in nature. An example, if a patient has a visible rash on an arm, this is something that can be seen, the size of the rash can be measured, and spreading of the rash can be observed. This is all information that falls under objective data.

Treatment/Compliance

Compliance is adhering to laws, regulations, and guidelines that apply to a person or medical practice's operation. Compliance maintains safety, prevents potential violations in areas such as HIPAA, and provides the patient with the best care possible.

Making Corrections

If an error is made on a medical record that needs to be corrected, the following steps should be taken: the erroneous information should be marked through with a **single line.** The new entry in the medical record should be **signed, dated, and timed.** The new entry may need to be directed to from the erroneous information, such as "see opposite page". The erroneous information must not be erased or removed in any way.

Patient Screenings/Wellness Assessments

Preventative care is extremely important in maintaining health and helping to prevent infections, diseases, and conditions. While not always 100% effective, preventative care can severely lessen the chances of certain disorders from arising.

Cancer Screening

Cancer screening is performed to check a person for cancer, even if symptoms are not present. Examples of cancer screening procedures include mammograms, Pap smears, CT scans, ultrasound, observation, and palpation of certain areas.

A **mammogram** is a procedure used to detect **breast cancer** in patients who are not showing any symptoms. It uses an **X-ray** to view the internal breast tissue. A mammogram is typically performed by placing the breast between **two glass plates** that **compress** the tissue. Compressing the tissue allows the X-ray to view all of the breast without missing anything.

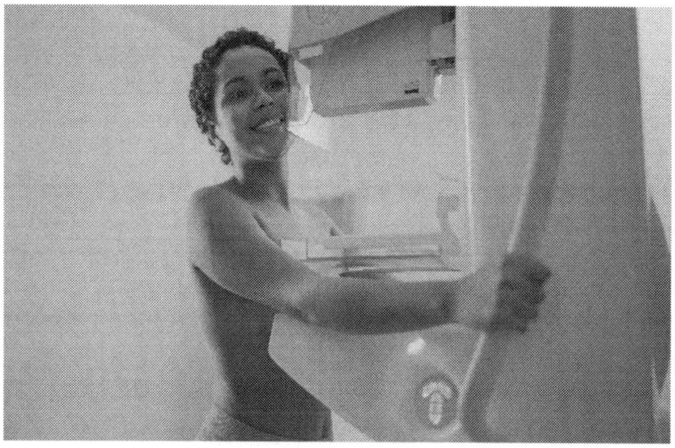

Sexually Transmitted Infections

Sexually transmitted infections, such as chlamydia and syphilis, are preventable and precautions should be taken when engaging in sexual intercourse to ensure infection does not occur. **Latex condoms** should be used to establish a barrier between skin and to prevent the transfer of fluids. Certain infections may be immunized against, examples being human papilloma virus and hepatitis B. The best way for a person to ensure there is no chance of obtaining a sexually transmitted infection is to practice abstinence.

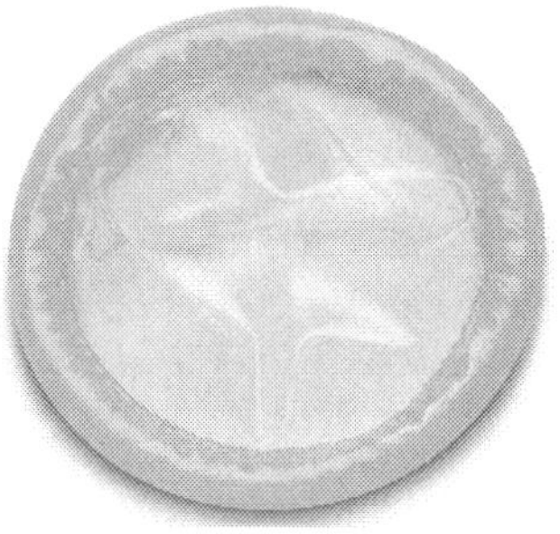

Nicotine Risks and Cessation

Smoking carries several risks, including developing conditions such as lung cancer, chronic bronchitis, asthma, and emphysema. **Cessation** of smoking greatly reduces the risk of developing any of the aforementioned conditions, and may also help lower the risk of developing heart disease, or suffering a stroke.

Recognition of Substance Abuse

Substance abuse disorders may often be difficult to spot, but there are signs a person may be exhibiting certain signs of an addiction. Physically, a person may present with altered pupils(either dilated or constricted), be uncoordinated in movements, have altered speech, have difficulty sleeping, and display poor hygiene. Behaviorally, a person may display a more aggressive attitude, become lethargic, and seem depressed and disconnected. They may start performing tasks they would not normally perform.

The Substance Abuse and Mental Health Services Administration hotline can be reached at: 1-800-662-HELP(4357).

Domestic Violence Screening and Detection

Domestic violence is screened by using multiple factors, including visual injuries, the person's dependence on substances such as alcohol or opioids, and mental illnesses such as depression. Screening may be performed by utilizing a medical questionnaire, a verbal interview, and examination of any injuries the person may have. Injuries such as bruising, especially on the face, are uncommon accidental injuries and may be a sign of abuse.

Suicide Awareness and Response

If a patient expresses potentially suicidal thoughts, a suicide risk assessment questionnaire may be administered. These questionnaires ask questions to gauge a patient's risk for suicide. Examples of suicide risk assessment questionnaires include **PHQ9**, **SAFE-T**, **ASQ**, and **C-SSRS**. A person scoring highly on one of these questionnaires may be referred to a mental health specialist for treatment.

The National Suicide Prevention Lifeline can be reached at 1-800-273-TALK(8225).

Osteoporosis Screening/Bone Density Scan

Osteoporosis is a degenerative disorder affecting bones, in which the bones may gradually become thin and brittle, which can increase the chances of fracture. It is recommended that postmenopausal women specifically be tested for osteoporosis, as they are at the greatest risk of developing it. Osteoporosis is tested using a bone density scan. During a bone density scan, the person is X-rayed using a machine known as a **DXA(dual energy X-ray absorptiometry) machine**. This machine X-rays a person and helps determine how dense the bones are, which can give an indication if a person has osteoporosis.

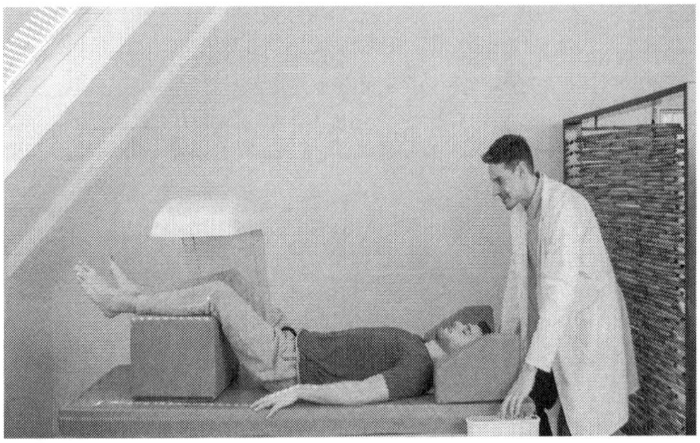

Depression Screening

Screening of depression may be difficult to perform due to certain symptoms being shared with other issues, such as substance abuse and addiction. Some signs of depression include a change in sleep habits, drastic weight fluctuations or changes, thoughts of self-harm, loss of interest in favorite activities, and lethargy. If suicidal thoughts are expressed, crisis intervention is required to help the patient.

Processing Provider Orders

Diabetic Teaching

Before a patient is discharged, they will be instructed on proper techniques and strategies to maintain a healthy lifestyle in regards to diabetes. Examples include healthy eating, being active daily, taking medication as prescribed, and consistently checking blood sugar levels. To monitor glucose, the patient may utilize a **continuous glucose monitor**, which reads the glucose content of the blood. The blood is most commonly collected via fingerstick.

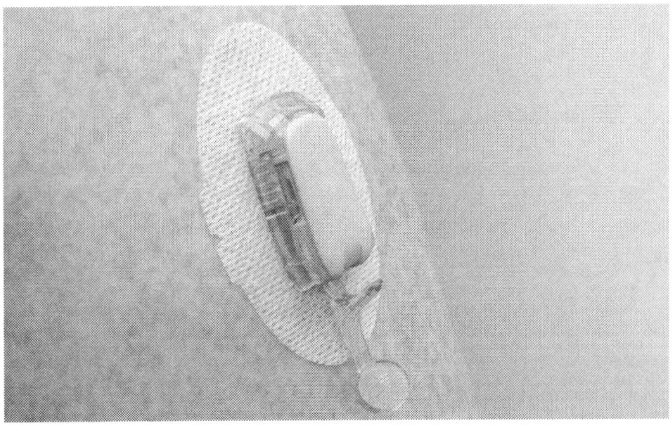

Assistive Devices

Assistive devices should be explained to the patient before discharge to ensure they are being used properly and safely. Assistive devices can include **crutches**, **walkers**, **wheelchairs**, and **canes**. These allow a patient to limit mobility in an area of the body to allow proper healing to take place.

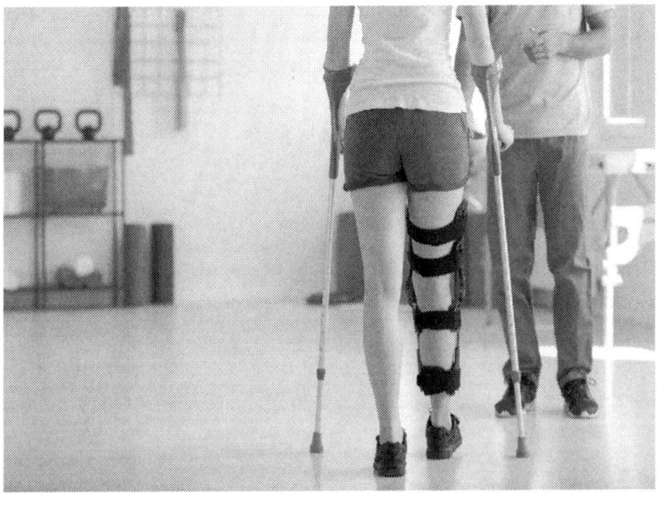

Pre-/Post Procedure/Treatment Instructions

Instructions provided to the patient pre- and post procedure are designed to help limit any complications, delays, or other issues that may arise from the procedure. Instructions are often given verbally and in written form, so the patient is able to recall instructions easier. After a procedure, instructions should be followed by the patient to prevent set-backs or complications such as infection, and to promote proper healing.

Patient-Administered Treatments

Patients often may be required to administer their own medications or treatments. Instructions should be given on proper administration, both verbally and in writing, and the competency of the patient should be evaluated to determine if they are able to self-administer. Examples of self-administered medication includes insulin injections, topical medication, and antibiotics.

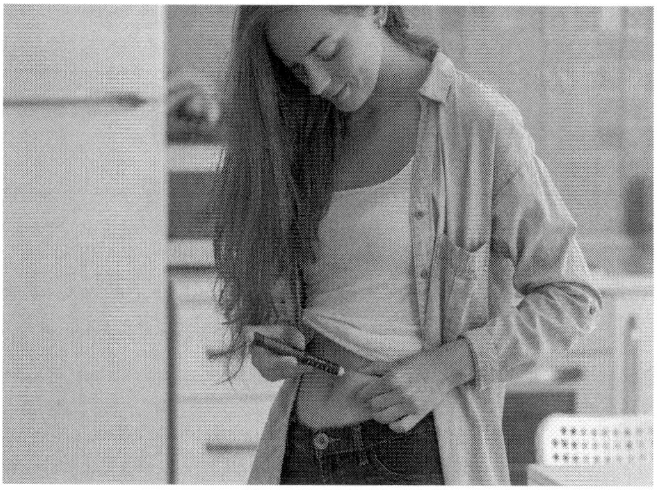

Home Monitoring

A patient may be required to monitor their blood pressure at home to give a detailed view of blood pressure throughout the day. Blood pressure monitors may be purchased over-the-counter, and utilized per instructions by the patient. The patient should record their blood pressure, food they are eating, and what time of day they are having their blood pressure read.

Alternative Medicine/Treatments

Alternative treatments may be sought for certain conditions, and may be preferred over medication or other procedures. Massage therapy is beneficial for many muscular disorders, is helpful in increasing lymph circulation, and can promote hormone regulation by stimulating the parasympathetic response. Other forms of alternative medicine or treatments include acupuncture, acupressure, meditation, yoga, and homeopathic treatments.

Nutrition Counseling

Nutrition is an important part of maintaining health and homeostasis in the body. There are seven main nutrients: protein, carbohydrates, fats, minerals, vitamins, fiber, and water.

Carbohydrates

Carbohydrates are the primary source of energy in human bodies. Carbohydrates include **sugars and starches**, which are found in many different food products. These foods include **fruits, vegetables, dairy products, wheats, and grains**. Simple carbohydrates, those found in foods such as fruits, are more easily digested than complex carbohydrates. Complex carbohydrates are digested more slowly, and found in foods such as **nuts, beans, and potatoes**.

Fats

Fat is an essential nutrient, helping to provide the body with **energy**. The body may create its own fat, or it may obtain fat from dietary sources such as **meats, fish, oils**, and certain fruits and vegetables like **avocados**. Fats that are considered healthier include omega-3 fatty acids, monounsaturated fatty acids, and polyunsaturated fatty acids. Fats that are considered unhealthy include saturated fat and trans fat.

Proteins and Amino Acids

Protein is one of the most important nutrients in the body. Most of the structures in the body are made of some type of protein. Protein is made from **amino acids**, some of which are produced naturally in the body, and others that must be consumed. Foods high in protein include **meat, seafood, beans, and eggs**.

Minerals and Electrolytes

Calcium is the most abundant mineral in the body. Calcium helps **strengthen bones**, and allows **muscles to contract**. Foods high in calcium include **spinach, kale, and salmon.**

Iron is vital in the body's ability to **transport oxygen and carbon dioxide**. Inside the cytoplasm of erythrocytes is a protein known as **hemoglobin**, which is made of iron. If there is an iron deficiency, a person may develop anemia. Foods high in iron include **beans, spinach, and lentils.**

Magnesium helps maintain **strong bones**, and regulates the heart beat by transporting ions that conduct nerve impulses in muscles. Magnesium deficiency may contribute to arrhythmia. Foods high in magnesium include **spinach, avocado, nuts, and wheat.**

Potassium aids in **muscle contraction** and **synthesizing protein**. Foods high in potassium include **bananas, avocados, beans, and tomatoes.**

Sodium aids the body in **maintaining pH balance**. It is also known as an **electrolyte**, because it aids in the transport of electric impulses traveling between nerves. Foods high in sodium usually only have sodium added to aid in preservation. Some of these foods include smoked or cured meats, such as ham.

Vitamins

Vitamin A is an important vitamin in regards to maintaining **healthy skin, mucous membranes, bones, and teeth**. Vitamin A can be found in orange and yellow fruits and vegetables. The most common type of Vitamin A is **beta-carotene.**

Vitamin B6 assists in the **production of hemoglobin and antibodies**. A deficiency in Vitamin B6 may result in anemia.

Vitamin B12 assists in the **production of erythrocytes**. Deficiency in Vitamin B12 may result in pernicious anemia.

Vitamin C assists the body's immune system and aids in **protection from free radicals**, unstable molecules that may damage cells. Vitamin C can be found in **citrus fruits, melons, broccoli, cauliflower, and strawberries.**

Vitamin D allows the body to **absorb calcium**. It is produced in the **skin** when the skin is exposed to the sun, but may also be fortified in foods(such as milk) to increase calcium absorption.

Vitamin K aids in **blood clotting**. It can be found in **leafy green vegetables** such as spinach and kale, as well as **fish, meat, and eggs.**

Fiber

Fiber is a form of **carbohydrate** arising from **plants** that, unlike most carbohydrates, is not broken down by the Digestive System into sugar. Fiber is categorized as either soluble or insoluble. Soluble fiber dissolves in water, while insoluble fiber does not. Fiber is extremely beneficial to maintaining optimal digestion, aiding food to move through the Digestive System easier. Foods high in fiber include **beans, lentils, leafy green vegetables, apples, and pears.**

Water

Water constitutes anywhere from **50% to 65%** of a person's body, depending on numerous factors, such as age, height, weight, level of physical activity, etc. Water is extremely important to body function, helping to **regulate the body's pH**, lubricate joints, nourish cells, eliminate waste by production of urine, aid in digestion, and more. There is no recommended amount of water to consume daily per the CDC due to different needs of each person, but regular plain water consumption is highly encouraged.

Function of Dietary Supplements and Herbs

Dietary supplements and herbs are used to **replace nutrients** that may be lacking in a person's diet, assuring the person is receiving adequate amounts of these nutrients. Examples of common supplements include iron, vitamin C, and zinc. A person should speak with their physician before taking supplements to ensure the supplements are appropriate, and that they do not interfere with any medications the person has been prescribed.

Special Dietary Needs

Weight control is an important aspect of nutrition. While a person's weight may be "higher" or "lower" than what is standard for an average person, it does not necessarily mean the person is not healthy. Excessive body fat, or extremely low body fat, may be unhealthy and should be properly managed with diet and exercise.

Diabetes is managed by keeping a consistent diet that promotes blood sugar levels staying in the appropriate range, while increasing exercise. A person with diabetes should generally focus on keeping blood glucose levels low. This can be accomplished by reducing carbohydrate intake, eating an adequate amount of fruit, vegetables, protein, and dairy, and avoiding foods with high sugar content.

Cardiovascular disease is commonly the result of an increased accumulation of plaque in the coronary arteries, which can reduce circulation to the heart muscle and lead to ischemia and necrosis of heart tissue. Reducing the amount of plaque build up in the coronary arteries is the main goal of treating cardiovascular disease. This can be accomplished by altering the diet to reduce the amount of saturated and trans fats being consumed, reducing carbohydrate intake, increasing protein intake, and reducing salt intake. Medication may be prescribed to help reduce the amount of plaque, or cholesterol, in the blood.

Much like cardiovascular disease, hypertension is commonly caused by an accumulation of plaque in the arteries. Reducing plaque can be accomplished by reducing intake of saturated and trans fat, carbohydrates, and sodium, while increasing intake of protein and vegetables. Medication may be prescribed to help manage hypertension and reduce cholesterol as well.

Proper nutrition is extremely important for a patient with cancer. During and after treatment, the patient may not feel the need to eat, or may feel ill due to the medication used. If a patient skips a meal as a result, the body may not receive sufficient nutrients to help treat the cancer. The patient should be eating healthy foods that are low in carbohydrates, incorporating high protein vegetables, meats low in fat, and citrus fruits into the diet.

Lactose sensitivity or intolerance is manageable, but nutrients need to be added elsewhere to make up for the loss of nutrients associated with lactose. Lactose is a sugar found in milk. Milk is often fortified with calcium. If milk and dairy products are removed from the diet, the person should add more leafy green vegetables to the diet to ensure they are receiving adequate amounts of nutrients such as calcium and iron.

A person with celiac disease may need to eliminate the protein gluten from their diet. Gluten can be found in many forms of grains, such as wheat or barley. Foods that contain high amounts of wheat, barley, and rye may need to be eliminated from the diet, such as bread. Certain grains, such as corn or flax, do not contain gluten, and may still be consumed.

Food allergies should be determined as early as possible. If a person has an allergy to a food, that food should be avoided. Common food allergies include nuts and shellfish. If these allergies are serious, a person may experience anaphylaxis, and be unable to breathe, which may lead to death.

When the kidneys stop functioning properly, a person is diagnosed with a form of kidney disease. There are many reasons a person's kidneys may not function optimally, usually associated with other medical conditions such as diabetes, and hypertension. The kidneys are responsible for filtering waste products from the blood, such as urea, ammonia, and other metabolic waste. The inability of the kidneys to remove these waste products leaves the waste in the body, creating a toxic internal environment that can become damaged and lead to many health complications, up to and including death.

Chronic kidney disease involves the kidney function decreasing over a longer period of time, and is most commonly the result of a person having both diabetes and hypertension simultaneously. Glomerulonephritis, polycystic kidney disease, and pyelonephritis are also contributing conditions that may damage the kidneys and influence their ability to filter waste properly over time.

Uremia is the result of a lack of waste being filtered by the kidneys. Increased amounts of urea and creatinine in the blood are markers of decreased kidney function, as well as an abundance of electrolytes such as sodium and potassium, and excessive water in the blood.

Kidney disease is commonly treated by treating the root cause, such as diabetes or hypertension. If these conditions are managed, and the kidneys have not experienced too large of a decrease in function, the kidneys may return to functioning properly. In advanced stages of kidney disease, dialysis may be performed to filter waste from the blood. Kidney transplants may be performed, in which another person's kidney and ureter are inserted into the body, attached to the external iliac artery and vein. The defective kidneys are left in the body to assist with filtration, even if they are functioning at a minimal level.

Food Label Interpretation

Food labels are utilized to give the consumer an overview of the nutritional contents of a food item. Information given on a food label will often give a recommended percentage of daily intake, including calories, fats, sugars, sodium, carbohydrates, fiber, cholesterol, and protein. Each person has a different dietary need in regards to these percentages, and the percentages given are only an average. Exact content of nutrients is also listed in grams.

Additional vitamins may be listed, if any are present in the food, such as vitamin A, vitamin C, vitamin D, along with other nutrients such as potassium, iron, and calcium. These are listed as a daily percentage.

Nutrition Facts

6 servings per container
Serving size
1 cup (230g)

Calories **per serving** **245**

Amount/serving	**% Daily Value***	**Amount/serving**	**% Daily Value***
Total Fat 12g	**14%**	**Total Carbohydrate** 34g	**12%**
Saturated Fat 2g	**10%**	Dietary Fiber 7g	**25%**
Trans Fat 0g		Total Sugars 5g	
Cholesterol 8mg	**3%**	Includes 4g Added Sugars	**8%**
Sodium 210mg	**9%**	**Protein** 11g	

Vitamin D 4mcg 20 · Calcium 210mg 16% · Iron 3mg 15% · Potassium 380mg 8%
Thiamin 13% · Riboflavin 9% · Niacin 12%

*The % Daily Value (DV) tells you how much a nutrient in a serving of food contributes to a daily diet. 2,000 calories a day is used for general nutrition advice.

Eating Disorders

A person may develop certain psychological disorders that influence their consumption of food. These are known as eating disorders. The three most common forms of eating disorders are anorexia nervosa, bulimia, and binge eating.

Anorexia nervosa occurs when a person intentionally **restricts** the nutrients they are consuming to **unhealthy levels** in an effort to become thinner. This has a severe impact on the overall health of the person, as they are depriving their body of important nutrients needed to live and function, such as protein, fat, carbohydrates, and important vitamins and minerals such as vitamin C, calcium, and potassium.

Bulimia most commonly involves a person ingesting large amounts of food, and then vomiting afterward. This is known as **purging bulimia.** Purging bulimia may result in damage to the esophagus, pharynx, oral cavity, and teeth due to the excessive presence of acids from the stomach. **Non-purging bulimia** involves a person eating large quantities of food, followed by excessive exercise, the use of laxatives and/or diuretics, or fasting. These activities, especially the use of laxatives and/or diuretics, do not allow the nutrients to remain in the body long enough to be effectively absorbed in the small intestine, leaving the person malnourished.

Binge eating is often associated with depression and stress, and involves a person **consuming unhealthy amounts** of food. This can lead to other disorders such as obesity, diabetes, and hypertension.

Clinical Workflow Matching

______: Device used to measure oxygen saturation in the blood

______: Mineral that helps maintain strong bones and regulate heart beat by transporting ions that conduct nerve impulses in muscles

______: Vitamin that aids in maintaining healthy skin, mucous membranes, bones, and teeth, found in orange and yellow fruits and vegetables

______: A person eating an unhealthy amount of food

______: Procedure used to detect breast cancer utilizing x-rays

______: Physical examination of a child

______: Dual energy X-ray absorptiometry is used to test for this condition

______: Device used to read blood sugar content

______: Instrument used to detect sound at the anterior elbow in a blood pressure reading

______: Pulse read at the proximal anterior thigh

______: Vitamin assisting in blood clotting, found in green leafy vegetables, fish, meat, and eggs

______: Regularity of a heart beat

______: Form of alternative medicine beneficial for muscular disorders, increasing lymph and blood circulation, and hormone regulation

______: Sugars and starches that are converted into energy in the body

______: Substance constituting 50-65% of a person's body

______: Measurement of body fat based on height and weight of an adult

______: Mineral vital to the body's ability to transport oxygen and carbon dioxide

______: Eating disorder marked by purging of food via vomiting after ingestion

______: Substances used to replace nutrients that may be lacking in a person's diet

______: Acknowledging a patient's behaviors to help the patient feel understood and empathized with

A: Continuous glucose monitor
B: Massage therapy
C: Heart rhythm
D: Water
E: Iron
F: Binge eating
G: Carbohydrates
H: Affirming
I: Femoral
J: Dietary supplements
K: Pediatric exam
L: Pulse oximeter
M: Vitamin A
N: Bulimia
O: Mammogram
P: Stethoscope
Q: Magnesium
R: Body Mass Index
S: Osteoporosis
T: Vitamin K

Answer Key on Page 292

Clinical Workflow Crossword

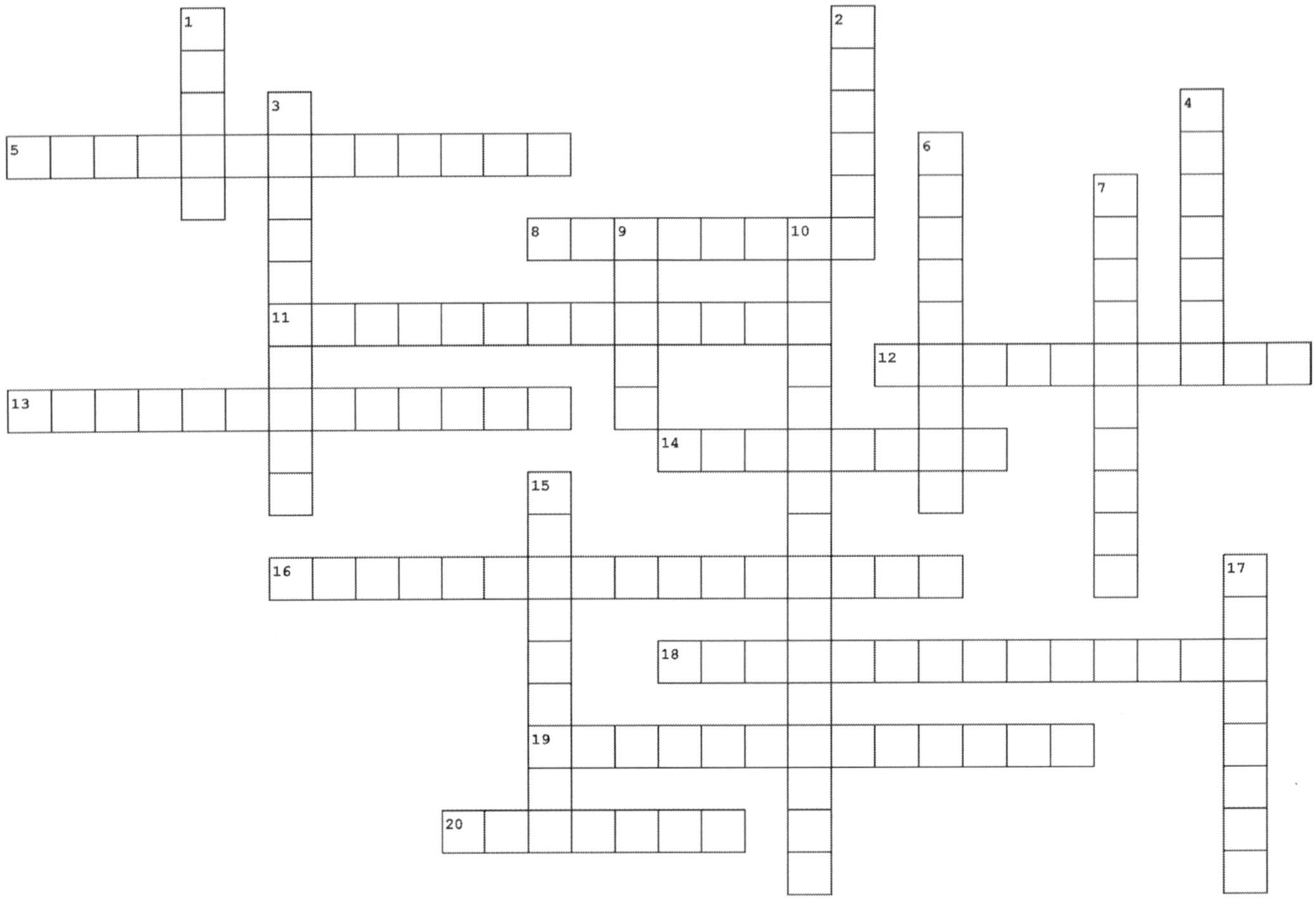

Across

5. Device used to measure oxygen saturation of the blood
8. Pulse read on the medial side of the arm
11. Primary source of energy in human bodies
12. Adhering to laws, regulations, and guidelines that apply to a medical practice's operation
13. Data that can be physically measured
14. Pressure felt in arteries as blood passes through
16. Device used to measure blood pressure
18. Primary reason a patient has come in for treatment
19. The amount of breaths a person takes during a one minute span
20. Most abundant mineral in the body

Down

1. Form of carbohydate arising from plants that is not broken down into sugar
2. Most common pulse location used
3. Device used to test for osteoporosis
4. Made from amino acids, found in meat, seafood, beans, and eggs
6. Pressure felt in arteries when blood is not passing through
7. Temperature read by placing thermometer under the tongue
9. Temperature read utilizing the tympanic membrane
10. Crutches, walkers, wheelchairs, and canes
15. Gives an overview of nutritional content in a food item
17. Vitamin that allows the body to absorb calcium, produced by the skin after sunlight exposure

Answer Key on Page 293

Clinical Workflow Practice Test

1. Aural temperature is read by using a thermometer in which location
A. The armpit
B. The forehead
C. The tympanic membrane
D. The rectum

2. An insight into a patient's daily life can best be gained by asking a patient for which of the following
A. Medication history
B. Social and occupational history
C. Family history
D. Past medical history

3. Sugars and starches are forms of
A. Proteins
B. Fiber
C. Fats
D. Carbohydrates

4. Blood oxygen saturation is measured using the following instrument
A. Spirometer
B. Sublingual thermometer
C. Pulse oximeter
D. BMI machine

5. Which of the following is the pulse point found on the foot
A. Popliteal
B. Dorsalis pedis
C. Apical
D. Femoral

6. Subjective data is best described as
A. Information a patient provides about themselves
B. Diagnostic testing information
C. Recommendations for future treatments or procedures
D. Information that is measured by a physician

7. A DXA machine is used to
A. Separate solids from liquids
B. Screen for osteoporosis
C. Filter toxic substances from the blood and return the cleaned blood to the body
D. View the internal anatomy of the stomach and small intestine

8. Which of the following is one of the primary functions of vitamin D
A. Allows the body to absorb calcium
B. Aids in blood clotting
C. Assists the immune system in protection from free radicals
D. Assists in production of hemoglobin and antibodies

9. Peak flow rate is a measurement of
A. The maximum amount of blood being pumped out of the heart by the left ventricle
B. The maximum amount of movement produced by a ball-and-socket joint
C. The maximum amount of urine being produced by the kidneys
D. The maximum speed a person is able to exhale

10. Helping a patient identify why they are hoping to achieve specific goals
A. Focusing
B. Engaging
C. Evoking
D. Planning

Answer Key on Page 295

What we face may look insurmountable, but what I learned is that we are always stronger than we know.

- Arnold Schwarzenegger

Medical Terminology

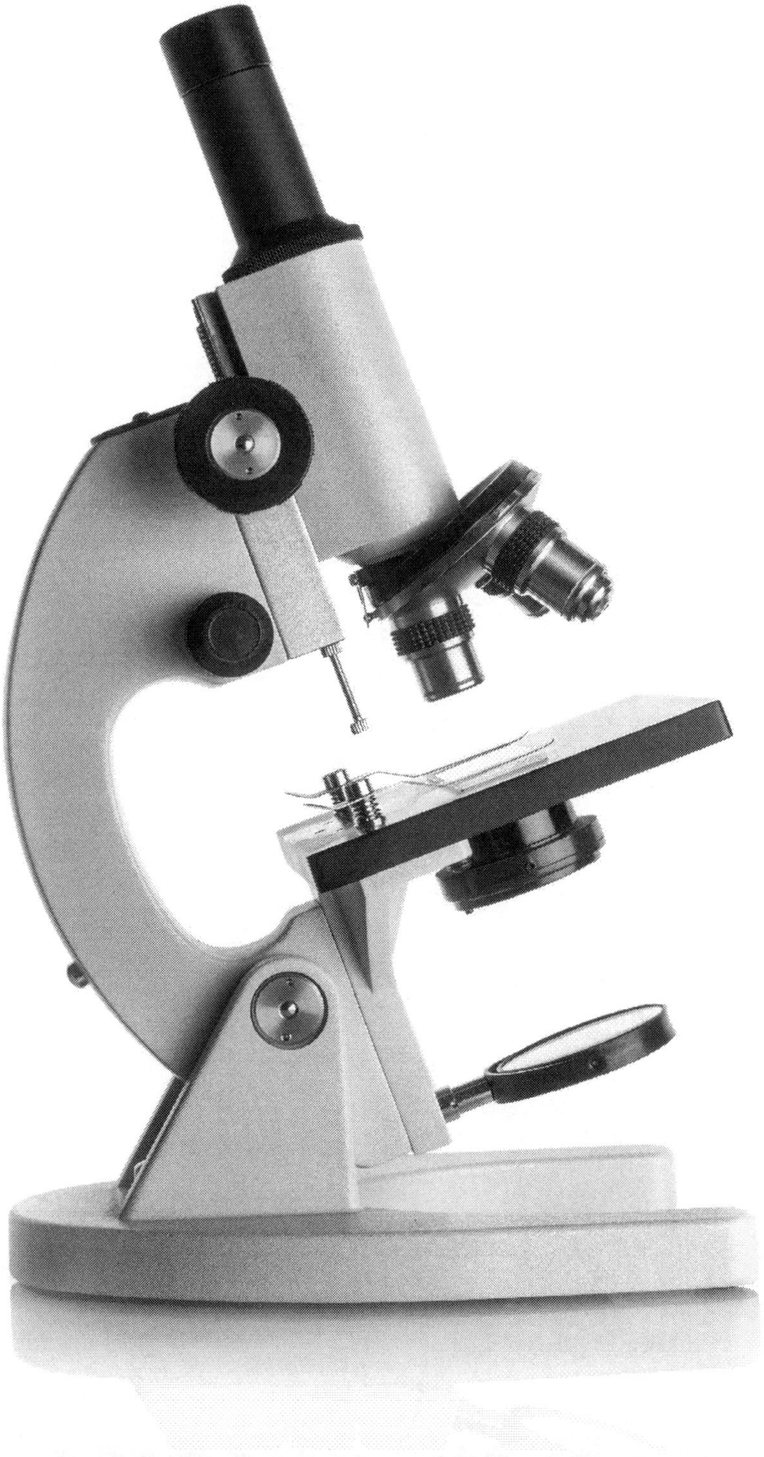

Medical Terminology

Medical terminology can be divided into three primary components: word roots, prefixes, and suffixes.

The word root of a medical term is the primary structure involved. It gives us a starting point when breaking down a word. An example is the word root "hepat/o", which means "liver".

A prefix is used to modify a word root, and is attached at the beginning of the word root. An example is "a-", which means "without". A disease that uses "a-" is "arrhythmia", which means "without rhythm".

A suffix is used to add description to, or alter, a word root, and is attached at the end of the word root. An example is "-itis", which means "inflammation". A disease that uses "-itis" is "hepatitis". As stated before, the word root "hepat/o" means "liver". If we attach "-itis", it becomes "inflammation of the liver".

Many different medical terms, prefixes, suffixes, and word roots have the same meaning. The reason for different terms having the same meaning can be traced back to the origin languages. Modern medical terminology originated in both Latin and Greek, with the majority of the words being Greek. When people like Celsus, a Roman physician, began creating medical terminology, they often used Greek terms, but conformed them to be Latin in origin. This is the reason for many terms sharing the same definition.

Medical terminology is especially useful when studying not only anatomy and physiology, but pathology as well. Knowing medical terminology can help you figure out what the general medical condition is just by looking at the name. First start by identifying the word root. We'll use the term "bursitis". The word root in "bursitis" is "burs/o", which means "bursa/bursa sac". This way, we know the condition has something to do with a bursa sac. Then we try to identify any prefixes. "Bursitis" does not contain any prefixes. Therefore, we move to suffixes. We know that "-itis" is a suffix, and it means "inflammation". We can then combine the two meanings together, and reach the conclusion that "bursitis" is inflammation of a bursa sac.

Word Roots

Cardiovascular Word Roots

angi/o: vessel(ex: **Angio**plasty)
aort/o: aorta(ex: **Aort**ic arch)
arteriol/o: arteriole(ex: **Arteriolo**sclerosis)
arteri/o: artery(ex: **Arterio**sclerosis)
ather/o: fatty plaque(ex: **Athero**sclerosis)
atri/o: atrium(ex: **Atri**al fibrillation)
bas/o: alkaline(ex: **Baso**phil)
cardi/o: heart(ex: Echo**cardio**gram)
chrom/o: color(ex: **Chromo**some)
eosin/o: rose colored(ex: **Eosino**phil)
erythr/o: red(ex: **Erythro**cyte)
granul/o: granule(ex: **Granulo**cyte)
hemangi/o: blood vessel(ex: **Hemangi**oma)
hem/o: blood(ex: **Hemo**globin)
kary/o: nucleus(ex: **Karyo**type)
leuk/o: white(ex: **Leuko**cyte)
morph/o: form(ex: **Morph**ology)
nucle/o: nucleus(ex: **Nucleo**lus)
phleb/o: vein(ex: **Phleb**itis)
poikil/o: irregular(ex: **Poikilo**cytosis)
reticul/o: mesh(ex: **Reticulo**cyte)
scler/o: hard(ex: Athero**sclero**sis)
sider/o: iron(ex: **Sidero**blastic anemia)
sphygm/o: pulse(ex: **Sphygmo**manometer)
thromb/o: clot(ex: **Thrombo**cyte)
vascul/o: vessel(ex: A**vascul**ar)
ven/o: vein(ex: **Ven**ipuncture)
ventricul/o: ventricle(ex: **Ventriculo**megaly)

Digestive Word Roots

append/o: appendix(ex: **Append**ectomy)
appendic/o: appendix(ex: **Appendic**itis)
bucc/o: cheek(ex: **Bucc**inator)
cheil/o: lip(ex: **Cheil**itis)
chol/e: bile(ex: **Chole**cystitis)
cholangi/o: bile vessel(ex: **Cholangi**tis)
col/o: large intestine(ex: **Col**itis)
colon/o: large intestine(ex: **Colono**scopy)
dont/o: teeth(ex: Perio**dont**al abscess)
duoden/o: duodenum(ex: **Duoden**al ulcer)
enter/o: small intestine(ex: Gastro**enter**itis)
esophag/o: esophagus(ex: **Esophag**itis)
gastr/o: stomach(ex: **Gastr**itis)
gingiv/o: gums(ex: **Gingiv**itis)
gloss/o: tongue(ex: Hypo**gloss**al nerve)
hepat/o: liver(ex: **Hepat**itis)
ile/o: ileum(ex: **Ileo**cecal sphincter)
jejun/o: jejunum(ex: **Jejuno**stomy)
labi/o: lip(ex: **Labio**mental groove)
lingu/o: tongue(ex: Bi**lingu**al)
odont/o: teeth(ex: **Odonto**blast)
or/o: mouth(ex: **Or**al cavity)
pancreat/o: pancreas(ex: **Pancreat**itis)
pharyng/o: pharynx(ex: **Pharyng**itis)
proct/o: anus(ex: **Procto**logy)
pylor/o: pylorus(ex: **Pyloro**stenosis)
rect/o: rectum(ex: **Recto**rrhagia)
sial/o: saliva(ex: **Sialo**rrhea)
sigmoid/o: sigmoid(ex: **Sigmoid**ectomy)
stomat/o: mouth(ex: **Stomat**itis)

Endocrine Word Roots

aden/o: gland(ex: **Aden**oma)
adren/o: adrenal glands(ex: **Adren**aline)
adrenal/o: adrenal glands(ex: **Adrenal**ine)
calc/o: calcium(ex: Hyper**calc**emia)
gluc/o: sugar(ex: **Gluc**agon)
glyc/o: sugar(ex: Hyper**glyc**emia)
gonad/o: gonads(ex: **Gonado**tropin)
home/o: same(ex: **Homeo**stasis)
kal/i: potassium(ex: Hyper**kal**emia)
thyr/o: thyroid(ex: Hyper**thyro**idism)
toxic/o: poison(ex: In**toxic**ation)
thalam/o: thalamus(ex: **Thalamo**tomy)

Integumentary Word Roots

adip/o: fat(ex: **Adip**ose)
albin/o: white(ex: **Albin**ism)
cirrh/o: yellow(ex: **Cirrh**osis)
cutane/o: skin(ex: Sub**cutane**ous)
cyan/o: blue(ex: **Cyan**osis)
derm/o: skin(ex: Sclero**derm**a)
dermat/o: skin(ex: **Dermat**itis)
erythem/o: red(ex: Lupus **erythem**atosus)
hidr/o: sweat(ex: Hyper**hidr**osis)
hist/o: tissue(ex: **Hist**ology)
ichthy/o: scaly(ex: **Ichthy**osis)
jaund/o: yellow(ex: **Jaund**ice)
kerat/o: hard(ex: **Kerat**in)
lip/o: fat(ex: **Lip**oma)
melan/o: black(ex: **Melan**oma)
myc/o: fungi(ex: Onycho**myc**osis)
onych/o: nail(ex: **Onycho**mycosis)
pil/o: hair(ex: Arrector **pili**)
phyt/o: plant(ex: Dermato**phyt**osis)
seb/o: sebum(ex: **Seb**aceous cyst)
squam/o: scale(ex: **Squam**ous suture)
sudor/o: sweat(ex: **Sudor**iferous gland)
trich/o: hair(ex: **Tricho**moniasis)
ungu/o: nail(ex: Tinea **ungu**ium)
xanth/o: yellow(ex: **Xanth**oma)
xer/o: dry(ex: **Xer**ophthalmia)

Lymphatic Word Roots

adenoid/o: adenoids(ex: **Adenoid**ectomy)
immun/o: immune(ex: **Immun**ology)
lymph/o: lymph(ex: **Lympho**ma)
lymphang/o: lymph vessel(ex: **Lymphang**itis)
phag/o: eat(ex: **Phago**cytosis)
splen/o: spleen(ex: **Splen**ectomy)
tonsill/o: tonsils(ex: **Tonsill**itis)
thym/o: thymus(ex: **Thym**ectomy)

Muscular Word Roots

adhes/o: stick to(ex: **Adhes**ion)
duct/o: carry(ex: **Duct**openia)
erg/o: work(ex: **Ergo**nomic)
fasci/o: fascia(ex: Tensor **fasci**ae latae)
fibr/o: fiber(ex: **Fibro**myalgia)
fibros/o: fiber(ex: **Fibros**is)
flex/o: bend(ex: **Flex**ion)
is/o: same(ex: **Iso**metric)
kinesi/o: movement(ex: **Kines**thetic)
lei/o: smooth(ex: **Leio**myoma)
lev/o: lift(ex: **Lev**ator scapulae)
metr/o: length(ex: Iso**metr**ic)
quadr/i: four(ex: **Quadri**ceps)
rect/o: straight(ex: **Rect**us abdominis)
ten/o: tendon(ex: **Teno**periosteal)
tendin/o: tendon(ex: **Tendin**itis)
tens/o: strain(ex: **Tens**or fasciae latae)
ton/o: tension(ex: Iso**ton**ic)
tort/i: twisted(ex: **Torti**collis)

Nervous Word Roots

astr/o: star(ex: **Astro**cytoma)
ax/o: axon(ex: **Axo**n)
cephal/o: head(ex: En**cephal**itis)

cerebell/o: cerebellum(ex: **Cerebell**um)
cortic/o: cortex(ex: **Cortico**steroid)
crani/o: skull(ex: **Crani**um)
dendr/o: tree(ex: **Dendr**ite)
dur/o: dura mater(ex: Epi**dur**al)
encephal/o: brain(ex: **Encephal**itis)
esthesi/o: sensation(ex: An**esthesi**c)
gangli/o: ganglion(ex: **Gangli**on cyst)
gli/o: glue(ex: **Glio**blastoma)
lex/o: word(ex: **Lex**icon)
lob/o: lobe(ex: **Lob**otomy)
mening/o: meninges(ex: **Mening**itis)
ment/o: mind(ex: **Ment**ality)
mot/o: move(ex: Loco**mot**ion)
myel/o: canal(ex: Osteo**myel**itis)
narc/o: stupor(ex: **Narco**lepsy)
neur/o: nerve(ex: **Neur**algia)
olig/o: few(ex: **Oligo**dendrocyte)
phas/o: speech(ex: Dys**phas**ia)
phren/o: mind(ex: **Phren**ology)
psych/o: mind(ex: **Psych**osis)
spin/o: spine(ex: Semi**spin**alis)
synapt/o: point of contact(ex: **Synap**se)
tax/o: order(ex: **Tax**onomy)

Reproductive Word Roots

amni/o: amnion(ex: **Amnio**centesis)
andr/o: male(ex: **Andro**gen)
cervic/o: neck(ex: **Cervi**x)
colp/o: vagina(ex: **Colpo**scopy)
embry/o: embryo(ex: **Embryo**nic stage)
epididym/o: epididymis(ex: **Epididym**itis)
episi/o: vulva(ex: **Episio**tomy)
fet/o: fetus(ex: **Fet**al development)
galact/o: milk(ex: **Galacto**rrhea)
genit/o: genitalia(ex: **Genit**al herpes)
gynec/o: woman(ex: **Gyneco**logy)
hyster/o: uterus(ex: **Hyster**ectomy)
hymen/o: hymen(ex: **Hymen**ectomy)
lact/o: milk(ex: **Lact**ation)
mamm/o: breast(ex: **Mamm**ary gland)
mast/o: breast(ex: **Mast**ectomy)
men/o: menstruation(ex: **Meno**pause)
metr/o: uterus(ex: **Metro**rrhagia)
nat/o: birth(ex: Neo**nat**al)
o/o: egg(ex: **Oo**cyte)
oophor/o: ovary(ex: **Oophor**ectomy)
orch/o: testicle(ex: **Orchi**ectomy)
ovari/o: ovary(ex: **Ovari**an tumor)
pen/o: penis(ex: **Peno**scrotal fusion)
perine/o: perineum(ex: **Perineo**tomy)
prostat/o: prostate(ex: **Prostat**itis)
salping/o: fallopian tube(ex: **Salping**itis)
sperm/o: sperm(ex: **Sperm**icide)
spermat/o: sperm(ex: **Spermato**genesis)
test/o: testicle(ex: **Test**icular tortion)
uter/o: uterus(ex: **Uter**ine lining)
vagin/o: vagina(ex: Bacterial **vagin**osis)
vesicul/o: seminal vesicle(ex: **Vesicul**itis)
vulv/o: vulva(ex: **Vulv**itis)

Respiratory Word Roots

alveol/o: alveolus(ex: **Alveol**i)
anthrac/o: black(ex: **Anthra**x)
bronch/o: bronchus(ex: **Bronch**itis)
con/i: dust(ex: **Coni**dium)
embol/o: plug(ex: **Embol**ism)
emphys/o: inflate(ex: **Emphys**ema)
epiglott/o: epiglottis(ex: **Epiglott**itis)
laryng/o: larynx(ex: **Laryng**itis)
muc/o: mucous(ex: Sub**muc**osa)
nas/o: nose(ex: **Nas**al cavity)
ox/o: oxygen(ex: Hyp**ox**ia)
pector/o: chest(ex: **Pector**alis major)
phon/o: sound(ex: Dys**phon**ia)
phren/o: diaphragm(ex: **Phren**ic nerve)
pleur/o: pleura(ex: **Pleur**al membrane)
pneum/o: lung(ex: **Pneum**onia)
pulm/o: lung(ex: **Pulmo**nary edema)
rhin/o: nose(ex: **Rhin**itis)
sinus/o: sinus(ex: **Sinus**itis)
spir/o: breathe(ex: **Spiro**meter)
steth/o: chest(ex: **Steth**oscope)
thorac/o: chest(ex: **Thorac**ic vertebrae)
trache/o: trachea(ex: **Tracheo**tomy)

Skeletal Word Roots

acr/o: extremity(ex: **Acro**megaly)
acromi/o: acromion(ex: **Acromio**clavicular)
ankyl/o: crooked(ex: **Ankyl**osis)
arthr/o: joint(ex: **Arthr**itis)
brachi/o: arm(ex: Biceps **brachi**i)
calcane/o: calcaneus(ex: **Calcane**al tendon)
carp/o: carpals(ex: **Carpo**metacarpal joint)
chondr/o: cartilage(ex: Costo**chondr**itis)
clavicul/o: clavicle(ex: Sterno**clavicul**ar)
cleid/o: clavicle(ex: Sterno**cleido**mastoid)
condyl/o: condyle(ex: Epi**condyl**e)
cost/o: ribs(ex: Inter**cost**al)
dactyl/o: fingers/toes(ex: Poly**dactyl**y)
femor/o: femur(ex: Rectus **femor**is)
fibul/o: fibula(ex: Tibio**fibul**ar joint)
humer/o: humerus(ex: Gleno**humer**al)
ili/o: ilium(ex: **Ili**acus)
ischi/o: ischium(ex: **Ischi**al tuberosity)
kyph/o: hill(ex: **Kyph**osis)
lamin/o: lamina(ex: **Lamino**tomy)
lord/o: curve(ex: **Lord**osis)
metacarp/o: metacarpals(ex: **Metacarpo**phalangeal)
metatars/o: metatarsals(ex: **Metatarso**phalangeal)
orth/o: straight(ex: **Ortho**pedic)
oste/o: bone(ex: **Osteo**arthritis)
patell/o: patella(ex: **Patell**ar tendon)
ped/i: foot(ex: **Pedi**cure)
pelv/i: pelvis(ex: **Pelvi**c girdle)
phalang/o: phalanges(ex: Inter**phalange**al)
pod/o: foot(ex: **Pod**iatrist)
pub/o: pubis(ex: **Pub**ic symphysis)
rachi/o: spine(ex: **Rach**itis)
radi/o: radius(ex: **Radio**ulnar joint)
sacr/o: sacrum(ex: **Sacro**tuberous ligament)
scapul/o: scapula(ex: Sub**scapul**aris)
scoli/o: crooked(ex: **Scoli**osis)
spondyl/o: vertebrae(ex: **Spondyl**osis)
synov/o: synovium(ex: **Synovi**al fluid)
tal/o: talus(ex: **Talo**tibial joint)
tars/o: tarsals(ex: **Tarso**metatarsal)
uln/o: ulna(ex: Humero**uln**ar joint)
vertebr/o: vertebrae(ex: Inter**vertebr**al disc)

Urinary Word Roots

albumin/o: albumin(ex: **Albumin**uria)
azot/o: nitrogenous(ex: **Azot**emia)
cyst/o: bladder(ex: **Cyst**itis)
glomerul/o: glomerulus(ex: **Glomerulo**nephritis)
ket/o: ketone bodies(ex: **Ket**osis)
nephr/o: kidney(ex: **Nephr**ologist)
pyel/o: renal pelvis(ex: **Pyelo**nephritis)
ren/o: kidney(ex: Ad**ren**al glands)
ur/o: urine(ex: **Ur**ic acid)

ureter/o: ureter(ex: **Uretero**scopy)
urethr/o: urethra(ex: **Urethr**itis)
urin/o: urine(ex: **Urin**ation)
vesic/o: bladder(ex: **Vesico**ureteral reflux)

Oncology Word Roots

blast/o: germ cell(ex: **Blast**oma)
carcin/o: cancer(ex: **Carcino**gen)
cauter/o: burn(ex: **Cauter**ize)
chem/o: chemical(ex:**Chemo**therapy)
cry/o: cold(ex: **Cryo**therapy)
mut/a: genetic change(ex: **Muta**tion)
onc/o: tumor(ex: **Onco**logy)
rhabdomy/o: skeletal muscle(ex: **Rhabdomyo**lysis)
sarc/o: connective tissue(ex: Kaposi's **sarc**oma)

Miscellaneous Word Roots

aur/i: ear(ex: **Auri**cle)
bi/o: life(ex: Micro**bio**logy)
burs/o: bursa(ex: **Burs**itis)
cerat/o: horn(ex: Tri**cerat**ops)
chir/o: hand(ex: **Chiro**practor)
corac/o: crow-like(ex: **Corac**oid)
coron/o: crown(ex: **Coron**oid)
dextr/o: right(ex: Ambi**dextr**ous)
dors/o: back(ex: **Dors**al body cavity)
dynam/o: power(ex: **Dynamo**meter)
ect/o: outside(ex: **Ecto**pic pregnancy)
faci/o: face(ex: **Faci**al nerve)
glauc/o: gray(ex: **Glauc**oma)
hydr/o: water(ex: **Hydro**therapy)
irid/o: iris(ex: **Irido**cyclitis)
kerat/o: cornea(ex: **Kerato**scope)
lacrim/o: tear(ex: **Lacrim**al duct)
lapar/o: abdominal wall(ex: **Laparo**tomy)
myring/o: eardrum(ex: **Myring**itis)
omphal/o: navel(ex: **Omphalo**cele)
ophthalam/o: eye(ex: **Ophthalamo**scope)
phot/o: light(ex: **Photo**sensitivity)
py/o: pus(ex: **Pyo**derma)
pyr/o: heat(ex: Anti**pyr**etic)
therm/o: heat(ex: **Thermo**meter)
tympan/o: eardrum(ex:**Tympan**itis)
ventr/o: belly(ex: **Ventr**al body cavity)
viscer/o: internal organs(ex: **Viscero**ptosis)
zo/o: animal(ex: **Zoo**notic)

Prefixes

a-: without(ex: **A**vascular)
ab-: away(ex: **Ab**duction)
ad-: towards(ex: **Ad**duction)
af-: towards(ex: **Af**ferent)
allo-: other(ex: **Allo**patric speciation)
an-: without(ex: **An**emia)
ana-: against(ex: **Ana**phylaxis)
ante-: before(ex: **Ante**cubital)
anti-: against(ex: **Anti**biotic)
auto-: self(ex: **Auto**nomy)
bi-: two(ex: **Bi**ceps femoris)
brady-: slow(ex: **Brady**cardia)
circum-: around(ex: **Circum**duction)
contra-: against(ex: **Contra**indication)
de-: cessation(ex: **De**generation)
di-: double(ex: **Di**encephalon)
dia-: through(ex: **Dia**lysis)
dipl-: double(ex: **Dipl**opia)
dys-: difficult(ex: **Dys**pnea)
ec-: out(ex: **Ec**topic pregnancy)
echo-: repeated sound(ex: **Echo**lalia)
ecto-: outside(ex: **Ecto**morph)
ef-: away(ex: **Ef**ferent)
en-: within(ex: **En**docrine)
endo-: within(ex: **Endo**scopy)
epi-: above(ex: **Epi**dermis)
eso-: inward(ex: **Eso**teric)
eu-: good(ex: **Eu**phoria)
ex-: outside(ex: **Ex**cretion)
exo-: outside(ex: **Exo**crine)
extra-: outside(ex: **Extra**corporial)
hemi-: half(ex: **Hemi**plegia)
hetero-: different(ex: **Hetero**chromia)
homo-: same(ex: **Home**ostasis)
hyper-: excessive(ex: **Hyper**thyroidism)
hypo-: below(ex: **Hyp**oxia)
im-: not(ex: **Im**potence)
infra-: below(ex: **Infra**spinatus)
inter-: between(ex: **Inter**osseous)
intra-: inside(ex: **Intra**venous)
iso-: same(ex: **Iso**tonic)
macro-: large(ex: **Macro**phage)
mal-: bad(ex: **Mal**ignant)
meso-: middle(ex: **Meso**thelioma)
meta-: change(ex: **Meta**physis)
micro-: small(ex: **Micro**organism)
mono-: one(ex: **Mono**nucleosis)
multi-: many(ex: **Multi**ple sclerosis)
neo-: new(ex: **Neo**natal)
nulli-: none(ex: **Nulli**fy)
oxy-: sharp(ex: **Oxy**tocin)
pan-: all(ex: **Pan**demic)
para-: beside(ex: **Para**thyroid)
per-: through(ex: **Per**itoneum)
peri-: around(ex: **Peri**osteum)
poly-: many(ex: **Poly**cythemia)
post-: after(ex: **Post**partum)
pre-: before(ex: **Pre**patellar bursitis)
pro-: before(ex: **Pro**gesterone)
pseudo-: false(ex: **Pseudo**ephedrine)
quadri-: four(ex: **Quadri**ceps)
retro-: behind(ex: **Retro**peritoneal)
semi-: half(ex: **Semi**membranosus)
sub-: under(ex: **Sub**scapularis)
super-: above(ex: **Super**ior)
supra-: above(ex: **Supra**spinatus)
sym-: together(ex: Pubic **sym**physis)
syn-: together(ex: **Syn**ergist)
tachy-: rapid(ex: **Tachy**cardia)
torti-: twisted(ex: **Torti**collis)
trans-: through(ex: **Trans**dermal)
tri-: three(ex: **Tri**ceps brachii)
ultra-: excessive(ex: **Ultra**sound)
uni-: one(ex: **Uni**lateral)

Suffixes

-ac: referring to(ex: Hypochondri**ac**)
-acusis: hearing(ex: Hyper**acusis**)
-al: referring to(ex: Iliofemor**al**)
-algia: pain(ex: Fibromy**algia**)
-ar: referring to(ex: Alveol**ar**)
-ary: referring to(ex: Coron**ary**)
-ate: form of(ex: Acet**ate**)
-ation: process(ex: Replic**ation**)
-asthenia: weakness(ex: My**asthenia**)
-blast: germ cell(ex: Osteo**blast**)
-capnia: carbon dioxide(ex: Hyper**capnia**)
-cele: hernia(ex: Meningo**cele**)
-centesis: puncture(ex: Amnio**centesis**)
-cision: cutting(ex: In**cision**)
-clast: break(ex: Osteo**clast**)
-crine: secrete(ex: Endo**crine**)
-cusis: hearing(ex: Dysa**cusis**)
-cyte: cell(ex: Erythro**cyte**)
-derma: skin(ex: Sclero**derma**)
-duction: bringing(ex: Ab**duction**)
-dynia: pain(ex: Gastro**dynia**)
-eal: referring to(ex: Corpor**eal**)
-ectasis: dilation(ex: Bronchi**ectasis**)
-ectomy: removal(ex: Append**ectomy**)
-edema: swelling(ex: Lymph**edema**)
-emesis: vomiting(ex: Hyper**emesis**)
-emia: blood(ex: Leuk**emia**)
-esis: condition(ex: Cent**esis**)
-esthesia: sensation(ex: An**esthesia**)
-ferent: to carry(ex: Af**ferent**)
-gen: produce(ex: Carcino**gen**)
-globin: protein(ex: Hemo**globin**)
-gnosis: knowing(ex: Dia**gnosis**)
-gram: record(ex: Echocardio**gram**)
-graph: recording(ex: Electrocardio**graph**)
-lysis: dissolve(ex: Dia**lysis**)

-malacia: soften(ex: Chondro**malacia**)
-mania: frenzy(ex: Pyro**mania**)
-megaly: enlargement(ex: Acro**megaly**)
-meter: measuring(ex: Thermo**meter**)
-metry: measuring(ex: Tele**metry**)
-oid: resembling(ex: Corac**oid**)
-ole: little(ex: Arteri**ole**)
-oma: tumor(ex: Carcin**oma**)
-orexia: appetite(ex: An**orexia**)
-ory: referring to(ex: Circulat**ory**)
-ose: referring to(ex: Comat**ose**)
-osis: condition(ex: Atheroscler**osis**)
-ous: referring to(ex: Por**ous**)
-pathy: disease(ex: Neo**pathy**)
-penia: deficiency(ex: Hydro**penia**)
-phagia: eat(ex: Dys**phagia**)
-phasia: speech(ex: Dys**phasia**)
-philia: attraction(ex: Hemo**philia**)
-phylaxis: protection(ex: Ana**phylaxis**)
-physis: growth(ex: Epi**physis**)
-plasia: formation(ex: Hyper**plasia**)
-plasm: growth(ex: Neo**plasm**)
-plasty: repair(ex: Rhino**plasty**)
-plegia: paralysis(ex: Quadri**plegia**)
-pnea: breathing(ex: **Apnea**)
-poiesis: formation(ex: Hemato**poiesis**)
-porosis: porous(ex: Osteo**porosis**)
-rrhage: bursting forth(ex: Hemo**rrhage**)
-rrhea: discharge(ex: Dia**rrhea**)
-rrhexis: rupture(ex: Entero**rrhexis**)
-scope: examining(ex: Endo**scope**)
-spasm: twitch(ex: Myo**spasm**)
-scopy: visual exam(ex: Arthro**scopy**)
-stasis: standing still(ex: Homeo**stasis**)
-stenosis: narrowing(ex: Arterio**stenosis**)
-stomy: opening(ex: Colo**stomy**)
-tension: stretch(ex: Hyper**tension**)
-thorax: chest(ex: Pneumo**thorax**)
-tomy: incision(ex: Ana**tomy**)
-toxic: poison(ex: Neuro**toxic**ity)
-tripsy: crushing(ex: Litho**tripsy**)
-trophy: nourishment(ex: A**trophy**)
-uria: urine(ex: Hyper**uria**)
-y: condition(ex: Acromegal**y**)

General Medical Terms

A

ABC: References things to check before administering resuscitation efforts, Airway, Breathing, Circulation.
Abscess: A localized collection of pus.
Acute: Sudden, severe onset of a medical condition or disease.
Adhesion: Stuck together.
Ambulant/Ambulatory: The ability to walk.
Arrest: Cessation of bodily activity or function.
Aseptic: Sterile.
Autonomy: Being self-governed.

B

Benign: Does not spread.
Biopsy: Surgically removing tissue to examine microscopically.

C

Cachexia: Loss of appetite, weight, with muscle atrophy, usually associated with a serious medical condition such as cancer.
Carcinogen: A substance that may cause cancer.
Chronic: Disease/condition that persists over a period of time.
Collis: Neck.

D

Diagnosis: Determination of the cause of a disease.

E

Edema: An excessive accumulation of fluid in an area.
Etiology: The study of the cause of a disease.
Excision: Surgically removing a structure or tissue.

F

Febrile: Presence of a fever.
Fistula: Location where an organ has developed an opening into another organ.

I

Idiopathic: An unknown cause of disease.
Incision: Cutting in to, typically with a scalpel.
Incontinence: Loss of control of the bladder and/or bowels.
In Situ: "In original place", commonly references cancer that is still in its place of origin, such as the epithelium of the skin.
Intravenous: Inside a vein, usually referencing injections.
Ischemia: Lack of blood flow to an area, which may result in necrosis.

M

Malaise: General unwell feeling or discomfort.
Malformation: A structure that is not formed properly.
Malignant: Spreading of cancer from one area to another.

N

Necrosis: Death of tissue.
Neopathy: A new disease.

P

Pallor: General paleness.
Palsy: Paralysis.
Peptic: Referring to the stomach.
Phlegm: Secretions expelled from the lungs, also known as sputum.
Phobia: Fear of a person, thing, or situation.
Prognosis: Predicted outcome of a disease and recovery rate.
Pulse: Expansion of an artery as blood passes through.
Pyrogenic: Producing fever.

S

Sepsis: An infection.
Sign: Observable indications of an illness.
Sinus: A cavity.
Sputum: Secretions expelled from the lungs, also known as phlegm.
Symptom: A physical manifestation of an illness.
Syndrome: Groups of symptoms caused by a disease.

T

Transient: Short duration.

Diagnostic Procedures

Echocardiogram

An echocardiogram is a type of **ultrasound** performed on the **heart** in order to view all the **structures and chambers of the heart**. This can be used to determine if there are any issues with the heart, such as valve defects, how strong the heart muscle is, or if there are any abnormal holes in the heart.

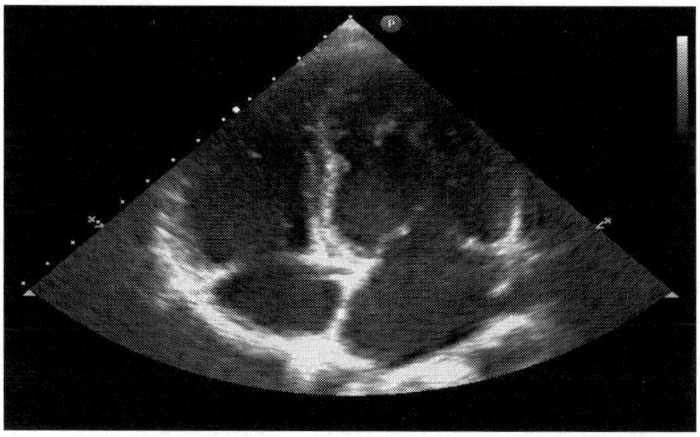

Mammogram

A mammogram is a procedure used to detect **breast cancer** in patients who are **not showing any symptoms**. It uses an X-ray to view the internal breast tissue. A mammogram is typically performed by placing the breast between two glass plates that compress the tissue. Compressing the tissue allows the X-ray to view all of the breast without missing anything.

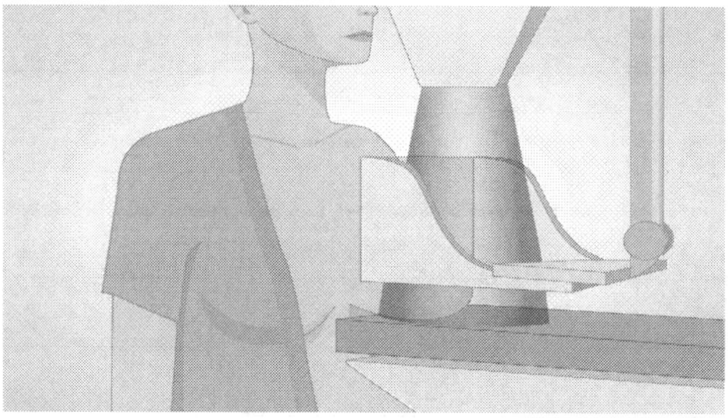

Electroencephalogram

An electroencephalogram is a test used to detect the **electrical activity of the brain**. It uses electrodes placed around the head that attach directly to the scalp to detect electric activity. Electroencephalograms are performed to help diagnose **brain disorders**, such as encephalitis, tumors, epilepsy, and damage to the brain from concussions.

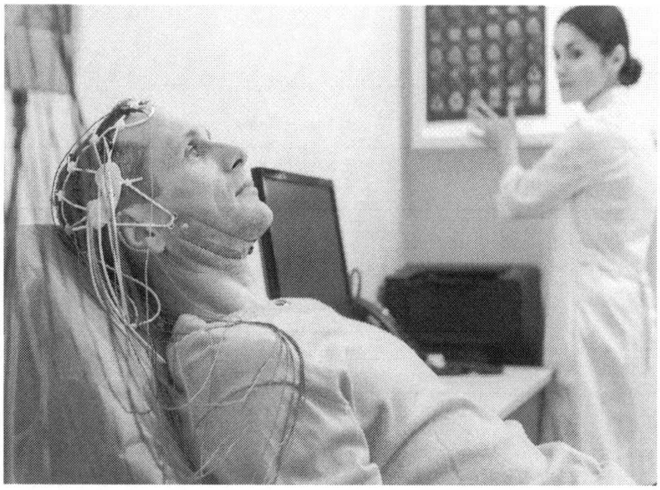

Electromyography

Electromyography is a test used to detect the proper functioning of **muscles and the nerves that innervate the muscles**. This is done to assess any **nerve or muscle damage** that may be present, or if communication between the nerve and muscle has been impaired. Electromyography is performed by several different means. A needle may be placed directly into the muscle to read electrical activity. Adhesive pads may be placed on the skin above the muscle to detect nervous conduction as well.

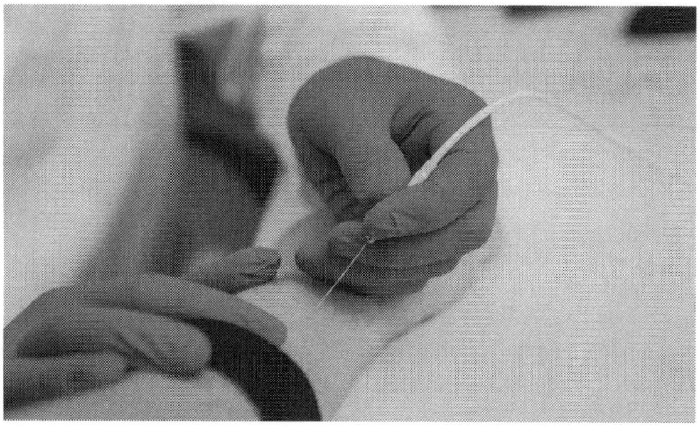

Myelogram

A myelogram is an imaging procedure used to view problems that may be occurring in the **spinal canal**. Special dyes are injected into the spinal column, and the patient is given X-rays, which allow the structures inside the spinal canal to be properly viewed. Myelograms are used to examine conditions such as herniated discs, infections such as meningitis, and tumors in the brain or spinal cord.

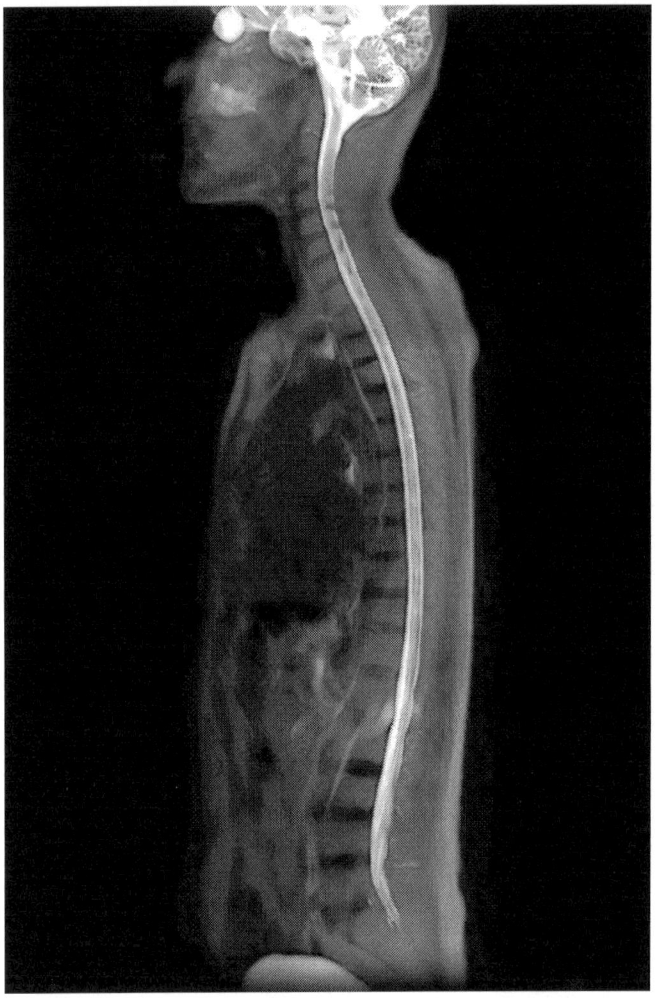

X-Ray

An X-ray is an imaging technique using radiation to view structures that light typically does not pass through. Structures most commonly seen using X-rays are **bones and metals**. X-rays allow visual examination of structures that may be broken, damaged, or infected.

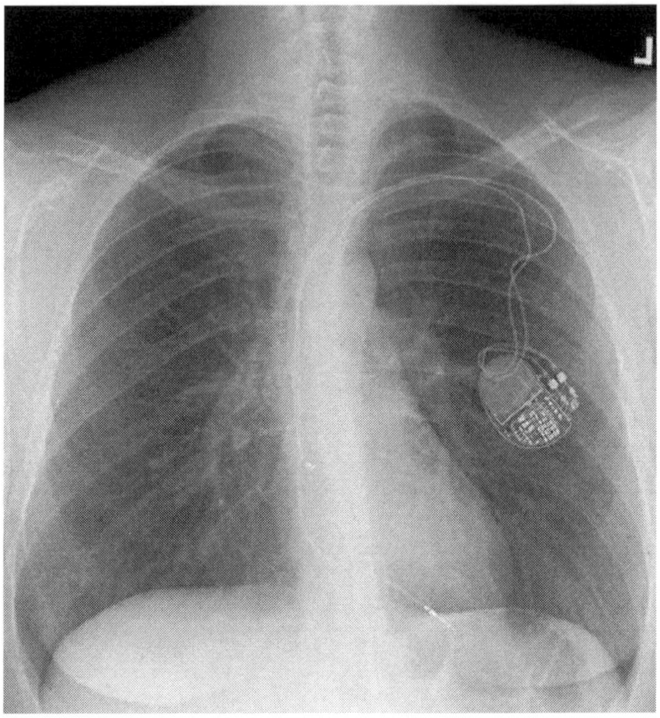

Surgical Procedures

Angioplasty

An **angioplasty** is a surgical procedure used to **open arteries**, most commonly the coronary arteries, that have been **blocked** by excessive accumulation of **plaque** on the walls of the arteries. The primary goal is to return or increase blood flow to structures that have seen a reduction in blood flow due to blockage. Balloon angioplasty involves inserting a small catheter with a balloon attached into an artery at the site of the blockage, and inflating the balloon. This presses the plaque against the walls and thins the plaque, allowing adequate blood flow to return. Insertion of a stent involves placing a circular metal mesh tube inside the artery at the site of angioplasty, preventing plaque from building on the location again.

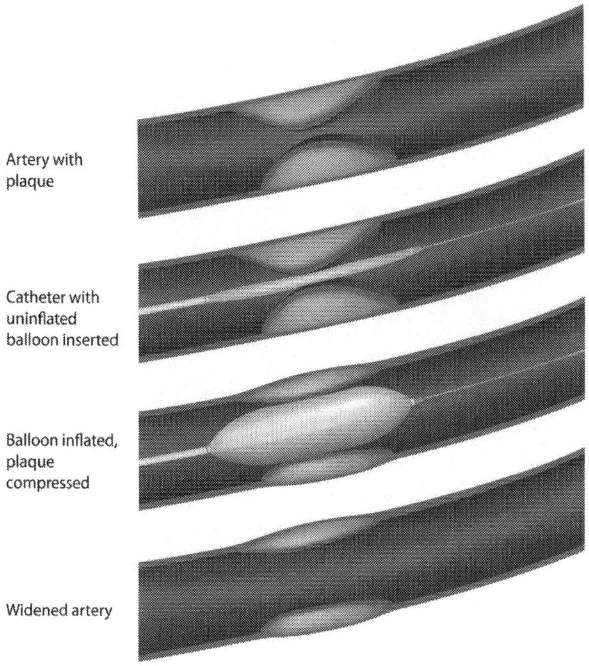

Appendectomy

Appendectomy is **surgical removal** of the **appendix**. When the appendix becomes inflamed and infected, it is an emergency medical situation, and the appendix must be removed. If the appendix is not removed, it may rupture, resulting in internal bleeding. An open appendectomy involves making an incision in the lower right abdomen and removing the appendix through this opening. Laparoscopic appendectomy involves creating three small incisions in the skin and inserting a tube with a camera and surgical instruments attached into one incision. Using the camera, the surgeon can guide the tools to the correct location, cut the appendix, and remove the appendix through another incision site.

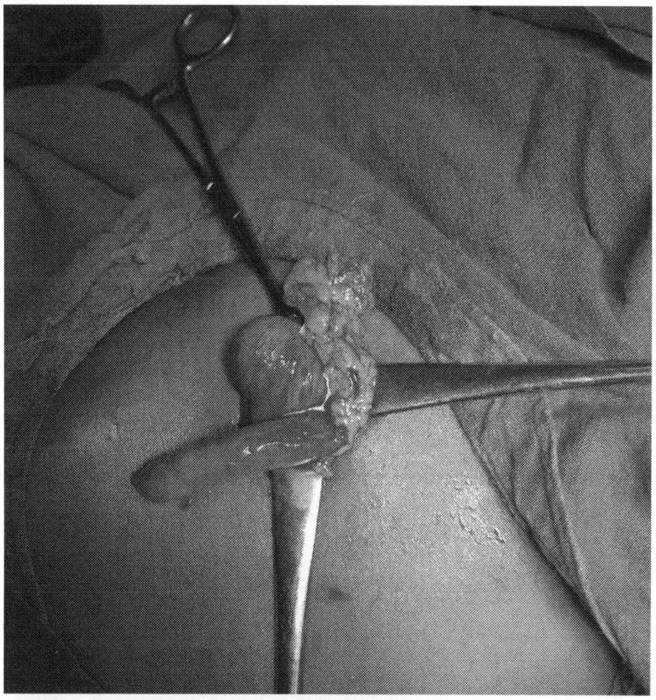

Arthroscopy

Arthroscopy is used to **view the inner structures of a joint**. It is performed by making a small incision, and inserting a **tube with a camera attached** directly into the joint. This allows a view of any structural damage that may occur, such as torn ligaments. If surgery is being performed, it may be performed arthroscopically, where all the instruments being used are inserted into the joint through small holes, without making a large incision.

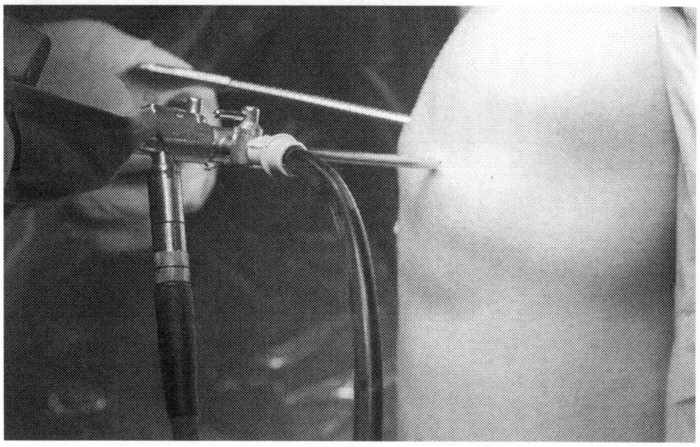

Biopsy

A **biopsy** is **removal of tissue for microscopic examination.** A biopsy is typically performed when there is an area of tissue that may be abnormal. These areas are commonly referred to as lesions, masses, or tumors. Biopsy may be performed by physically cutting out tissue using a scalpel, or by inserting a needle into a mass and extracting tissue with the needle. The tissue is then examined using a microscope to determine the type of tissue involved, if the growth is benign or malignant, or if the tissue is nothing to worry about.

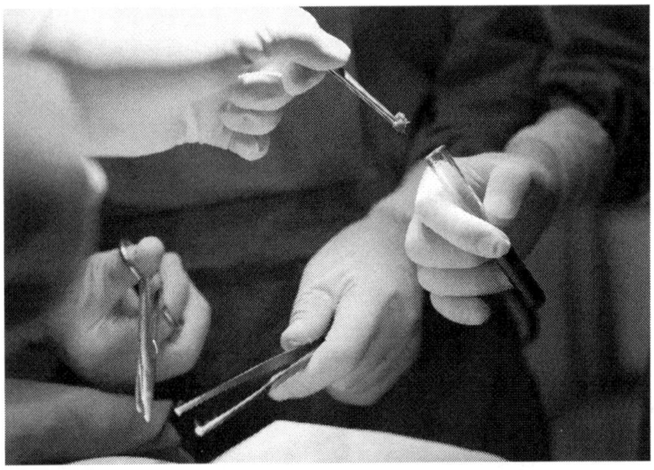

Bone Graft

A **bone graft**, similar to a skin graft, is the **removal of a small amount of bone tissue** from one part of the body, **placing the removed tissue on another bone** that may be lacking in sufficient tissue. This can be done if part of a bone is removed during surgery, or in cases such as joint replacements to help the new structures anchor in to the bone more securely. The new bone sets, and the area where the graft is located becomes stronger.

C-Section

C-section, also known as **Caesarian section/birth**, is delivering a baby via making an **incision in the mother's abdomen.** An incision is made in the uterus, and the baby is extracted. The uterus and abdomen are then surgically closed. C-sections are most commonly performed when there is the possibility of complications during childbirth that could harm the child, mother, or both.

Cataract Removal

A **cataract** is an area in the lens of the eye that has become **cloudy**. This can interfere with a person's vision, making it more difficult to do tasks such as reading, play sports, or perform tasks at the workplace. Cataract removal involves **removing the entire lens** of the eye, replacing it with an **artificial lens.** The lens may be removed by using an ultrasound to destroy the lens and allow it to be removed, or by removing the lens in one single piece.

Cholecystectomy

Cholecystectomy is **surgical removal** of the **gallbladder**. If the gallbladder has developed **gallstones**, the gallstones may block the bile duct, and cause bile to back up in the gallbladder. This can be a painful condition. If extraction of the gallstones or lithotripsy does not fix the issue, the gallbladder may be removed. Bile then drains from the liver directly into the duodenum.

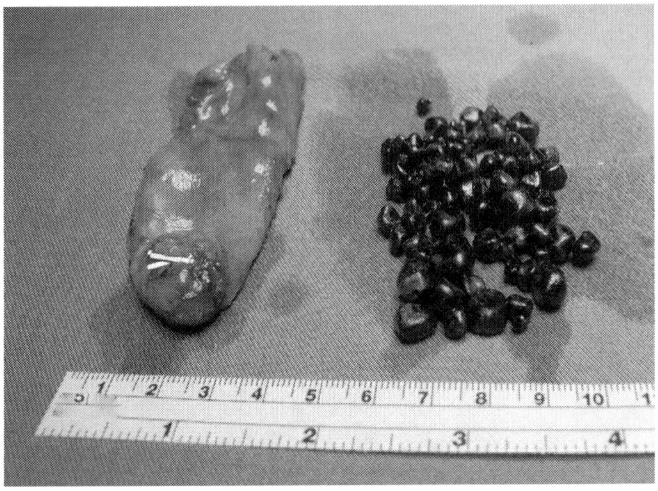

Coronary Bypass

If a person has a **blockage in the coronary arteries** that cannot be fixed by using angioplasty, or if a person is experiencing a myocardial infarction resulting from blockage of the coronary arteries, a **coronary artery bypass** can be used to re-establish blood flow into the heart. During this procedure, a portion of another artery or vein such as the great saphenous vein, radial artery, and mammary artery is removed and relocated to the base of the aorta. It is then attached to the coronary artery past the site of blockage, reintroducing blood flow into the heart tissue supplied with blood by the artery. A double coronary bypass involves two coronary arteries receiving bypass, triple involves three coronary arteries, and quadruple involves four coronary arteries.

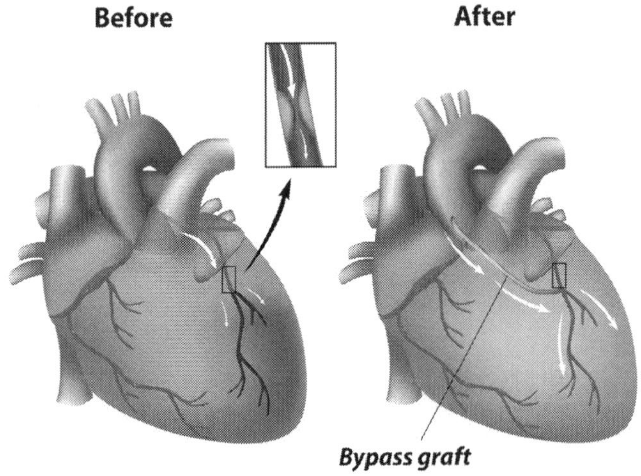

Debridement

Debridement is the process of **removing dead or damaged tissue** from a wound. Debridement is performed to **clean a wound** of any tissue that could cause bacterial growth, and to stimulate new tissue formation to help the wound heal. Debridement is often performed on ulcers that have developed due to poor circulation, such as decubitus ulcers or diabetic ulcers. After debridement, the wound is left with granulated tissue. The wound is covered by a bandage to prevent infection, and new tissue forms. Scarring of the area is likely, and secondary intention healing occurs, filling in the space of missing tissue with scar tissue.

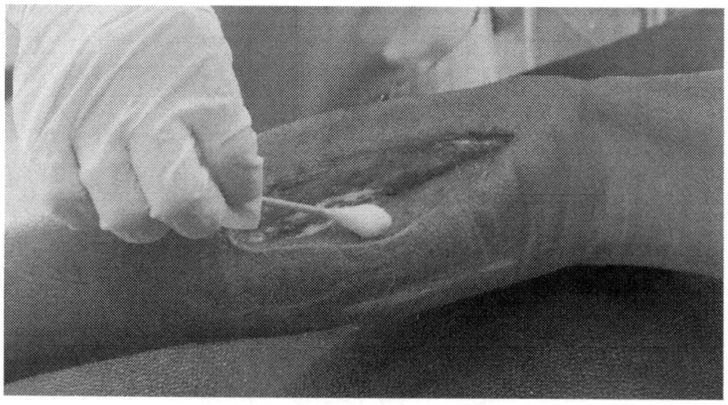

Dilation and Curettage

Dilation and curettage is a procedure used to **remove tissue from the uterus**. D&C is most commonly performed during miscarriage, abortion, or to diagnose certain medical conditions such as uterine bleeding. During the procedure, the **cervix is dilated**, and a **curette** is used to **remove tissue**. A curette is a small metal instrument designed to be used for scraping and removing tissue.

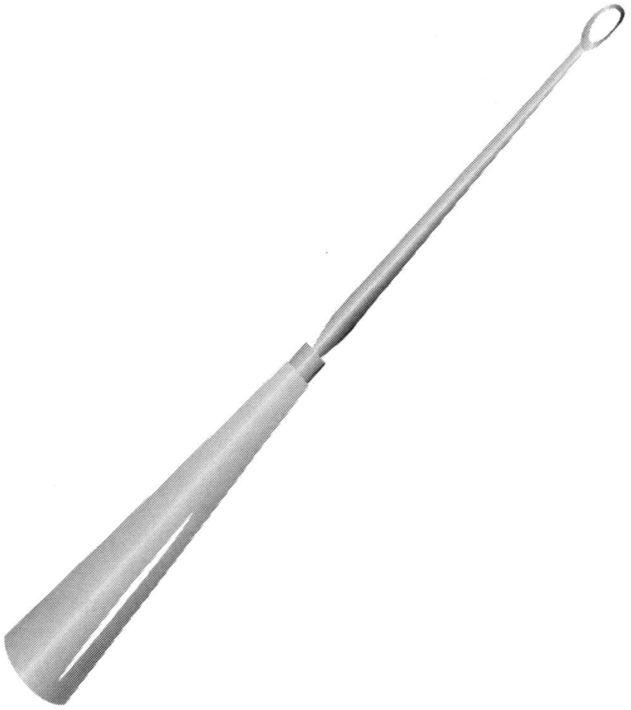

Epidural

An epidural is a medical procedure used to **block pain and sensation in the lower body**. It is performed by injecting analgesics and anesthetics around the **spinal cord in the lumbar region**. The medications are delivered via a catheter inserted into the site of injection. Epidurals are commonly used during labor to eliminate pain associated with child birth.

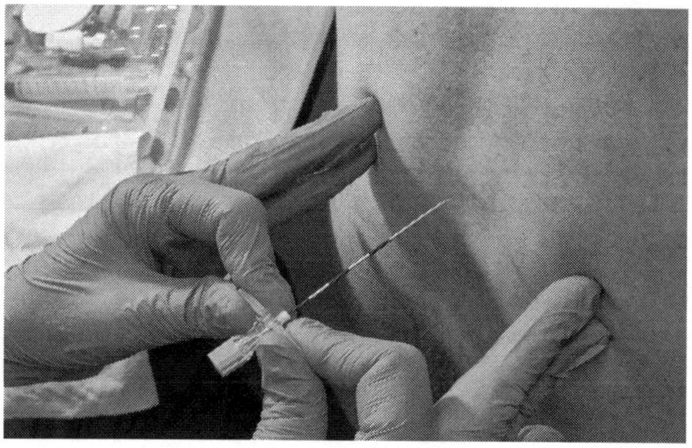

Hernia Surgery

Hernia surgery is performed to **return a structure or organ** that has protruded through its normal location back, and to **repair the area of protrusion**. These surgeries require an incision. Open hernia surgery involves a surgeon making one cut into the groin, and then repairing the hernia by stitching the area of herniation to prevent the hernia from occurring again. A synthetic mesh may be attached to help strengthen the area as well. Laproscopic hernia surgery involves making a small incision near the umbilicus. A tube containing a camera, light, and surgical tools is inserted into this incision, and is routed to the site of the hernia. A mesh is usually attached to the abdominal wall in laproscopic repair. Robotic hernia repair is similar to laproscopic repair, but instead of the surgeon physically handling the instruments, the surgeon controls tools via an electric console.

Hysterectomy

Hysterectomy is **surgical removal of the uterus**. Cancer, prolapse of the uterus, the development of uterine fibroids, endometriosis, and heavy periods are primary reasons a person may have the uterus removed. A partial hysterectomy removes only the upper portion of the uterus, leaving the lower portion of the uterus and cervix intact. In a total hysterectomy, the uterus and cervix are removed, leaving the fallopian tubes and ovaries. In a radical hysterectomy, the entire internal female reproductive system is removed.

Joint Replacement

If a person has developed severe joint issues, such as osteoarthritis, or has suffered fractures at locations such as the neck of the femur, joint replacement surgery may be performed. During the procedure, the **damaged bone and articular cartilage is removed**. The bone is then hollowed out to a point. **Prosthetics** are then placed inside the bone, and replace the structures that create the joint. For example, the neck/head of the femur is removed, and an artificial neck/head made of metal is attached in its place. An arthritic knee may require the surfaces of the femur and tibia to be removed, and metal replacements inserted to allow the joint to move without pain once again.

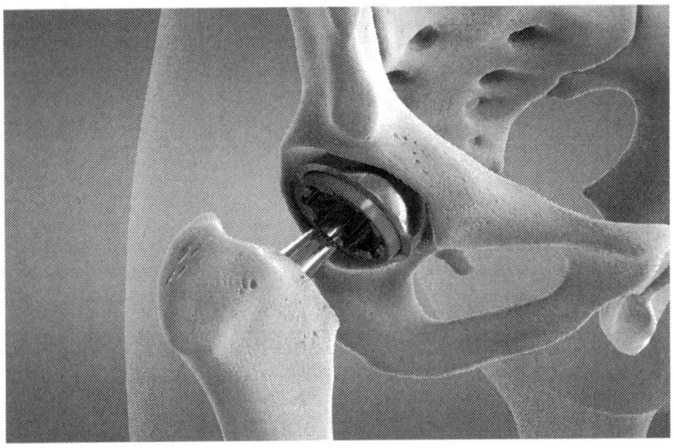

Lithotripsy

Lithotripsy is the use of **sound waves** administered via ultrasound to **break up or destroy deposits** building up in the body, such as **kidney stones and gallstones.** Lithotripsy is typically only performed if one of these deposits is too large to pass from the body on its own. The sound waves produced break up the deposit, and allow it to be passed normally. These sound waves are produced by a machine known as a lithotripter.

Mastectomy

Mastectomy is **surgical removal of breast tissue.** Mastectomy is most commonly performed if there is breast cancer, or chance of breast cancer occurrence. Total mastectomy is the removal of an entire breast, including the nipple, areola, and skin. Radical mastectomy removes the breast, nipple, areola, skin, pectoral muscles, and lymph nodes in the chest and axilla. Modified radical mastectomy removes the breast, nipple, areola, skin, lymph nodes in the chest and axilla, and the lining of the pectoral muscles. Patients who have a mastectomy may opt for reconstructive surgery afterwards.

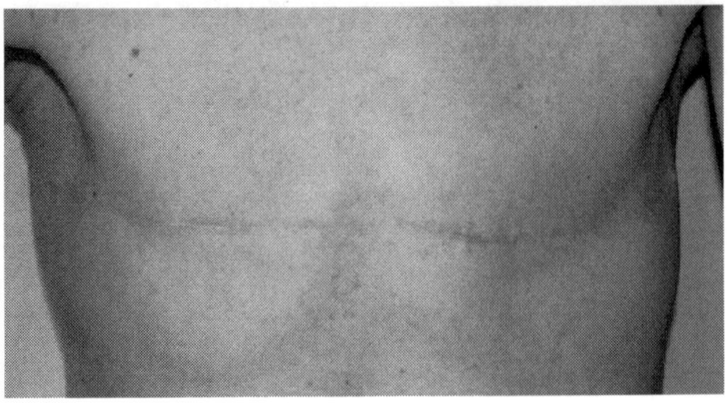

Prostatectomy

Prostatectomy is **surgical removal of the prostate.** The prostate may be partially or completely removed depending on the reason for the excision. Complete removal of the prostate is known as radical prostatectomy. Prostatectomy is most commonly performed to treat prostate cancer or benign prostatic hyperplasia, an enlargement of the prostate that can restrict the flow of urine. Prostatectomy is performed by making a small incision in the abdomen or perineum and removing the prostate through the opening.

Skin Graft

A skin graft is **transplanting skin from one location on the body to another** where skin has been lost, commonly from burns or injuries. A thin layer of epidermis is removed using a shaver(similar to a potato peeler), then placed on the area where skin is needed. The area is covered in bandages to allow healing. Over time, the skin adheres to the injured area and becomes new skin for the area.

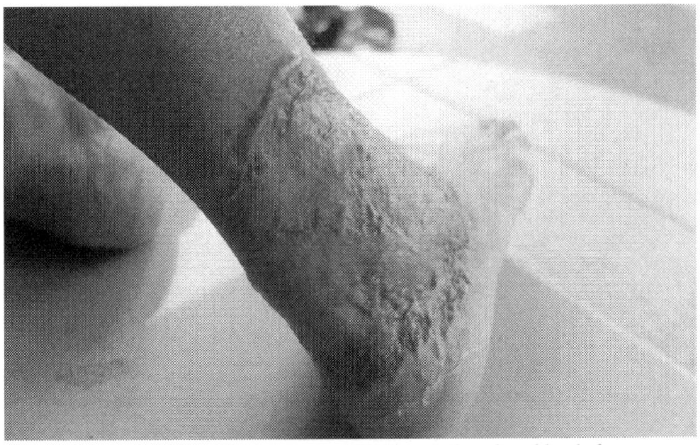

Area of skin where skin graft has been placed and healed

Tonsillectomy

Tonsillectomy is **surgical removal of the tonsils.** Tonsillectomy is commonly performed if infections of the throat are common that result in tonsillitis, or if a person has difficulty breathing during sleep. During a tonsillectomy, the tonsils are removed under general anesthesia, typically by use of electrocautery, dissection using a scalpel, or by using an ultrasound at high frequencies to cut the tonsils and stop the bleeding simultaneously.

Medical Terminology Matching

Word Roots		Prefixes		Suffixes	
_____: necr/o	_____: gloss/o	_____: auto-	_____: bi-	_____: -ferent	_____: -pnea
_____: leuk/o	_____: my/o	_____: a-	_____: macro-	_____: -blast	_____: -gen
_____: melan/o	_____: nephr/o	_____: tachy-	_____: brady-	_____: -duction	_____: -phagia
_____: cost/o	_____: brachi/o	_____: meta-	_____: torti-	_____: -crine	_____: -clast
_____: spondyl/o	_____: erythr/o	_____: syn-	_____: anti-	_____: -cision	_____: -edema
_____: gastr/o	_____: encephal/o	_____: homeo-	_____: iso-	_____: -trophy	_____: -osis
_____: derm/o	_____: hem/o	_____: hypo-	_____: circum-	_____: -algia	_____: -cyte
_____: chondr/o	_____: pneum/o	_____: inter-	_____: endo-	_____: -stasis	_____: -oid
_____: hepat/o	_____: phleb/o	_____: dia-	_____: ad-	_____: -emia	_____: -lysis
_____: cyst/o	_____: cardi/o	_____: micro-	_____: hyper-	_____: -derma	_____: -ectomy
A. Muscle	K. Vertebrae	A. Together	K. Large	A. Nourishment	K. Bringing
B. Liver	L. Stomach	B. Change	L. Towards	B. Blood	L. Germ Cell
C. Bladder	M. White	C. Without	M. Small	C. Production	M. Removal
D. Kidney	N. Vein	D. Two	N. Around	D. Swelling	N. Dissolve
E. Arm	O. Lung	E. Against	O. Twisted	E. Resembling	O. Cutting
F. Blood	P. Skin	F. Rapid	P. Excessive	F. Condition	P. Pain
G. Black	Q. Cartilage	G. Through	Q. Inside	G. Skin	Q. Eating
H. Tongue	R. Death	H. Equal	R. Below	H. Standing Still	R. Breathing
I. Brain	S. Red	I. Slow	S. Self	I. To Carry	S. Secrete
J. Rib	T. Heart	J. Same	T. Between	J. Break	T. Cell

Answer Key on Page 292

Medical Terminology Breaking Down/Building

Break down the following diseases by their word roots, prefixes, and suffixes, giving the definition of each part in the blank spaces.

1. Arteriosclerosis: __________/__________/__________
2. Pyelonephritis: __________/__________/__________
3. Encephalitis: __________/__________
4. Lymphedema: __________/__________
5. Hyperthyroidism: __________/__________/__________
6. Cholecystitis: __________/__________/__________
7: Hepatitis: __________/__________
8: Phlebitis: __________/__________
9. Torticollis: __________/__________
10. Dermatophytosis: __________/__________/__________
11. Acromegaly: __________/__________
12. Myocardial Infarction: __________/__________/__________
13. Insomnia: __________/__________
14. Neuralgia: __________/__________
15. Tenosynovitis: __________/__________/__________

Build the name of the following diseases just using their definition.
Remember, not every disease has a prefix or suffix!

1. Without blood: __________/__________
2. Fatty plaque hard condition: __________/__________/__________
3. Stomach inflammation: __________/__________
4. Black tumor: __________/__________
5. Fiber muscle pain: __________/__________/__________
6. Bone joint inflammation: __________/__________/__________
7. Bladder inflammation: __________/__________
8: Without breath: __________/__________
9. Nail fungus condition: __________/__________/__________
10. Skin inflammation: __________/__________
11. Above tension: __________/__________
12. Without rhythm: __________/__________
13. White blood condition: __________/__________
14. Hill condition: __________/__________
15. Cell inflammation: __________/__________

Answer Key on Page 294

Medical Terminology Crossword

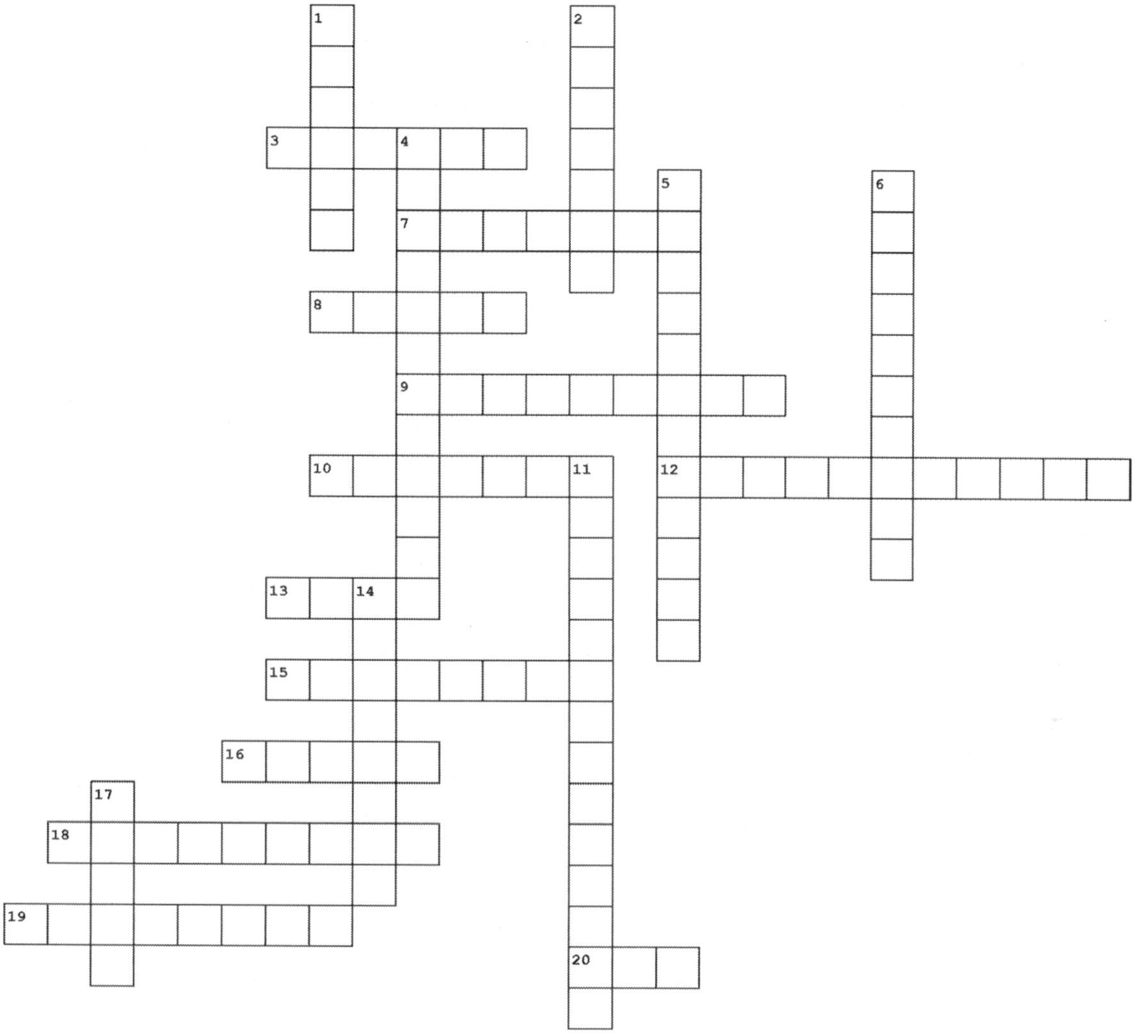

Across

3. intra-
7. Location where an organ has developed an opening into another organ
8. cardi/o
9. Imaging procedure used to view problems that may be occurring in the spinal canal
10. ecto-
12. Viewing the inner structures of a joint via use of a camera inserted into the joint
13. -algia
15. Loss of appetite, loss of weight, muscle atrophy associated with cancer
16. hepat/o
18. Predicted outcome of a disease and recovery rate
19. Procedure used to block pain and sensation in the lower body
20. pan-

Down

1. ren/o
2. a-
4. -itis
5. A structure that has not been formed properly
6. Surgical removal of breast tissue
11. Ultrasound performed to view all chambers and structures of the heart
14. Lack of blood flow to an area that may result in necrosis
17. encephal/o

Answer Key on Page 293

Medical Terminology Practice Test

1. "Removal of the gallbladder" is
A. Angioplasty
B. Cholecystectomy
C. Colostomy
D. Leiomyogram

2. The suffix "-emia" means
A. Blood condition
B. Production
C. Inflammation
D. Death

3. Procedure used to open arteries that have been blocked by excessive accumulation of plaque attached to the walls of the arteries
A. Arthroscopy
B. Debridement
C. Lithotripsy
D. Angioplasty

4. Which medication means "against life"
A. Antipyretic
B. Antibiotic
C. Antifungal
D. Antiviral

5. An ultrasound performed on the heart to view all structures and chambers of the heart
A. Electrocariogram
B. Electromyography
C. Myelogram
D. Echocardiogram

6. The term "endocrine" means
A. Secreting outside
B. Secreting above
C. Secreting inside
D. Secreting below

7. Of the following, which term refers to a cancer that is still found in its place of origin
A. Fistula
B. Sepsis
C. Malignant
D. In situ

8. Which of the following is "around the heart"
A. Epidural
B. Pericardium
C. Perineum
D. Epimysium

9. Removing tissue from the uterus is performed by utilizing
A. Hysterectomy
B. Debridement
C. Dilation and curettage
D. Biopsy

10. Which of the following describes a condition that involves the kidneys
A. Pyelonephritis
B. Osteoporosis
C. Gastritis
D. Cystitis

Answer Key on Page 295

Safety and Infection Control

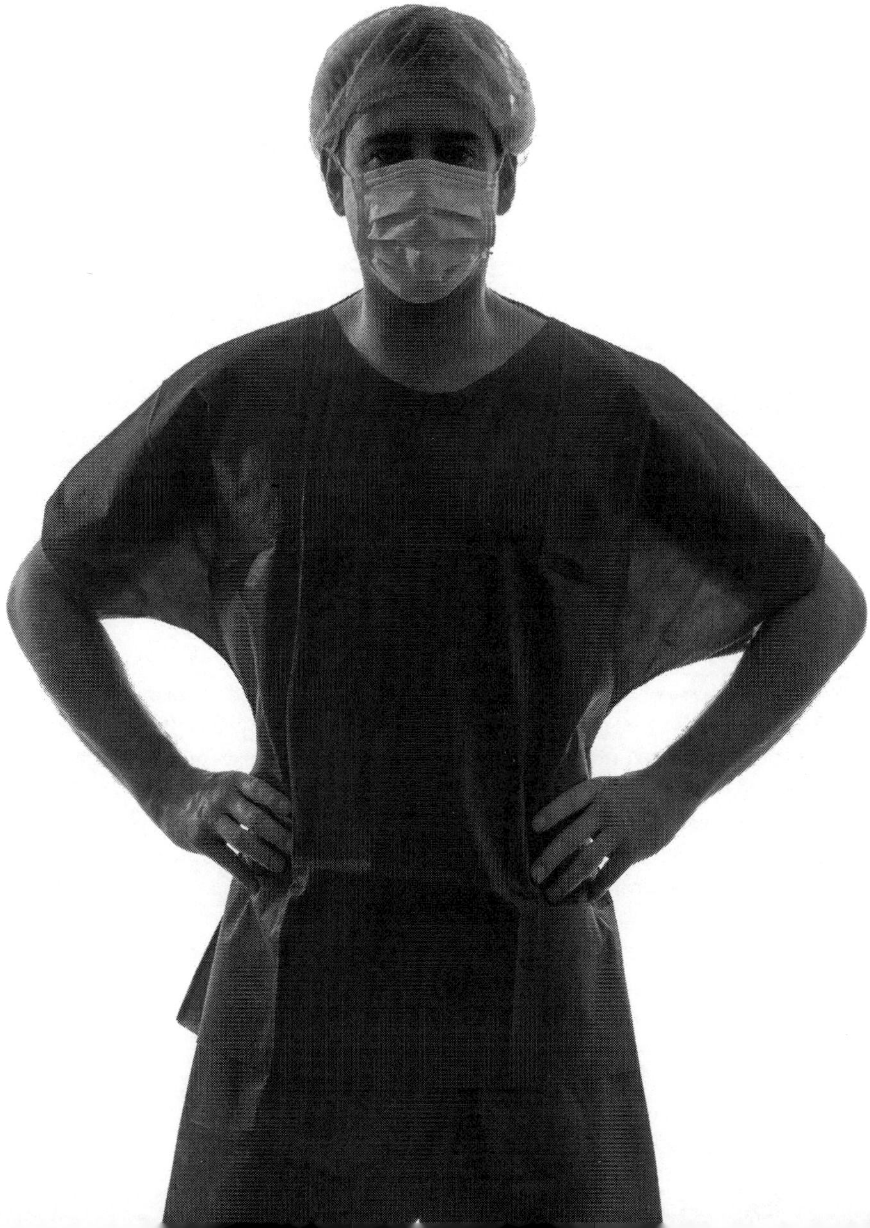

Infectious Agents

Infectious Diseases

An infection is an **invasion of a microorganism** inside the body in some way, which can range from localized and less serious, to systemic and life-threatening. These microorganisms are usually not inside the body, and therefore, the body does not have a knowledge of how to exactly combat the infection when first exposed. When there is an infection, the body develops antibodies, and these are used to destroy the invading microorganism.

There are four primary types of infections: bacterial, viral, parasitic, and fungal.

Bacterial Infections

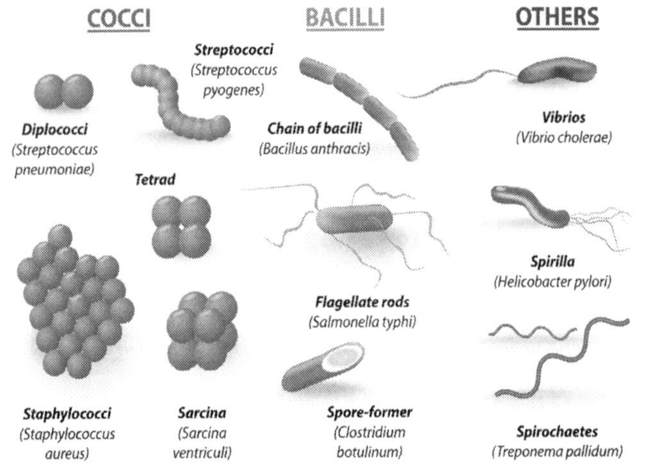

Bacteria are **single-celled organisms** that can only be seen under a microscope. They have a membrane surrounding the cell, and are able to freely reproduce via cell mitosis.

Bacterial infections are caused by an invasion of certain types of bacteria, such as H. pylori, staphylococcus, streptococcus, and salmonella. Bacteria come different shapes and sizes, some looking like rods(bacillus), and others looking like balls(borrelia) or spirals(spirilla). Bacterial infections make a person sick by **releasing toxic substances in their waste**. An overabundance of these toxins cause a person to become ill, depending on the severity. Bacteria are known to reproduce quickly, and treatment should be sought for serious bacterial infections such as pneumonia and strep throat. Treatment for bacterial infections involves taking a course of antibiotics, such as penicillin, which destroy the bacteria. Any course of antibiotics should be completed fully, as ceasing taking the prescribed dosage could result in any remaining bacteria becoming resistant to the antibiotics. It's in these cases where infections such as MRSA(methicillin-resistant staphylococcus aureus) may appear and become extremely difficult to treat, which may be life-threatening.

Viral Infections

Viral infections are caused by viruses, structures smaller than bacteria, that contain RNA or DNA in their core. They attach to healthy cells and **insert code into the cell** that changes the behavior in the cell and **causes the infected cell to create more virus particles.** These particles come together in the cell, creating new viruses. When too many of these viruses have formed, they break through the host cell and enter the body, infecting more healthy cells. This process is known as the **lytic cycle.**

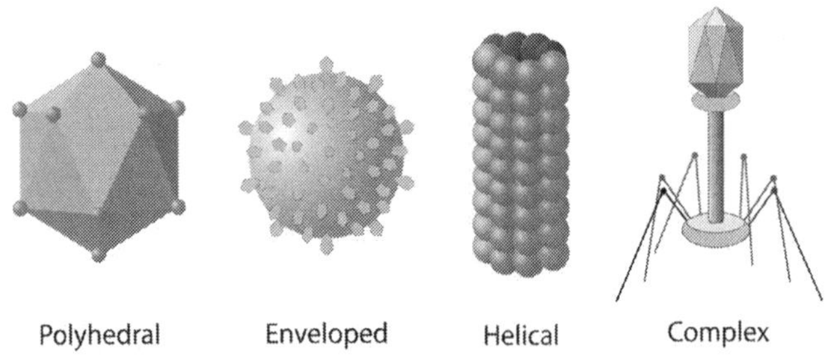

When the body detects a viral infection, it releases chemicals known as **pyrogens** into the body, which elevate body temperature. This increased body temperature, known as a fever, does not give the viruses an environment to thrive in, and ultimately the viruses die or fail to reproduce due to the extreme temperature change. Treatments for viral infections typically are used to treat the symptoms, as there is no way to destroy the virus itself. Vaccines can be used to introduce dead or weakened viruses into the body, which allow the body's immune system to develop antibodies for them, preventing future infections. Antiviral medications can be used to prevent a virus from reproducing, but cannot kill the virus.

Some viruses never leave a person's body and become dormant, not always causing problems. Others never leave the body and actively affect the body, such as HIV. Most of the time, in instances such as influenza, the body's immune system naturally fights off the virus over the course of a week or two.

Parasitic Infections

Parasitic infections are caused by small organisms that **use a host** in order to survive. These parasites may affect their host in some way, or they may not, depending on the type of parasite. The three types of parasites are protozoa, helminths, and ectoparasites.

Protozoa are single-celled organisms, and they live inside the host's body, multiplying beyond safe levels. A protozoa infection is considered serious, most commonly the result of drinking water that may contain the parasite.

Helminths are also known as **worms**, such as tapeworms, flukes, and roundworms. Worms most commonly enter the host's body through consuming a food or drink that contains the worm or worm larvae.

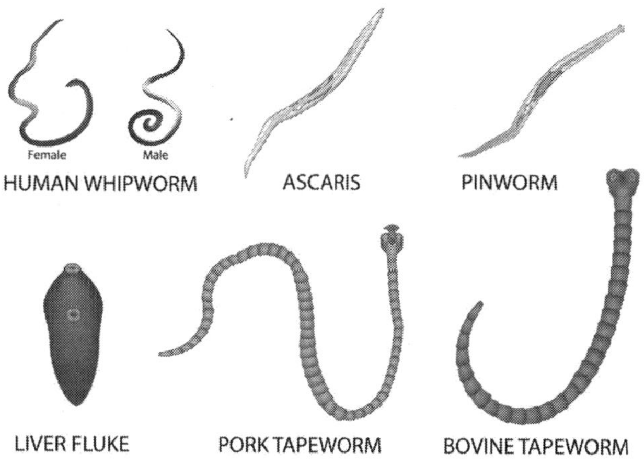

Types of Helminths

Ectoparasites are parasites that attach to the surface of the host, often feeding off the blood of the host to survive. Examples include mosquitoes, leeches, and ticks.

Some parasitic infections do not require treatment. If symptoms or infection appears, treatment should be sought. Common parasitic infection treatments include anti-parasitic medications used to destroy any parasites, and removal of the parasite if medication does not work.

Fungal Infections

Fungal infections are caused by a fungus **coming into contact with the skin** or entering into the body via means such as **inhalation.** Certain fungi thrive in specific environments that are **dark, warm, and humid**. Examples of these include athlete's foot and jock itch. Other fungi may attach to dead tissues, such as the nails or skin. An example of these include ringworm and onychomycosis.

Common forms of fungi that result in infection include candidiasis, aspergillosis, sporothrix, talaromyces, and histoplasma. These fungi can be found in various parts of the world, and can affect people differently depending on the strength of their immune system. Some fungi thrive in extremely moist environments, while other fungi may not need as much moisture to grow.

Fungal infections are treated with medications known as antifungals, which are designed to destroy fungus. These can be used directly on the skin as ointments or shampoos, orally in gel or liquid form, or inserted into a part of the body such as the vagina in cases such as yeast infections. Serious fungal infections may need to be treated with antifungals injected into the body.

Infection Cycle/Chain of Infection

Chain of Infection

The chain of infection specifically refers to a pathogen leaving its original location and infecting an organism, encompassing all the steps that lead to infection.

The infectious agent's normal habitat is known as a **reservoir.** Every microorganism has its own reservoir, and transmission may not necessarily come from exposure to the reservoir. Humans may be reservoirs for certain infections, such as staphylococci or streptococci infections. Animals may be reservoirs for several infectious agents, such as rabies, anthrax, and plague. Certain environments may also be reservoirs, such as soil. Dark and humid environments are reservoirs for fungi to grow.

Portals of exit refer to the manner in which an infectious agent **leaves its host**. For example, a virus such as influenza leaves its host through the respiratory tract, while hepatitis B leaves its host through the blood. As previously discussed, there are several different modes of transmission, and not every pathogen can be spread through every means.

Portals of entry refer to the manner in which an infectious agent **enters its new host**. Portals of entry and portals of exit are often the same with each pathogen. For example, hepatitis B leaves the host through blood, but does not enter the new host unless it is also mixed with that host's blood.

Body Barriers

The body contains many different barriers to prevent infections from entering the body or harming the body. The body's **first line of defense** is the **skin and mucous membranes**. These surfaces are exposed to pathogens constantly, but provide a thick layer of tissue that does not permit passage into the body, or contains chemicals that help to destroy the pathogens once introduced into the body. The skin provides a thick barrier. The cilia and mucous in the nose, throat, and lungs helps to trap debris that enters the body, preventing it from harming structures like the lungs. The stomach produces acids that can destroy harmful bacteria.

The body's **second line of defense** is the **immune system**, and includes the inflammatory response. This allows the body's immune system, and cells such as neutrophils, to destroy any invading pathogen or debris that may cause the body harm. The body may increase in temperature and produce a fever, which helps to destroy pathogens that cannot survive in higher temperatures. The second line of defense is also known as **innate immunity**, because it does not differentiate between different pathogens and treats them all the same way.

The body's **third line of defense** is also the **immune system**, but it is the responsibility of **T-cells** to recognize specific pathogens that have entered the body, and antibodies to neutralize the infection. This takes place after an infection has already been seen in the body before, and the body has developed an immunity to the pathogen. The third line of defense is also known as **adaptive immunity**, because it adapts to the presence of pathogens in the body and produces antibodies to combat future infections.

Modes of Transmission

There are various different ways a pathogen may enter the body. **Direct contact transmission** occurs when one person comes into direct contact with a person who is infected, in instances such as touching, kissing, sexual contact, or blood exposure. **Indirect contact transmission** occurs when an infected person does something such as sneezes, which sends the pathogen into the air. The pathogen is contained in **droplets** of fluid in the air, which can then be inhaled by another person, causing that person to become infected as well. If an infection can be spread through breathing, it is known as an **airborne illness**.

Standard Precautions and Exposure Control

Whenever there is any type of exposure to any body fluid, **standard precautions** should be utilized. Standard precautions assume any type of bodily fluid or substance is **contaminated** or contains contagious substances, and should be treated and cleaned as such.

Body fluids may be defined as any of the following: blood, saliva, vomit, urine, feces, semen, vaginal secretions, tears, sweat, oil, and mucous. **Secretions** are substances created by **glands**, such as **oil and mucous**. **Excretions** are **waste products** that the body expels, such as **urine and feces**. While neither a secretion or an excretion, blood may also exit the body due to some sort of trauma to the body such as a cut. Blood is especially dangerous because it may contain certain viruses, such as HIV, Hepatitis B, and Hepatitis C, which can all survive outside the body for an extended period of time.

Mucous membranes are membranes that produce mucous. These membranes can be found throughout the body, such as the entire digestive tract, mouth, nasal cavity, pharynx, larynx, and lungs.

Occupational Safety and Health Administration

The **Occupational Safety and Health Administration**, also known as **OSHA**, is an agency responsible for enforcing **occupational safety and health standards**. OSHA was developed in 1970, designed to ensure employers provide safe working environments for their employees. Employers are required to provide information to employees about any hazardous materials or conditions they may be exposed to, properly train employees in matters of workplace safety, provide personal protective equipment, keep records of illnesses or injuries sustained on the job, and not discriminate against an employee who has used their rights.

Workers are allowed to file reports or complaints to OSHA, be provided with a safe working environment, be properly trained regarding hazardous workplace environments, and are protected from retaliation for being a whistleblower in regards to unsafe working conditions.

Personal Protective Equipment

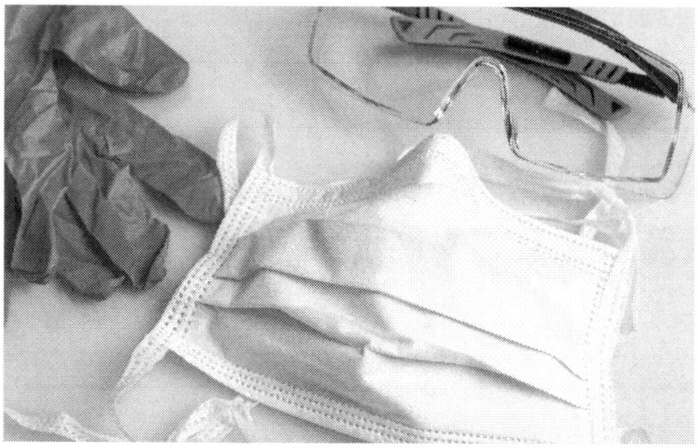

In the case of exposure, personal protective equipment is utilized to ensure there is no risk of infection to the person cleaning the fluid or substance. The amount of personal protective equipment required is dependent on the amount of fluid, and whether or not there is a risk of fluid being splashed around, such as with sewage.

Gowns are used to cover a person's clothing. Gloves are worn to protect the hands. Masks are used to prevent any airborne pathogens from being inhaled. Caps are used to protect the hair and prevent fluids from contaminating the hair. Eye protection, such as glasses, are used to prevent fluids from entering the eye.

One of the most important ways for a medical professional to ensure the environment is as sterile as possible is to utilize **hand washing** whenever possible. Hand washing with antibacterial soap helps eliminate a large portion of bacteria and microorganisms on the medical professional's hands. Any time a medical professional comes into physical contact with the patient or an instrument that will be used on a patient, the hands should be washed.

Hand washing is extremely important in reducing contamination and preventing infection from occurring. Before any form of medical treatment, the hands must be washed for a minimum of 15 seconds, utilizing soap and hot water. The soap should be lathered and rubbed on the hands and between the fingers. If there is dirt or debris under the fingernails, it may be cleaned out with the use of a bristle brush. Once the hands have been washed, they should be dried, and a paper towel or cloth should be used to turn the water off and open any doors to prevent the hands from being recontaminated.

If hand washing is not an option, the medical professional should use an **alcohol-based hand rub.** These typically come in a gel or foam, and contain isopropyl alcohol that destroys microorganisms on the skin. A dime-sized amount should be used, spread around the hands and between the fingers to cover all areas.

Coughing and sneezing etiquette is also extremely important in reducing the chance of infection. When a person coughs or sneezes, they expel not only air, but saliva and potentially harmful airborne illnesses. To reduce the chance of infection, a person should not cough or sneeze into their hands, but into either a tissue, or if a tissue is unavailable, the **upper sleeve/elbow**.

Post-Exposure Protocol

In any work-place environment where exposure to body fluids and blood is expected, a **post-exposure plan** is required. Post-exposure plans are used to protect employees who come into direct contact with body fluids during the course of work, providing them with structured directions in regards to safely cleaning the fluid, disposing of the fluid and any materials used to clean the fluid, proper sanitization and disinfection, and ensuring the employee is able to be tested for any blood-borne pathogens if exposure has occurred. Post-exposure plans like these are a requirement of OSHA.

Sharps/Needle Safety

Sharps are any form of **needle** that has been injected into the body. A common form of sharps are insulin needles. Sharps should be disposed of in a **sharps container**, which is a box that is used to hold only needles. This box is usually strong plastic, and prevents anyone who comes into contact with the box from being punctured by a needle that has already been used.

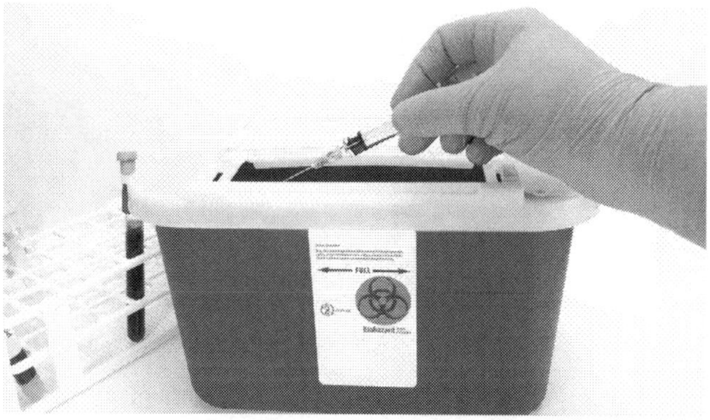

Medical Asepsis

Asepsis refers to a **lack of bacteria, virus, or microorganisms** present in a location or on an object. Asepsis is especially important in the medical field, and a way to protect not only the patient but the medical professional from possible infections.

Sterilization and Disinfection

To **sterilize** an object is to **reduce the number of microorganisms** on the object to a safe enough level or make that object usable without the risk of infection spreading. To **disinfect** an object means to **completely destroy all microorganisms** on the object. In cases such as blood exposure, the surface that has been exposed to the blood would be disinfected to ensure that no viruses or bacteria survive. Common forms of chemicals that can both sanitize and disinfect are ammonia and bleach. The amount of one of these substances being diluted with water determines if the object will be sanitized or disinfected. The more of a substance like bleach is used, the more it will be disinfected as opposed to sanitized.

Cleaning

Sanitization of the reception area is vital in not only providing comfort for the patient, but it instills confidence in the patient that the practice is of high quality. **Cleaning services** may be employed or contracted with, but it may be the job of the medical assistant to ensure the reception area is clean. Surfaces should be cleaned with antiseptic wipes, anything that has been moved out of its normal location, such as magazines left on a chair, should be placed back where they belong. Trash should be emptied regularly.

Biohazard Disposal/Regulated Waste

Disposal of any form of biohazard waste is extremely important. Failure to properly dispose of biohazard waste may be extremely dangerous and lead to contamination, infections, and accidental sticks.

Blood and body fluid must be disposed of by placing the substances in a container that can be closed and prevent fluids from potentially leaking during storage or transport. These containers must be **color-coded** to reflect which type of fluid or other potentially infectious material is inside. These are in accordance with OSHA guidelines.

When a spill occurs, ranging from blood to other hazardous material, a **spill kit** may be utilized to safely clean the spill. Spill kits contain the necessary tools for properly and safely cleaning a spill, including protective clothing such as gowns, gloves, and goggles, materials to absorb the spill such as paper towels, a dustpan and broom for cleaning in case of things like broken glass, disposable bags, and a container that holds the waste. Certain containers may also contain substances that control acid spillage such as sodium bicarbonate.

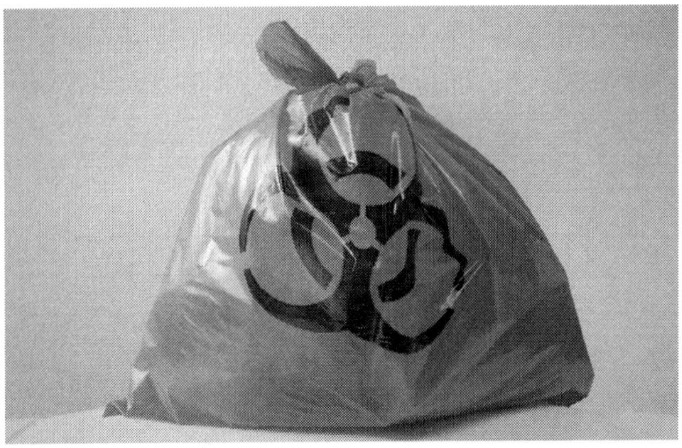

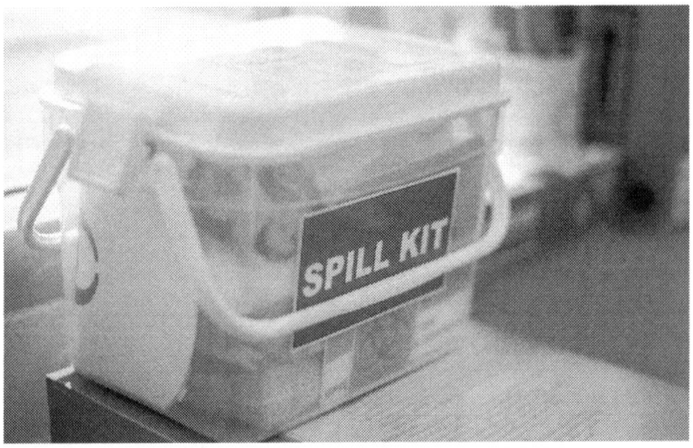

Safety Resources

Safety Signs, Symbols, and Labels

Safety signs, symbols, and labels are all useful, and in many cases required to prevent injuries in the workplace. Below are common signs, symbols, and labels that may be found in a workplace.

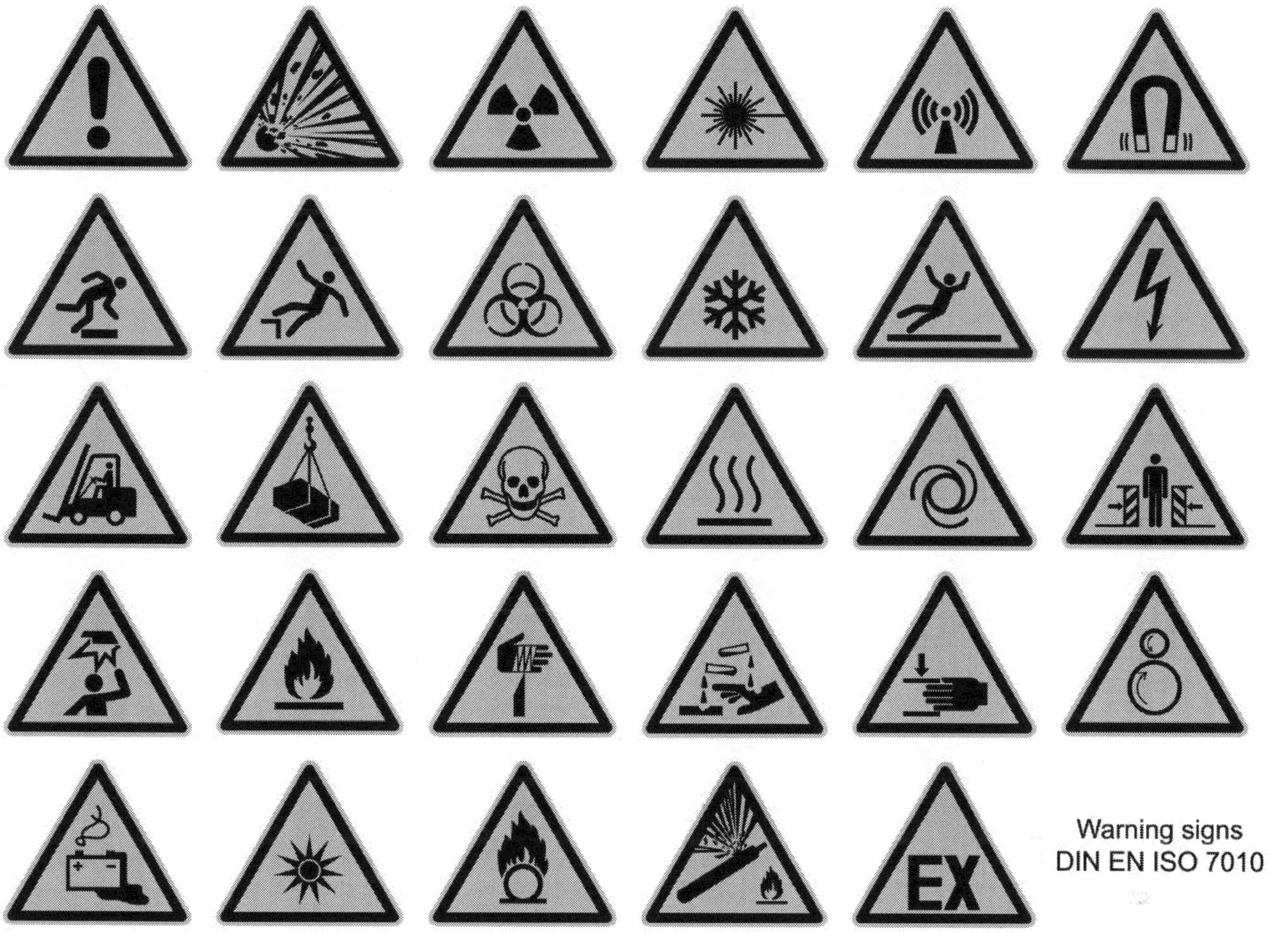

The reception area in a medical office should be **well-lit** and arranged in a way to allow a patient to safely exit the reception area if an emergency arises. **Exit signs** are required to be clearly visible. **Smoke detectors** are required to be placed in the office, and should be tested frequently. **Security systems** should be added to the office, as there is sensitive information, material, and possible medications that could be accessed easily without security devices installed.

Safety Data Sheets(SDS) and GHS

Safety data sheets(SDS) are required for manufacturers of chemicals or other potentially harmful substances to provide, which gives information on safely handling hazardous materials, health risks associated with handling the hazardous materials, and safely transporting and storing the material.

The **United Nations** developed a system used to **classify chemicals and their hazards**, and specifying information required to be included on hazardous chemical labels, safety data sheets, and in safety training. This allows the hazards of handling and working with chemicals to be easily understood.

Safety and Emergency Procedures

Workplace Accident Prevention

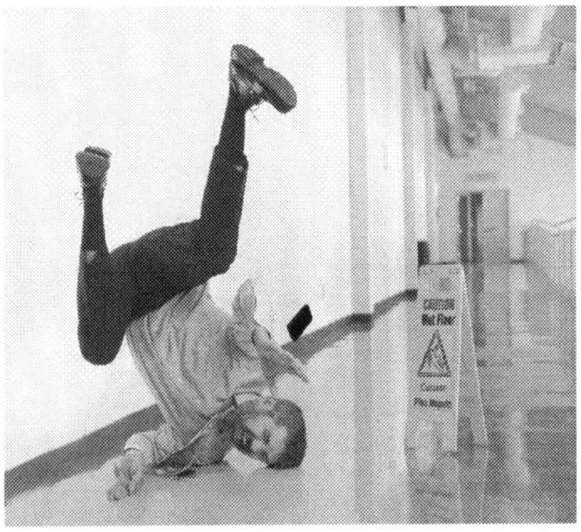

Slips occur when there is a **lack of friction** between a person's foot and the surface they are walking on. Common reasons a person may slip include slick or slippery floors, spills of wet substances, and floor mats that are not secure on the floor. Slips can be prevented by cleaning any spillage as quickly as possible, and a "Wet Floor" sign should be placed in the location to bring awareness to those walking through the area.

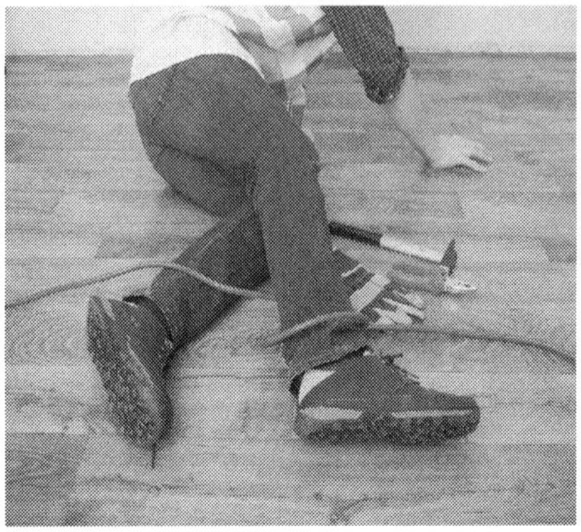

Trips occur when a person's foot gets **caught on an object**, causing the person to lose their balance. The person may stumble, or they may fall. Common reasons a person may trip include the foot getting caught on uncovered cables, edges of rugs or carpet, and objects sticking out in the path of where the person is walking. Trips can be prevented by removing any clutter or obstructions from a person's walking path, replacing any carpet or rugs a person may catch their foot on, and cover any wires that may be tripped over.

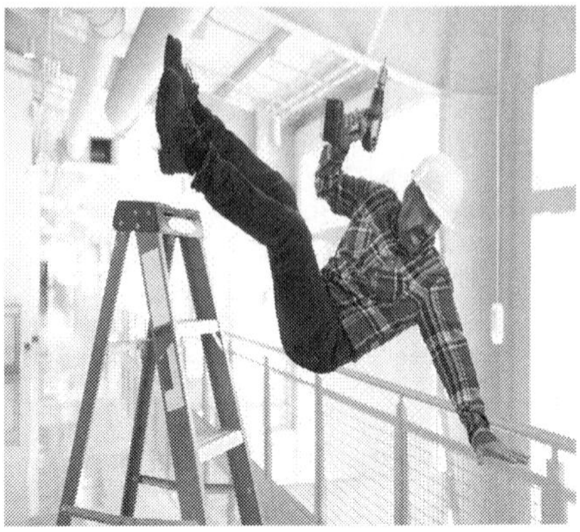

Falls occur when a person encounters an **unstable surface** that causes them to fall, other occupational structures such as ladders that are not secure and stabilized, and holes that a person may fall in to. Falls can be prevented by wearing appropriate footwear for the job being performed, making sure objects being used such as ladders are secure and stabilized, and any hole a person may fall in to are covered. If the hole cannot be covered, signs should be posted notifying those in the area of the hole to prevent falling.

Electrical Safety

Whenever there is possible exposure to electricity, safety should be taken to prevent shock or electrocution. Any areas or objects that have the potential to cause harm via electricity should be marked with appropriate signs warning of the danger. If works needs to be performed dealing with electrical wiring, electricity should be turned off beforehand. Personal protective equipment should always be worn. This equipment includes rubber gloves, safety glasses, safety shoes, hard hats, and flame-resistant uniforms.

Emergency Response Plan

When an emergency arises in a hospital or office setting, such as natural disasters, exposure to hazardous materials, and fires, an emergency response plan is needed. An emergency response plan contains guidelines for what each person is responsible for and how to act in case of an emergency. This can include preparation of a medical triage, instructions for quarantining an area or person, coordinating with local and government agencies, and in some cases, developing an evacuation plan. An evacuation plan details designated routes a person or persons should be directed to in order to effectively exit the premises without encountering danger.

Crash Cart

In cases of medical emergencies in office, a crash cart may be utilized to help treat the patient and the emergency. A crash cart is a mobile cart that contains several pieces of equipment. On a typical crash cart, there contains several medicines such as epinephrine, lidocaine, dopamine, diazepam, and nitroglycerin. Crash carts also contain monitors and an AED, in case of cardiac arrest.

Automated External Defibrillator

An Automated External Defibrillator, or **AED**, is a **portable defibrillator** used to send electric shocks to the heart in a person who is suffering from **sudden cardiac arrest**. The person will have two sticky pads attached to their skin that connect to the AED, one pad placed on the chest and one on the left side of the trunk. The AED sends a shock to the person through the pads, directly into the heart, which can help return the heart to its normal rhythm.

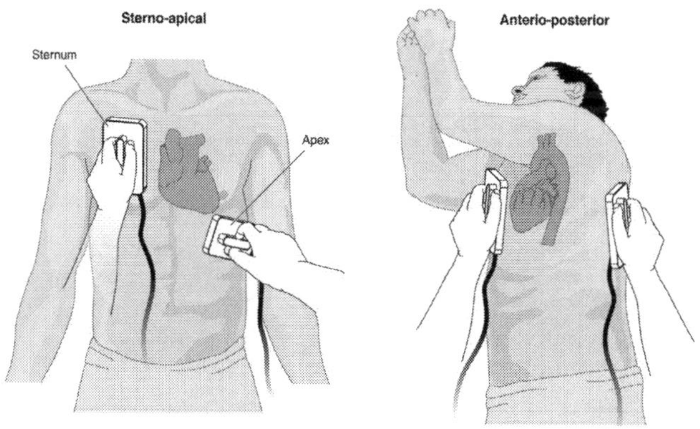

Fire Prevention

Fire extinguishers are a requirement of any workplace, per OSHA regulations. Fire extinguishers must be placed in an **easy to find** location, and must not be placed in a location that can increase susceptibility to injury on the part of the employee. Extinguishers should be located **within 75 feet** of an employee at all times.

Fire extinguishers must be maintained and inspected once a month. Training must be administered by the employer to all employees upon hiring and once every year afterwards.

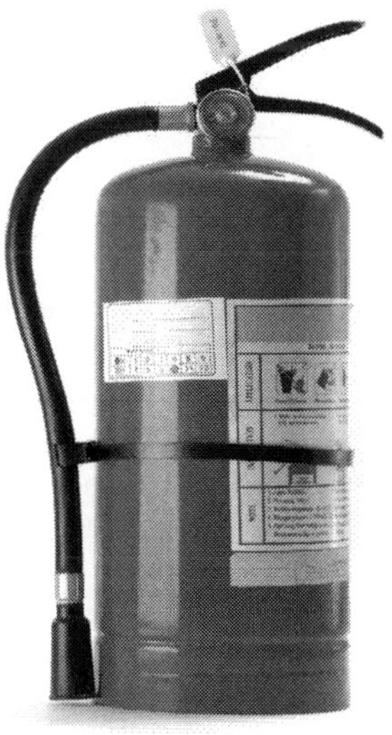

Emergency Management, Identification, and Response/Basic First Aid

There are many different ways to care for a person with a medical emergency, depending on the type of injury and the severity. When using first aid, **universal precautions** should be administered. Universal precautions are treating every person and fluid as if they were **contaminated or infectious**. Universal precautions are extremely important in containing blood-borne pathogens. Any time there is exposure to any type of bodily fluid, **gloves and other personal protective equipment** should be worn, and contact with blood should be avoided at all costs.

The **emergency triage** is used in emergency departments to assess incoming patients. It is usually performed by a **triage nurse**, who will assess the **severity** of the patient's injuries, the **urgency** of treatment required, and the **location** of the treatment needed. This helps determine the order in which a patient is seen, with more severe cases being seen before those with less severe cases.

CAB refers to the initial assessment steps that should be taken when coming into contact with an unconscious person. **Circulation** should be checked using pulse points. If no circulation is detected, the **airway** should be checked to determine if there is an obstruction that is causing the person to be unable to **breathe.** If there is an obstruction, it should try to be removed using a gentle finger swipe. If there is no circulation, the airway is not blocked, and the person is not breathing, CPR should be performed and EMS should be notified.

Bleeding Control

If a person is bleeding, a **sterile bandage** should be placed on the wound to promote **blood clotting**, which stops bleeding. If the bleeding is severe, a **tourniquet** may be applied, which should significantly reduce the bleeding. The person should lie down and be kept warm using a blanket, if available.

Burns

Treatment of burns depends on the severity of the burn. Minor burns on the skin are treated by running the burn under cold water for ten minutes. Lotion that contains aloe vera or cocoa butter should be applied afterwards to help keep the area from drying. The wound should be bandaged. If a blister forms, it should not be popped.

Major burns are considered medical emergencies, and should be treated as such. The area of the burn should be protected, and the person who has suffered the burn should be removed from any danger. If there is any jewelry in the area of the burn, it should be removed. The burn should be covered and raised above the heart.

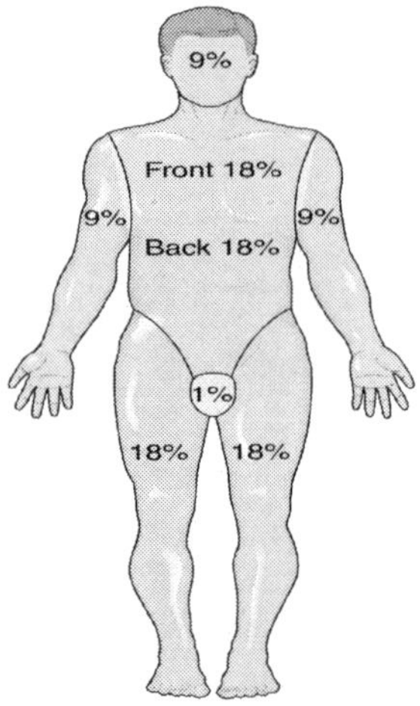

The Rule of 9's is used to determine the extent of burns by the total body area involved. Each percentage represents the percentage of the body damaged by burns:

- Head and Neck: 9%
- Right Arm : 9%
- Left Arm: 9%
- Right Leg: 18%
- Left Leg: 18%
- Thorax: 18%
- Abdomen: 9%
- Lower Back: 9%
- Groin: 1%

Cardiac and Pulmonary Arrest

If a person is suspected of suffering from cardiac arrest, CPR should be performed immediately. CPR, which stands for **Cardiopulmonary Resuscitation**, is extremely important to know and understand how to perform. CPR consists of alternating **chest compressions and breathing support** in cases where cardiac arrest has occurred. Refer to American Red Cross guidelines for appropriate instruction, techniques, and requirements.

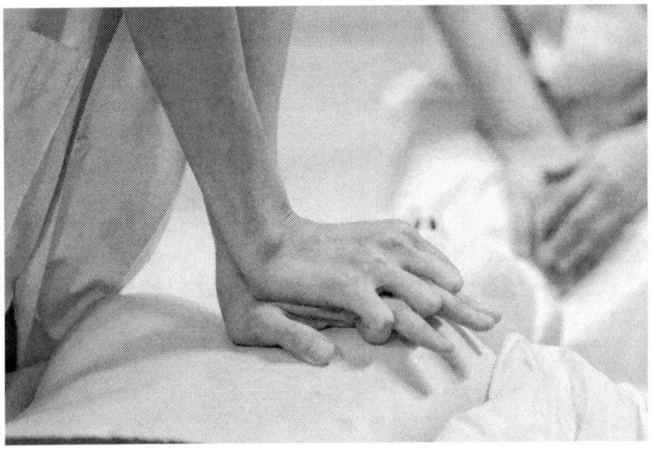

Foreign Body Obstruction

If a person swallows an object, usually it will not cause problems. However, if the object becomes lodged in the esophagus, it may cause internal damage, and should be removed quickly.

If a swallowed object or piece of food enters the **larynx or trachea**, **choking** will occur. A person who is choking may have extreme difficulty in coughing or talking, and may place their **hands to their throat** to indicate they are choking. This person should be treated immediately, utilizing **five blows to the back**, followed by **five abdominal thrusts**. This process should be repeated until the object is dislodged. If the person loses consciousness, they should be placed on the ground, and the throat should be checked for blockages. If the blockage is able to be removed without pushing it further into the respiratory tract, a **finger sweep** should be utilized. If not, CPR should be performed until paramedics arrive.

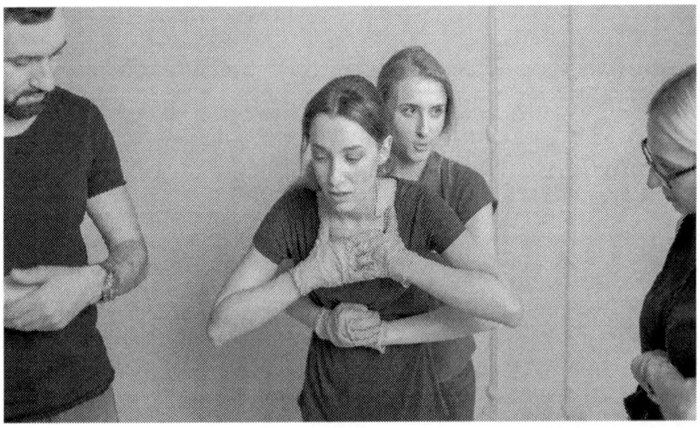

Diabetic Ketoacidosis

Diabetic ketoacidosis occurs when a **diabetic** person has **too many ketones** in the body, caused by **hyperglycemia.** A person may have problems breathing, be fatigued, exhibit pain in the abdomen, and experience nausea and vomiting. If this person is unconscious as a result, EMS should be notified immediately. If they are not breathing, CPR should be administered until paramedics arrive.

Insulin Shock

If a person has **diabetes**, they need to take insulin to help manage their body's blood sugar. If **blood sugar levels fall too far**, it is known as **hypoglycemia**, and may result in **insulin shock.** A person may develop insulin shock for several reasons, such as injecting too much insulin, not increasing blood sugar levels, not eating, or exercising without increasing carbohydrate consumption. **Mild drops in blood sugar levels** can be treated quickly by **ingesting high carbohydrate food or liquid.** Severe hypoglycemia may result in insulin shock, however, and a person may develop seizures, muscle tremors, or they may become unconscious. If a person loses consciousness, EMS should be notified immediately. If a shot of glucose is available, it should be administered immediately.

Bone Fractures

Tending to a broken bone depends on the severity of the fracture. All fractures should be seen by a medical professional right away. If a fracture breaks through the skin, bleeding should be stopped. The area of the fracture should be **immobilized**, as movement in the area may cause damage to other structures in the body. The person may **develop shock**, and wrapping them in an **insulating blanket** may help. An ice pack may help reduce inflammation and pain in the area. The person should be taken to a hospital to have the bone reset, and the ensure there isn't major damage to other structures such as blood vessels inside the body that may cause internal hemorrhaging.

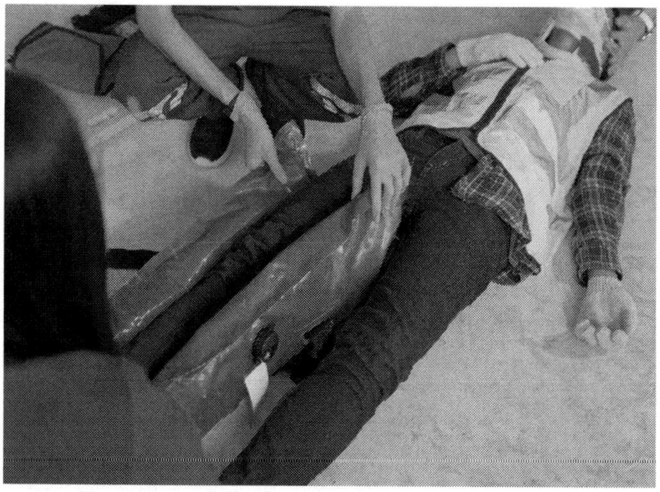

Poisoning

Poisoning may occur in several different ways. Poisoning via **inhalation**, such as **carbon monoxide poisoning**, may require the person be given an **antidote**, or require **breathing support** by way of an **oxygen mask. Injection poisoning** introduces harmful substances into the body via **needles, insect stings, sharp objects**, or **bites.** The poison usually requires the use of an **antidote** to treat. **Absorption** of poison typically includes exposure to substances such as **pesticides.** The area affected should be cleansed thoroughly with water.

Ingestion is introducing harmful substances through **swallowing.** Depending on the substance ingested, the person may be required to **induce vomiting**, or need to **drink milk or water.**

Seizure

If a person is having a seizure, the seizure should be **allowed to run its course.** Afterwards, the patient should be placed into a **seated position**, where they can rest and recover. If the seizure lasts for **five minutes or longer**, it is the person's **first seizure**, or the person is **unable to effectively walk or breathe** afterwards, **EMS should be contacted.**

Shock

If a person is in shock, **EMS should be notified immediately.** The person should **lie down**, keeping the **head flat.** A **blanket** or other clothing should be applied to keep the person's body temperature up. If the person is **vomiting**, they should be **placed on their side** to prevent choking. If any injuries are apparent, they should be treated.

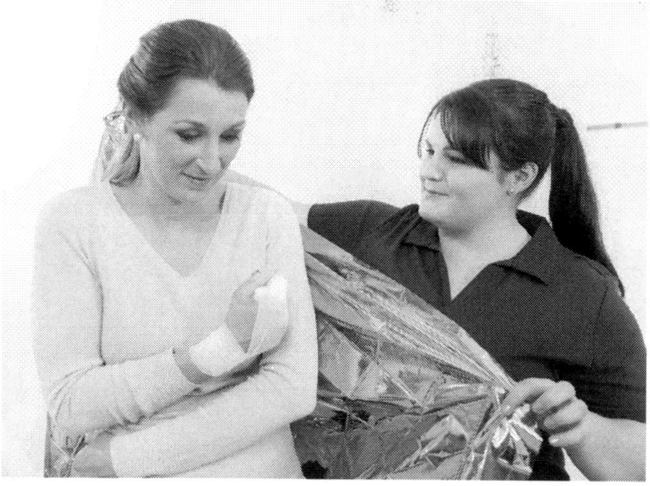

Cerebral Vascular Accident

If a person is suspected of suffering a cerebral vascular accident, they may be exhibiting symptoms commonly seen with **strokes**, including **drooping face, difficulty speaking, weakness in the arms** that occurs suddenly, **sudden headache**, and sudden problems with **vision. EMS should be notified immediately**, as a cerebral vascular accident is a life-threatening condition. If the person is unconscious and not breathing, CPR should be performed. If the person is still conscious, they should be kept as calm as possible. They should not be given food or drink, to avoid vomiting.

Syncope

Syncope, also known as **fainting**, is usually not a serious condition. It is caused by the brain very **temporarily losing blood flow**. However, **injuries caused by falling** may occur. If a person has fainted, any restrictive clothing should be removed, and the legs should be elevated at least one foot above the heart. If the person is unconscious and not breathing, EMS should be notified, and CPR should be performed. If the person has not regained consciousness after one minute, EMS should be notified. Injuries sustained during a fall should also be treated, such as bleeding.

Wounds

An **abrasion** is a **scraping off of layers of the skin**, such as a skinned knee from falling. An **avulsion** is when the skin or another structure, such as a finger or toe nail, is **pulled and ripped**. An **incision**, such as produced during surgery, is a **clean cut through tissue**. A **laceration** is a cut that produces **jagged edges**. A **puncture** is caused by an object **piercing the skin**, producing a hole.

Wounds should be cleaned with soap and water. Pressure and sterile bandages, gauze, or cloth should be applied to wounds to stop bleeding. The injured area should be raised above the heart if bleeding persists.

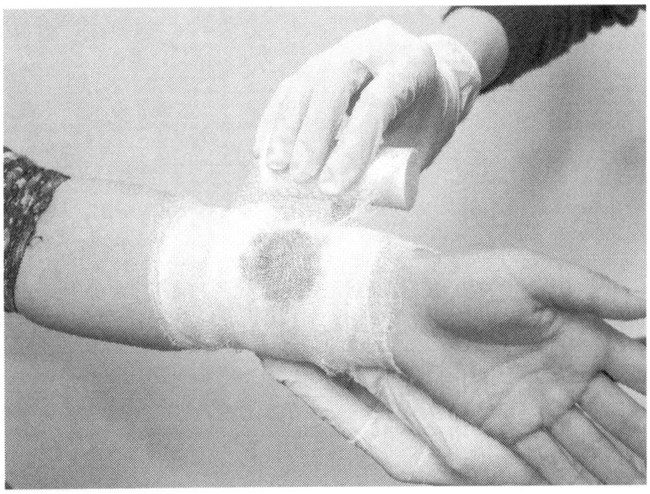

Cold Injuries

There are two main types of cold injuries: hypothermia and frostbite. **Hypothermia** is caused by the **body temperature dropping below 90 degrees**. This can be potentially fatal. **Frostbite** is caused by a **formation of ice crystals in soft tissues**, typically the fingers, toes, and parts of the face such as the nose and ears. If the tissues are frozen for too long, they experience **necrosis**.

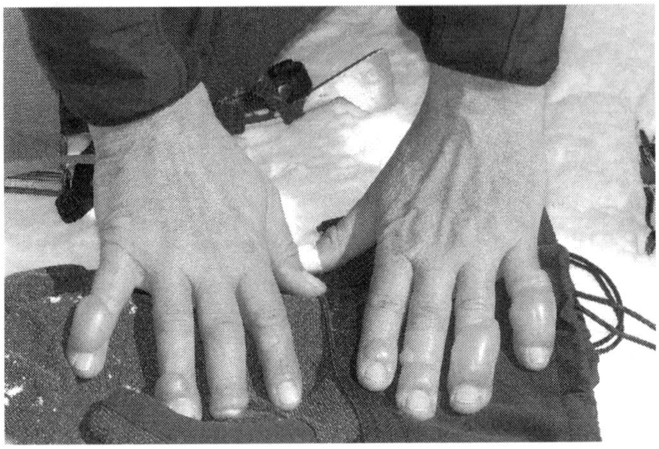

Heat Injuries

There are three main types of heat injuries that don't involve burns: heat exhaustion, heat cramps, and heat stroke. **Heat exhaustion** is caused by a person having a **high body temperature with excessive sweating**. Sweating is a product of homeostasis, which is trying to cool the body. If the person continues to sweat, it means the body isn't properly cooling down. This can lead to **heat cramps**, which cause **tightening and involuntary spasms** of the muscles due to **dehydration and loss of electrolytes**, such as sodium and potassium. **Heat stroke** is when a person has an **extremely high body temperature**, with a **lack of sweating**. This occurs when a person is **severely dehydrated**, and has no more fluid to use as sweat to try cooling the body down. This can be potentially fatal.

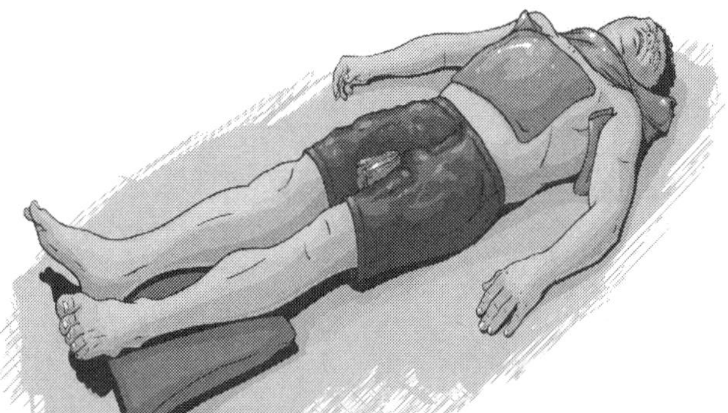

Orthopedic Injuries

Strains, sprains, and dislocations are all forms of **orthopedic injuries**. Strains and sprains are primarily treated with the use of **PRICE: Protect, Rest, Ice, Compression, Elevation**. The damaged area should be protected from further injury, rested to allow proper healing, iced to reduce inflammation, compressed to help further reduce inflammation, and elevated to assist in proper circulation and reduce inflammation. If a bone is **dislocated**, it should be **relocated if possible**. If not, the area should be **stabilized and protected**. If a fracture has taken place in conjunction with the dislocation, the fracture should be treated as normal, and the person should be taken to a hospital for treatment.

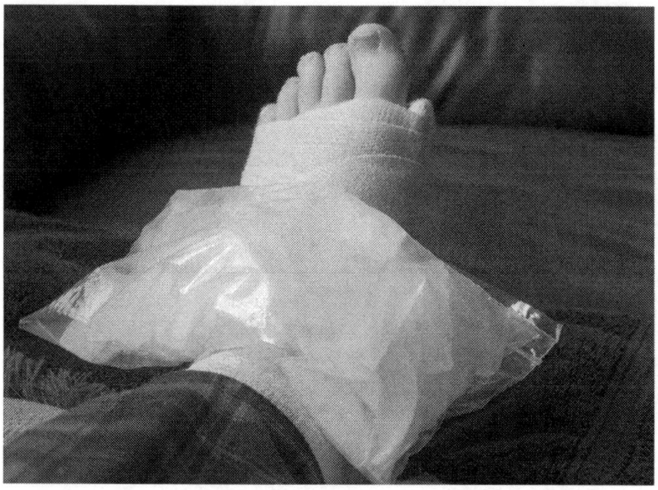

Asthma Attack

During an asthma attack, a person may have **extreme difficulty breathing** due to constriction of the bronchial tubes. The person may be **unable to effectively speak**, and the lips and fingers may turn a blueish color. Constrictive clothing should be removed or loosened. If the person has an **inhaler**, it should be utilized. The person should be taken to a hospital for treatment, as an asthma attack may actually worsen despite symptoms seemingly disappearing, such as wheezing.

Hyperventilation

Hyperventilation is a **psychological disorder** that causes a person to **breathe extremely rapidly or deeply**. This creates a **surplus of carbon dioxide** in the body, as the person is **not effectively exhaling**. Because hyperventilation is a common symptom of **panic attacks**, helping the person calm down is the primary treatment. Using a calm, reassuring tone can help a person regain proper breathing. The person should try holding their breath, as this may help reset the breathing pattern. If hyperventilation persists, EMS should be notified.

Vertigo

Vertigo is **dizziness** a person may experience for many different reasons, but commonly a problem with the **inner ear**. If a person becomes dizzy, they should be **seated**, or **lie down**. Preventing movement is the most important step in treating vertigo. If vertigo lasts for an extended period, EMS should be notified.

Animal Bites

If an **animal bite** occurs that results in a **puncture**, **bleeding should be forced** from the wound to try clearing out as much bacteria as possible. The area should be **cleansed with soap and water**, and a **sterile dressing** should be applied to control bleeding and allow for proper healing.

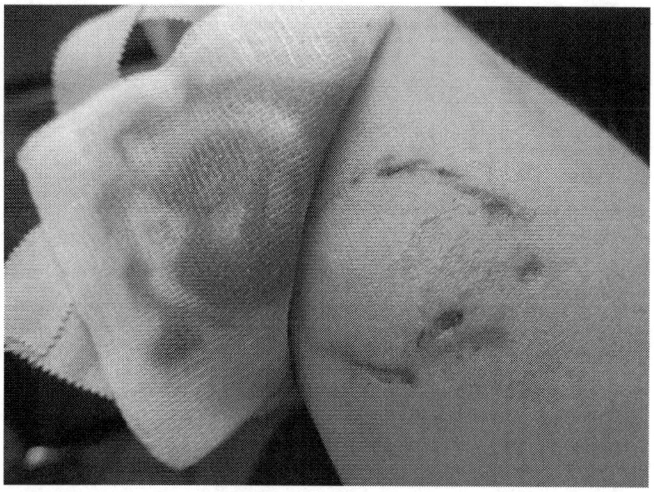

Insect Stings

Insect stings, such as from bees, should be **scraped with a sharp flat surface to remove any stinger** left behind that may be in the skin. The area should be **cleansed with soap and water**. If asphyxiation is suspected, EMS should be contacted immediately.

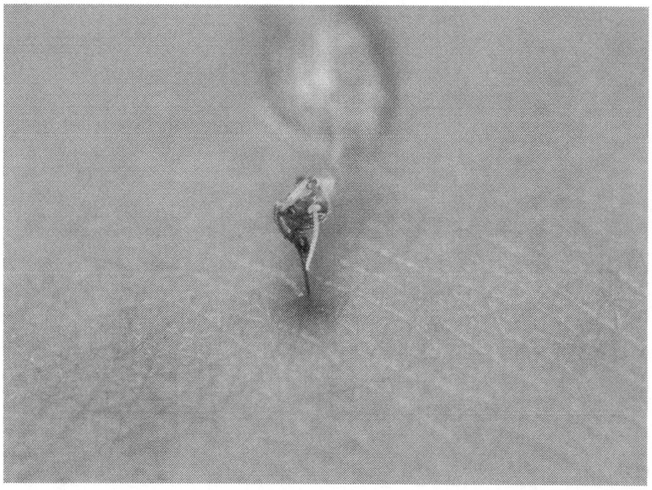

Snake Bites

Snake bites should be **cleansed with soap and water.** The **area of the bite should be immobilized below the heart** to decrease the ease of blood flow to the heart from the area that contains venom. EMS should be notified.

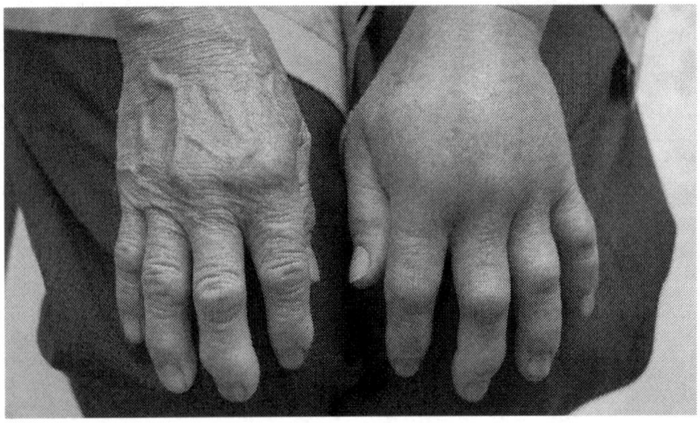

Spider Bites

Spider bites should be **cleansed with soap and water.** The **area of the bite should be immobilized below the heart.** The patient should be advised to seek medical attention.

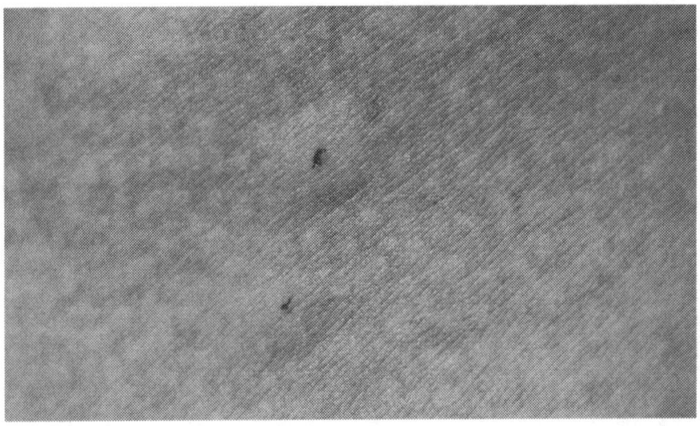

Scorpion Stings

Scorpion stings should be **cleansed with soap and water.** The **area of the sting should be immobilized below the heart.** The patient should be advised to seek medical attention.

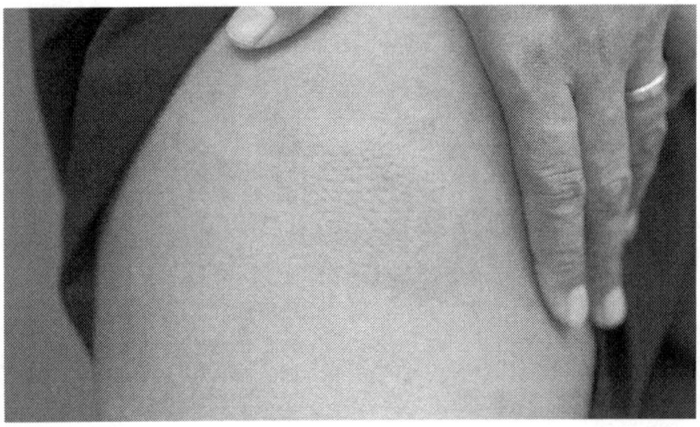

Head Trauma

A **concussion** occurs when there is a **blow to the head** that causes an **injury to the brain.** While a concussion is not always obvious, if a person suffers a head injury, assuming a concussion has occurred is recommended. The person should **keep the head and neck immobilized**, and **simple questions** should be asked to **determine cognitive function.** These questions can include asking the person their name, their age, and their location.

If the person is unconscious, CAB should be checked. If the person is not breathing, the throat should be checked for an obstruction. If there is an obstruction, it should try to be removed using a gentle finger swipe. If there is no obstruction, CPR should be performed and EMS should be notified.

Chemical Exposure

Chemical exposure can occur in many different ways, such as **inhalation, ingestion**, and **direct contact.** In cases where a patient has inhaled a chemical, it is vital that they are moved into an area of clean, breathable air. The patient may be encouraged to cough to help remove the chemical from the lungs. If the patient stops breathing, CPR should be performed. In cases where a patient has ingested a chemical, a poison control center should be contacted immediately. If cases where a patient's eye has come into contact with a chemical, eye irrigation should be utilized to wash the chemical from the surface of the eye. In cases where a patient's skin has come into contact with a chemical, the chemical should be washed off, and depending on the chemical involved, the area should be cleaned with soap and water.

Ergonomics

Ergonomics is all about making the workplace more efficient for the employee. If the job is physically strenuous, it may be considered an unsafe environment if the employee, and employer, don't take necessary steps to reduce the amount of physical stress being experienced. Factors employees face that deal with ergonomics include the **height of the desk** or work space, the **placement of a computer monitor** in relation to the employee's head, the **posture** of an employee while sitting or standing, and the ability of the employee to physically move throughout the day. All of these factors should be taken into account to allow the employee to work in a comfortable environment and reduce the chances of physical stress.

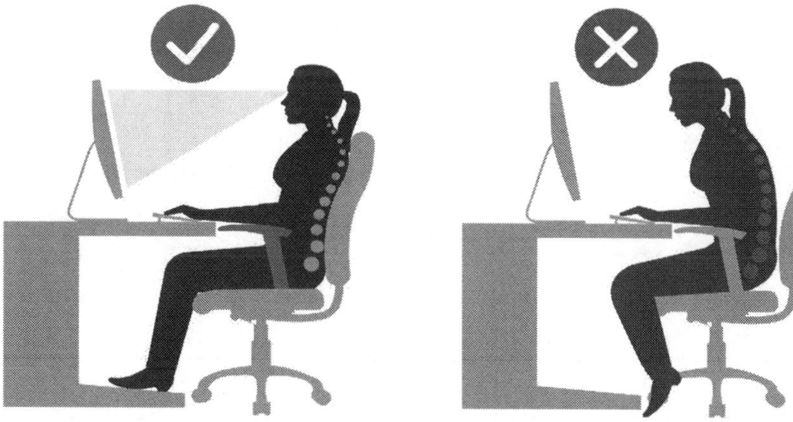

Risk Management, Quality Assurance, and Safety Procedures

Reporting Unsafe Activities and Behaviors

Unsafe activities and behaviors should be reported to appropriate agencies to ensure the behavior is corrected. An example of these agencies includes OSHA. Reporting these activities can be done confidentially or anonymously. If a report is submitted confidentially, the person submitting the report also submits their name, but the name is not released. Confidential reporting makes the report official, and provides federal whistleblower protection to the person reporting. Anonymous reporting does not provide these same protections, as the person reporting does not include their name.

Conflicts of Interest

A conflict of interest is when a person's **decisions** may be **influenced** due to **personal biases**. These decisions are often made to benefit the person, and don't necessarily take into account the overall well-being of others. This can be an issue in the medical professional/patient dynamic, as the patient looks to the medical professional for guidance in care. An example, if a doctor has a hand in developing a new form of treatment that they make money on whenever a patient receives the treatment, the doctor may have a conflict of interest if they suggest this treatment to a patient. This does not necessarily mean that the doctor doesn't have the patient's best interests in mind, but encouraging the patient to take the treatment, and being expected to receive payment for the treatment, means that the doctor could be influenced by the potential payment.

Patient Safety Variance Reporting

Variance reporting is utilized when there is any circumstance that occurs that is **out of the normal**, such as equipment failure, injuries the patient has sustained while in care, death of the patient while under care, unusual events occurring during surgery, and any potential criminal events. Reporting these incidents helps prevent these issues from occurring in the future, and holds certain parties responsible.

Safety and Infection Control Matching

______: Invasion of a microorganism inside the body

______: Reducing the number of microorganisms on an object to a level safe enough to make the object usable without the risk of infection

______: A person's decisions being influenced due to personal biases

______: Treating every person and fluid as if they are contaminated and infectious

______: Blow to the head causing an injury to the brain

______: Primary treatment for strains and sprains

______: Person who assesses severity of a patient's injuries, urgency of treatment required, and location of treatment needed in emergency departments

______: Provides employees with structured directions in regards to safely cleaning and disposal of body fluids, sanitization, and blood-borne pathogen testing

______: Container used to hold needles

______: Chemical released by the body when a virus is detected to elevate body temperature

______: Single-celled organisms that live inside of a host's body and multiply beyond safe levels

______: Lack of bacteria, virus, or microorganism present in a location or on an object

______: Touching, kissing, sexual contact, and blood exposure can result in this mode of transmission

______: Means in which an infectious agent enters its new host

______: The body's second line of defense against pathogens, which includes inflammation

______: Reporting when there is a circumstance that is considered out of the normal such as equipment failure, injuries and death a patient suffers under care, and unusual events during surgery

______: Agency responsible for enforcing occupational health and safety standards

______: Condition arising from a person having too many ketones in the body

______: Completely destroying all microorganisms on an object

______: Parasites that attach to the surface of a host

A: Variance reporting
B: Infection
C: Disinfection
D: Portals of entry
E: Post-exposure plan
F: Pyrogen
G: Diabetic ketoacidosis
H: Universal precautions
I: Asepsis
J: Sterilizing
K: Direct contact
L: Conflicts of interest
M: Ectoparasites
N: OSHA
O: Sharps container
P: Immune system
Q: Triage nurse
R: PRICE
S: Protozoa
T: Concussion

Answer Key on Page 292

Safety and Infection Control Crossword

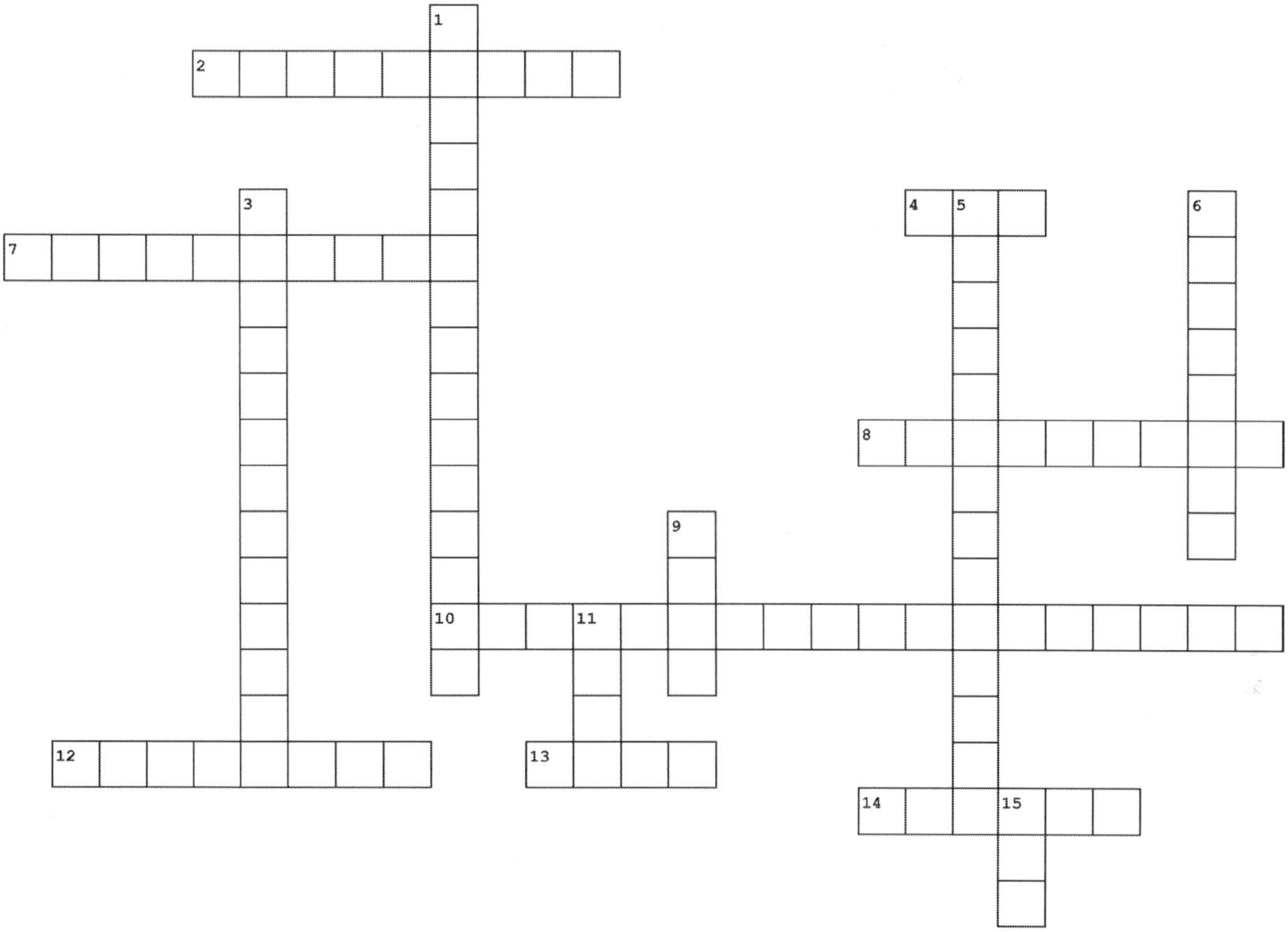

Across

2. Tapeworms, flukes, and roundworms are categories as these
4. Portable defibrillator used to send electric shocks to the heart in a person suffering from sudden cardiac arrest, abbv.
7. The process of a virus infecting a cell and reprogramming it to replicate viral particles
8. Mobile cart containing pieces of equipment to treat patients in emergency situations
10. A person's decisions being influenced due to personal biases
12. Sign required to be placed in public spaces that is clearly visible showing how to leave an area safely
13. Lack of friction between a person's foot and the surface they are walking on results in this
14. Candidiasis, sporothrix, and talaromyces are all forms of

Down

1. Sneezing and coughing are considered which form of infectious transmission
3. Mosquitoes, leeches, and ticks are categorized as these
5. Plan detailing designated routes a person should be directed in order to effectively exit a premises in cases of emergencies
6. Staphylococcus, H. pylori, and salmonella are all forms of
9. A person's foot getting caught on an object results in this
11. A person encountering an unstable surface may result in this
15. System developed by the United Nations to classify chemicals and their hazards, abbv.

Answer Key on Page 293

Safety and Infection Control Practice Test

1. Drooping face, sudden weakness in the arms, sudden headache, and difficulty speaking are all signs of
A. Syncope
B. Diabetic ketoacidosis
C. Cerebral vascular accident
D. Concussion

2. The normal habitat of an infectious agent
A. Reservoir
B. Portal of exit
C. Host
D. Portal of entry

3. Lack of friction between a person's foot and the surface they are walking on may produce
A. Trips
B. Falls
C. Stumbles
D. Slips

4. Reducing the number of microorganisms on an object to a safe enough level or make the object usable without the risk of spreading infection
A. Sanitization
B. Sterilization
C. Disinfection
D. Cleaning

5. All of the following are appropriate ways to help control bleeding except
A. Apply a tourniquet
B. Apply direct pressure on the wound
C. Run the wound under water
D. Place a sterile bandage on the wound

6. Device used to send electric shocks to the heart in cases of cardiac arrest
A. Crash cart
B. Autoclave
C. Holter monitor
D. Automated external defibrillator

7. Orthopedic injuries such as strains and sprains are best treated using
A. PRICE
B. SPLINT
C. PPALM
D. SOAP

8. All of the following are examples of direct contact transmission except
A. Exchanging saliva with an infected person
B. Inhaling droplets infected with a pathogen
C. Exposure to blood infected with a pathogen
D. Touching an area of skin that contains a contagious pathogen

9. Needles that have been used must be discarded in
A. Spill kits
B. Biohazard bins
C. Biohazard bags
D. Sharps containers

10. The body's third line of defense
A. Skin
B. T-cells
C. Inflammatory response
D. Mucous membranes

Answer Key on Page 295

Procedures/Examinations

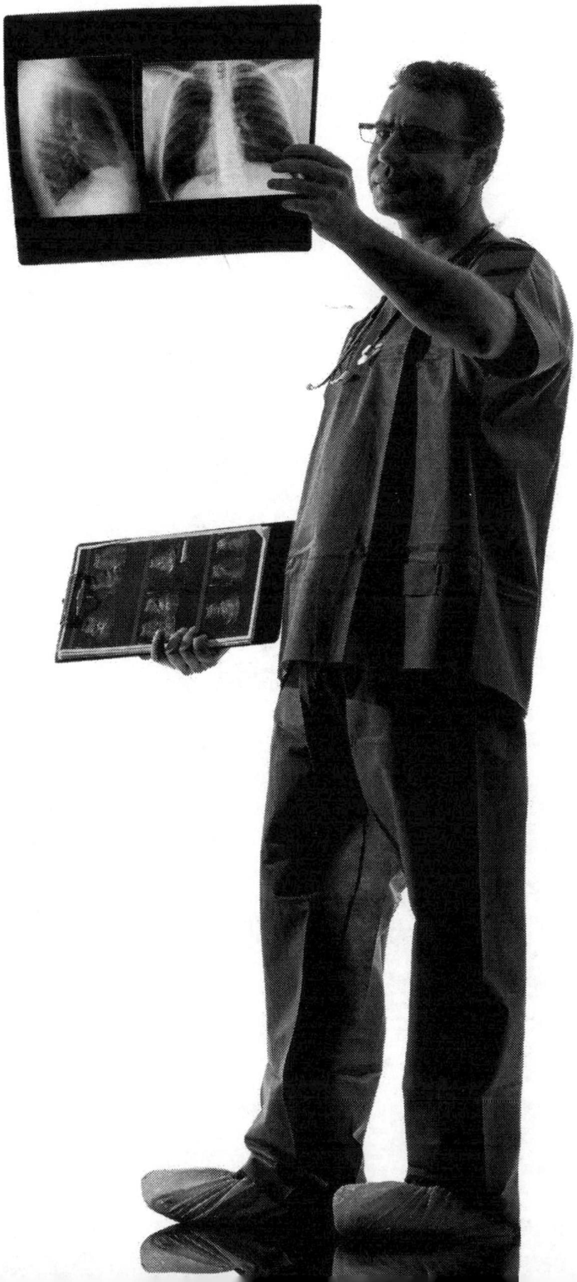

Prepare Patients for Examinations, Procedures, and Treatments

Auscultation

Auscultation is **listening to internal body sounds** produced by the heart, lungs, or other organs such as the stomach. Sounds observed include the heart beat, heart murmurs, wheezing in the lungs, and digestion. Auscultation is usually performed by using a **stethoscope.** Sounds may also be heard by using sonography.

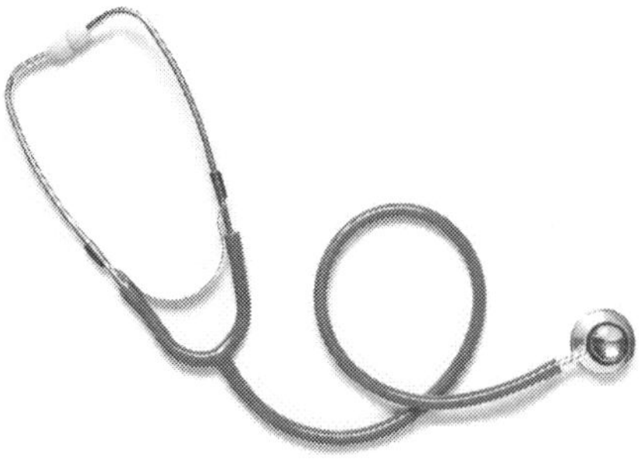

A stethoscope is an **auditory** instrument used to **listen to the internal body**, most commonly the heart and lungs. It consists of two ear plugs connected to metal tubes, which then connect to rubber tubing. At the end of the tubing are two structures, the diaphragm and the bell. The diaphragm transmits higher frequency sounds to the ears, while the bell transmits low frequency sounds.

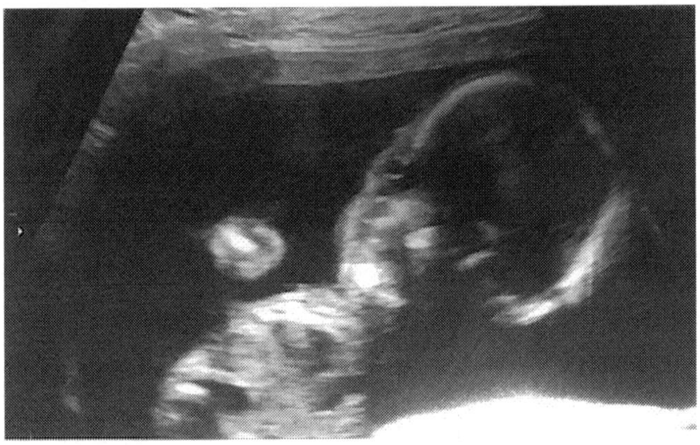

An **ultrasound**, also known as **sonography**, is an **imaging technique** utilizing **sound waves** to produce pictures of structures inside the body. Commonly, ultrasound is used to view the development of a fetus during pregnancy, but may also be used to examine infections inside the body, liver and gallbladder function, and heart conditions. The part of the machine that is used to perform the scanning is known as the **transducer**.

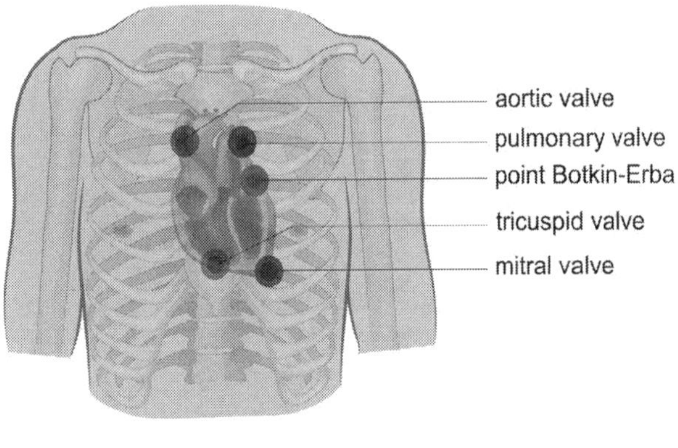

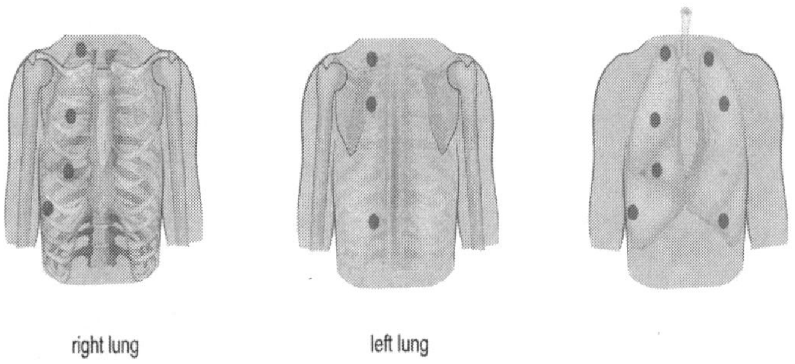

Inspection

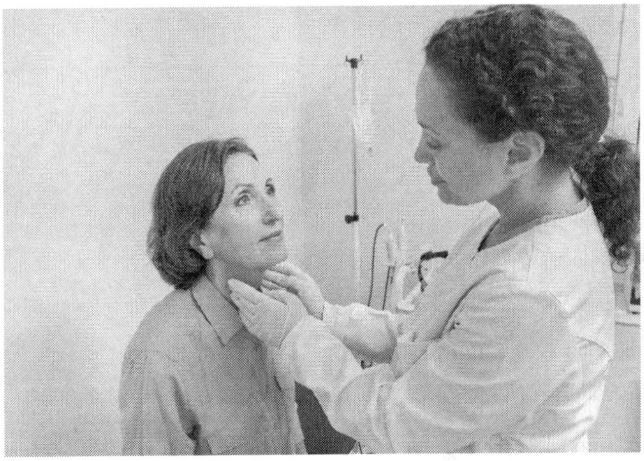

During inspection, the medical professional is **observing and examining** a patient uninterrupted. This allows the examination to be thorough, and for the medical professional to determine if there are any abnormalities in a person using the naked eye. These inspections are usually performed to screen for any medical conditions the patient may have.

Manipulation

Manipulation is the use of the **hands** to **physically move, adjust, or alter** the location of a structure in the body. Manipulation is commonly used in joint relocations, re-setting fractures, and turning a fetus.

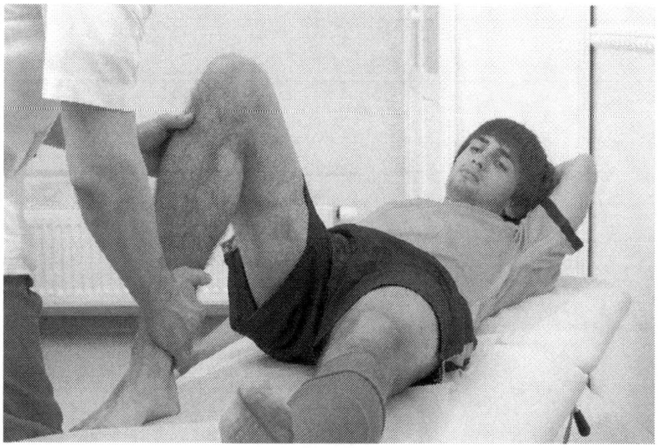

Palpation

Palpation is the use of **touch** to assess or examine an area or structure. Palpation can be used to examine areas of inflammation, tenderness in areas such as the abdomen, fractures, dislocations, sprains, strains, fever, reduced circulation, and more.

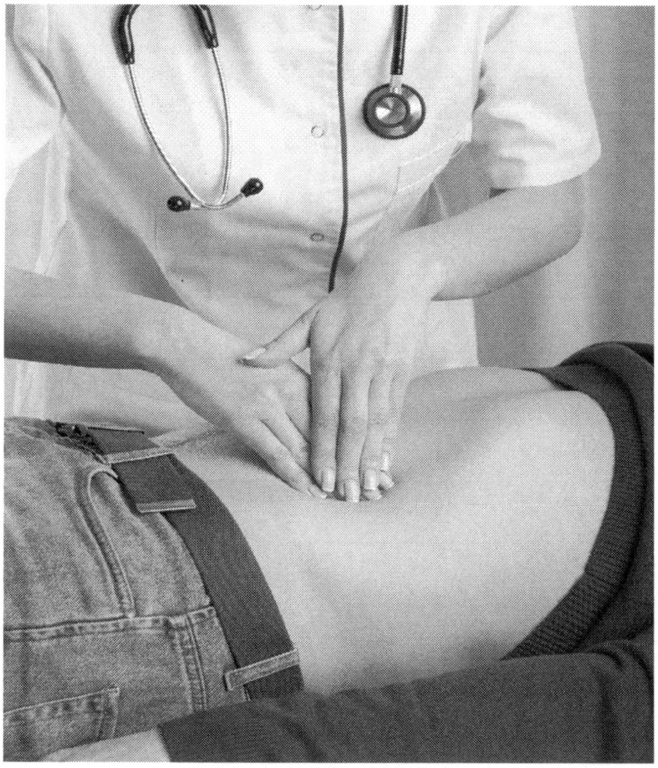

Mensuration

Mensuration is performed by **measuring** certain structures or areas of the body. This can help determine if there is deformity in an area, an increased amount of fluid causing edema, if there are any structural abnormalities, or to establish a normal measurement.

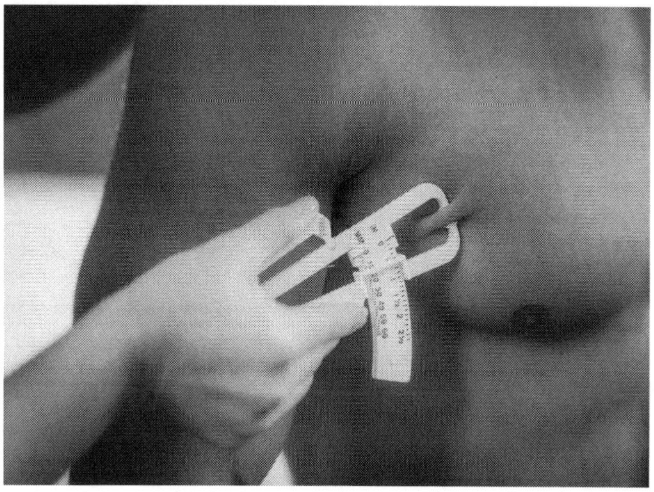

Percussion

Percussion is performed by **tapping** on areas of the body. This allows examination of the presence of fluid in an area, or the size and location of an organ. Certain areas may sound hollow, like the lungs or abdomen, while others may sound solid, like bones.

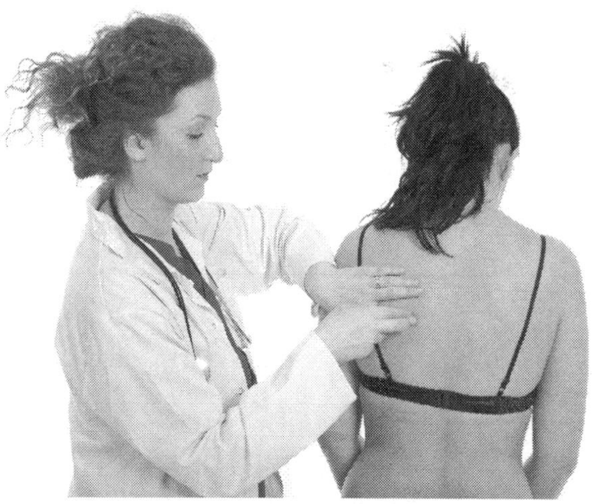

Body Positions and Draping

Sims' Position

Sims' position is the main body position used for **rectal exams, enemas, and treatments**. Proper Sims' position includes the patient lying on their left side, with the left lower limb straightened. The right hip and knee are flexed. The right lower limb is resting on a pillow to allow for comfort.

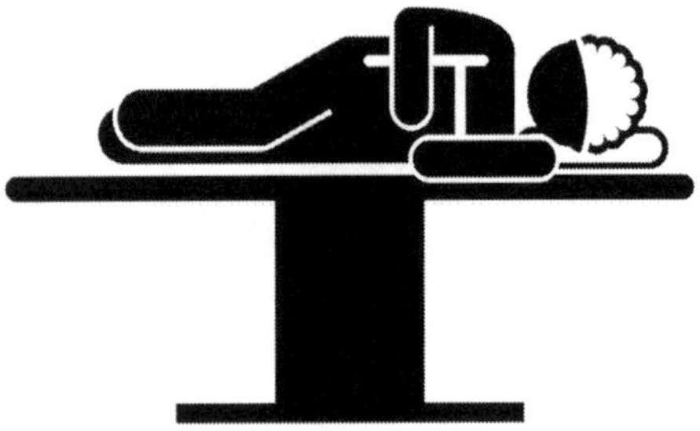

Fowler's Position

Fowler's position simply requires the patient to be **seated**, with the seat back set at an angle of **45 to 60 degrees**. High Fowler's position allows the seat back to be set as high as 90 degrees, while low Fowler's position allows the seat back to be completely reclined to zero degrees, with the head only slightly elevated.

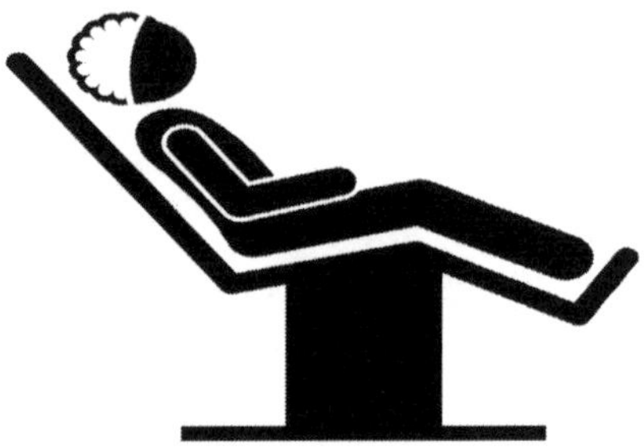

Supine Position

Supine position is performed by having a person lie **face up** on a table. A pillow under the head can be used for comfort, and a bolster may be placed under the knees to take pressure off the lower back.

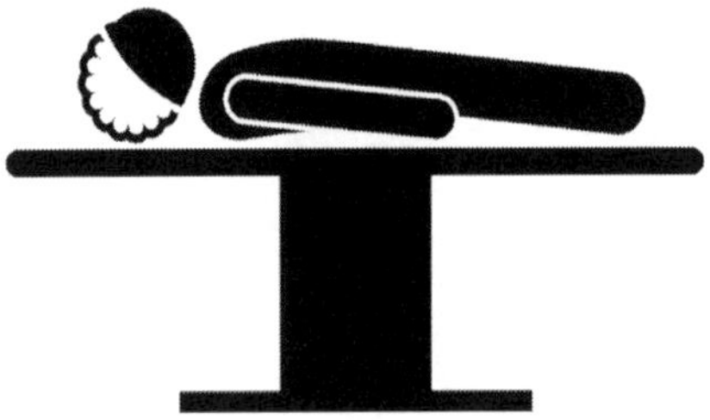

Prone Position

Prone position requires nothing more than the patient to lie **face down** on the table. The head may be turned to one side, or placed in a head rest if one is available. The arms are placed either off the side of the table, or beside the patient. A bolster may be placed under the ankles to take pressure off the lower back.

Knee-Chest Position

Knee-chest position is performed by the patient lying prone on the table, with the knees and chest coming into contact with the table, and the abdomen and hips raised off the table. The patient is using flexed elbows on the table to support their weight. Knee-chest is used in **rectal or gynecological examination.**

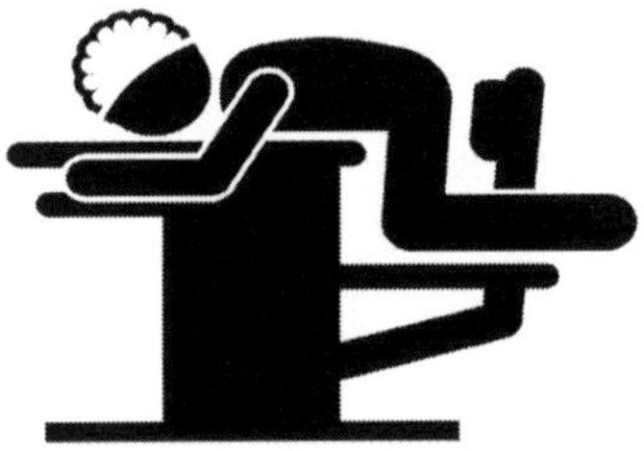

Lithotomy Position

Lithotomy position is used during **childbirth**, or during surgery on the pelvic region. It requires the patient to lie flat in a supine position, with the legs and feet placed into stirrups that separate them.

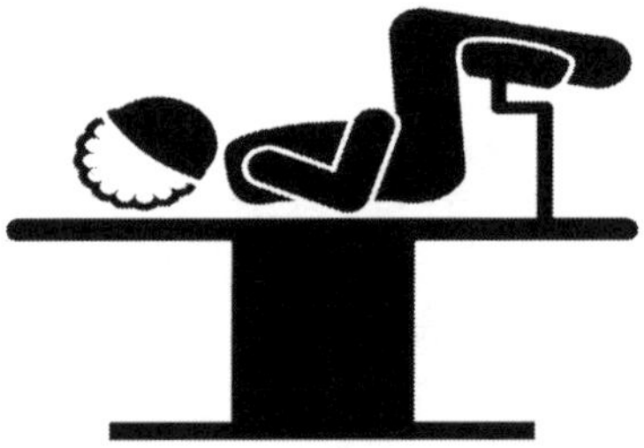

Dorsal Recumbent Position

Dorsal recumbent position is similar to lithotomy, in that the patient lies flat on their back in a supine position, with the legs and feet separated. However, the legs and feet rest on the table itself, and are **not placed in stirrups**. This allows **pelvic examination** to take place.

Pediatric Exam

A **pediatric exam** is a physical examination of a **child.** This examination is performed to ensure the child is growing at a normal rate, both in height and weight, and developmentally. Each age has certain milestones that are likely for a child to have met, and each are examined and tested.

A **growth chart** is used to measure the **physical growth** of a child. Growth encompasses height, weight, and head circumference. These measurements are compared to the general population, and this gives an overall view of the child's growth rate compared to the majority of other children.

OB/GYN Exam

Obstetricians and gynecologists are doctors who specialize in **women's reproductive health.** An obstetrician focuses on reproductive health during and after pregnancy, while a gynecologist focuses primarily on just reproductive health without the pregnancy aspect. OB-GYNs are doctors who are trained in all facets of reproductive health.

OB-GYN exams are performed to check the reproductive health of a woman who may be experiencing menopause, pregnancy, or may screen for certain types of cancer.

A **pelvic exam** is a physical examination of a woman's **vagina, cervix, uterus, fallopian tubes, ovaries, and vulva.** Visual inspection is performed on the vulva and vagina, where the doctor is looking for possible infection or inflammation in the area. After the areas are examined, a vaginal speculum is used to dilate the vaginal canal, which allows the doctor to visually inspect the cervix. Further examination requires the doctor to insert two fingers that are lubricated into the vaginal canal and press on the abdomen, which helps check for any issues or abnormalities in the uterus.

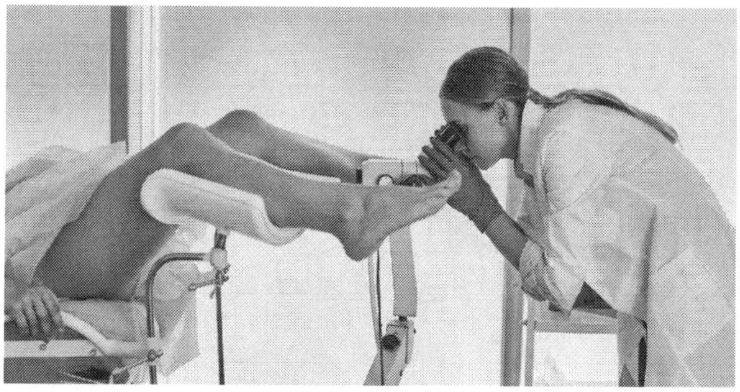

While examining the cervix, the doctor may perform a **Pap smear** to test cervical cells for potential **cervical cancer.** During a Pap smear, the cervix is swiped by a small tool that looks similar to a spatula, and the cells are sent to the lab for examination.

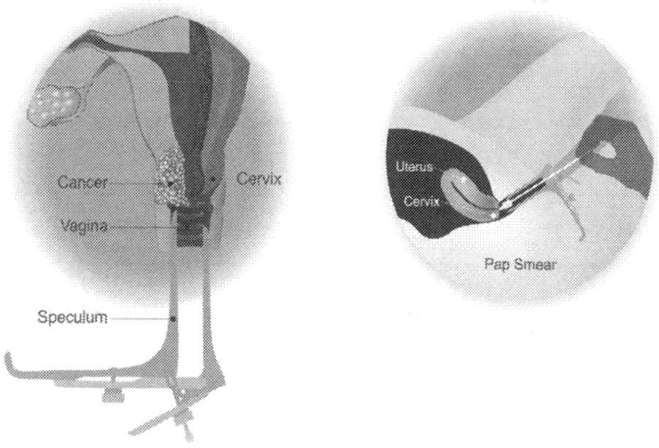

Prenatal and Postpartum Exams

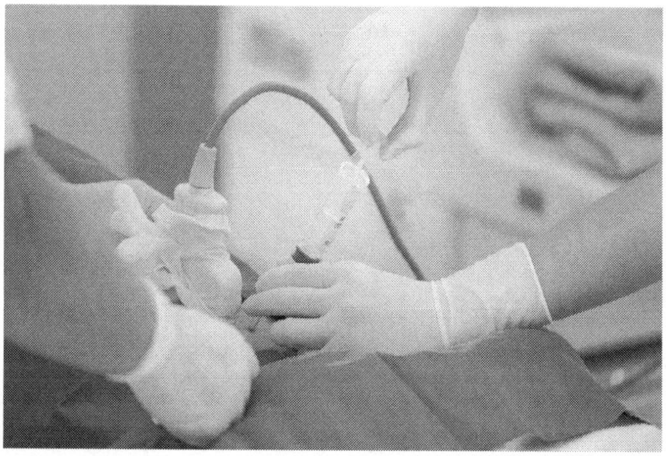

Prenatal exams are performed **during pregnancy** and **before birth** to help determine the health of the fetus. Examples of these tests include amniocentesis, ultrasound examination, and urine testing. Amniocentesis is performed by inserting a small needle into the amniotic sac and drawing out a small amount of amniotic fluid that is tested for certain genetic markers indicative of conditions such as Down syndrome and cystic fibrosis. Ultrasound examinations are used to measure the growth of the fetus and proper development of the organs. Urine tests are performed to test the mother's overall health and check for conditions that may affect fetal development, such as diabetes and preeclampsia.

Postpartum exams are performed to check the health of the mother **after delivery**. These exams are usually performed six weeks after delivery, which should give the body enough time to recover physically. Blood pressure is checked, the abdomen is inspected and palpated for tenderness, and if a C-section was performed, the surgical site is examined for potential infections and proper healing. A pelvic exam is performed to ensure the reproductive organs are healed or healing. In addition to a physical examination, the doctor will check on the emotional health and well-being of the mother, as postpartum depression may be present.

Supplies, Equipment, Techniques, and Patient Instruction

Eye Irrigation

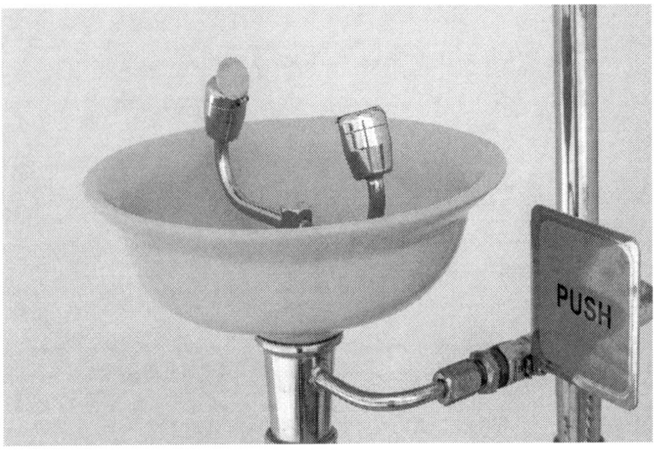

If an irritant gets into the eye that has potential to cause damage to the eye, the eye should be irrigated. Irrigation helps remove the substance, or dilute the substance, which reduces the chances of damage occurring. The patient should lie supine on a table. Using sterile gauze, the eyelids should be cleaned to remove any substance on the eyelids that could contribute to damaging the eye. A bowl or kidney dish should be placed on the patient's cheek to catch fluid, and the patient should slightly lean to the same side so the fluid properly drains into the dish. Using a large syringe, saline is placed in the center of the eye and the corners of the eyelids, which performs irrigation and helps remove any foreign objects. The saline solution also helps to dilute any substances that enter the eye.

If there is an introduction of substances that are highly acidic or highly alkaline, the patient should utilize an emergency eye irrigation system. These resemble drinking fountains, and provide a constant stream of water that the patient should run their eye through for several minutes.

Ear Irrigation

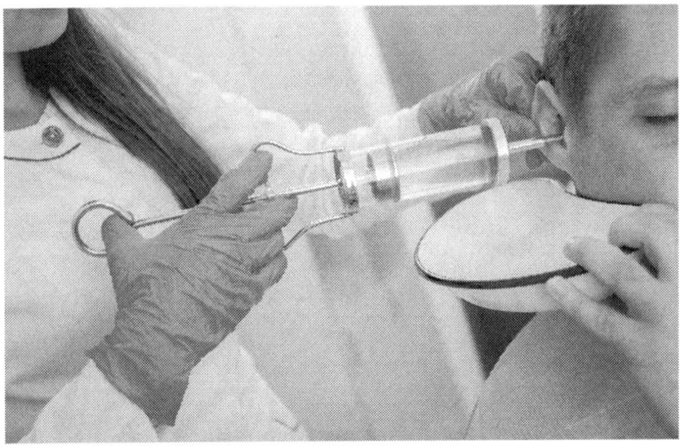

The ears produce a substance known as cerumen, or ear wax. Normally, the body manages to keep the amount of ear wax in the ear to a minimum, but in some circumstances the ear may produce too much ear wax, or the ear wax may harden and become stuck in the ear. If either of these occur, or if a foreign object becomes stuck in the ear, the ear may need to be irrigated. Similar to an eye irrigation, an ear irrigation requires the use of a large syringe, which injects a saline solution into the ear to flush out the obstruction. The solution is collected with a bowl or kidney dish.

Suture/Staple Removal

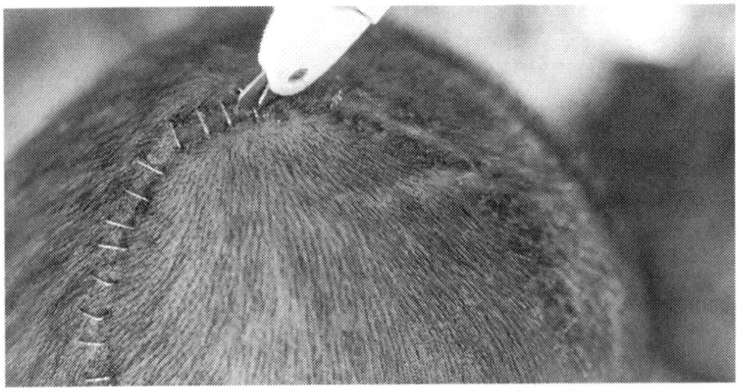

Removing sutures and staples are relatively simple and similar in nature. Removal of sutures or staples should generally be performed after waiting at least two weeks from the date they were put in, which gives the body enough time to form adhesions between the two wound edges, and prevents infection from opening the wound early. The time frame is left up to the physician. Before any suture or staple is removed, the area should be cleaned to prevent infection. To remove a suture, the knot is grasped with tweezers and lifted, and a pair of scissors is used to cut the suture. The suture is then pulled out from the body.

Removal of a staple requires a surgical staple remover. The staple remover is placed close to the skin and slides gently under the staple. The staple remover grasps the staple and gently pulls the staple out. After all staples are removed, the area is cleaned again, and if needed, a bandage is applied to the area.

Cast Care

Casts are utilized when a patient has suffered a **fracture**, and the bone must be **stabilized** to properly heal. Casts are made of **plaster** or **fiberglass.** Plaster is easily molded into the shape of the injured area, and allows the bones to set in the correct location and for bone repair to occur without potential deformity. Plaster is most commonly utilized when bones need to be reset after fracture has occurred. Fiberglass casts are commonly utilized when a bone does not need to be reset into its proper position. Beneath any cast is a layer of cotton, which helps to protect the skin. The cast, and the area beneath the cast, should be kept free from moisture. When a patient bathes, they should cover the cast in plastic to avoid introducing moisture into the cast.

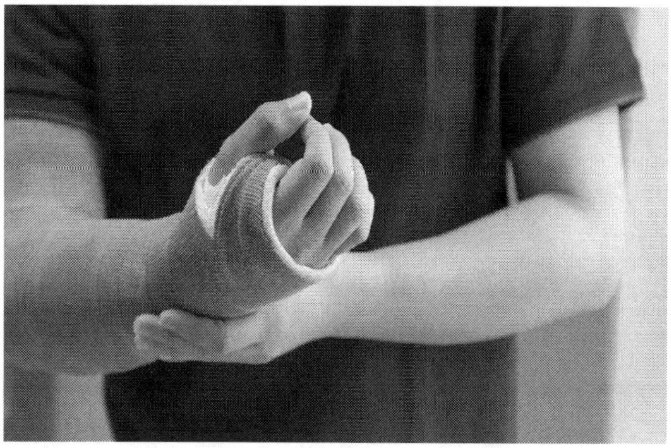

Splints

Splints are used to provide a means of **immobilization**, often before a cast is placed. This may allow inflammation in the area to subside, allowing physicians a better look at the injury, giving a better determination of treatment options. Splints immobilize an area and prevent the area from suffering increased damage. Splints can also be safer than casts in the short term, allowing the affected area to swell to a safer degree than is offered by a cast. This swelling, if under a cast, may develop into compartment syndrome. When the swelling after surgery has began to subside, the risk of compartment syndrome drops significantly and a cast is then able to be placed on the area.

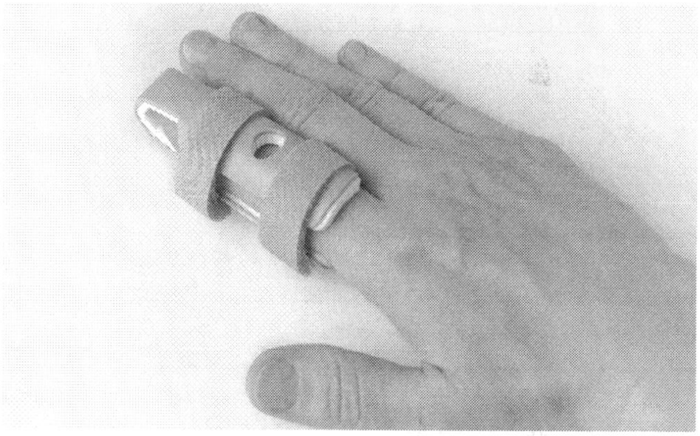

Slings

Slings are used to **immobilize**, or significantly reduce movement, in the **shoulder and/or wrist** when an injury occurs in or around these joints. Severe sprains of the acromioclavicular or sternoclavicular joints, dislocation of the shoulder, fracture of the clavicle, and similar injuries may not require surgical repair, and may heal over time if the area is only immobilized with a sling. Slings are usually adjustable, and hold the upper limb to the body by wrapping around the chest, opposite shoulder/neck region, and back. Slings hold the upper limb in a medially rotated position, which provides more support for the limb.

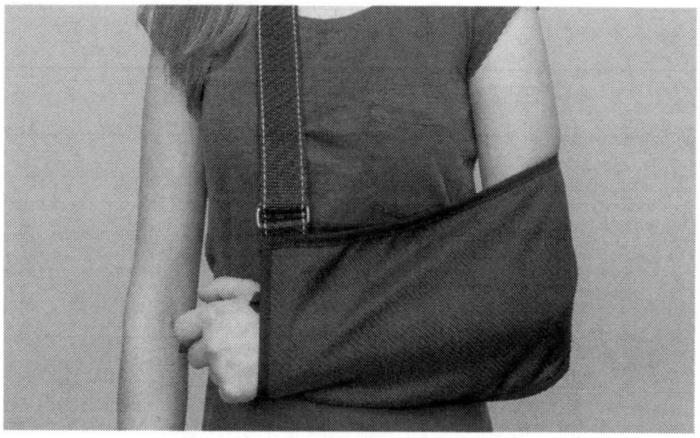

Compression Devices

Compression devices are used to **mimic the Lymphatic System** by **rhythmically compressing the legs** to increase the flow of lymph. This can decrease lymphedema. Typical compression devices may also include compression socks, and cuffs that wrap around the legs.

Surgical Assisting

Surgical Asepsis

Surgical assisting is a vital step in maintaining a sterile environment in an operating room. A surgical assistant helps by dressing the patient in sterile surgical drapes, creating sterile field boundaries. Surgical assistants may also help with surgical tray setup, and help other members of the operating team apply gowns, caps, gloves, and goggles.

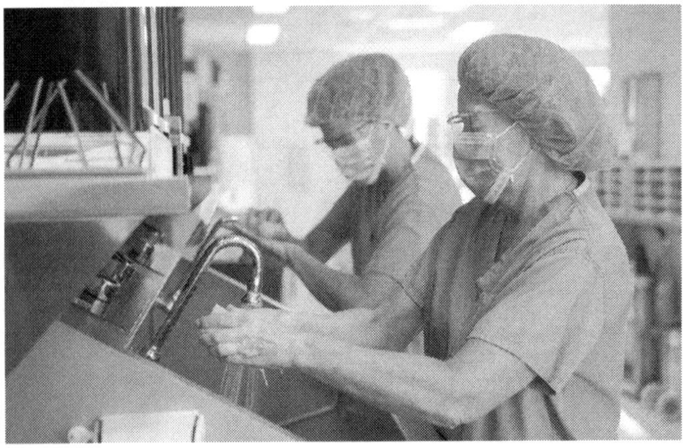

When surgery is being performed, the environment and surgical tools need to be as sterile as possible. Opening any portion of the body runs the risk of introducing pathogens into the body, which can quickly turn into infection. As discussed, hand washing should always be performed to sanitize the hands, but when surgery is to be performed, the medical professional will perform a **surgical scrub**. Surgical scrubs are performed in one of two methods: the numbered stroke method, or the timed method. In the **numbered stroke method**, each portion being scrubbed will have a **set amount of strokes** used to ensure the area is as clean and possible. During the timed method, the area is continuously scrubbed for **three to five minutes**, cleaning from the hand to the arm.

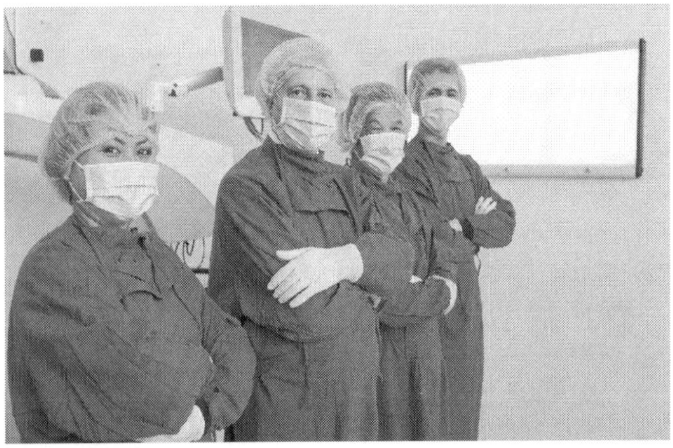

Medical dress during surgery also reduces the instance of microorganism exposure. Covering the hands are **surgical gloves**. Tucked inside the gloves is the **gown**, which is tied from behind. **Surgical glasses** are worn to protect the medical professional from fluids entering the eye. **Surgical caps** are worn over any hair the medical professional has to prevent hair or skin particles from falling onto the patient. **Face masks** are used to prevent fluids from entering the mouth and to help prevent airborne illnesses from infecting others. **Shoe covers** are used to prevent the spreading of microorganisms via the shoes into a sterile environment. All of these are considered **personal protective equipment**, and should be utilized any time there may be exposure to blood or other body fluids.

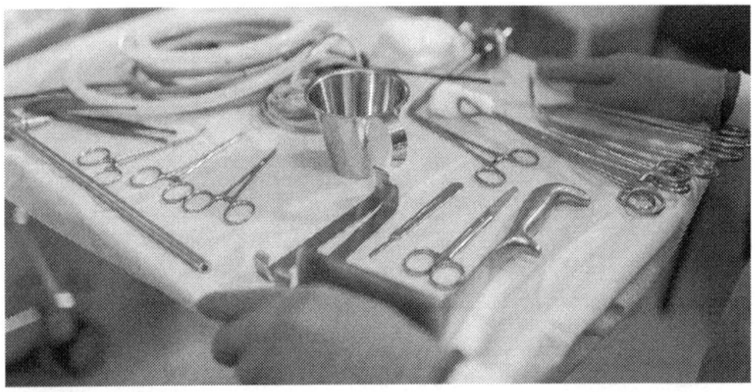

It is extremely important that surgical instruments remain sterile before a surgical procedure. Failure to use sterile equipment can introduce harmful microorganisms into the body and result in infection. To prevent contamination of the surgical tray prior to surgery, the tray should be covered by a sterile surgical drape. Once the drape is uncovered, re-gloving the hands should be done before handling individual instruments. If any instruments become contaminated, a new surgical tray will need to be set up.

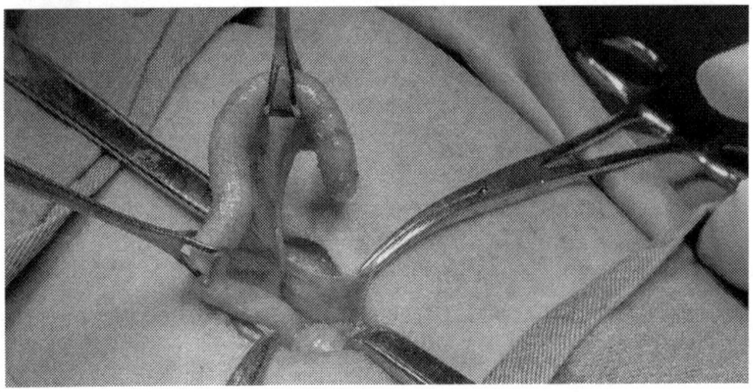

Sterile field boundaries are required for surgical procedures to establish aseptic barriers. This reduces the chance of infection. Areas being operated on are able to be exposed, but any area not being operated on should be covered by a sterile surgical drape. The surgical drape may also cover equipment being used and any furniture that may become contaminated.

Before surgical procedures are performed, the skin should be sterilized to prevent infections post-operation. The medical professional's hands should be washed and gloves should be worn during prep. The area of the skin should be cleaned utilizing either an aqueous or alcohol-based substance. Examples of these substances include providone-iodine, chlorhexidine, and isopropyl alcohol. The area is scrubbed using these substances, which destroy bacteria and other microorganisms in the process, helping to significantly reduce the chances of infection.

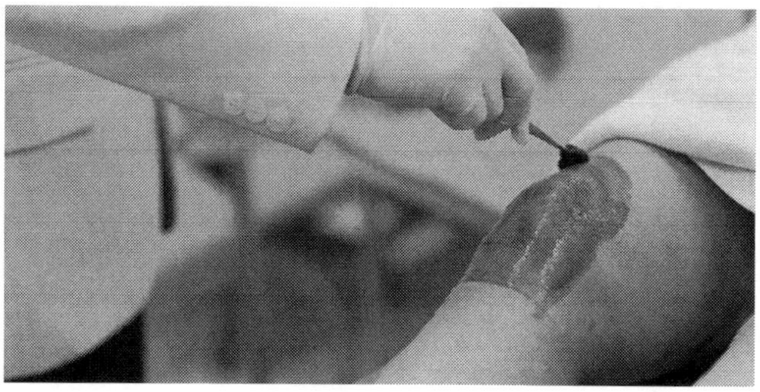

Wound Care

Chronic/Non-Healing Wound

If a person has a wound that has not healed over the course of **eight weeks or longer**, it is considered a **chronic or non-healing wound**. These wounds pose an increased risk of **infection**. Several treatment options are available depending on the severity of the wound. Dead tissue is removed in a process known as debridement, leaving healthy tissue untouched. This allows the wound the chance to begin healing properly. Different forms of debridement may be utilized, such as manually removing dead tissue using tweezers, scalpels, or curettes. Maggots may also be utilized to clean the wound, as maggots will only eat dead tissue. These maggots are grown in laboratories, and are specifically bred only to clean wounds. The maggots are placed on the wound, then covered by a bandage. After several days, the bandage and maggots are removed, revealing a clean wound free of dead tissue.

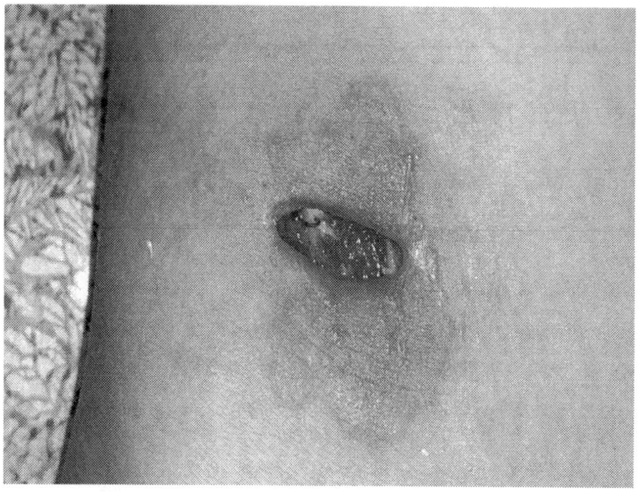

Chronic wounds are more likely to occur in patients who suffer from forms of neuropathy or poor circulation, such as patients who are diabetic.

Bandaging/Dressing Change

Dressing changes are important to provide a **sterile environment** over a damaged area of the skin, which helps **prevent infection** for occurring. In order to properly change a dressing, gloves should be worn. The dressing should be gently removed from the edges, using moist gauze where needed to prevent the tape from hurting the skin. Once completely removed, the dressing should be discarded, and the wound should be cleaned. Gloves should be changed, and the wound should be cleaned utilizing saline or another sterile solution. After the wound and the skin around it have been properly cleaned, the gauze used for cleaning and drying the wound should be discarded. The skin around the wound should be dried, and a new dressing is ready to be applied. The dressing should be opened from the corners, and the area coming into contact with the wound should not be touched to prevent introducing bacteria into the wound. The dressing is placed over the wound, and secured to the body using tape. Gloves are removed and the hands are washed.

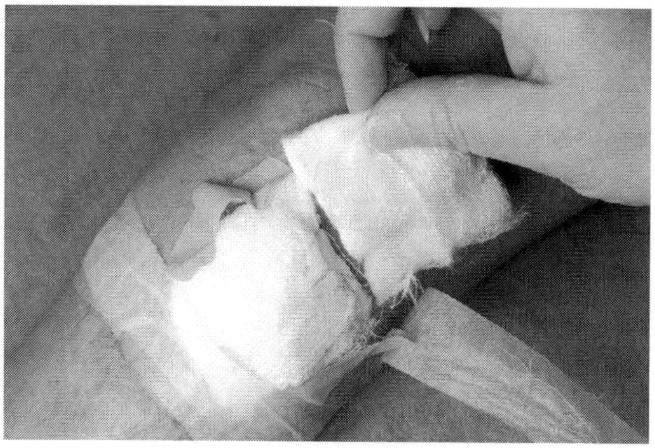

Post-op/Incision Care

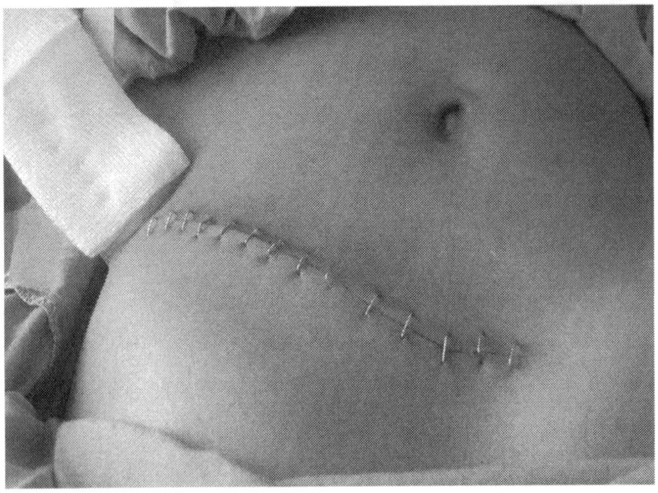

Incisions are most commonly closed by either **sutures** or **staples**, and caring for the area around the incision is vital in **preventing complications or infections** from occurring. After being closed, the incision is covered by a sterile dressing to prevent excessive bleeding in the area. The dressing should be changed regularly to prevent the wound from becoming septic, and to allow the wound the best chance to heal properly.

Incision sites may have accompanying **drains** to collect fluid and prevent fluid, such as blood, lymph, and serous fluid, from building up in the area. The fluid should be drained in regular intervals, and the amount of fluid being drained should be recorded to assess healing and potential complications post-op.

Ostomy Care

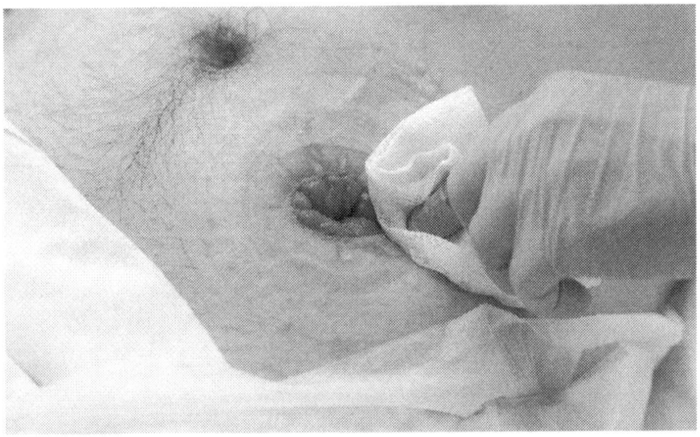

If a patient has colostomy, ileostomy, or urostomy, **urine** and **feces** is collected in a **bag** located outside the body that connects to the abdomen. These are utilized when a person has a problem with an organ that is not functioning properly, and bypasses that organ entirely to allow waste to leave the body. The area of the stoma, the hole in the abdomen in which waste leaves the body, must be cleaned and cared for. The amount of waste being removed in these instances, especially with an ileostomy, should be recorded. In the case of an ileostomy, because the waste does not move through the large intestine, the patient may become dehydrated if they are producing excessive waste.

Instruments

There are various surgical instruments, each used for a specific purpose. Categories of surgical instruments include instruments that cut, instruments that hold or grasp tissues or structures, and instruments that retract and allow viewing.

Cutting Instruments

A **scalpel** is a surgical instrument used for **cutting, dissecting, and removing tissue**. Scalpel blades come in differing sizes, which are used to perform different tasks. Some scalpels may be single-use, and are disposed of after one use. A scalpel that is **double edged** is known as a **lancet**.

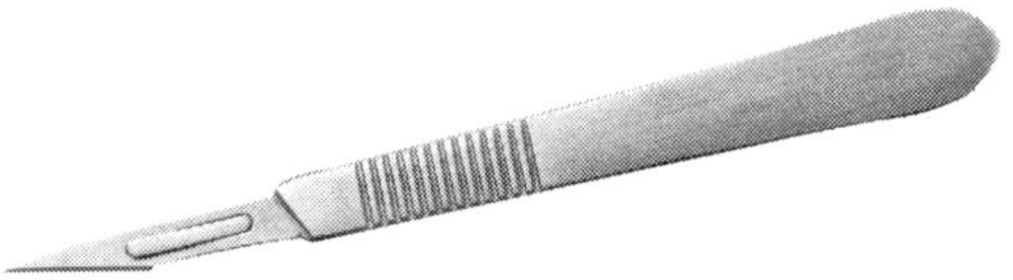

Scissors are instruments used for **cutting and separating structures**. These structures range from tissue in the body to bandages and dressings. Fine tip scissors are useful for cutting in very fine locations and minimally damage tissue. Curved tip scissors are useful in avoiding cutting of underlying tissues.

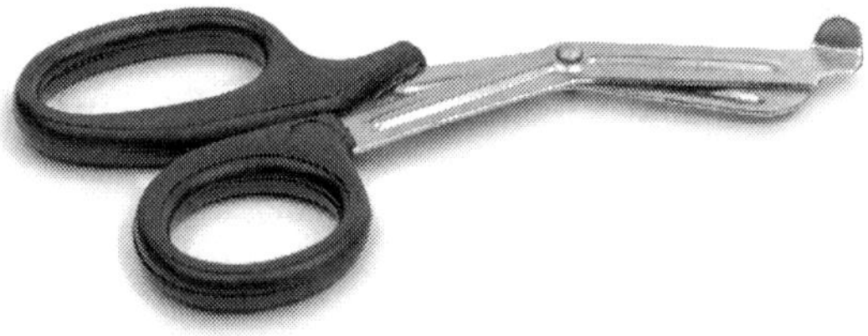

Grasping Instruments

Forceps are a medical instrument used to **grasp small objects.** These are often used when an object needs to be grasped that is too small for fingers. Forceps vary in size and type. Forceps may also be used to aid in childbirth, guiding the baby's head through the birth canal.

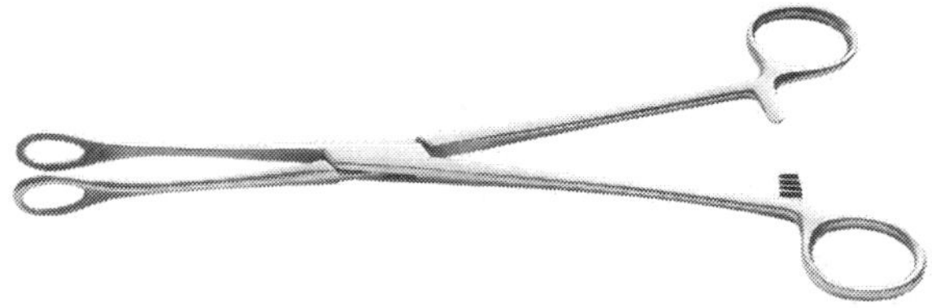

Retracting Instruments

Retractors are instruments used to **hold tissues open during surgery.** They may even be used to keep organs from intruding on a surgical procedure. Commonly, retractors are metal instruments with hooks at the end. These may need to be held in place by hand, or can be set without having to be held in instances such as rib spreaders.

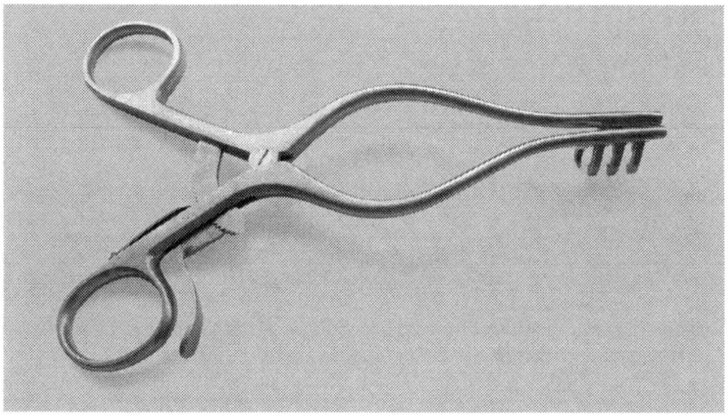

A **speculum** is an instrument used to **open the walls of a cavity.** A vaginal speculum is used by gynecologists to examine the vagina and cervix, and also allows access to the cervix for tissue collection performed in a Pap smear. A nasal speculum(pictured) is used by otorhinolaryngologists to easier view into the nasal cavity.

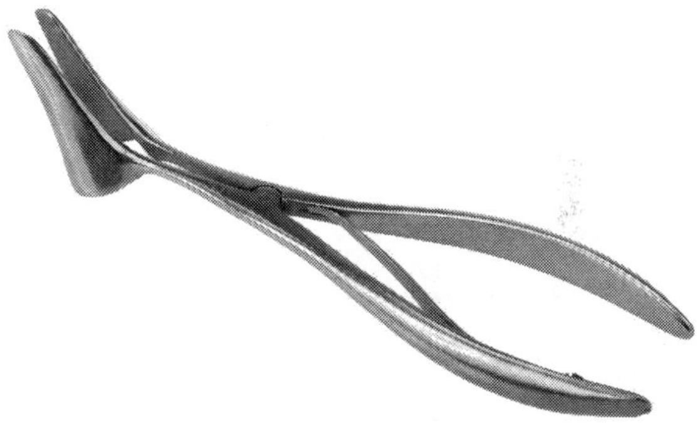

Other Instruments

An **anoscope** is an instrument used to examine the **anus and rectum.** The anoscope is lubricated and inserted into the anus. A light on the anoscope illuminates the anal canal, and a camera attached to the anoscope allows viewing of the anus.

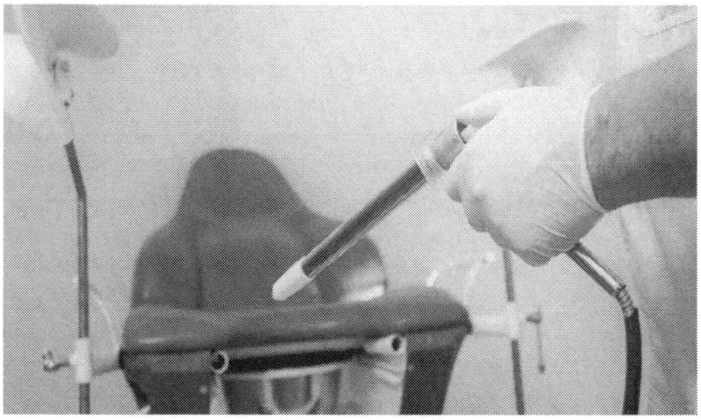

A **catheter** is a small tube inserted in to a part of the body to **help fluid drain.** The most common form is a urinary catheter. These are inserted into the urethra and into the urinary bladder. From there, fluid is able to drain freely from the bladder. Pictured is a Foley catheter.

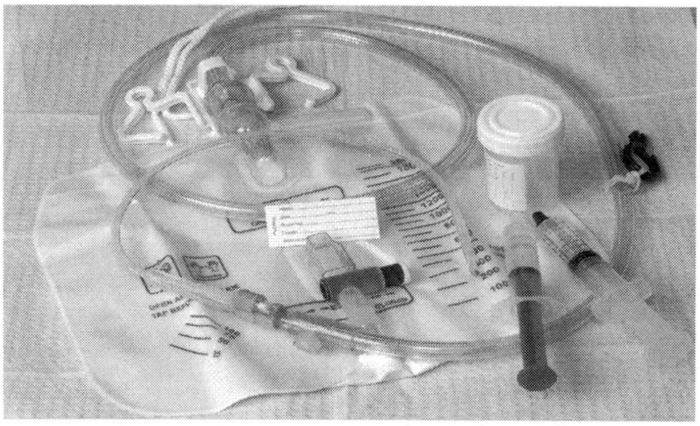

Dressings are used on **wounds** to prevent introduction of microorganisms. Dressings vary depending on the type of wound. Examples include cloth such as gauze, foam, and hydrogel.

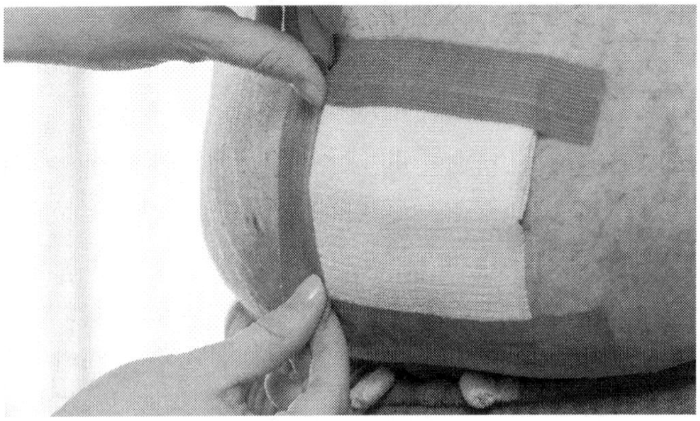

A **laryngoscope** is an instrument used to **view the larynx**, also known as the voice box. In addition, laryngoscopy may be performed to **intubate the trachea**. The laryngoscope allows direct line of sight of the glottis, the opening of the larynx, by moving the tongue and epiglottis from view. A mirror may be used if it is difficult to see the larynx.

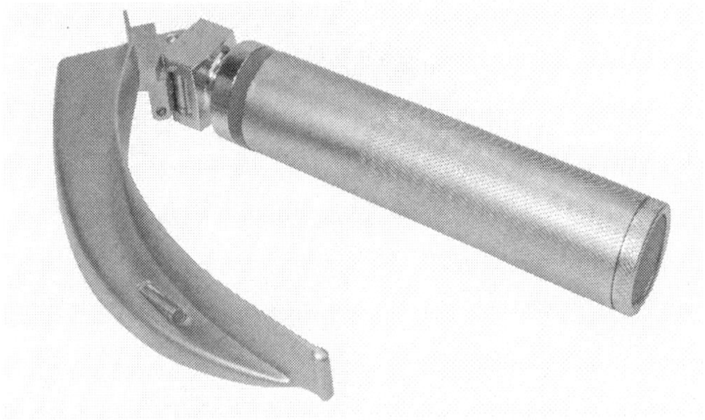

An **endoscope** is a device that contains a **camera and light source** used to **view inside organs**. Commonly, an endocopy is performed to view the esophagus, stomach, and small intestine. An endoscopy performed to view the large intestine is known as a colonoscopy.

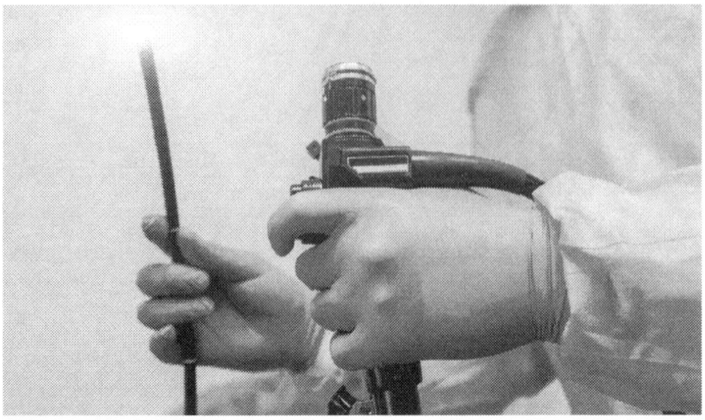

A **proctoscope** is an instrument used to examine the **anus, rectum, and sigmoid colon**. The proctoscope is lubricated and inserted into the anus, rectum, or large intestine. A light on the proctoscope illuminates the area being viewed, and a camera attached to the proctoscope allows viewing of the area.

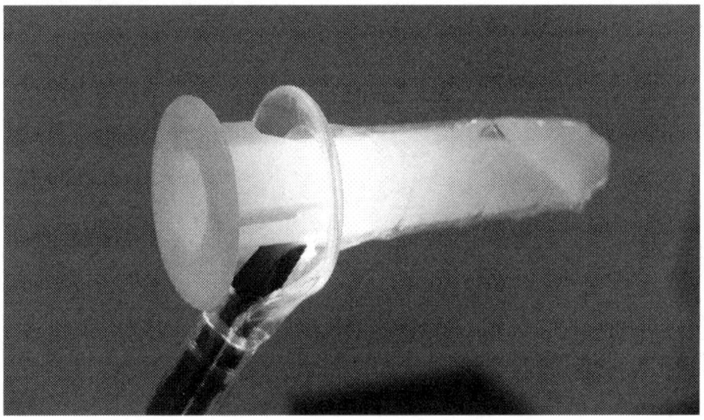

Sterilization Techniques/Autoclave

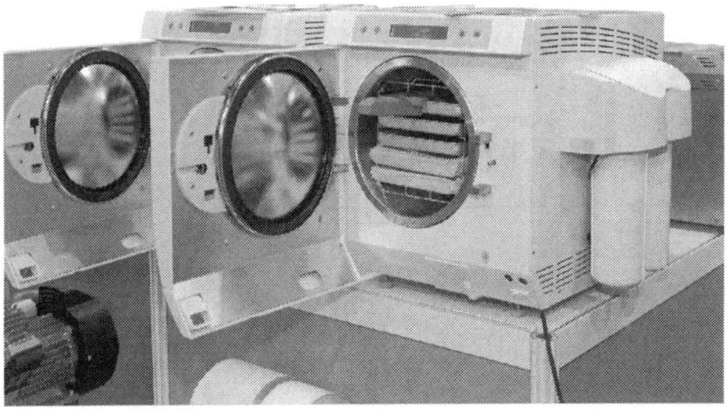

An **autoclave** is a device used to **sterilize medical equipment**. An instrument is placed inside the autoclave, and the door is closed. The air inside the machine is removed, as air does not help the sanitization process. The outer chamber of the autoclave increases the pressure inside, and the inner chamber sterilizes by utilizing steam. The steam reaches temperatures above 250 degrees Fahrenheit. This high temperature, combined with the pressure from the outer chamber, destroys the cell membranes, killing the cells.

Certain instruments should not be used in an autoclave, such as instruments that are sensitive to heat. Other instruments should be wrapped in autoclave paper to prevent oxidation of the instruments from coming into contact with the stainless steel surface of the autoclave. When using the autoclave, a label should be created that details the instruments being sterilized, and the date the autoclave is being used.

Sterilization indicators should be used in an autoclave. These indicators are small strips placed inside the autoclave that change color when exposed to temperatures above 250 degrees Fahrenheit. These indicate that the autoclave has been used, and the instruments inside the autoclave have been sterilized. If the color on the strip does not change, it means there was an issue with the autoclave that prevented it from functioning properly, and therefore, the instruments have not been sterilized.

Specimen Collection Techniques

Blood Collection

The primary mode of collecting blood is through **venipuncture**. Venipuncture is performed by puncturing a vein with a **needle**, which allows blood to enter a collecting tube. Venipuncture is most commonly performed at the median cubital and cephalic veins, located in the arm. However, other sites may be chosen for various reasons, including scarring in the area, hematomae in the general area, IV therapy, and blood transfusions. If these veins are not able to be utilized, the basilic vein on the dorsal forearm or the dorsal veins on the hand may be utilized.

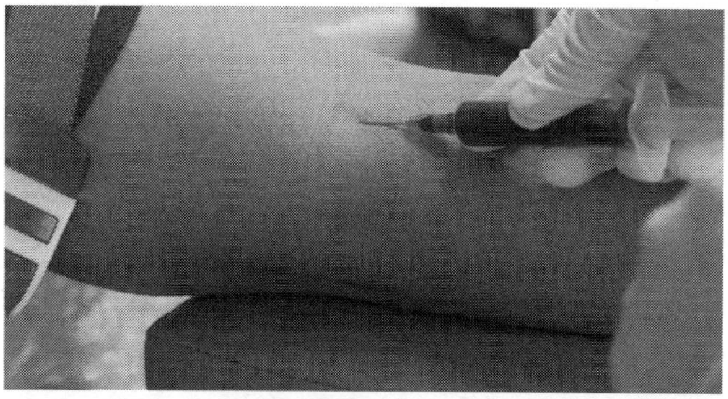

In preparation for venipuncture, the site should be cleaned using **70% isopropyl alcohol** and should be air dried. A **tourniquet** is applied roughly four inches above the venipuncture site, which fills the vein with blood and makes it larger and easier to puncture. The patient should make a fist without squeezing the hand. When it is time to perform the venipuncture, the skin should be pulled taut and the vein should be anchored using the thumb. The needle is then inserted into the vein at a 15-30 degree angle. The tourniquet is then removed, and a sample is collected.

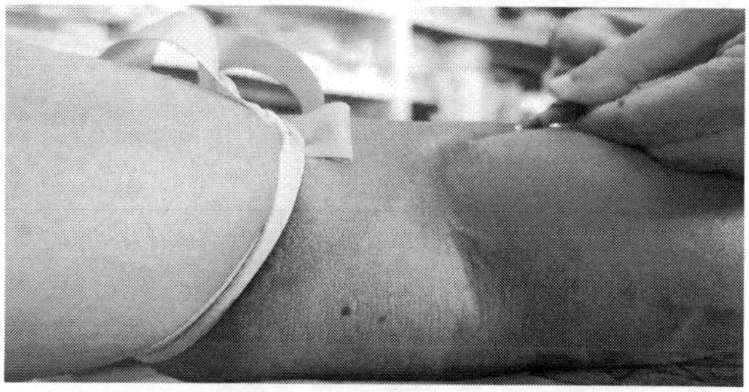

Evacuated collection tubes are used to collect blood, and are only able to hold a set amount of blood in each tube. These tubes contain no air, and pull the blood from the veins by using a vacuum effect. After the collection tube has been filled with blood, the needle is removed from the vein, and **gauze** is applied and pressure is applied on the area to encourage blood clot formation and to prevent hematomae to form. Materials should be properly discarded, the specimens should be labeled and stored or examined immediately.

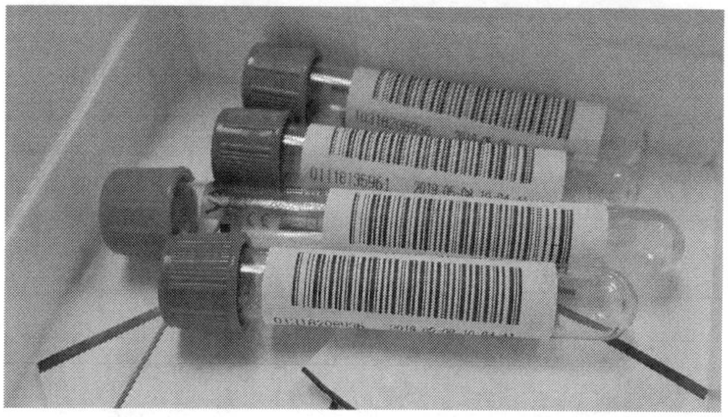

Collection tubes vary due to the presence of different additives in each tube. These additives are used to either clot the blood, or prevent the blood from clotting. Each tube contains a **colored rubber stopper** at the top, and the color is used to indicate which type of additive is present in the tube. Examples of additives used include heparin to prevent blood clotting in the tube, and sodium citrate to remove calcium.

Tubes that **clot the blood** will have caps colored **red**, **gold**, **orange**, **royal blue**, or a **red/gray mixture.** These tubes contain clot activators that will clot the blood when the tube is inverted.

Tubes that **prevent clotting** will have caps colored **light green**, **light blue**, **green**, **gray**, **lavender**, **yellow**, **tan**, and **pink.** These tubes contain anticoagulants that will prevent the blood from clotting when the tube is inverted.

Another way to collect blood is by using a **capillary** or **dermal puncture**. These are performed when only a small amount of blood needs to be collected, and only punctures the capillaries. In an adult, the most common location is on a finger, known as a **fingerstick**. In a child or infant, the most common location is on the heel of the foot, known as a **heelstick**. Rarely, the ear lobe may also be used. Capillary punctures are commonly used to test iron content in the blood, or to test the metabolic functioning in an infant.

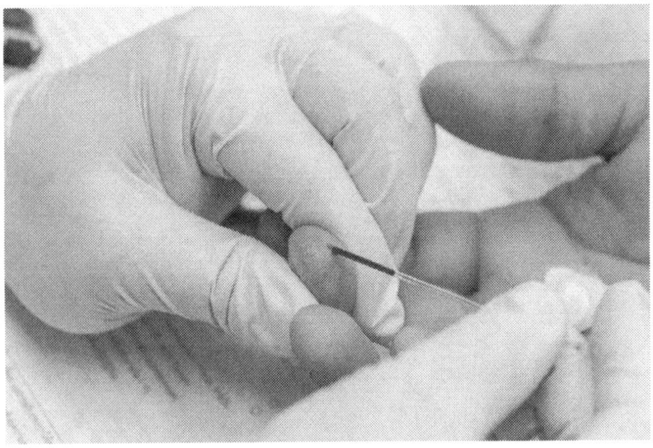

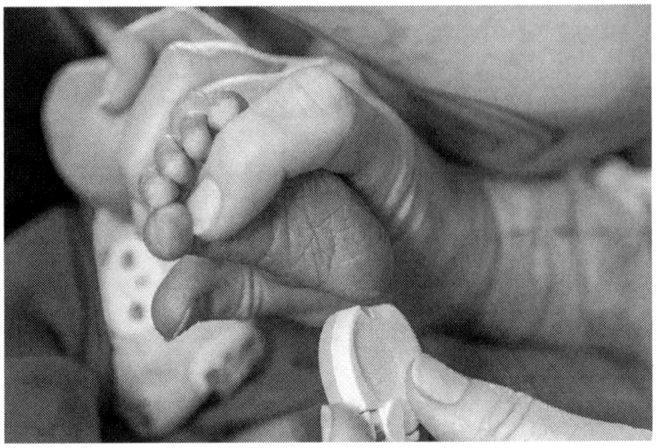

Urine Collection

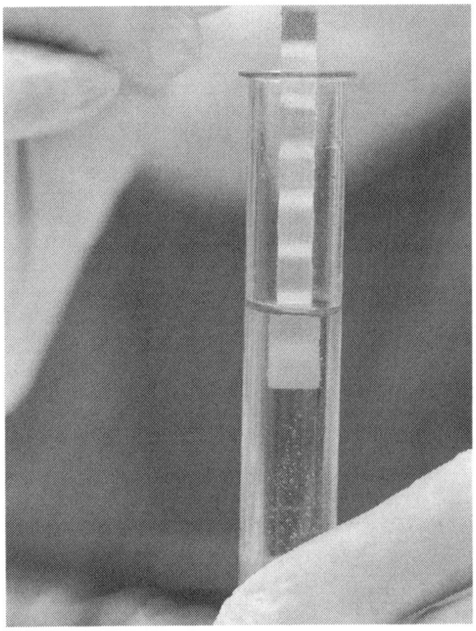

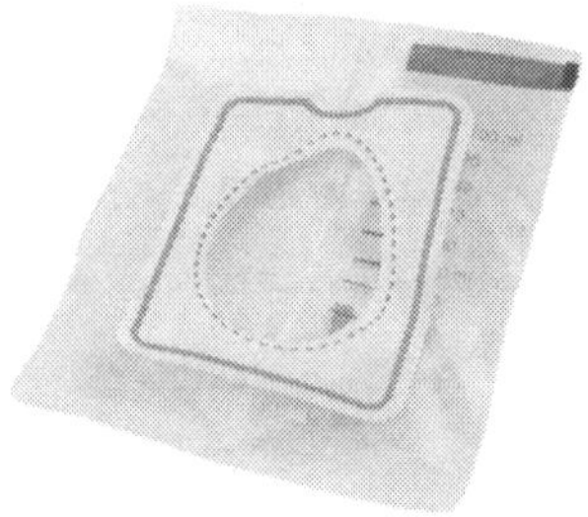

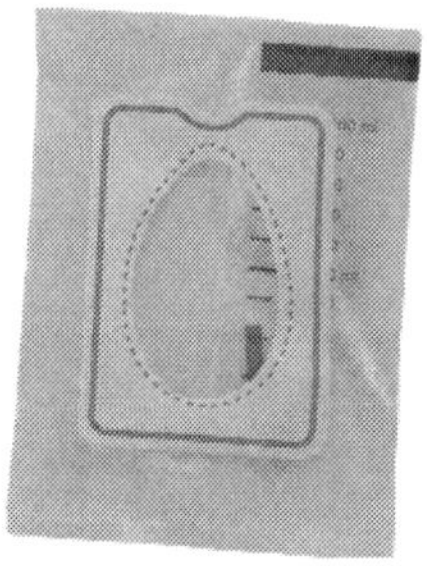

Urine samples are obtained and examined for a number of reasons. Examination of urine is known as **urinalysis**. Examining the urine can reveal several things about the internal chemistry of a person, from protein to electrolytes and more.

Random urine collection is performed for urinalysis, and may be collected at any time. While convenient, random specimens may be diluted or contaminated, as they are not as controlled as other collection means.

Midstream/clean catch is the most preferred type of urine collection, as it is the most controlled, and least likely to be contaminated. The patient will first clean the exit of the urethra using a sanitizing towelette. This will reduce the amount of bacteria at the exit of the urethra. The patient will then void the first portion of urine from the body into a toilet. After this is done, the rest of the urine is collected into a cup. Voiding the first portion of urine instead of collecting it is to help further cleanse the area and prevent contamination.

Timed 24-hour collection is performed by having the patient first empty the bladder. After the bladder is emptied, the 24 hour time clock begins, and any urine produced during the 24 hours is collected and examined. This gives a greater view of the long-term functioning of the body and its production of urine. Timed 24-hour collection is useful in testing levels of substances such as creatinine, protein, and sodium.

If a child or infant needs to have urine collected, a **pediatric urine collector** it utilized. The pediatric urine collector is a small bag that is placed around and adhered to the urethral opening. As the child urinates, the urine is collected in the bag. The urine is then transferred into a cup.

A **catheter** is a small tube inserted in to a part of the body to help **fluid drain**. The most common form is a urinary catheter. These are inserted into the urethra and into the urinary bladder. From there, fluid is able to drain freely from the bladder. If a patient is bedridden or unable to urinate properly, a Foley catheter is inserted into the urinary bladder and urine is then collected.

Fecal Collection

Fecal specimens are obtained from a patient, where a patient will **defecate** into a bag and then **scoop** a small portion of the feces into a storage container. If the feces is not able to be transferred immediately to the laboratory, the sample should be refrigerated. The sample should be free of contaminants like urine. Fecal specimens are used to detect **parasites** that may be in the digestive tract, such as tapeworms, hookworms, and roundworms.

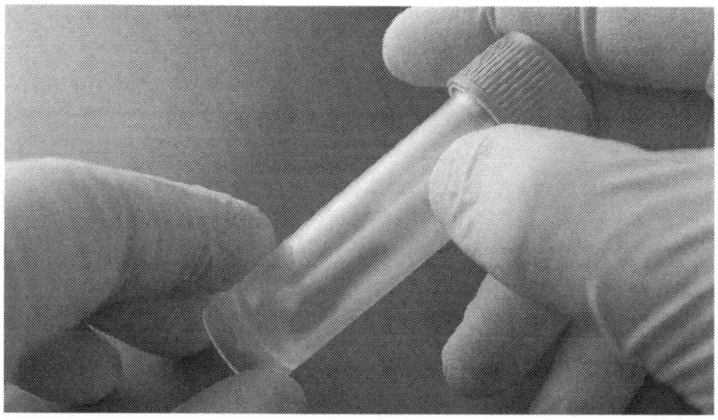

Throat Swab

Throat swabs are used if there is a suspected **bacterial infection** in the throat, such as **strep throat or tonsillitis.** The swab is completed by the medical professional applying gloves, depressing the patient's throat with a tongue depressor. A sterile cotton swab is gently moved over the area of suspected infection, such as the base of the tonsils. Gagging may occur, so it should be performed quickly. The swab is then taken to a laboratory, where it is placed onto a plate known as a petri dish. The bacteria is allowed to grow, and the culture is examined to determine the type of infection.

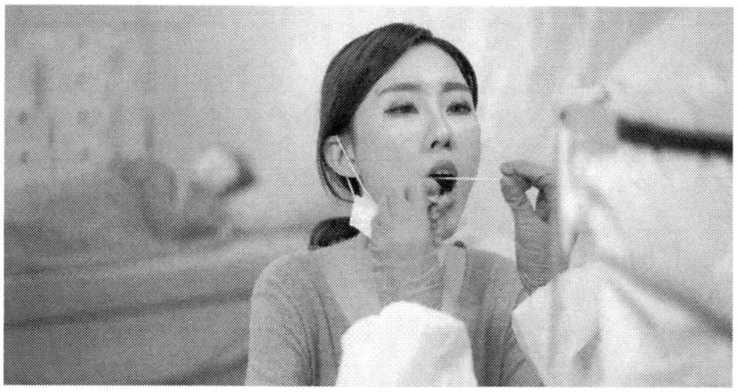

Sputum Collection

Sputum is **phlegm in the lungs**. Sputum collection is typically performed when a patient is suspected of having an infection such as **tuberculosis or pneumonia.** Sputum is collected by having the patient **cough** hard enough from the chest for phlegm to dislodge from the lung. After the sputum has entered the mouth, it is spit into a collecting container. Often times, numerous specimens are obtained over several days. Before each specimen is collected, the patient should rinse the mouth to reduce the amount of bacteria that may also be collected. After the specimen is collected, it should be sealed in the container and either submitted to a laboratory or refrigerated until it can be examined.

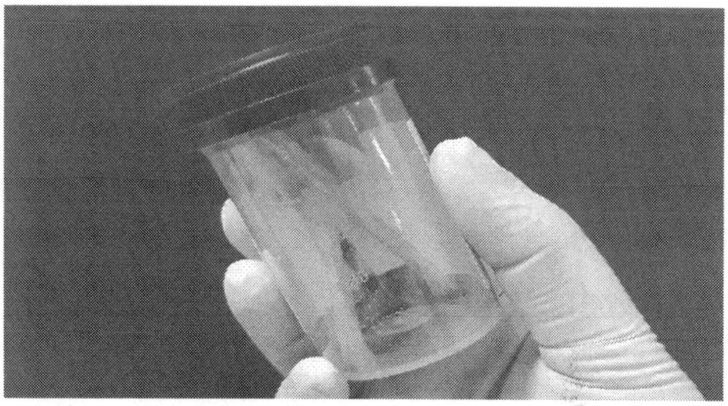

Nasopharyngeal Swab

Nasopharyngeal swabs are used to determine if a patient has any **respiratory infections**, such as **influenza**. The swab is performed with the patient sitting upright, and the head tilted back. The medical professional applies gloves, then inserts the swab directly into the nasal passage. The sterile cotton swab is placed against the nasopharynx at the back of the nasal cavity and rotated to collect material for testing. The swab is removed and placed into a container, and immediately tested.

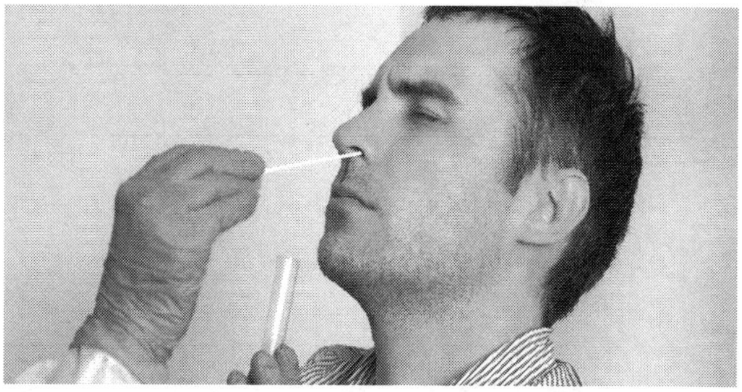

Wound Swab

Wound swabs are performed in order to determine if there is any type of **infection** in an **open skin lesion**, or if there is infection already present, to determine what kind of bacteria is causing the infection. To perform a wound swab, the medical professional will put on gloves, and utilizing a sterile cotton swab that has been dampened with sodium chloride, the wound is swabbed. The location of the swab should be a part of the wound that is not necrotic or showing signs of infection, as these materials may compromise the examination. After the clean portion of the would is swabbed, the sample is placed in a container and examined. Wound swabs should ideally be performed before medications have been prescribed or taken, because antibiotics can interfere with the growth of the bacteria.

Preparing, Processing, and Examining Specimens

When collecting specimens for examination, collecting tubes should always be labeled properly. This prevents any mistakes in regards to who the specimen came from, what the specimen is used for, and ensures that retesting is not necessary. Every label should include all of the following: the patient's name, the patient's medical record number, the patient's location, the date and time the specimen was collected, the type of specimen collected, what the specimen is being tested for or the specific test being utilized, and the name or the physician who ordered the test to be performed.

Specimens have the potential to be contaminated by numerous means. Introduction of bacteria, fungus, or other debris is an extremely common form of contamination that can influence the specimen being tested. When collecting a sample, if possible, the area of the body the sample is being collected(for example, the antecubital region when performing venipuncture) should be sterilized with use of isopropyl alcohol to eliminate as much bacteria in the area as possible before specimen collection. Damage to equipment, such as collection tubes, can introduce foreign substances into the sample and contaminate the sample. If equipment is not properly sanitized using machines such as an autoclave, contamination may result.

Preservation

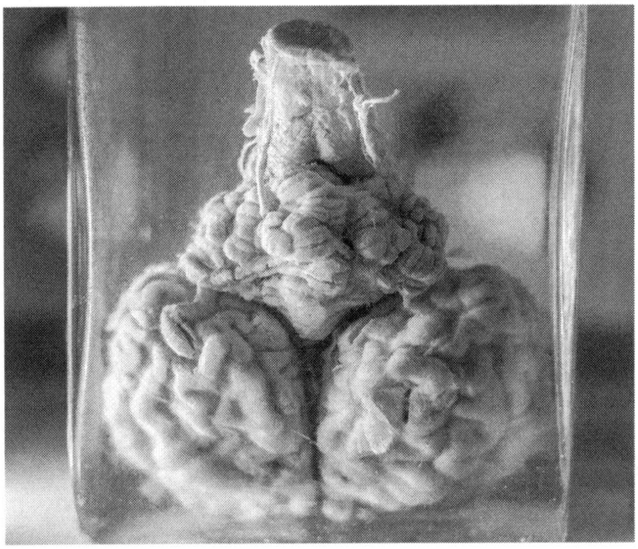

If unable to be immediately tested, specimens should be preserved for testing at a later date. **Refrigeration** is utilized to preserve blood and serum samples until they are able to be tested, usually stored between 2-8 degrees celsius. If a specimen is taken that needs to be completely preserved over a long period of time, without degradation, **fixative preservation** is used. These samples are typically used in microscopic examination, and are cells or tissue. A specimen is collected, and is preserved through different means, depending on what the specimen is. The specimen may be immersed in a substance such as formaldehyde, or heated to kill the organism being tested.

Incubator

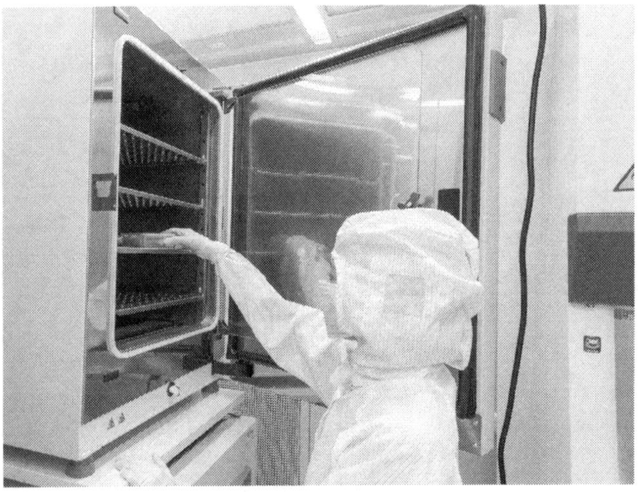

When collecting a sample of a microorganism or cells, an **incubator** may be used not only for **preservation**, but to allow the specimen to **grow.** An incubator provides a **constant temperature**, with desired **humidity**, that allows these organisms to grow. Incubators are commonly used to allow bacterial or fungal samples to grow, which helps determine the type of microorganism collected.

Inoculating a Culture

An inoculation is **introducing a bacteria or fungus into a liquid.** This liquid is then introduced **into the body.** This introduces an antigen into the body, allowing the body to develop an immunity to it.

In the first steps of inoculation, the bacteria or fungus must be given an environment to grow. The microorganism is obtained from an **agar plate**, and mixed with **Luria broth** in a collecting tube. The tube is sealed, and placed in a shaking incubator. This allows the microorganism to properly grow.

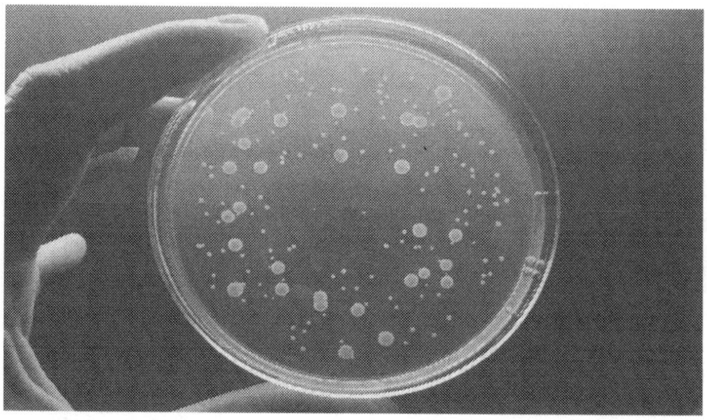

Centrifuge

A **centrifuge** is a medical device used to **separate solids from liquids.** This is especially useful in separating plasma from the blood cells in blood. Centrifuges accomplish this by **spinning** in circles extremely fast, forcing the solids in a substance to move to the bottom of the collection tube, and the liquids move to the top.

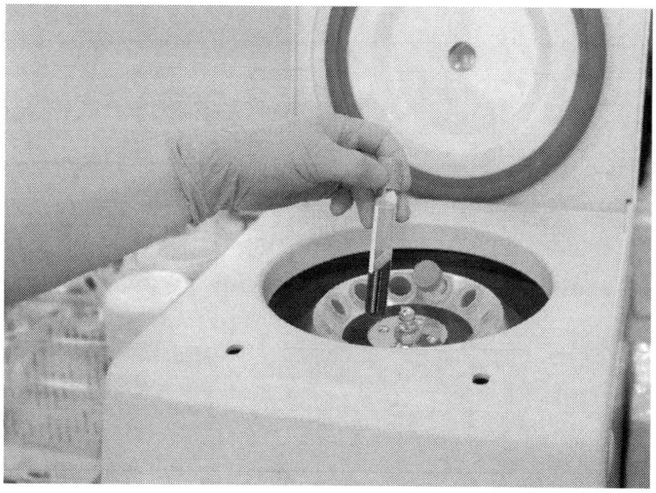

Microscope

A **microscope** is a device used to view things that are **too small** to be seen with the naked eye. The most common type is an **optical microscope**. Optical microscopes require the use of **slides** with a substance placed on them, viewed through a lens that zooms in on the object. **Light** is produced below the slide, which allows the structures to be viewed. **Dry mount** is observing microorganisms or structures on a slide without adding fluid to the slide. An example of a structure used on a dry mount is hair. **Wet mount** is observing microorganisms on a slide by adding fluid to the slide. This is used most commonly when trying to observe structures or cells that are still living, such as bacteria. **Saline** is commonly used to preserve living organisms in a sample, while **potassium hydroxide(-KOH)** is used to kill all bacteria in a sample. KOH slides are commonly utilized to test for yeast infections, because the potassium hydroxide kills bacteria, but does not kill yeast.

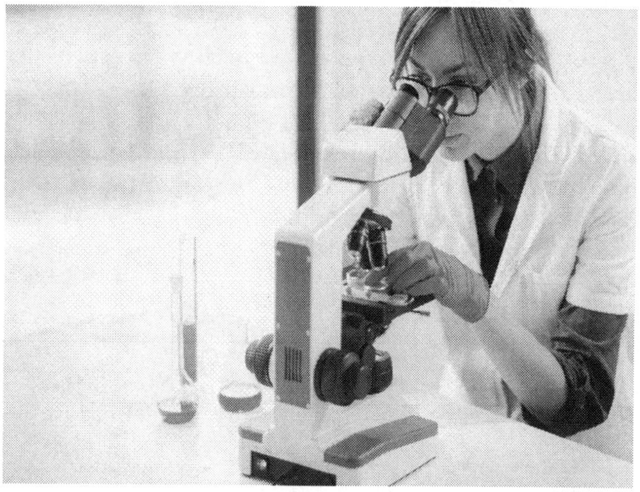

Laboratory Quality Control

Clinical Laboratory Improvement Act

The **Clinical Laboratory Improvement Act**, also known as **CLIA**, regulates all **laboratory testing** performed on humans to ensure the testing is up to **quality standard**. These tests can include health assessments, diagnoses, and treatments of diseases.

Testing Records and Performance Logs

Testing records are required to be maintained for all laboratory tests. These records are used to examine the results of the test when compared to a control test. Performance logs are used to establish which medical personnel performed the test, and analyze the results of the test each day. This helps trace any errors that occur with specific personnel, and holds the personnel and facility accountable for the test and results.

Equipment Calibration and Maintenance

Medical equipment is required to be calibrated on a consistent basis to ensure it is functioning properly. If equipment is not functioning properly, maintenance should be performed on the equipment to repair it. If the equipment cannot be repaired, it should be replaced, and the defunct equipment should not be used. Calibration and maintenance of equipment is required to be documented.

Quality Control Testing

Control tests are used to test consistency of tests versus a control. These ensure that certain variables are not influencing the test.

Monitor and Document Temperature Controls

Collected specimens that are required to be stored are kept in environments with specific temperature settings, such as refrigerators and incubators. These pieces of equipment, and their temperature settings and controls, are required to be monitored by all medical personnel. Temperature is required to be documented to ensure no specimens are influenced by inappropriate temperature settings.

Laboratory Panels and Selected Tests

Urinalysis

Urinalysis is the process of **analyzing urine** and its contents. Urinalysis is commonly performed to test for **infections** of the urinary tract, **diabetes**, or any issues the kidneys may have. **Physical urinalysis** is used to analyze the urine based on its physical appearance, such is its **color** or whether or not it is **cloudy. Chemical urinalysis** is used to analyze the urine based on its chemical content, which involves many different substances. These substances can include **blood, protein, ketones, glucose, and bilirubin**. The **acidity** of the urine may also be tested, also known as its **pH level**.

Microscopic urinalysis is performed to observe any **cells** or substances in the urine that can't be seen with the naked eye. This is used to observe **blood, bacteria, cancerous cells, crystals**, and regular **epithelial cells** from the urinary tract.

If a urinary tract infection is suspected, a **culture** may be acquired to determine the exact cause of the infection. The most common method of obtaining a culture is using **midstream/clean catch**, or by using a **urine collection bag** with children. A **catheter** may be used to obtain a urine culture, or in some rare cases, **suprapubic aspiration** may be used to obtain urine, in which a doctor removes urine from the bladder using a **needle**.

Hematology Panel

Hematology panels are performed to test the blood for blood-related disorders such as anemia, leukemia, and hemophilia. Blood is most commonly collected with the use of venipuncture.

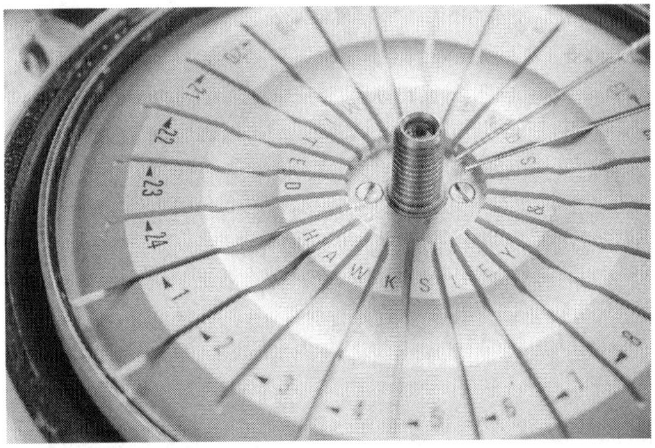

Hematocrit is the **percentage of blood** that consists of the **red blood cells.** Hematocrit testing is performed by a machine that measures the **complete blood count(CBC)**. This gives an accurate percentage of the blood content. A centrifuge may also be used for small quantities of blood, measuring the amount of blood at the bottom of the tube after it has been separated from the plasma and leukocytes. **Low hematocrit levels** in a person means they have some form of **anemia.**

Hemoglobin is tested, commonly in conjunction with hematocrit, to determine if a person is **anemic** in some way. The blood is cycled through a machine, which gives an accurate reading of hemoglobin content in the blood.

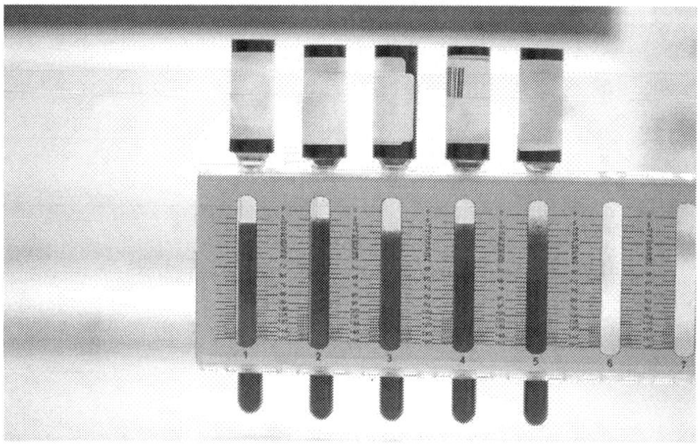

Erythrocyte sedimentation rate is used to measure the amount of **systemic inflammation** in the body. During this test, blood is collected, and **set vertically** for one hour. After the initial hour, the amount of plasma that is seen at the top of the tube is measured and recorded. This determines how quickly the erythrocytes are settling at the bottom of the tube. When there is **inflammation** in the body, there is an increased amount of **fibrinogen and c-reactive protein** in the blood. These substances cause erythrocytes to settle more rapidly.

Automated cell counts are used to measure the total amount of living and dead cells in the blood. This helps determine if there are any atypical blood cell counts, blood disorders such as anemia, or other imbalances in cells such as leukemia. These cell counts are performed by a machine that reads the blood, determining levels of each type of blood cell.

Platelets are also measured, which helps determine if there is a problem with blood clotting. A **prothrombin time test(PT)** is a test that measures the amount of time it takes for a blood clot to form. If a person is taking blood thinners, a certain ratio of prothrombin time will be established using the **international normalized ratio(INR)**. This allows comparison of testing results to be performed between different laboratories.

Chemistry/Metabolic Testing

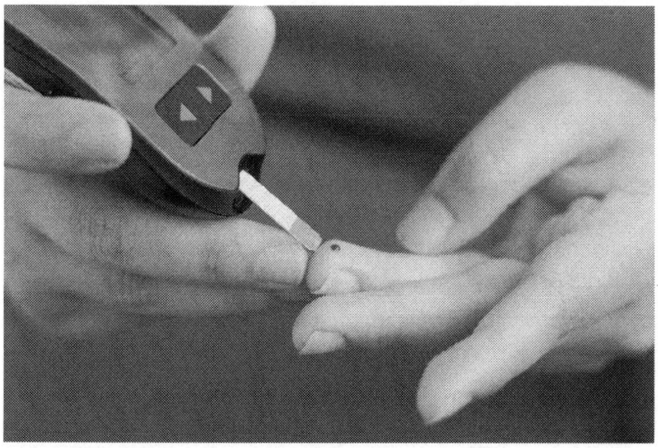

Chemistry in the body is tested through collection of blood and urine. These substances are then tested, and certain substances are observed and measured to obtain a view of body and organ function.

Glucose, the amount of **sugar in the blood**, is measured using blood and urine. If glucose is high, it may mean a person has a condition such as **diabetes**, or may be suffering from other disorders such as **kidney failure**. If a person has diabetes, they will need to constantly check their blood glucose, which is most commonly performed by doing a **finger stick**, which produces a small amount of blood that is read by a monitor. This monitor reads the amount of glucose present in the blood.

Kidney function tests are performed to measure the functioning of the kidneys. These tests include **Albumin to Creatinine Ratio(ACR)** and **Glomerular Filtration Rate(GFR)**. ACR is performed by extracting a sample of urine. The urine is tested for albumin levels. Albumin is a protein that should be in the blood, not the urine. Albumin in the urine may be a sign that the kidneys are not properly filtering waste from the body, and may be damaged in some way. GFR is a blood test that measures the amount of creatinine in the blood. Creatinine is a substance that is normally removed from the blood by the kidneys. If the kidneys are not functioning properly, there may be too much creatinine in the blood. The Glomerular Filtration Rate takes into account a person's age, height, weight, sex, and race, along with the amount of creatinine in the blood, to determine a view of proper kidney functioning.

Liver function tests are performed to measure the functioning of the liver. These tests specifically measure the amount of **enzymes, proteins, and bilirubin** in the liver. The liver may also be biopsied to test the liver tissue itself.

Lipid profiles are performed to test **lipid levels** in the blood. Lipid panels are specifically designed to measure the amount of **HDL(high density lipoprotein)**, **LDL(low density lipoprotein)**, and **triglycerides** in the blood. These tests are performed to determine if a person has high or low amounts of lipids, or cholesterol, in their blood, which can be an indicator of risk for developing cardiovascular disease.

Hemoglobin A1c is a test designed to give an **average range of blood sugar** over the past **three months**. Hemoglobin that has glucose attached to it is tested, and it is this which is counted and measured. This is primarily performed on people who are **diabetic**, and is another step in monitoring blood glucose levels.

Electrolytes are **minerals** that are essential to bodily function. Major electrolytes include **sodium**, **potassium**, **magnesium**, **calcium**, **phosphorus**, and **chloride.** Electrolytes can assist in regulation of homeostasis, hydration, muscle contraction, and pH levels. Electrolytes can be lost from the body through sweat, or removed from the body in the urine if there are too many electrolytes in the blood. An electrolyte panel is performed to read electrolyte levels in the blood, which helps to determine if there is an electrolyte imbalance. Blood is collected via venipuncture. Electrolyte panels are often performed as one part of a full metabolic panel.

If the thyroid is not functioning properly, a metabolic panel may be performed to determine if the thyroid is producing adequate amounts of **thyroid hormone.** If the thyroid is not producing adequate thyroid hormones, a person is diagnosed with hypothyroidism. Complications of hypothyroidism include weight gain, sensitivity to cold, hair loss, fatigue, and goiter development, among others.

Specialized Testing

Mononucleosis tests are performed to detect **antibodies** in the body that are used to directly combat mononucleosis. This is an indicator of a mononucleosis infection. Blood is collected and observed under a microscope after being mixed with a chemical that the antibodies react to. If the desired reaction occurs, then a person is considered to have contracted mononucleosis.

Rapid Group A Streptococcus tests are performed if a person is suspected of having **strep throat**. During this test, the tongue is depressed, and the **tonsils** and **back of the throat are swabbed.** The swab is placed in a collecting tube and sent to a lab for testing. After strep throat is verified, the person will be prescribed antibiotics to combat the infection.

C-reactive protein(CRP) tests are performed when **systemic inflammation** is suspected. CRP is made in the liver, and is distributed into the blood stream when there is inflammation. High levels of CRP in a blood sample may indicate inflammation. Analysis of the blood typically takes a few days.

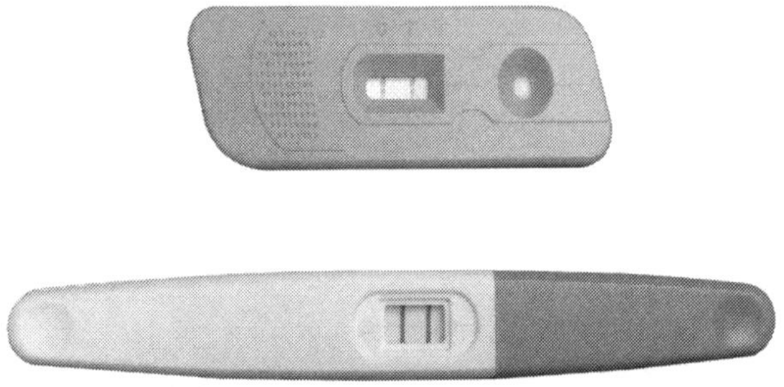

hCG pregnancy tests are used to determine if a woman is pregnant or not. These tests are performed by urine or blood collection. hCG is a hormone produced by the **placenta. High levels** of hCG is indicative of **pregnancy**. An hCG pregnancy test can be performed at home using an over-the-counter pregnancy test. The person will **urinate** onto a strip, and the hCG reacts to chemicals on the strip, which will then indicate pregnancy.

H. pylori tests are performed if there is a suspected infection of the Helicobacter pylori bacterium, which is a major contributing factor towards the development of peptic ulcers. These tests include collecting a **stool sample**, a **urea breath test**, or in more serious cases, performing **endoscopy and biopsy of the stomach.** The urea breath test consists of a person drinking urea, which is then broken down into carbon dioxide by H. pylori. After 15 minutes, the person's breath is measured for increased amounts of carbon dioxide, which can indicate an infection.

Influenza tests are performed to determine if a person is infected with a strain of **influenza.** Commonly, a **swab of the nasopharynx** is performed, but a nasal aspirate may be performed, in which a saline mixture is inserted into the nose and then suctioned out into a collecting tube. This fluid, which contains mucous, is tested for presence of influenza.

Genetic/hereditary tests are utilized to test for variants in a person's **genome** that may cause **disease**, or the risk of **developing** a disease in the future. Genetic risk assessments are primarily performed to test for specific forms of **cancer.** Different forms of cancer have different percentages associated with developing these cancers, as some cancers are more common than others, especially in regards to family history.

An **absolute risk** is the probability that a person will eventually develop a disease or condition based on their genetic profile and patterns in their lifestyle or behavior. These risks are always given as a percentage. For example, if 20 out of 100 individuals are at risk of developing skin cancer at some point in their life, the absolute risk is listed as 20%.

A **relative risk** is used when **comparing two demographics** in relation to probability that the disease will develop. For example, the risk of developing Crohn's disease is greater in people of Jewish descent than people of non-Jewish descent. This means the relative risk of developing Crohn's disease is higher for people of Jewish descent than those who are not.

Tuberculosis is a bacterial infection of the lungs, and if left untreated, may lead to severe lung damage and potential death. Tuberculosis is spread through droplets in the air. Testing for suspected cases of tuberculosis is performed by using the **Mantoux tuberculin skin test**. During this test, a small amount of a fluid known as **tuberculin(also known as purified protein derivative) is injected** into a small area of the forearm, which leaves a **circular raised bump**. After two or three days, the patient returns, and the bump and area are examined. If the area is over 15mm wide, the person is considered infected. The bump may feel hard, and it may be red, but the redness is not an indicator of infection.

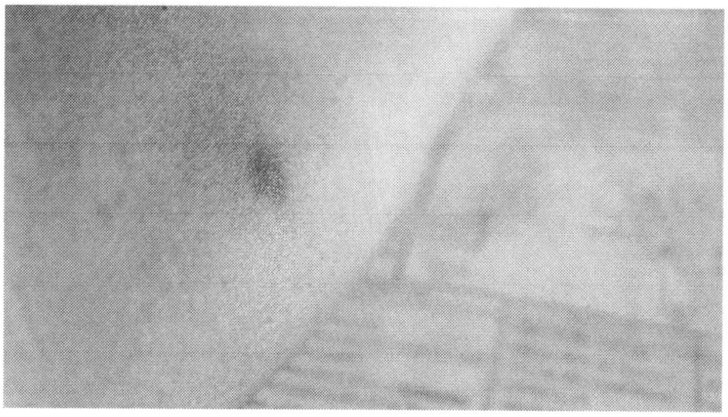

Fecal occult blood testing is performed to determine if there is blood in a person's stool. Blood in the stool can be indicative of problems such as ulcerations, infections, and even cancers. A stool sample must be collected. Once the specimen is submitted, a **guaiac test** is commonly performed. During a guaiac test, a **card** with **two or three separate sections** on it is used. Each section is designed to test stool collected on different days. The stool from each day is placed on a different section of the card and allowed to dry. The samples are then examined to determine the amount of blood, if any, is in the stool.

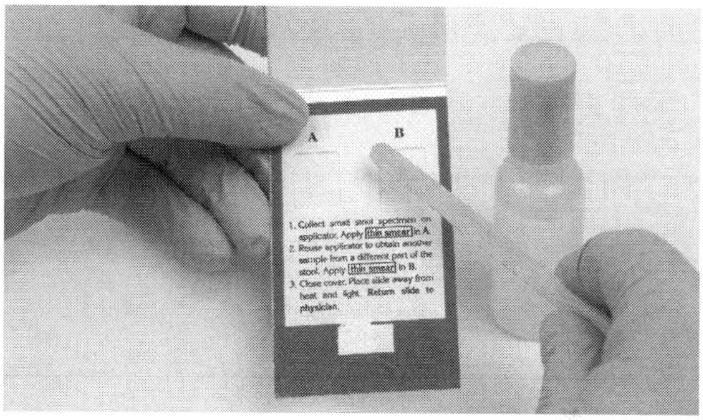

Cardiovascular Testing

Electrocardiogram(ECG/EKG)

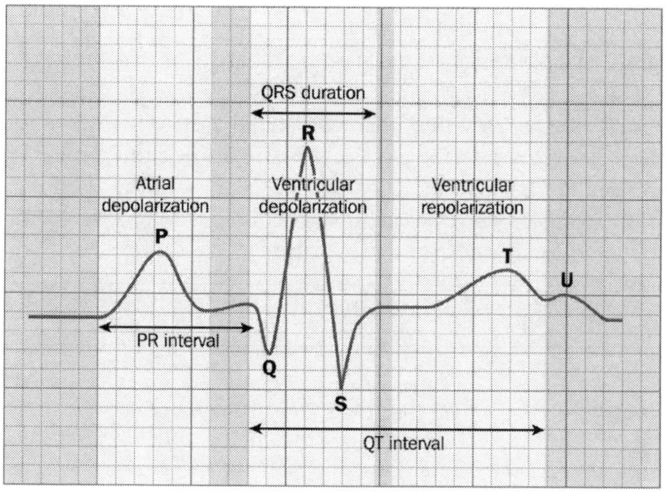

If a doctor feels as if a patient needs to have their heart rhythm monitored, they may administer an ECG/EKG. During this procedure, **ten pads attached to electrodes** are attached to the patient's bare skin on specific points around the trunk. The ECG/EKG picks up the electrical activity of the heart, and produces a visualization that shows **each wave of electrical activity**. The first wave seen is known as the **P wave**, and shows the contraction of the atria. Next is the **QRS wave**, which shows the depolarization and contraction of the ventricles. Following that is the **T wave**, which represents re-polarization of the ventricles.

To get an accurate reading, the patient's skin needs to be prepared properly. The skin should be clean and dry, the area should be swabbed with alcohol, and any hair in the area should be shaved. Ideally, the patient should recline at a 45 degree angle and the room should be a comfortable temperature.

In a typical 12 lead ECG/EKG, the leads should be placed at the following locations:

V1: The fourth intercostal space, located at the right sternal border
V2: The fourth intercostal space, located at the left sternal border
V3: Halfway between V2 and V4 leads
V4: The fifth intercostal space, located at the midclavicular line
V5: The left anterior axillary line, located at the same transverse plane as V4
V6: The left midaxillary line, located at the same transverse plane as V4 and V5
RA: The right arm at the inside wrist
LA: The left arm at the inside wrist
RL: The right leg at the inner ankle
LL: The left leg at the inner ankle

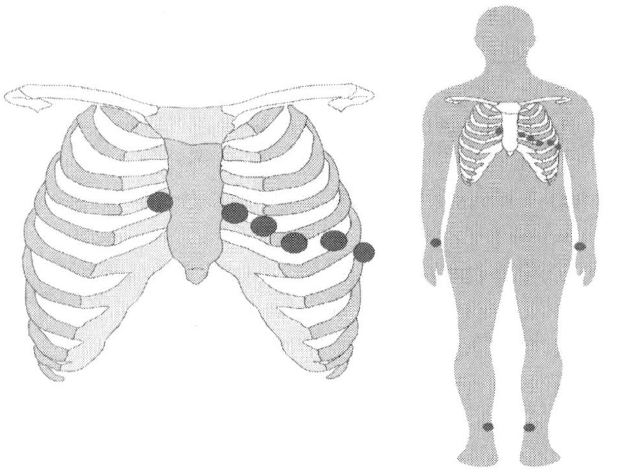

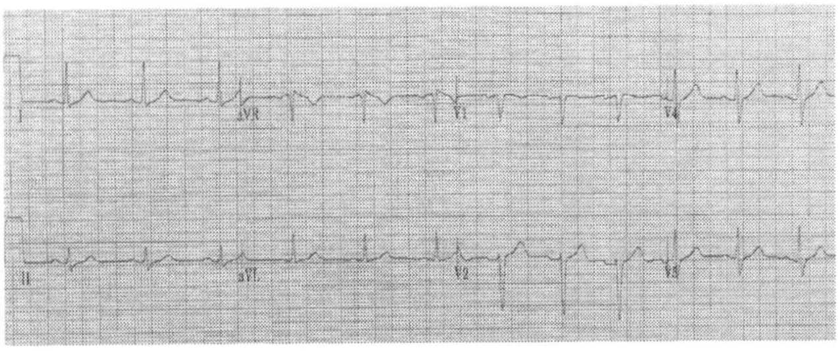

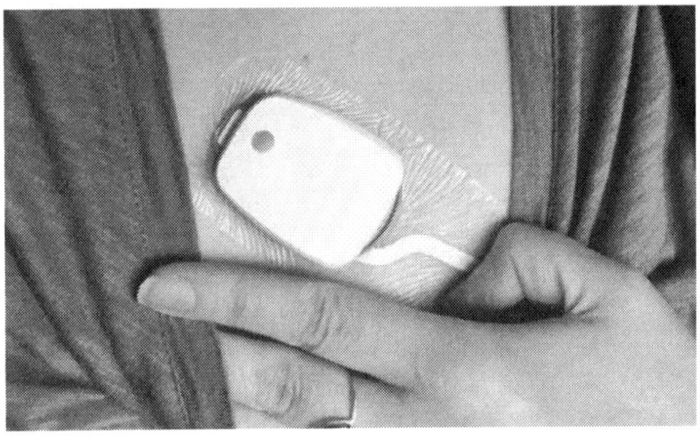

Occasionally, artifacts may appear on an ECG/EKG reading. **Artifacts** are **abnormalities** in the reading caused by **non-cardiac origins**. An **intentional artifact** may be caused by a **pacemaker**.

When an artifact appears on a rhythm strip during an ECG/EKG, it should be identified and attempts should be made to eliminate the artifact. Most commonly, an issue with a connection between the skin and the ECG/EKG pads. The skin should be shaved if hair is present. The skin should be rubbed with isopropyl alcohol, or soap and water to reduce the amount of oil or dirt on the skin. After cleaning and/or shaving the area, the skin should be rubbed and dried via gauze to ensure no liquid residue interferes with the ECG/EKG.

Heart rhythm using an ECG/EKG is visually displayed on **rhythm strips**. Rhythm strips show the heart rhythm as it beats over a **set time**, allowing interpretation of an entire set of heart beats. The rhythm strip details time and voltage produced by the heart. Rhythm strips are utilized to establish heart rhythms, view heart rhythms over time, and to identify any irregularities a person may have in their heart rhythm. These irregularities are known as arrhythmias. Arrhythmias may be caused by many different dysfunctions, such as atrial fibrillation causing the atria to contract at irregular times.

In some cases, a person may need to have heart activity recorded over 24-48 hours. In these cases, a **Holter Monitor** is used. These are **portable machines** that remain attached to a patient, continuously recording heart activity. These can be used if a person has irregular heart rhythms that come and go, and aren't present during an initial ECG/EKG reading.

Cardiac stress test may be administered to measure the function of the heart during physical activity. During this exam, the patient has an EKG attached to their body, and they perform some form of **exercise**. This causes the heart to increase in rate and force, which the EKG can measure to detect any abnormalities.

Atrial Fibrillation

Atrial fibrillation results from the atria receiving signals that occur at irregular times, causing the atria to beat rapidly and unsynchronized. This results in the walls of the heart quivering, also called fibrillating.

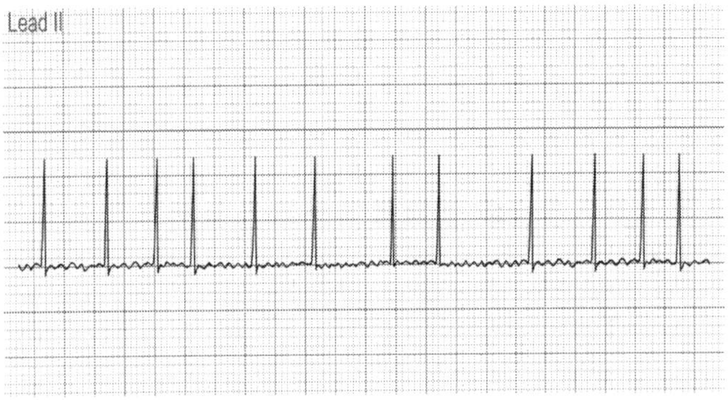

Atrial Flutter

During atrial flutter, the heart's atria beat too quickly. The rhythm of the beats is constant, but the beating of the atria is too rapid. The contractions of the atria can increase to over 240 beats per minute. Blood is able to pool in the atria due to incomplete filling of the atria before a contraction, which may lead to the development of clots.

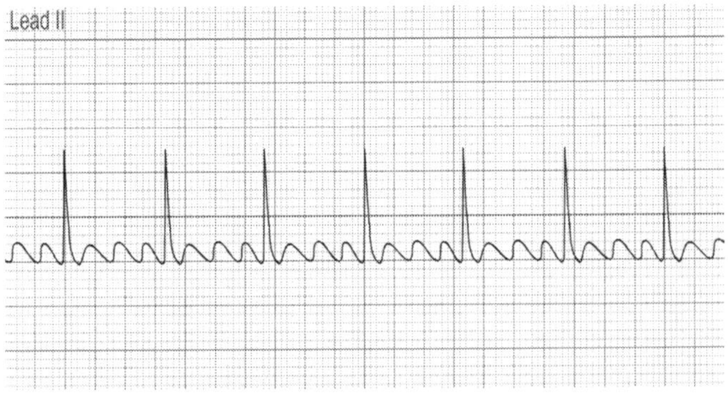

Bigeminy PVC

Bigeminy premature ventricular contractions occur due to factors such as medications, alcohol, and caffeine, and cause the ventricles to prematurely contract and feel like the heart skips a beat. This occurs every other beat, as opposed to trigeminy PVC, which occurs every third beat.

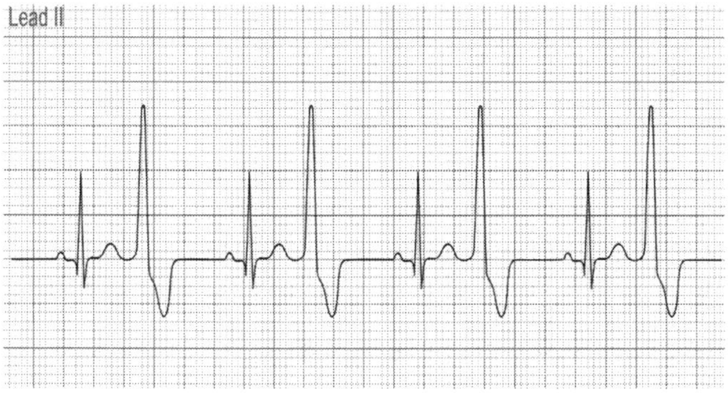

Cardiac Asystole

Cardiac asystole results from the heart stopping beating. Without medical intervention such as cardiopulmonary resuscitation or the use of an AED, cardiac asystole results in death.

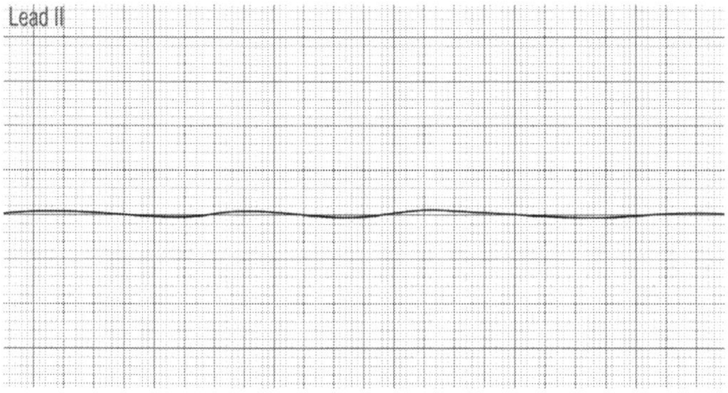

Complete Heart Block

Also known as a third-degree AV block, can be caused by damage to the AV node, resulting in signals from the AV node not passing from the atria to the ventricles. A pacemaker or implantable cardioverter defibrillator is used to control heart rhythm of a person with a complete heart block.

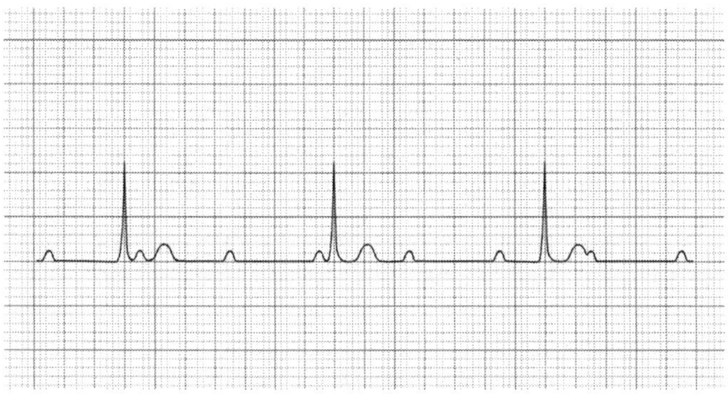

Couplet PVC

A couplet premature ventricular contraction is when the premature ventricular contraction occurs twice in a row. This is commonly found with use of alcohol and certain medications.

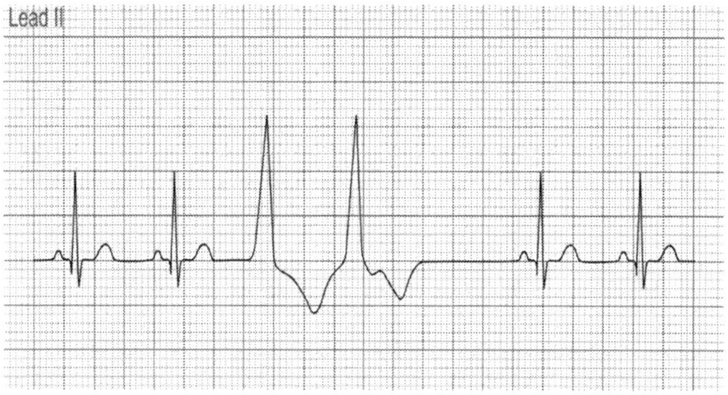

First-degree AV Block

First-degree AV block occurs when there is a slowing of the electrical signal through an AV node. The impulse still makes its way to the atria and ventricle, it just takes longer than usual to do so.

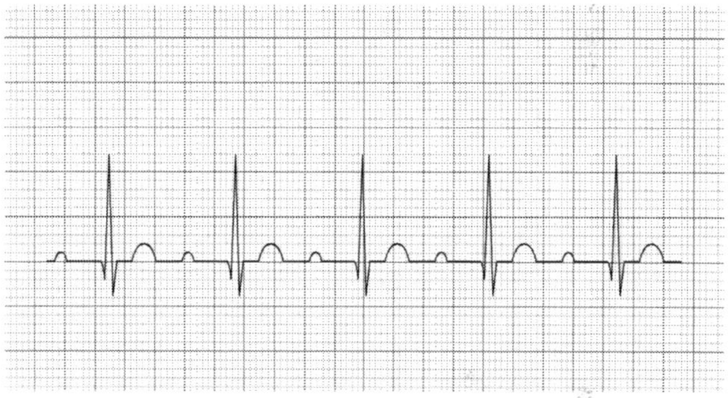

Premature Atrial Contraction(PAC)

Premature atrial contraction results from an impulse telling the atria to contract early. This results in the atria contracting when there may not be sufficient blood in the chamber.

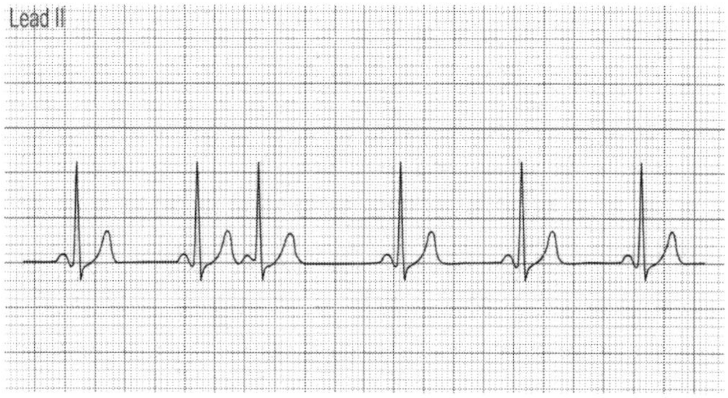

Premature Ventricular Contraction(PVC)

Premature ventricular contraction is similar to premature atrial contraction, resulting from an impulse telling the ventricle to contract early. This results in the ventricles contracting when there may not be sufficient blood in the chamber. When this occurs in the left ventricle, it may result in the body not receiving adequate oxygen in each wave of blood flow. Premature ventricular contraction can cause the heart to feel as if it is skipping a beat or fluttering.

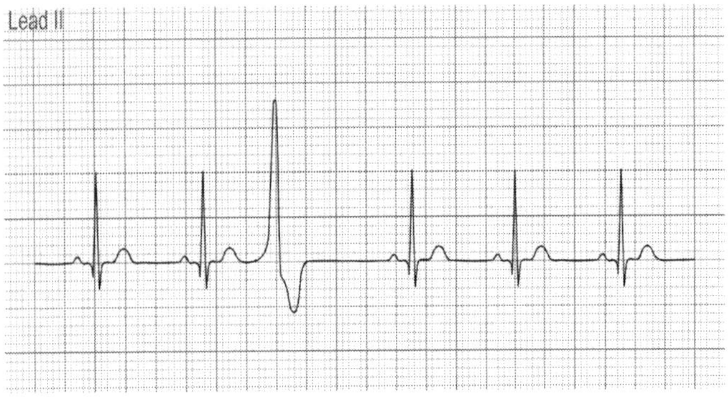

Second-degree AV Block

Second-degree AV block is similar to a first-degree AV block in that the electrical impulse from the AV node is slowed, but with a second-degree AV block, the impulse may not reach the ventricle.

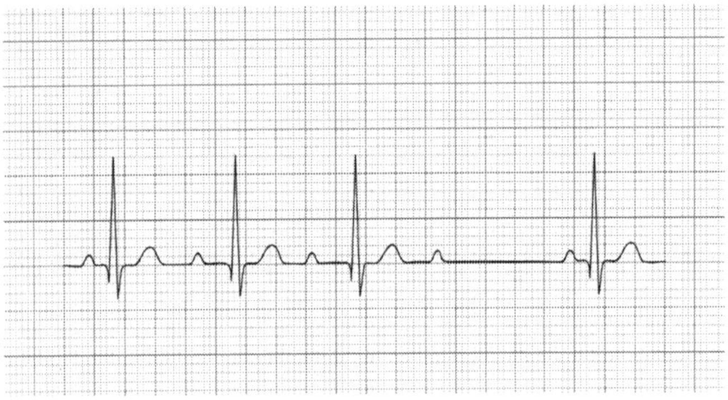

Sinus Arrest

Sinus arrest is cessation of activity in the sinus node that typically only lasts for a short time. Symptoms a person may experience include chest pain, dizziness, fatigue, and shortness of breath. Causes of sinus arrest include hyperkalemia, sleep apnea, certain medications, and SA node disorders.

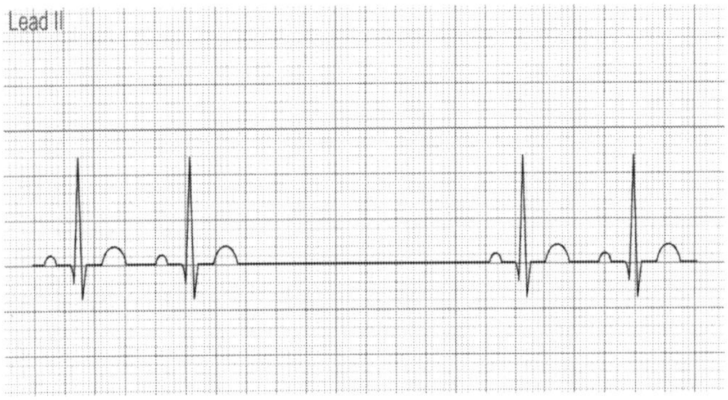

Sinus Bradycardia

Sinus bradycardia is marked by a slowed heart rhythm, resulting from the SA node sending signals at a rate much slower than usual, typically 60 beats per minute or lower.

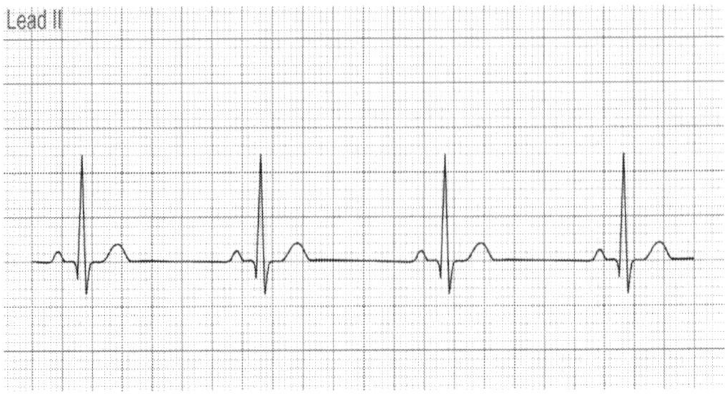

Sinus Tachycardia

Sinus tachycardia is marked by rapid heart rhythm, resulting from the SA nodes sending signals at a rate much faster than usual, typically 100 beats per minute or above.

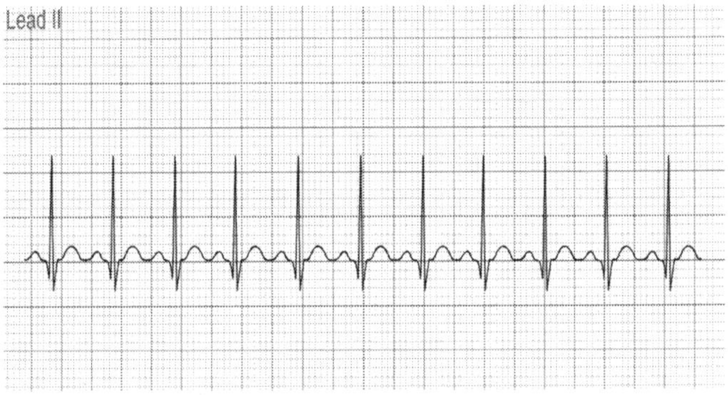

ST Depression

ST depression, typically resulting from ischemia in the heart, is marked by an ST segment that is unusually low in relation to the baseline in an EKG.

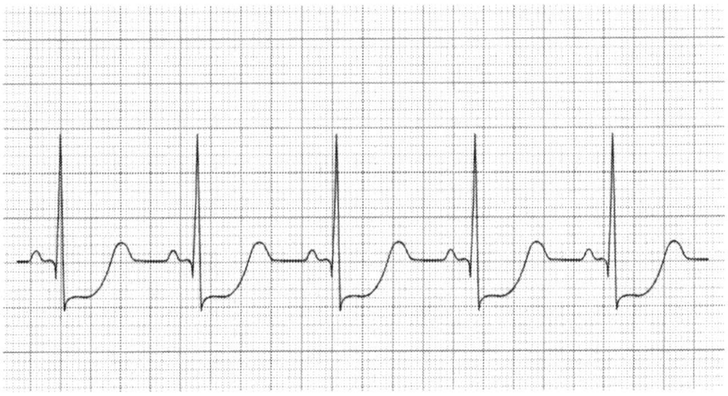

ST Elevation Myocardial Infarction

ST elevation myocardial infarction(STEMI) results from ischemia in the heart, resulting in myocardial infarction. In an EKG, this is marked by an ST-segment that is elevated. An ST-segment typically has no electrical activity. An ST elevation indicates that part of the heart muscle, typically the ventricle, is dying.

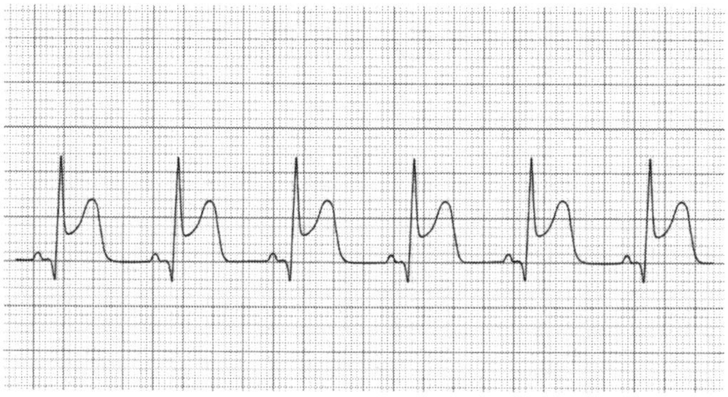

Supraventricular Tachycardia(SVT)

Supraventricular tachycardia results from the atria contracting at an abnormally rapid rate. This can cause the heart to beat over 100 times per minute. This causes a person to potentially experience a fluttering sensation in the chest, fatigue, chest pain, and shortness of breath.

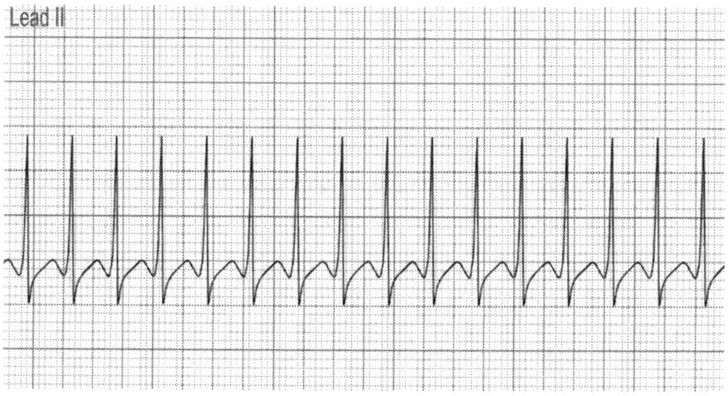

Trigeminy PVC

Trigeminy premature ventricular contractions occur due to factors such as medications, alcohol, and caffeine, and cause the ventricles to prematurely contract and feel like the heart skips a beat. This occurs every third beat, as opposed to bigeminy PVC, which occurs every other beat.

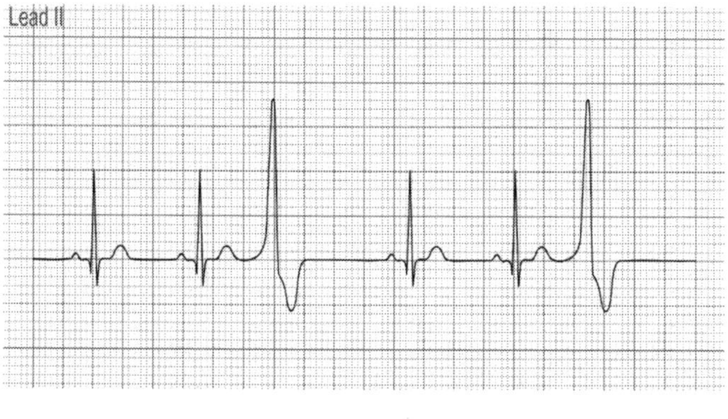

Ventricular Fibrillation

Ventricular fibrillation results from impulses being sent to the ventricles at abnormal times, causing the ventricles to twitch and be unable to contract normally. Ventricular fibrillation is a medical emergency, because the ventricles are unable to sufficiently pump oxygen-rich blood to the body. The most common cause of cardiac arrest is ventricular fibrillation. Unconsciousness commonly occurs, and a person may require cardiopulmonary resuscitation or an AED for emergency treatment. If treatment is successful, devices such as pacemakers may be implanted to help regulate the heart rhythm and prevent future episodes.

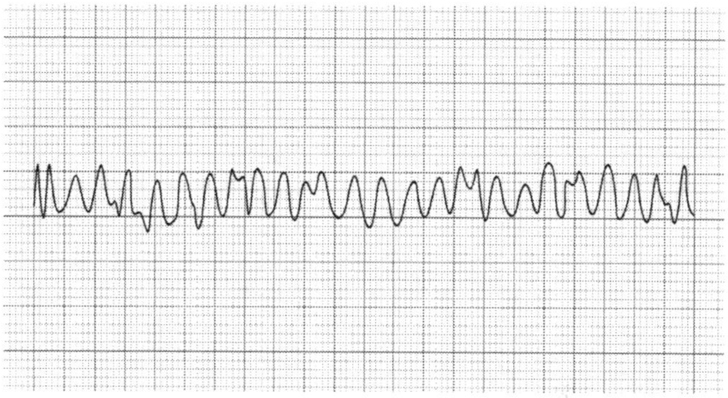

Ventricular Tachycardia

Ventricular tachycardia is when there are three premature ventricular contractions in a row. This causes the heart to beat rapidly. Due to the rapid beating, the ventricles may not effectively fill with oxygen-rich blood. Therefore, a person may not receive adequate oxygen with each pump of blood. A person may feel lightheaded or lose consciousness as a result.

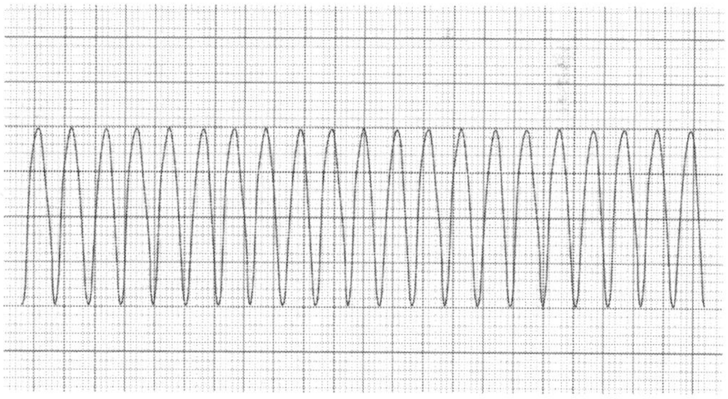

Vision Testing

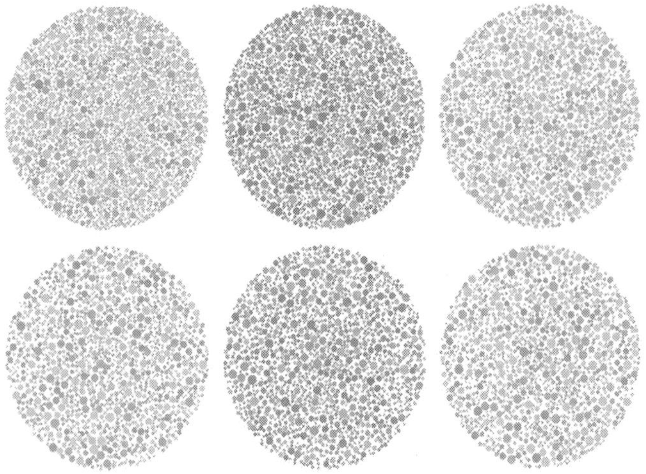

Color blindness is most commonly tested using the **Ishihara test**. Developed by Dr Shinobu Ishihara in 1917, the test consists of **plates with dotted patterns** on them. The patterns are colored in such a way that a person who is color blind may not be able to see the patterns on the plates. These patterns may be abstract, or may be numbers. People who are not colorblind will see the designs. Some plates are designed where only people who are colorblind can see the pattern. Other plates contain multiple designs, with one design being visible by people who are not color blind, and another design being visible by people who are color blind.

Visual Acuity

Visual acuity tests are used to determine the **sharpness** of a person's vision. Visual acuity is measured by using eye charts, read at a specific distance. This determines how sharp a person is able to see with an object that is further away, or how sharp a person can see with an object closer to the eyes.

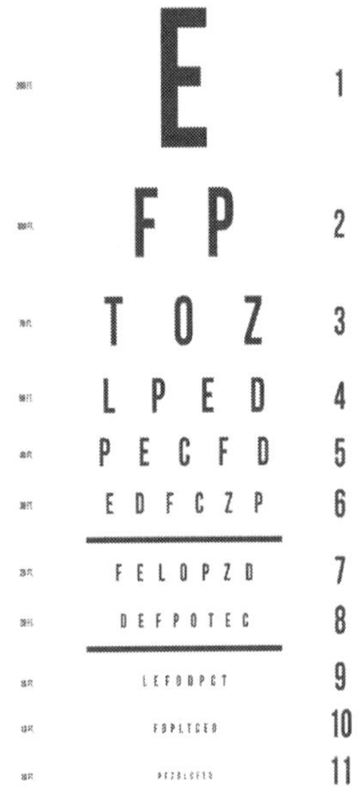

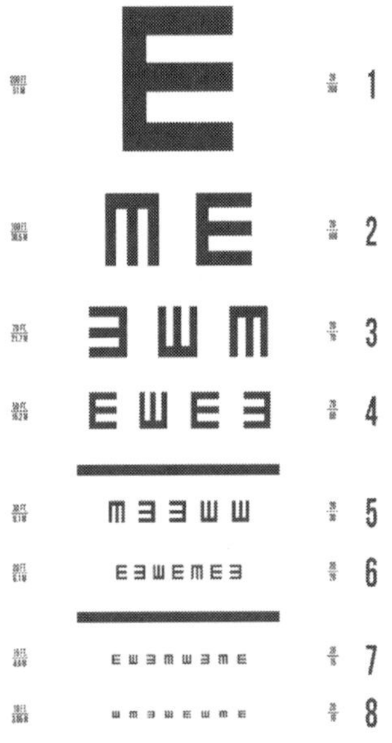

Herman Snellen, a Dutch ophthalmologist, developed the **Snellen chart** in 1862. On the original chart, which has since been improved upon and is known as a **LogMAR chart**, letters and numbers are placed on a 5x5 grid, with the top line being the largest size, and the bottom line being the smallest. The distance the person is asked to read the chart is typically 20 feet away.

For people who do not know or understand the Latin alphabet, an **E chart** may be utilized. This chart, which is similar in design to the Snellen chart, only contains the **letter E**. The E is **randomly rotated**, with the limbs of the E pointing to the right, left, up, or down. This allows people to demonstrate which direction the limbs are pointing, which shows acuity.

A **Jaeger chart** is a chart held by the patient, consisting of **paragraphs of text** written in **different sizes**. The smallest text a person can read on a Jaeger chart helps determine the person's visual acuity.

Ocular Pressure/Tonometry

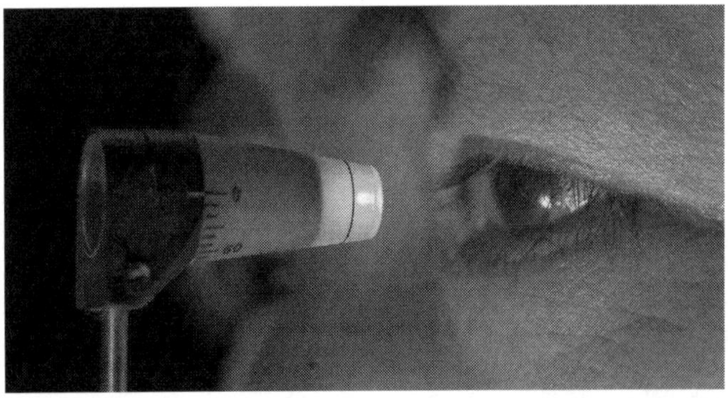

Ocular pressure is measured to help determine if a patient is at risk for the development of **glaucoma**. The preferred method of measuring ocular pressure is with the use of a **tonometer**. During this measurement, the eye is numbed with special eye drops. Once the eye is numb, a tonometer is used to gently press against the cornea. This allows a measurement of the amount of resistance from the cornea. Another measurement may be taken by blowing air onto the eyeball for a short period of time. This also determines the amount of pressure pushing back on the air.

Visual Fields

Visual field tests are used to determine a person's entire **field of view**, or how much they can actually see. These tests help diagnose vision loss based on how much a person can see in their **peripheral vision** while focusing on one specific object or point in front of them. This is often performed by the patient covering one eye, and the medical professional holding up fingers in the patient's peripheral area, then asking how many fingers are visible.

Audiometric Testing

Hearing tests are performed to ensure the ears and hearing are functioning optimally. If hearing loss occurs, a person may be given hearing aids to assist in picking up audio.

Pure tone audiometry is a type of test given to determine the hearing threshold of a person that helps develop a diagnosis for hearing loss. This diagnosis can include the degree of hearing loss and the type of hearing loss. It is usually performed by placing headphones on that will play a high pitched beep on one side at a time. This is used to determine the quietest sound a person is able to hear.

Speech and word recognition may be used to assess the ability of a person to hear. This is done by the patient wearing **headphones**, with the audiologist saying words through the headphones. The patient will then repeat the word spoken by the audiologist. This also helps determine the quietest sound a person can hear, and is similar to pure tone audiometry in this regard.

Speech recognition threshold(SRT) is the minimum level of hearing required for a patient to recognize **50% of speech.** This test is commonly utilized to assess the lowest decibel level a patient can identify speech at, which is useful in establishing settings for hearing aids.

Speech detection threshold(SDT) is utilized to test if a patient can detect the **presence of speech 50% of the time**. The patient only needs to **acknowledge hearing sound**, and does not need to be able to understand what is being spoken.

Tympanometry is used to measure the **mobility of the tympanic membrane**, which can help determine if there is hearing loss in conjunction with pure tone audiometry. Tympanometry is performed by first examining the tympanic membrane with an **otoscope**. Then, a **probe tipped with flexible rubber** is placed into the ear, which changes **air pressure** in the ear. This change in pressure should produce a low-pitched tone in the ear, similar to changes felt and heard when changing altitude.

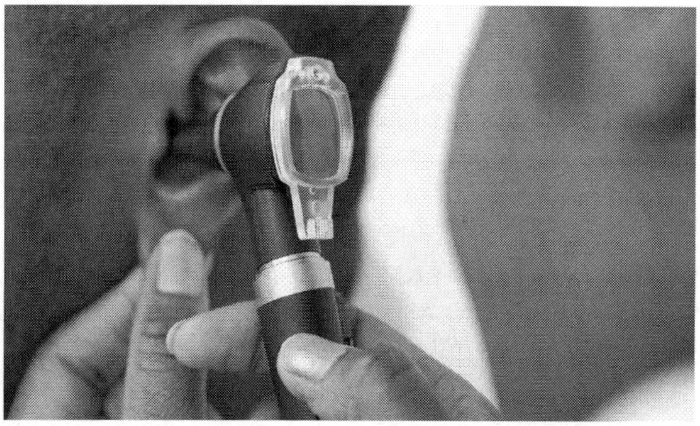

Allergy Testing

If a person is suspected of having an allergy to a substance, an allergy test may be administered to determine the exact allergen. This can help determine how the body reacts to the allergen and what the specific allergen is. This helps establish a treatment plan, and whether exposure to the allergen is manageable or not. Allergy testing can be done to help determine many different conditions, including asthma, dermatitis, food allergies, bee allergies, and hay fever.

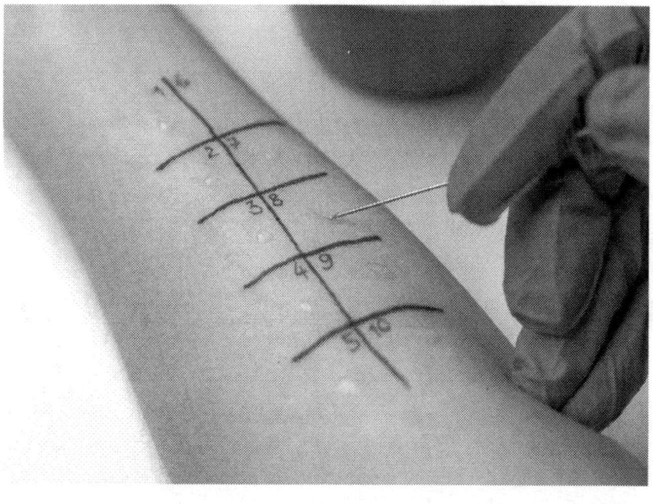

Scratch testing, also known as **skin prick testing**, is used to check for **rapid development of allergies** with specific substances. A mark is made on the skin, and the substance is placed on the skin in liquid form using a dropper next to the mark. The skin is then slightly punctured where the allergen is located, which introduces it into the body.

After about 15 minutes, the area is observed to determine any allergic reactions. Typically, other substances are also tested at the same time to determine in the skin is reacting normally to other substances that aren't suspected to be allergens.

Intradermal skin testing is performed by **injecting the allergen** into the dermis. Intradermal skin testing is primarily performed to check for allergies related to **penicillin** or **insect venom**. The site of injection is observed for around 15 minutes, after which the allergic reaction should be visible in the skin.

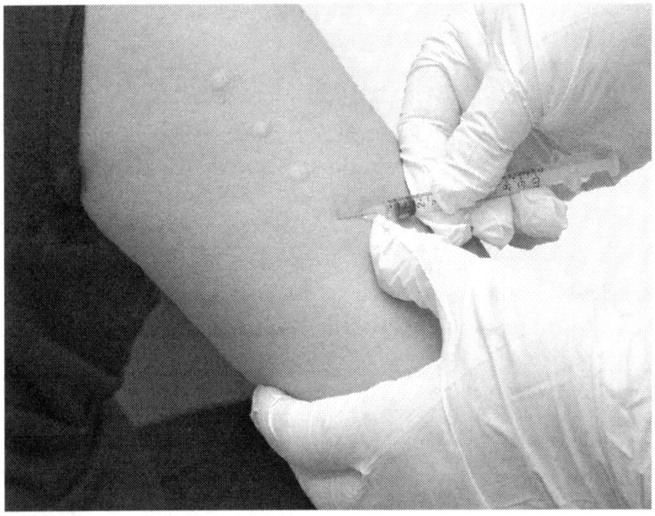

Patch testing is used to test for allergic reactions that may have **delayed responses**. In a patch test, allergens are placed onto **patches**, and these patches are placed directly **on the skin**. The most common location for these patches is on the back. The patches are kept on the skin for up to 48 hours. After the patches are removed, the skin is examined. If there is any area that appears irritated or inflamed, it may indicate an allergy of some sort.

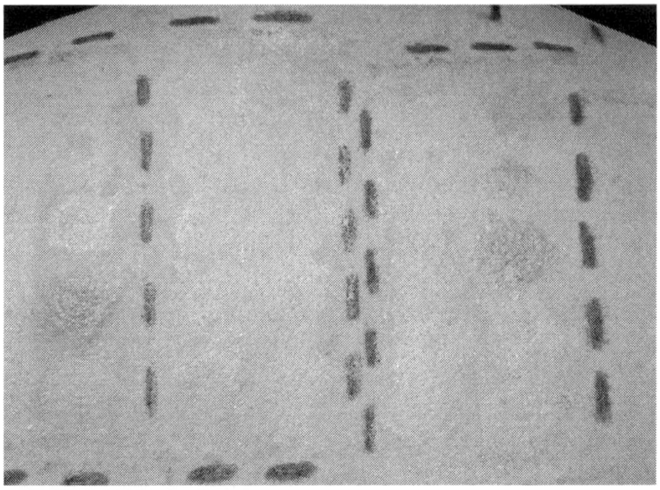

When a person experiences an allergic reaction in the body, the body releases immunoglobin E antibodies, also known as IgE. **Radioallergosorbent tests**, also called **RAST**, are performed by **collecting blood** and measuring the concentration of **IgE antibodies** in the blood. Allergens that are tested using RAST include food, medications, mold, and dust. When reading RAST outcomes, the lower the number given, the less likely it is that the person will experience an allergic reaction to a substance.

Respiratory Testing

Pulmonary function tests(PFTs) are used to determine the rate of **breathing, gas exchange, and lung volume**. This can show if there is some sort of obstruction of air flow, or if there is a restriction in the flow of air. **Obstructive air flow** includes medical conditions such as asthma, bronchitis, and emphysema. **Restrictive air flow** includes medical conditions such as scoliosis and obesity, which can restrict the functioning of the lungs by reducing the amount of expansion the lungs may produce upon inhalation.

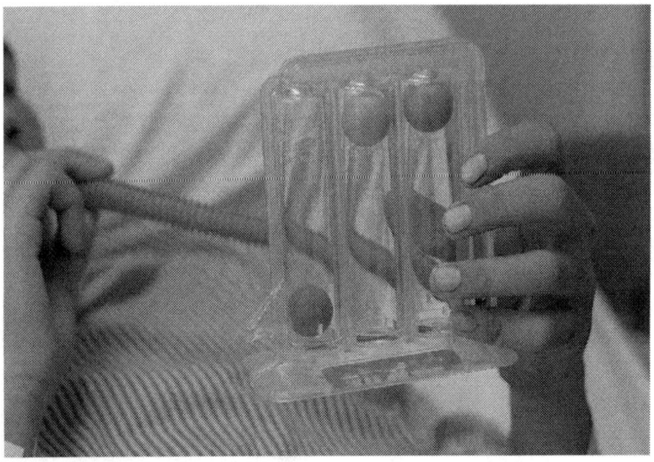

Spirometry is used to measure the amount of air being **inhaled**, the amount of air being **exhaled**, and **how quickly** the air is moved out of the lungs. This is performed by the patient breathing into a tube attached to a machine known as a **spirometer**. A clip is usually placed on the nostrils to prevent air flow from occurring through the nose. A baseline is taken for normal breathing, then the patient will inhale quickly and deeply, then exhale as long as they can. This is performed three times to get an average of lung function, as one test may be compromised in some way, such as the seal around the tube not being as strong as it should be and air leaking out. Medication may be administered, and then the test may be repeated again after 15 minutes to determine if medication helps improve lung function.

Peak flow rate is the **maximum speed** a person is able to **exhale**. Peak flow rate is measured to help determine if a patient with a condition like asthma should utilize medication more frequently or not.

Diagnostic Imaging

Nuclear Imaging

Nuclear imaging is a form of radiology in which small amounts of radioactive substances, also known as **radionuclides**, are absorbed by specific organs. These substances, of which there are many, are administered most commonly by intravenous injection, but may also be administered orally. The radionuclide will give off radiation, and the organ that contains the substance is viewed using a gamma camera. This allows the function of organs, and the diagnosis of certain diseases, to be achieved. Diseases or conditions that can be viewed using nuclear imaging include infections, cysts, tumors, heart disease, kidney disease, thyroid disease, and enlarged organs.

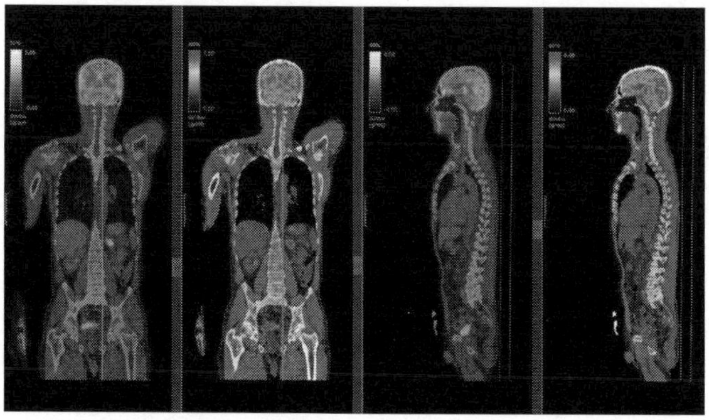

Computerized Axial Tomography

Computerized Axial Tomography, also known as CT or CAT Scan, is an imaging technique in which a **snapshot** is taken of a part of the body on a **given body plane**. This allows viewing of structures in the body from differing points of view. CT is extremely similar to MRI, but uses **X-ray** to produce images instead of magnetic fields.

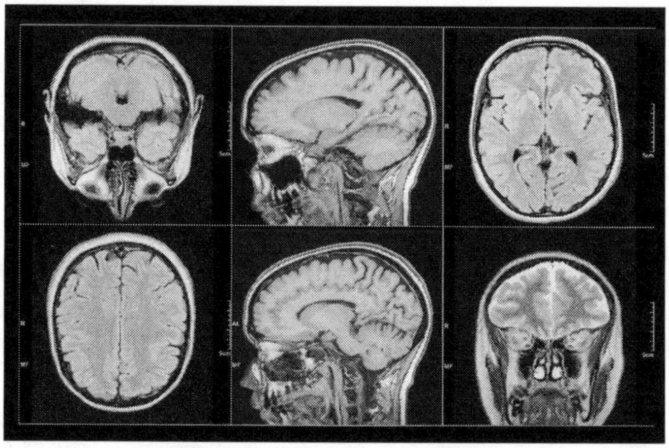

Magnetic Resonance Imaging

Magnetic Resonance Imaging is the use of **high powered magnetic fields** to help **produce images of structures and organs** inside the body. These images are typically much more detailed than X-rays, especially when viewing organs. MRI is used to help diagnose conditions such as tumors, issues with the Digestive System, and issues with the heart and blood vessels. The MRI machine is a large tube in which a person lies for an extended period of time, which allows a detailed image to be produced.

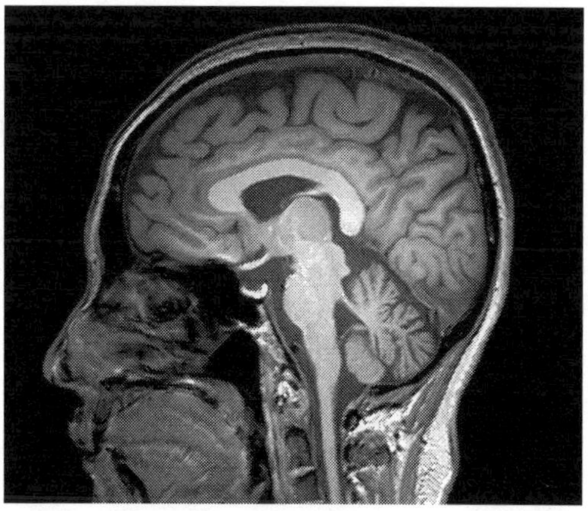

Ultrasound

An ultrasound, also known as **sonography**, is an imaging technique utilizing **sound waves** to produce pictures of structures inside the body. Commonly, ultrasound is used to view the development of a fetus during pregnancy, but may also be used to examine infections inside the body, liver and gallbladder function, and heart conditions. The part of the machine that is used to perform the scanning is known as the transducer.

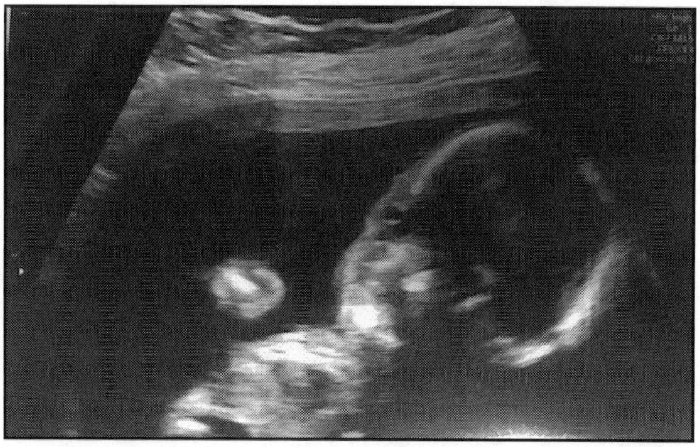

Diagnostic tests have normal ranges for healthy function that results are measured against. When diagnostic test results fall outside of these normal ranges, the results must be noted and reported. Abnormal testing results can have numerous effects on the patient's body, and in some cases, the person may be experiencing a severe medical crisis that should be treated immediately.

Procedures/Examinations Matching

______: Material used to create a cast

______: Most preferred type of urine collection for urinalysis

______: A wound that has not healed over the course of eight weeks or longer

______: Introducing a bacteria or fungus into a liquid

______: Percentage of blood that consists of red blood cells

______: The use of hands to physically move, adjust, or alter the location of a structure in the body

______: Device used to sterilize medical equipment utilizing steam and pressure to destroy microorganisms

______: Instruments used to grasp small objects

______: Form of swab performed if there is a suspected respiratory infection

______: Substance applied to the skin to sterilize the area before a surgical procedure is performed

______: Test performed when there is a suspected tuberculosis infection

______: Listening to internal body sounds produced by the heart, lungs, or other organs

______: The atria receiving signals that occur at irregular times, causing the atria to beat rapidly and unsynchronized

______: Medical dress item used to prevent fluids from entering the mouth and prevent airborne illnesses from infecting others

______: Device used to preserve a specimen, or to allow a specimen to grow

______: A double edged scalpel

______: Device used to immobilize the shoulder or wrist when an injury occurs in or around these joints

______: Test performed when systemic inflammation is suspected

______: Instruments used to hold tissues open during surgery

______: The heart ceasing function

A: Incubator
B: Cardiac asystole
C: Face masks
D: Forceps
E: Sling
F: Providone-iodine
G: Nasopharyngeal swab
H: CRP test
I: Manipulation
J: Atrial fibrillation
K: Retractors
L: Chronic/non-healing wound
M: Lancet
N: Hematocrit
O: Fiberglass
P: Autoclave
Q: Inoculation
R: Auscultation
S: Midstream/clean catch
T: Mantoux tuberculin skin test

Answer Key on Page 292

Procedures/Examinations Crossword

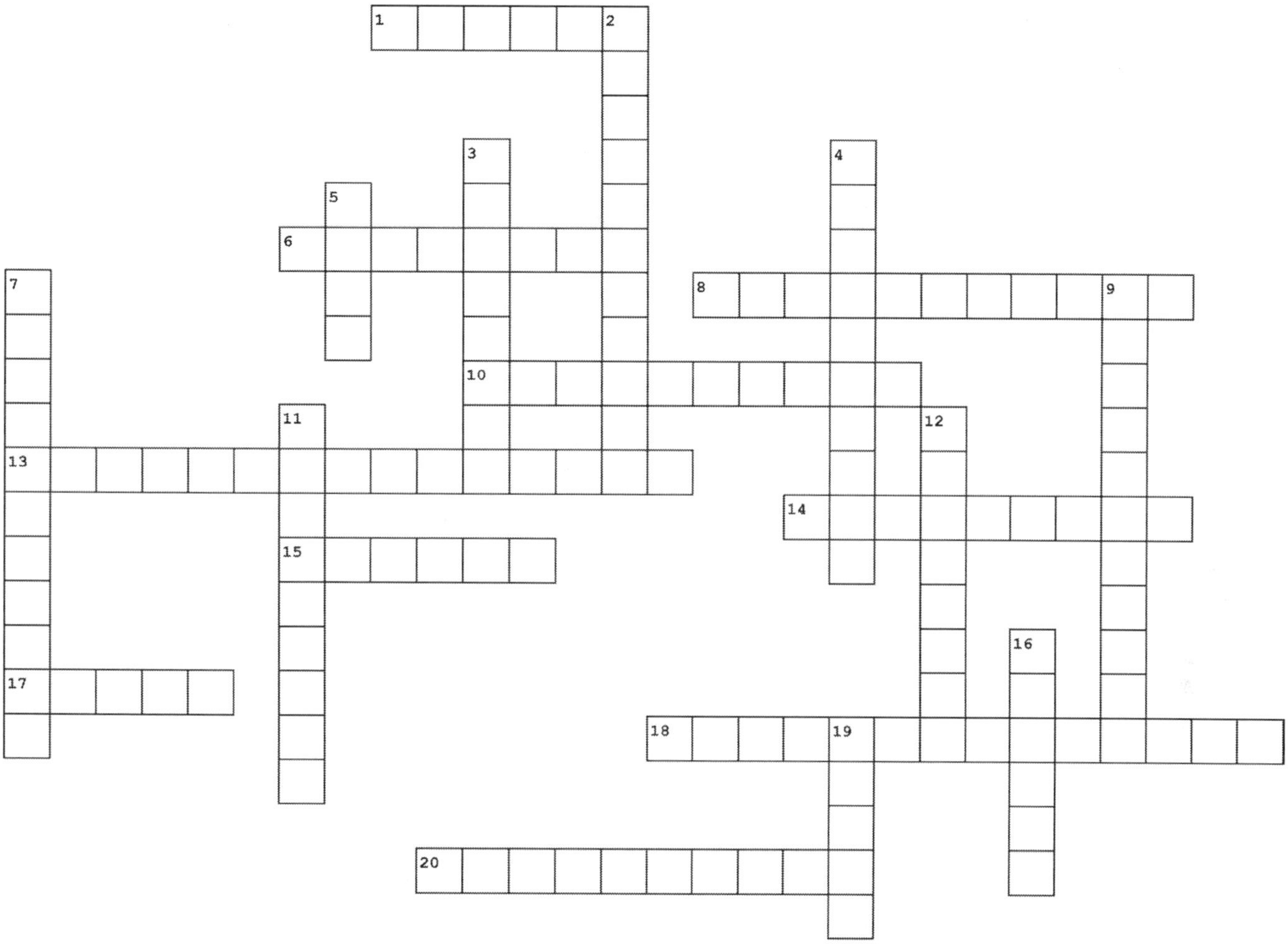

Across

1. Form of urine collection that may be performed at any time
6. Small tube inserted into a part of the body to help fluid drain
8. The use of ice or cold in a treatment to reduce inflammation
10. Substance a microorganism is mixed with in a collecting tube during inoculation
13. Position in which a patient lies flat on the back with the legs and feet separated, used for pelvic examinations
14. The use of touch to assess or examine an area or structure
15. Position in which a person lies face up on a table
17. Doctor who specializes in women's reproductive health
18. Exam performed to check the health of a mother after delivery
20. Tapping on areas of the body to examine the presence of fluid in an area

Down

2. Measuring certain structures or areas of the body
3. Instrument used to open the walls of a cavity such as the nasal cavity or vagina
4. Swab performed if there is a suspected bacterial infection such as tonsillitis or strep throat
5. Used to stabilize a bone after fracture to allow healing to occur
7. Method used in surgical prep in which hands and arms are continuously scrubbed for three to five minutes
9. Instrument used to examine the anus, rectum and sigmoid colon
11. Items used on wounds, such as gauze, foam, or hydrogel, to prevent introduction of microorganisms
12. Swiping the cervix to test cervical cells for potential cervical cancer
16. Phlegm in the lungs
19. Position in which a person lies face down on a table

Answer Key on Page 293

Procedures/Examinations Practice Test

1. During venipuncture, which of the following is applied to fill the vein with blood, making venipuncture easier to perform
A. 70% isopropyl alcohol
B. Tourniquet
C. Sterile gauze
D. Providone-iodine

2. Form of arrhythmia caused by damage to an AV node, resulting in signals from the AV node not passing from the atria to the ventricles
A. Complete heart block
B. Ventricular tachycardia
C. Sinus bradycardia
D. Cardiac asystole

3. Albumin to Creatinine Ratio and Glomerular Filtration Rate are both tests used to measure the function of
A. Stomach
B. Liver
C. Pancreas
D. Kidneys

4. A QRS Complex represents which of the following
A. Depolarization of the right ventricle and left ventricle
B. Conduction of an electrical impulse from the bundle of His through the ventricles
C. Repolarization of the right ventricle and left ventricle
D. Contraction of the atria due to firing of the SA node

5. Which of the following describes Sims' body position
A. The patient lies prone on the table with the knees and chest coming into contact with the table, and the abdomen and hips raised off the table
B. The patient lies supine on the table with the legs and feet placed into stirrups that separate them
C. The patient is seated with the seat back set at an angle of 45-60 degrees
D. The patient lies on their left side with the left lower limb straightened and the right hip and knee flexed

6. Evacuated collection tubes have different colored rubber stoppers at the top which indicate
A. How much blood is to be contained in each tube
B. The time required to preserve the blood in a refrigerator
C. What additive is inside each tube
D. If the blood is from an artery or a vein

7. Nasopharyngeal swabs may be used to determine if a patient is suffering from
A. Tonsillitis
B. Strep throat
C. Sinusitis
D. Influenza

8. Introducing a bacteria or fungus into a liquid is known as
A. Indigestion
B. Incubation
C. Inoculation
D. Immunization

9. Which of the following visualizes the time it takes for a nerve impulse to travel from the SA node through the atria into the ventricles
A. PR Interval
B. P Wave
C. ST segment
D. QRS Complex

10. Hemoglobin A1c is a test designed for what purpose
A. Determine the ability for the blood to properly clot
B. Determine if the kidneys are properly filtering waste from the blood
C. Determine an average range of blood sugar over the past three months
D. Determine lipid concentration in the blood

Answer Key on Page 295

Anatomy and Physiology

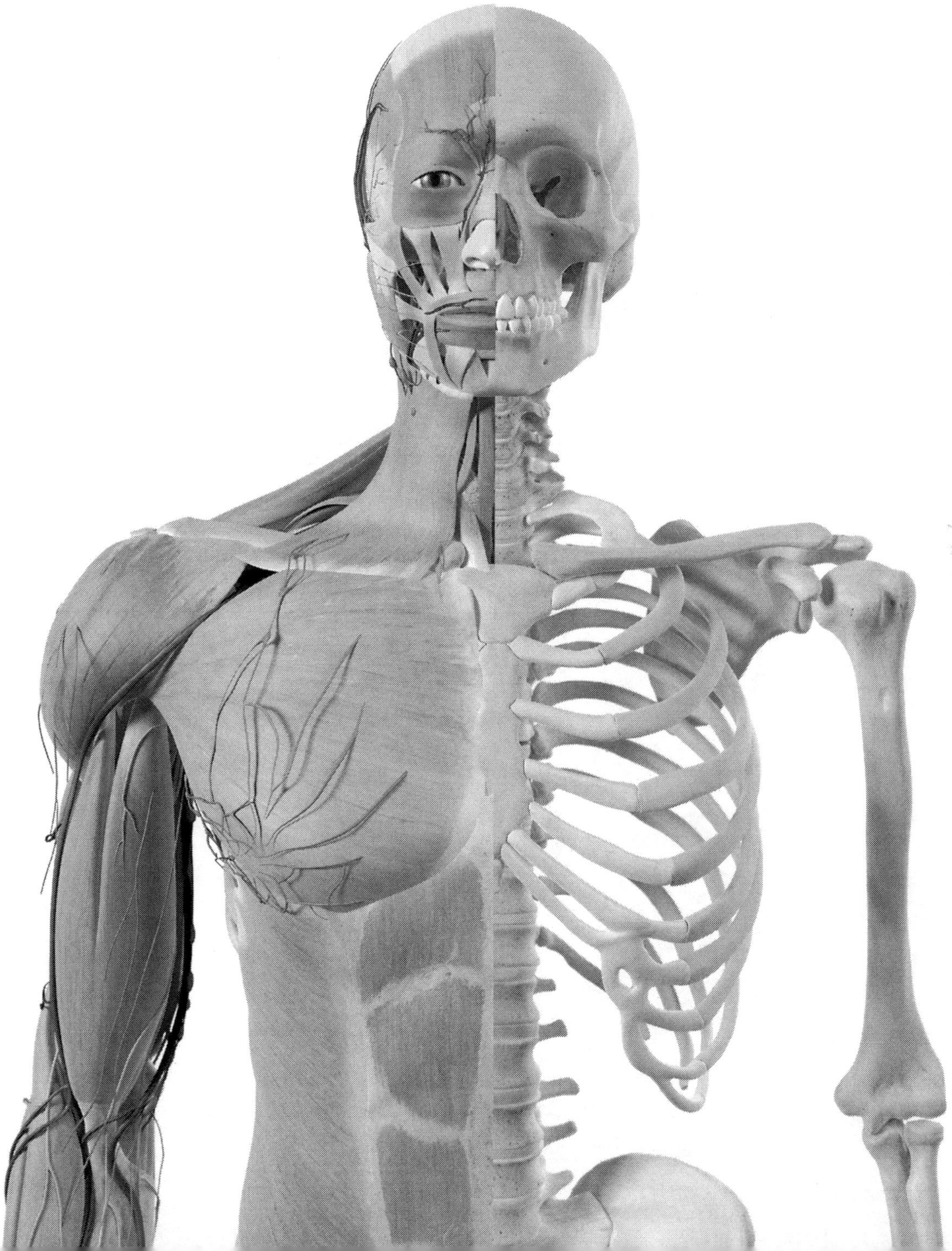

Anatomy and Physiology

Anatomy is the study of the **structure** of the human body. All of the parts that make up the body constitute anatomy, from bones, muscles, and nerves, to cells, tendons, ligaments, and everything in between.

Physiology is the study of the **function** of the body. How do the parts of the body that make up the body's anatomy function? What do they do? This is physiology. Anatomy and physiology go hand-in-hand.

Homeostasis

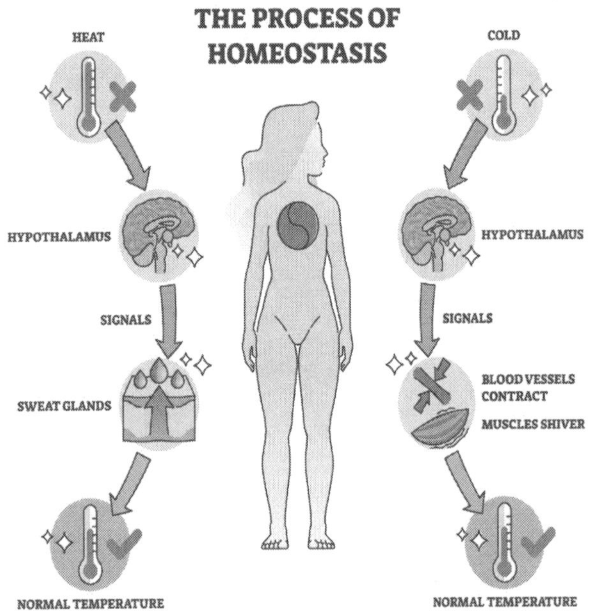

Homeostasis is the existence and maintenance of a **constant internal environment**. The body's internal environment is constantly changing and responding to various stimuli. Examples of stimuli are temperature, hormones, diet, and the body's pH level. These stimuli that change the body's internal environment in some way are known as **homeostatic variables.** As the variables change, so too does the internal environment.

The body responds to these changes by utilizing **homeostatic mechanisms**, such as sweating and shivering. An example, when body temperature gets too high, the body mechanically (physically) responds by sweating. Sweat evaporates off the skin, which cools the body down, lowering body temperature. When the body becomes too cold, the body responds by mechanically increasing the amount of twitching in the skeletal muscles. This increased twitching, which is normally undetectable, results in shivering, which produces body heat and raising body temperature.

The body's internal environment is constantly changing, and the body constantly adjusts certain aspects of itself to respond to these changes. If temperature is an example, the **set point**(normal range) of a body's temperature is 98.6 degrees Fahrenheit. The internal body temperature is never set right at 98.6 degrees. It is constantly fluctuating around it, maintaining a normal range of optimal body function.

Regional Anatomy

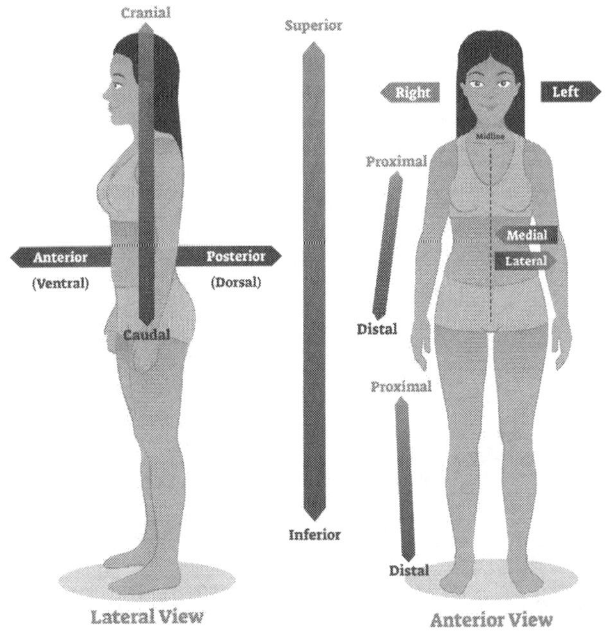

Regional Anatomy is the study of the structures of the body, broken down into different parts. When describing the position of one structure in the body in relation to another structure or structures, we use **directional terms**. An example, using the term "medial condyle" instead of just "condyle" lets us communicate effectively which condyle is being discussed.

The main directional terms are:

- **Superior**: Above.
- **Inferior**: Below.
- **Anterior**: Front.
- **Posterior**: Back.
- **Proximal**: Closer to the midline.
- **Distal**: Further from the midline.
- **Medial**: Middle.
- **Lateral**: Side.
- **Deep**: More internal.
- **Superficial**: Towards the surface.

Body Planes

Body planes are important for viewing structures from different aspects. These can be used when doing simple visual assessment, or in instances such as surgery or cadaver dissection.

There are four main body planes: A **midsagittal**, or **median plane**, runs down the **midline of the body**, splitting the body into **equal left and right sides.** This is the only location for a midsagittal plane.

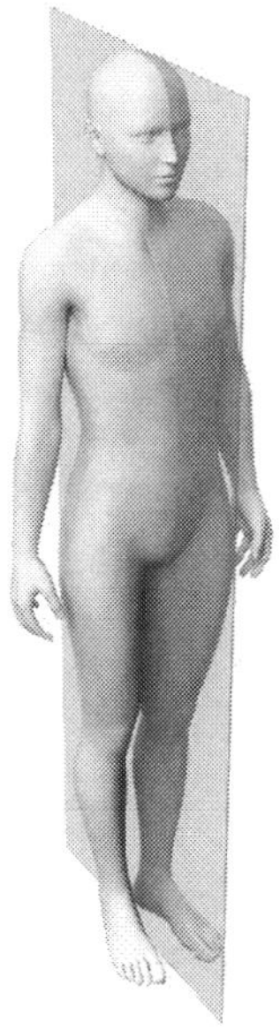

A **sagittal plane** also splits the body into left or right sides, but **not equally**. It can be located anywhere along the body except down the midline. Pictured is a **midsagittal plane**, splitting the body into equal left and right sides.

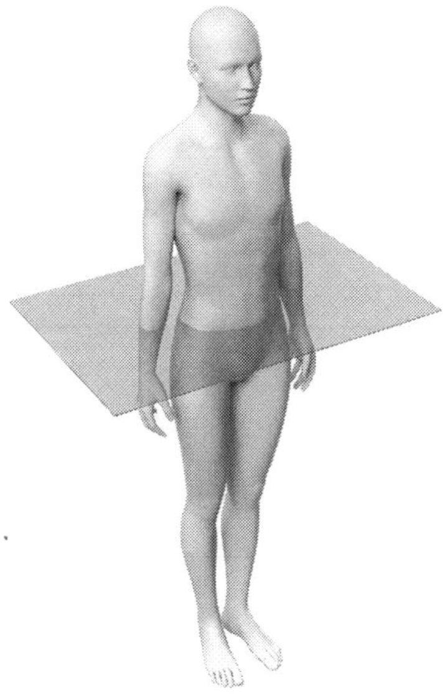

A **transverse**, or **horizontal plane**, splits the body into **superior and inferior** portions. It does not have to be at the waist. It can split the body into superior and inferior at any point along the body.

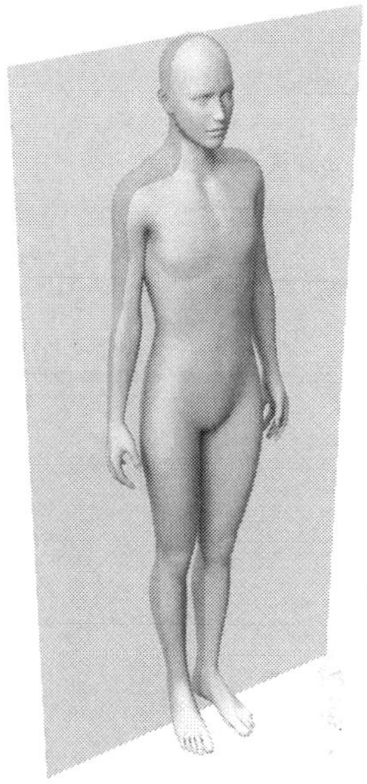

A **frontal**, or **coronal plane**, splits the body into **anterior and posterior**. If a person wanted to dissect the heart and make all four chambers visible, they would cut the heart into a frontal or coronal plane. See photo on page 97.

Body Regions

The body can be broken down into different parts, or regions. There are three main body regions: the central body region, the upper limb, and the lower limb.

The **central body region** contains all of the structures located in the **center of the body**: the **head**, the **neck**, and the **trunk**. Take away the arms and legs, and you're left with the central body region.

The **trunk** can be further divided into three regions: the **thorax**, or **chest**, the **abdomen**, and the **pelvis**. The thorax contains the heart, lungs, esophagus, thymus, and major blood vessels connecting to the heart. The abdomen contains the majority of our digestive organs, including the stomach, liver, gallbladder, pancreas, small intestine, and large intestine. It also contains the kidneys and ureters. The pelvis contains the urinary bladder, urethra, and reproductive organs.

The **upper limb** can be broken down into four regions: the **arm**, **forearm**, **wrist**, and **hand**. The arm contains the humerus. The forearm contains the radius and ulna. The wrist contains the carpals. The hand contains the metacarpals and phalanges.

The **lower limb** can also be broken down into four regions: the **thigh**, **leg**, **ankle**, and **foot**. The thigh contains the femur. The leg contains the tibia and fibula. The ankle contains the tarsals. The foot contains the metatarsals and phalanges.

The abdomen specifically can be divided into **four quadrants**, or **nine regions**. Dividing the abdomen into these quadrants or regions helps pin-point exact locations a person may be experiencing pain or discomfort, or identify what structures are in a given area.

The four quadrants are the upper right, upper left, lower right, and lower left.

The **upper right quadrant** contains the liver, gallbladder, pancreas, right kidney, small intestine, and large intestine.

The **upper left quadrant** contains the stomach, spleen, pancreas, left kidney, small intestine, and large intestine.

The **lower right quadrant** contains the small intestine, large intestine, uterus, ovary, and urinary bladder.

The **lower left quadrant** contains the small intestine, large intestine, uterus, ovary, and urinary bladder.

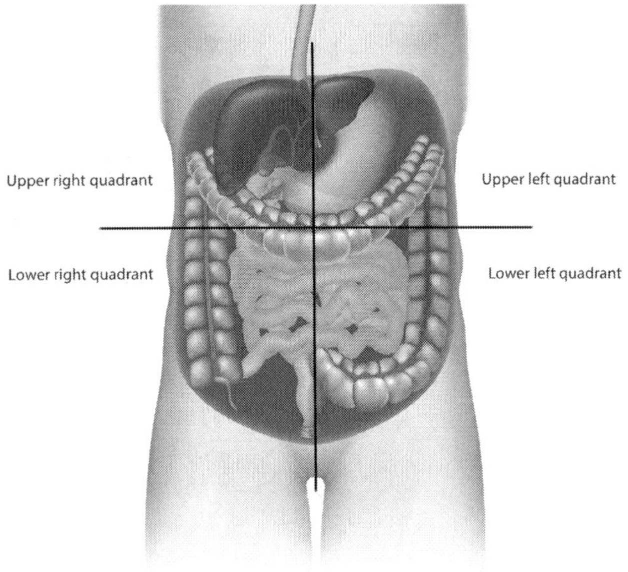

The nine regions of the abdomen are the **right hypochondriac, epigastric, left hypochondriac, right lumbar, umbilical, left lumbar, right iliac, hypogastric, and left iliac.** These regions are smaller than the quadrants and allow very specific locations to be utilized.

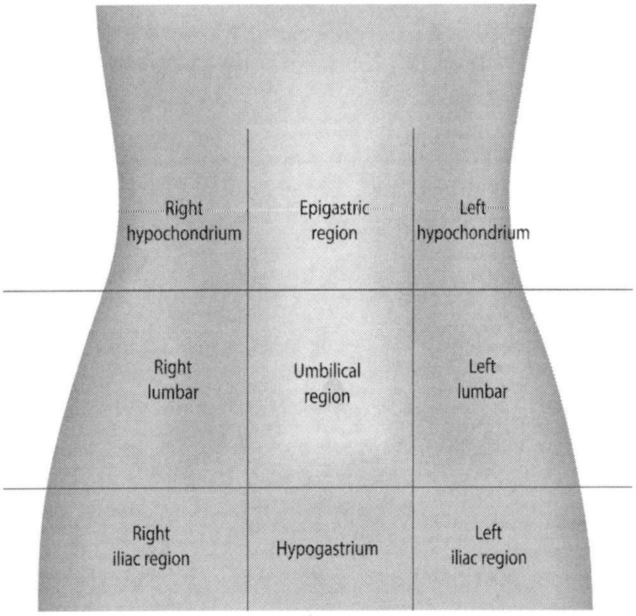

Body Cavities

The **dorsal body cavity** is created by the **cranium and the vertebral column.** Its responsibility is to **protect the brain** via the bones of the cranium(frontal, parietal, temporal, occipital), and to **protect the spinal cord** via the vertebrae. The spinal cord passes through the spinal canal, a passageway created by the vertebral column. The brain and spinal cord are vital in body function, and are thus protected by bones to maximize their safety.

The **ventral body cavity** is divided into two separate cavities, the **thoracic cavity** and the **abdominopelvic cavity.** The thoracic cavity holds three more cavities inside of it, the pleural cavity, the mediastinum, and the pericardial cavity. The **pleural cavity** contains the **lungs.** The **mediastinum** is the area located **between the lungs** that contains major blood vessels such as the aorta and superior vena cava, the pulmonary arteries, the trachea, and the esophagus. The **pericardial cavity** contains the **heart.**

The **abdominopelvic cavity** can also be split into smaller cavities, the abdominal cavity and the pelvic cavity. The **abdominal cavity** houses all major digestive organs such as the stomach, liver, pancreas, gallbladder, small intestine, and large intestine, and also contains the kidneys. The **pelvic cavity** contains all internal reproductive organs and the urinary bladder.

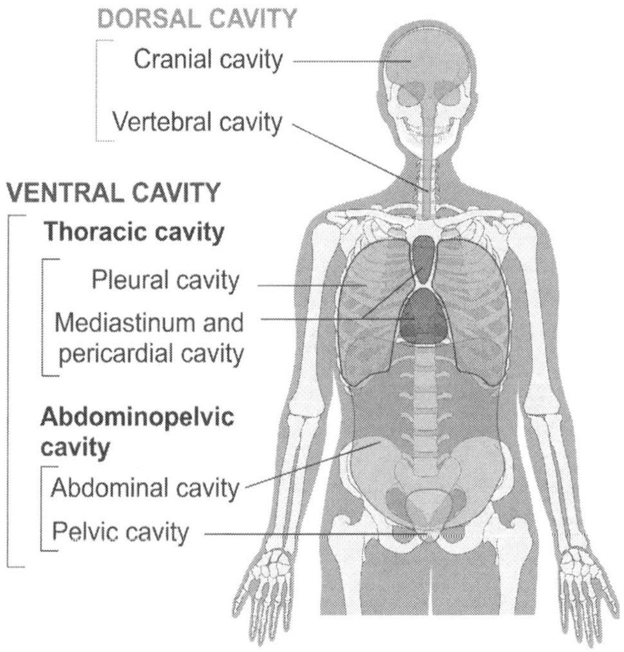

Cells

Cells are the **functional units** of all tissues. Cells are responsible for performing all essential life functions, from synthesizing nutrients to destroying pathogens and debris. Cells **divide** via a process known as **mitosis.** During mitosis, the cell splits from one single mother cell into two separate daughter cells. These daughter cells then divide further into daughter cells of their own, and the cycle repeats until enough cells are present to form a tissue.

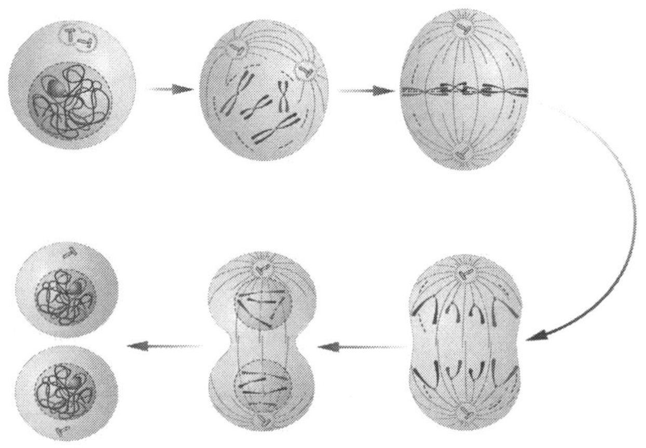

Mitosis

Inside each cell are **organelles**, structures that help regulate function of the cell.

The **nucleus** regulates the **overall function** of the cell. Inside the nucleus is **DNA**(deoxyribonucleic acid), which is the building block for life. Also inside the nucleus is the **nucleolus**, which contains **RNA**(ribonucleic acid). RNA is vital in transmitting signals from DNA to ribosomes for protein synthesis.

Golgi apparatus allows proteins and lipids to be bundled and **transported** within the cell itself.

Lysosomes are responsible for **breaking down** several different substances inside the cell, including protein and waste products.

Mitochondria are responsible for the production of **adenosine triphosphate(ATP)**, the molecule that provides **energy** to the body by transporting chemical energy to parts of the body that require it.

Ribosomes, which contain protein and RNA, are responsible for **synthesizing cell proteins.**

Smooth endoplasmic reticulum is responsible for synthesizing **carbohydrates and lipids** for use in producing new cell membranes.

Cytoplasm is found inside the cell, and is a **gel-like substance.** It allows organelles, nutrients, and waste products to move throughout the cell.

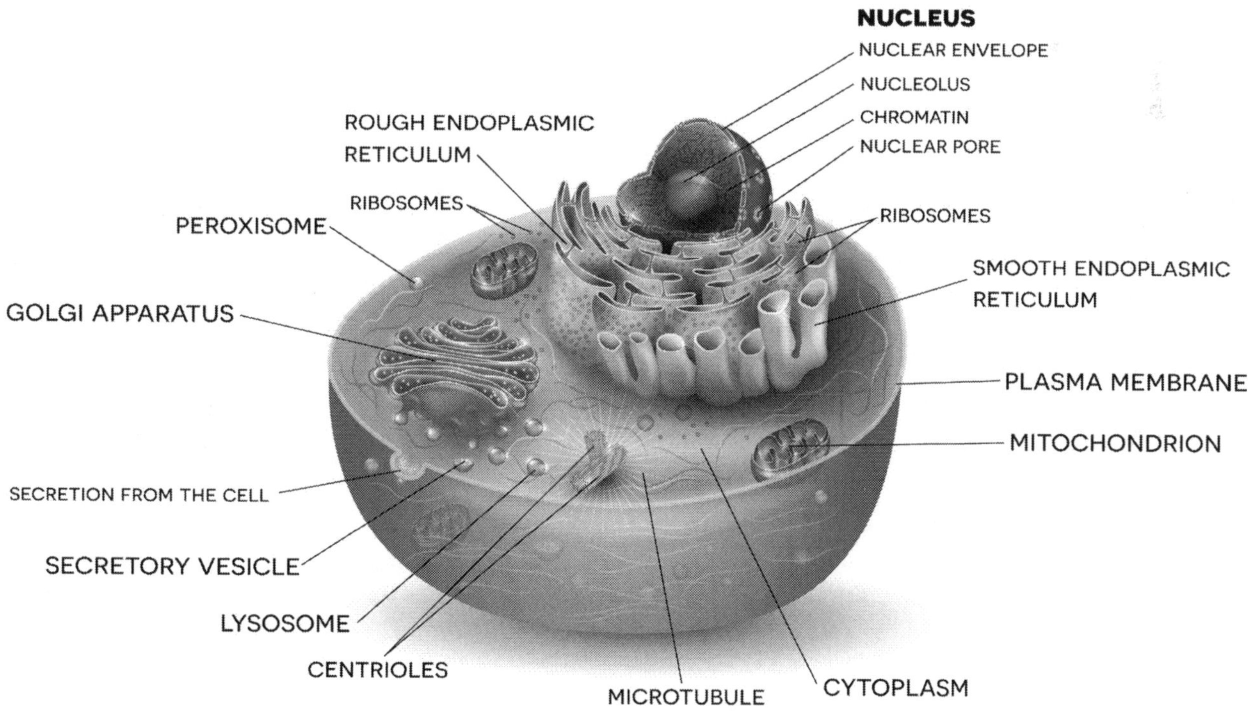

Tissue

The body is constructed by smaller parts making bigger parts, until we have an organism. The organization of the body is: cells > tissues > organ > organ system > organism. A **tissue** is made of a **group of cells** with **similar function and structure.** When these cells, all formed roughly the same way, which perform the same action, come together, they form a tissue. There are **four** types of tissue in the human body: epithelial, muscular, nervous, and connective.

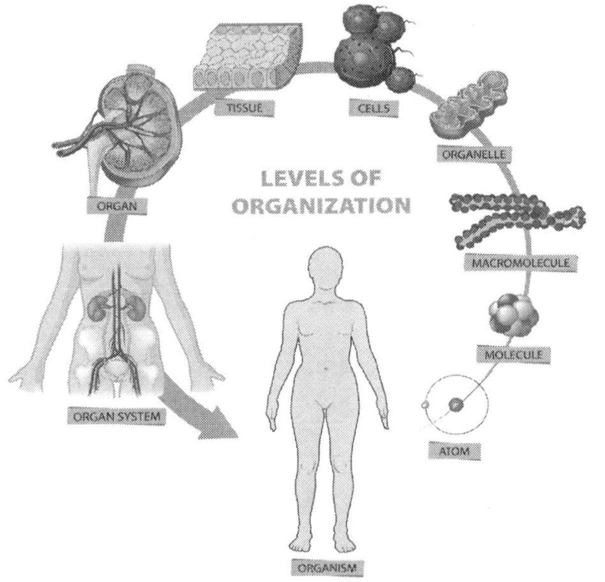

Epithelial Tissue

Epithelial tissue forms most **glands**, the **digestive tract**, the **respiratory tract**, and the **epidermis**. Anywhere there is a mucous membrane, there is epithelium. Epithelial tissue is responsible for **protection**(the epidermis protects the body from pathogens and trauma), **secretion**(glands secrete substances, from hormones to mucous), and **absorption of nutrients**(the linings of the small intestine are made of epithelium, which allows nutrients to be absorbed into the blood stream). Epithelial tissue is also **avascular**, which means there is no direct blood supply to the tissue. This is what allows layers of the epidermis to be peeled away without any bleeding.

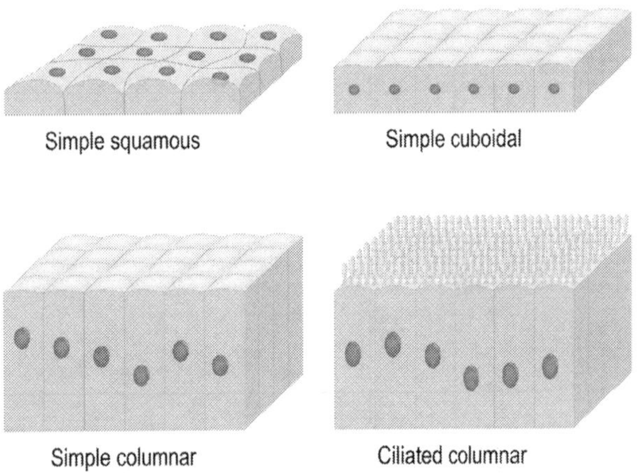

Muscular Tissue

Muscular tissue creates **muscles.** There are three types of muscles: skeletal muscles, so named because they connect to the skeleton, cardiac muscles, which create the heart, and smooth muscles, which are abundant in several locations in the body.

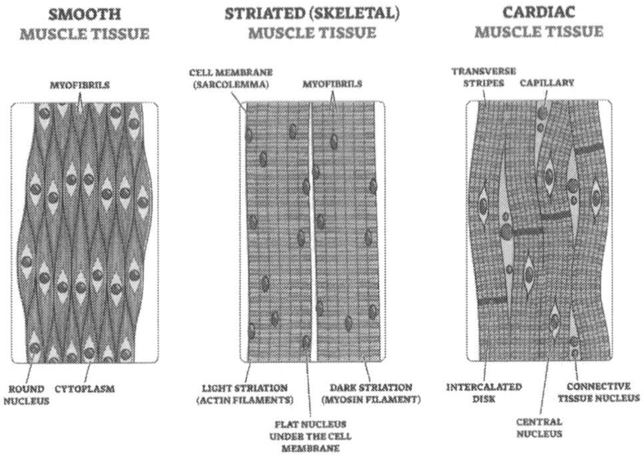

Skeletal muscles attach to the **skeleton.** Another name for skeletal muscle is "**striated**" muscle, due to its appearance under a microscope. These muscles are **voluntary**, meaning they can be controlled. When these muscles contract, they pull on the bones they attach to, which allows movement.

Skeletal muscles are always in a state of **twitching**, even if it can't be felt. It's this twitching, very fine contractions, that produces **body heat.** When body temperature drops, the skeletal muscles increase the amount of contraction, which produces high body temperature, with the twitching of the muscles becoming more apparent. This is what happens when a person shivers.

Cardiac muscle is the muscle that makes the **heart.** Another name for cardiac muscle is "**branching**" muscle, due to its appearance under a microscope. Cardiac muscle is **involuntary**, meaningit cannot be controlled. Cardiac muscle is powerful, shooting **blood** out of the heart with each contraction. The only function of cardiac muscle is to send blood from one place to another.

Smooth muscle is found in several locations throughout the body. Another name for smooth muscle is "**non-striated**" muscle, due to its appearance under a microscope. Smooth muscle is **involuntary**, meaning it cannot be controlled. Because smooth muscle is found in several different regions of the body, it has several different functions. Smooth muscle can be found in the **walls of hollow organs** such as the stomach and intestines. When these muscles contract, they force food through the Digestive System, which is known as **peristalsis.**

Other locations smooth muscle can be found are in the skin, and in the eyes. In the skin, smooth muscle attaches to hair.

When these muscles contract, they stand hair up, producing goosebumps. These muscles are known as the **arrector pili** muscles. In the eyes, smooth muscles help to dilate the iris and pupil.

Nervous Tissue

Nervous tissue forms the **brain**, **spinal cord**, and **nerves**. The primary cell of nervous tissue is known as a **neuron**. Neurons process nervous impulses, sending these impulses to other tissues, such as muscles, or between other neurons.

Neurons receive **action potentials**(electric impulses), which are brought into the cell by **dendrites**, branch-like projections coming off the cell body of the neuron. Once the nucleus processes the information coming into the cell, it sends the impulse out of the cell to its destination by way of the **axon**, a long projection coming off the cell body. The axons terminate at other neurons, or help innervate muscles.

Surrounding the axons are sheaths of protein and fat known as **myelin**. Myelin sheaths allow efficient and rapid transmission of impulses traveling along an axon, and help provide protection for the axon. Myelin sheaths in the peripheral nervous system are produced by **Schwann cells**.

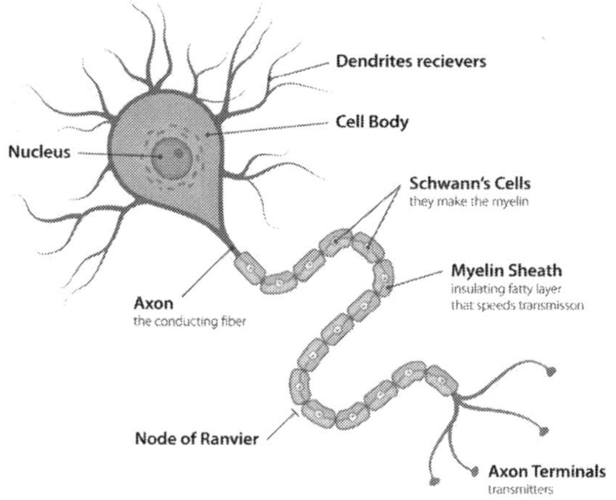

Connective Tissue

Connective tissue is the most abundant form of tissue in the body. There are several different structures made by connective tissue, including **tendons**, **ligaments**, **fascia**, **bones**, **lymph**, **cartilage**, **and blood**. Connective tissue is responsible for **connecting** tissues. In addition to connecting tissues, it helps to **separate** tissues, as seen in serous membranes and cartilage.

Connective tissue contains two specific types of cells known as blast cells and clast cells. These cells play a very important role in the health of connective tissue. **Blast cells** are germ cells that are responsible for **building connective tissue**. Blast cells divide and build tissue until the structure is complete. Once the structure is complete, the blast cells mature, and stop dividing. **Clast cells** are responsible for **breaking down tissue**, which is very important in keeping the tissue healthy. If a person suffers an injury such as a sprain or a fracture, clast cells will enter the area and destroy the dead tissue, cleaning the area, which allows blast cells a clean surface to build new tissue on.

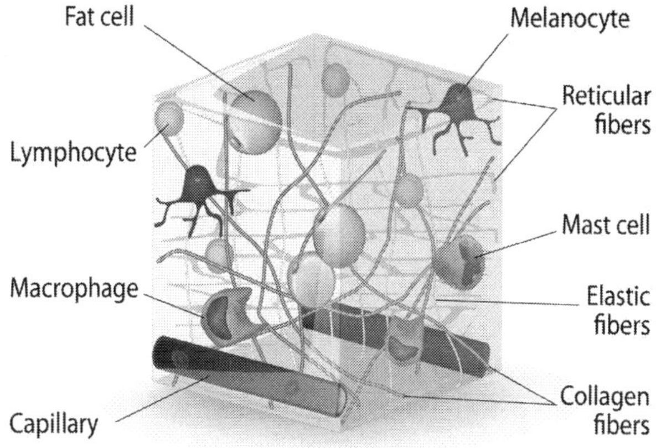

Blood

Blood is the **most abundant** form of connective tissue in the body. Blood is mainly a mode of **transportation** for blood cells, hormones, nutrients, and waste products. There are four parts of blood: erythrocytes, leukocytes, thrombocytes, and plasma.

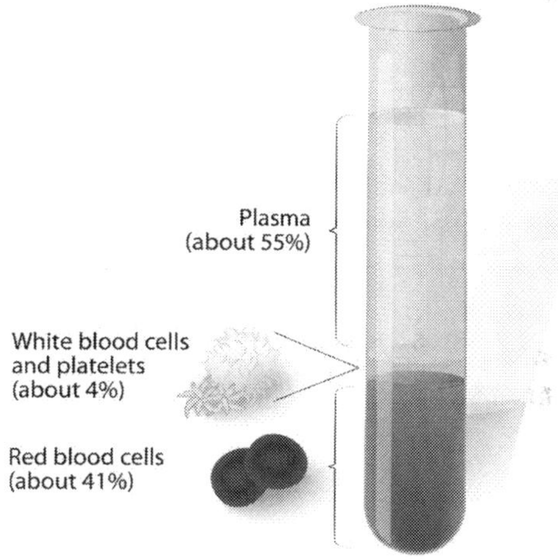

Erythrocytes, also known as **red blood cells**, are responsible for **transporting oxygen and carbon dioxide** throughout the body. The cytoplasm of erythrocytes is made of a protein known as **hemoglobin**, which is primarily made of iron. Hemoglobin is what oxygen and carbon dioxide attach to. In the lungs, when the erythrocytes are exposed to the alveoli, carbon dioxide detaches from the erythrocytes, and oxygen then attaches in its place. This is how gas exchange occurs in erythrocytes.

Leukocytes, also known as **white blood cells**, are the body's primary **defense against pathogens**. There are several different types of leukocytes, ranging from T-cells to basophils. These cells eat pathogens(such as bacteria), dead cells, and debris floating in the blood stream. **Thrombocytes**, also known as **platelets**, have one function: to **clot the blood**. This is vitally important when a person is bleeding. If the blood does not clot, the person could continue bleeding until they lose too much blood.

Plasma is the **fluid** portion of blood. The majority of blood, around 56%, is made of plasma. Plasma is what allows all of the blood cells, hormones, nutrients, and waste to move throughout the body. Without plasma, these substances would go nowhere.

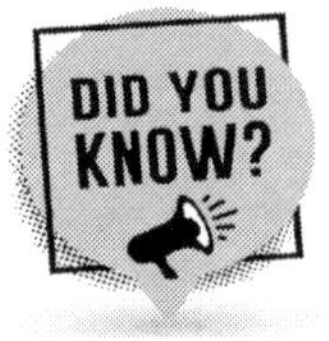

Leukocytes have an average lifespan of 2-3 weeks, and are then destroyed by the Lymphatic System!

Serous Membranes

Serous membranes are forms of connective tissue that are used to **separate organs from one another**, preventing friction. They accomplish this by surrounding the organ or body cavity.

Inside the thorax, there are two serous membranes: the **pericardium**, which **surrounds the heart**, and the **pleural membranes**, which **surround the lungs.** These membranes help protect these organs from injury.

Inside the abdomen and pelvis, there is one serous membrane: the **peritoneum.** This membrane keeps the organs inside the abdomen and pelvis from being injured, and provides a pathway for many blood vessels, lymph vessels, and nerves to travel.

Inside of a serous membrane is a thick fluid, known as **serous fluid.** This fluid helps the membranes absorb shock. Holding the fluid in place are two walls. The **inner wall**, which comes into contact with the organs, is known as the **visceral serous membrane.** The **outer wall**, which comes into contact with other structures such as bones or other organs, is known as the **parietal serous membrane.**

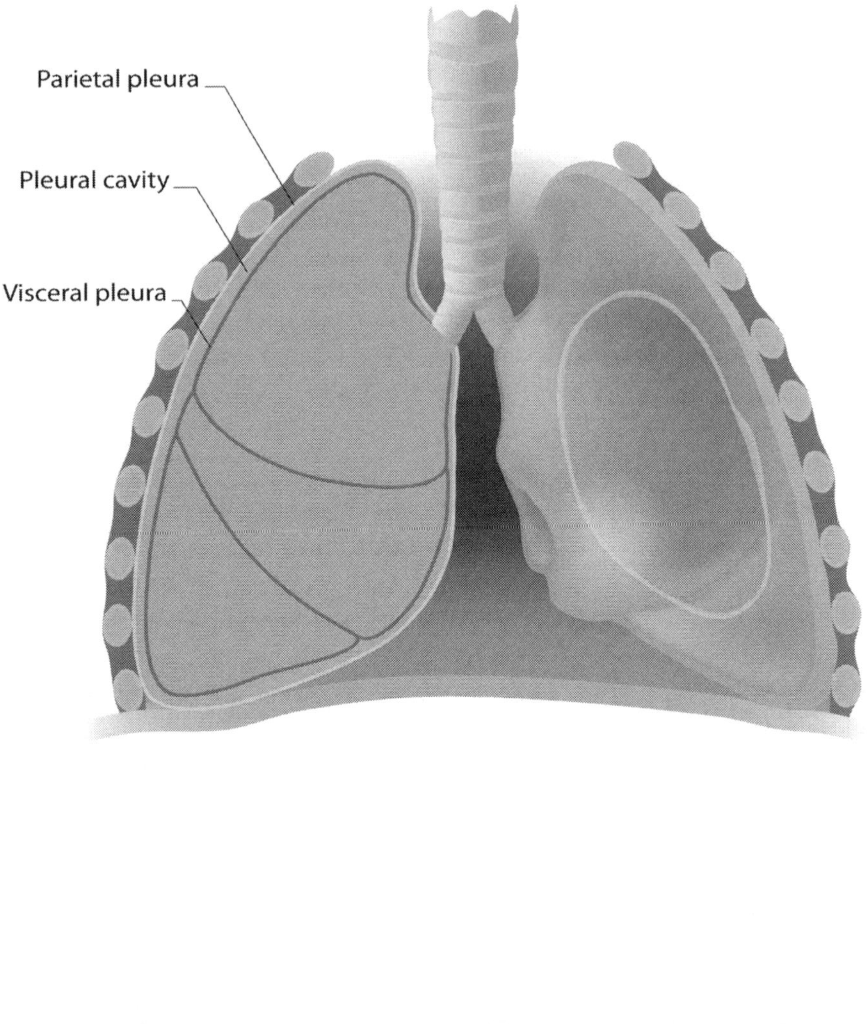

Cardiovascular System

The Cardiovascular System is one of the most important organ systems in the body, responsible for **transportation** of nutrients such as oxygen and hormones to tissues. It also allows for waste to be moved to areas of the body where it can be eliminated, such as the lungs, liver, and kidneys. Wastes include carbon dioxide and urea.

Heart

The primary organ of the Cardiovascular System is the heart. The heart, a large, powerful muscle, has one function: to **pump blood** throughout the body.

Blood is sent to the body to exchange oxygen and carbon dioxide. When gas exchange occurs, oxygen detaches from the erythrocytes, and carbon dioxide takes its place. Deoxygenated blood is returned to the heart via the **largest veins** in the body, the vena cavae(1). The **superior vena cava** returns blood to the heart from the head and upper limbs, while the **inferior vena cava** returns blood to the heart from the trunk and lower limbs. When blood first enters the heart, it is deoxygenated, and enters into the **right atrium**(2). It then passes through the **tricuspid valve**(which separates the right atrium from the right ventricle), into the **right ventricle**(3). The cardiac muscle in the right ventricle contracts, and it sends the deoxygenated blood out of the heart to the lungs through the **pulmonary arteries**(4[main pulmonary artery], 5[left and right branches]). Despite carrying deoxygenated blood, these vessels are still called arteries because they carry blood away from the heart. After blood cycles through the lungs, exchanging oxygen and carbon dioxide, the blood returns back to the heart through the **pulmonary veins**(6[left and right branches]). Again, despite carrying oxygenated blood, these vessels are called veins because they carry blood towards the heart. The blood re-enters the heart into the **left atrium**(7). It passes through the **bicuspid/mitral valve**(which separates the left atrium and left ventricle), into the **left ventricle**(8). An extremely powerful contraction occurs in the left ventricle, which shoots blood out of the heart to the rest of the body through the **aorta**(9), the **largest artery** in the body. The aorta has three branches that emerge from the **aortic arch**(10), sending blood to regions such as the head and upper limbs.

The pathway of blood flow through the heart

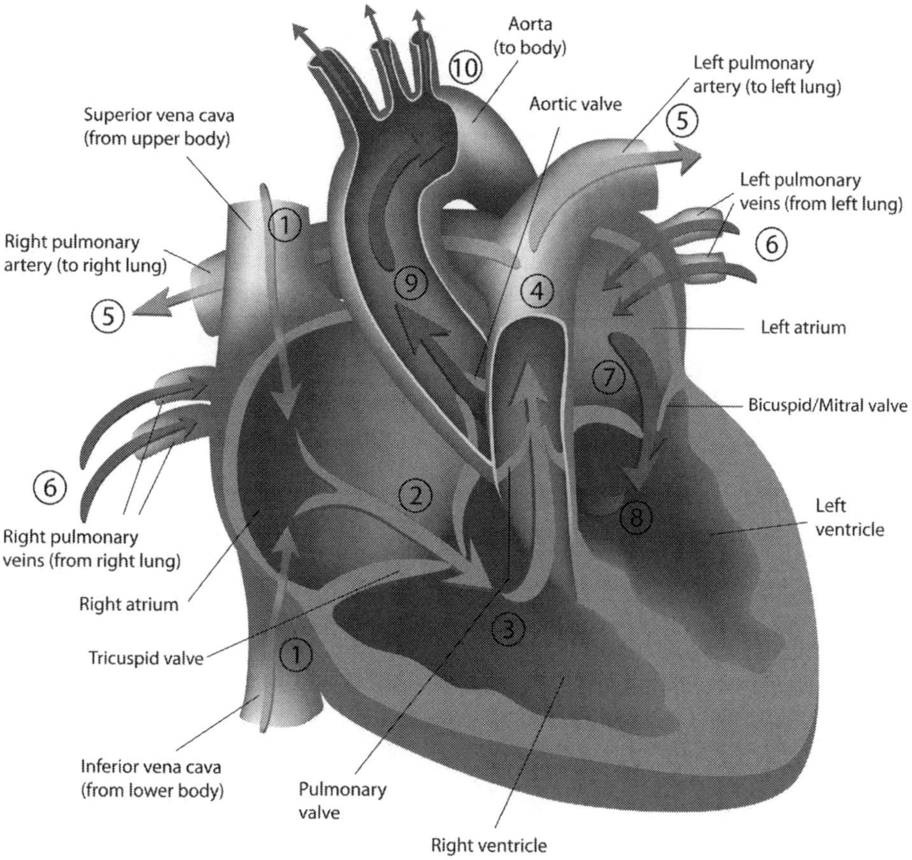

Easy to Remember: Each side of the heart is made of the same structures, just with different names! Remember "VAVVA": Vein, Atrium, Valve, Ventricle, Artery!

Blood Vessels

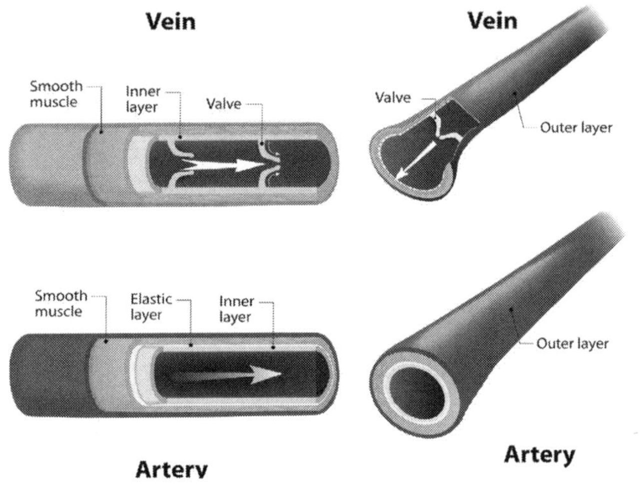

Blood vessels are the main mode of transportation for not only blood, but other substances, such as hormones. These substances are carried throughout the body in blood vessels. The largest types of blood vessels are known as arteries. **Arteries** primarily carry oxygenated blood **away from the heart**, to tissues. Arteries are the deepest blood vessels due to their size and importance. Tissues surrounding the arteries help to protect them from damage, which could result in severe bleeding and loss of oxygen.

Veins are blood vessels that primarily carry deoxygenated blood **towards the heart**, where it can replace carbon dioxide with oxygen. Veins are much more superficial than arteries, often visible under the skin, whereas most arteries cannot be seen.

Capillaries are microscopic arteries, and are where gas exchange takes place between blood vessels and tissues. Capillaries branch off from arterioles, exchange gas, and then return blood to veins through the smallest type of vein known as a **venule**.

Major arteries and veins are often named after their location in the body, such as the brachial artery/vein(in the arm), femoral artery/vein(in the thigh), abdominal aorta(in the abdomen), etc.

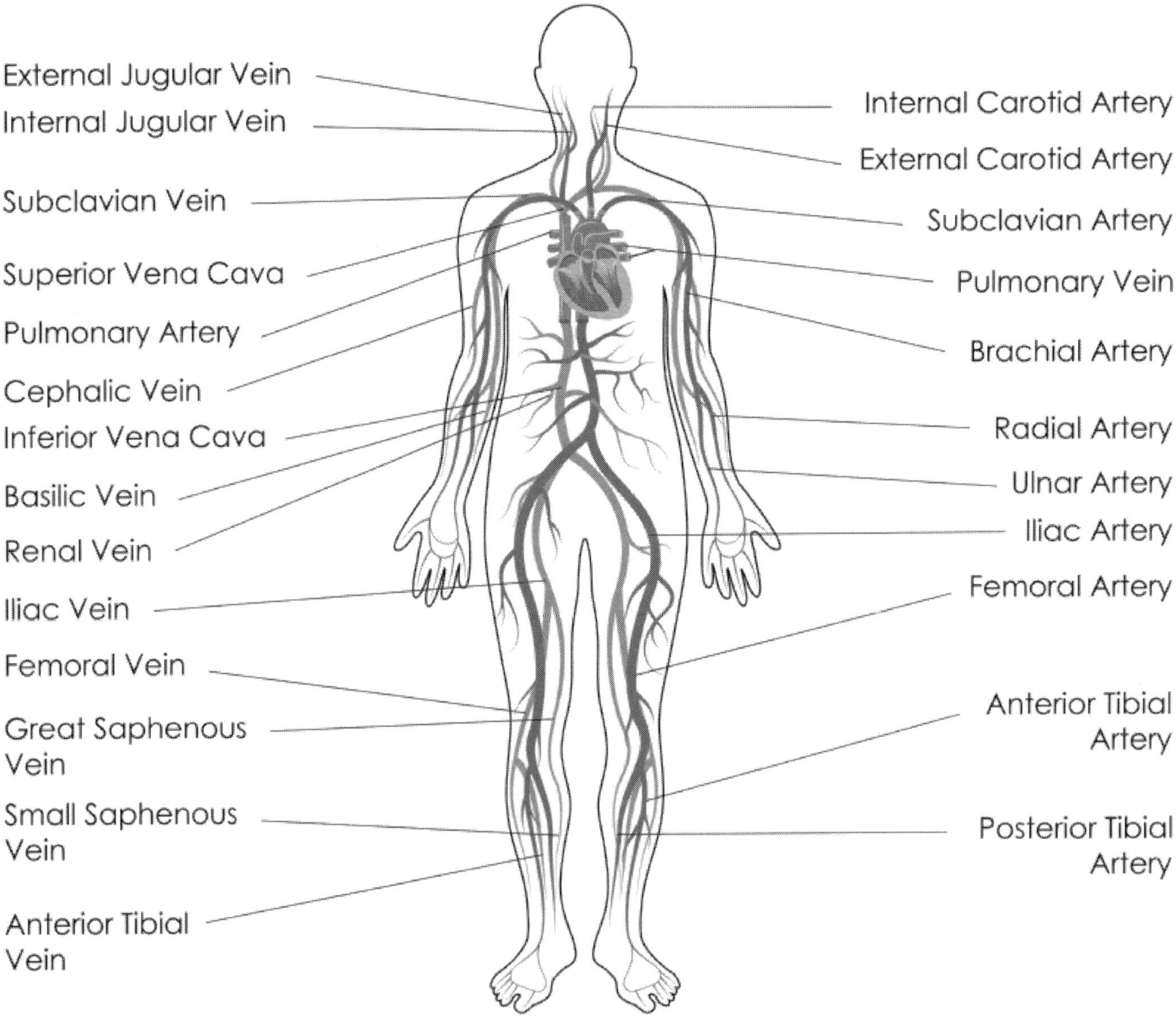

Digestive System

The Digestive System has many structures, organs, and functions. It is one of the most important systems in the body, responsible for **bringing nutrients into the body**, **digestion of food**, **absorption of nutrients** into the body's tissues, and **elimination of waste products**.

Structures of the Digestive System include the mouth, pharynx, esophagus, stomach, liver, gallbladder, pancreas, small intestine, and large intestine.

Digestion

The **mouth**, also known as the **oral cavity**, is the first place digestion begins taking place. The **teeth** manually break down food by **chewing**, or **mastication**. The food mixes with **saliva**, which contains digestive enzymes such as **amylase**, that help to break down carbohydrates. The **tongue** assists with mastication by pressing food against the teeth. Once food has been properly chewed, it is swallowed.

After food is swallowed, it moves from the mouth into the **pharynx**, also known as the **throat**. The pharynx is simply a passageway for food, water, and air on the way to their respective destinations. Food leaves the pharynx and enters the esophagus.

The **esophagus** is a long tube that runs from the pharynx inferiorly, passes through the diaphragm, and connects to the **stomach**. The esophagus, much like the pharynx, has one function: transporting food. The esophagus, and every hollow organ of the Digestive System, is lined with smooth muscle. When the smooth muscle rhythmically contracts, it forces food further along in the organ. This is known as **peristalsis**.

Once food reaches the **stomach**, both ends of the stomach close off, and the stomach begins **digesting** the food. Powerfully, it churns the food, breaking it down manually. Stomach acids like **hydrochloric acid** and **pepsin** mix with the food inside the stomach and further help to break down the food. Once food is properly digested, the stomach opens at the pylorus, the bottom of the stomach, and food exits the stomach and enters into the small intestine.

The small intestine is where the majority of absorption of nutrients occurs. Accessory organs produce substances that help aid the small intestine in digestion. These accessory organs are the liver, gallbladder, and pancreas.

The **liver**, the heaviest internal organ, mainly acts as a **blood detoxifier**. It filters harmful substances from the blood. However, it aids in digestion by **producing bile**, a yellowish substance that aids in the emulsification of fats. Connecting to the liver is the gallbladder. Once the liver produces bile, it empties the bile into the gallbladder, where it is stored until it is needed.

The **gallbladder** has one function: to **store bile** and empty bile into the small intestine through the bile duct, which connects to the duodenum, the first section of the small intestine.

The **pancreas** creates **pancreatic juice**, which aids in the digestion of proteins, lipids, and carbohydrates. These substances empty into the small intestine through the same path as bile, the bile duct.

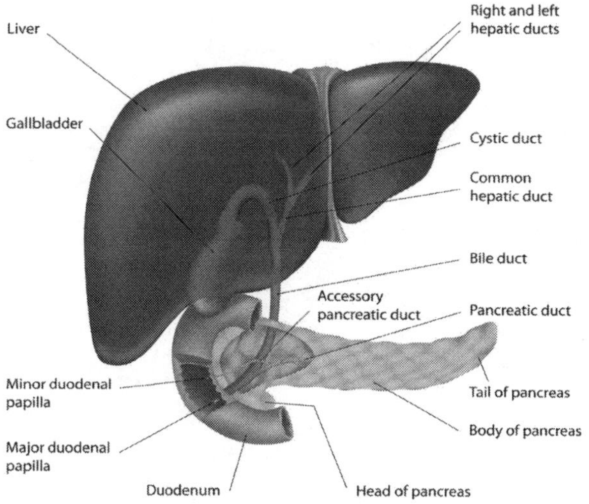

Food moves from the stomach into the **small intestine**. The first section of the small intestine is known as the **duodenum**. The duodenum is the last section of the Digestive System that digestion of food takes place. Bile and pancreatic juice mix with food in the duodenum and further break down substances. Peristalsis forces the food from the duodenum further into the small intestine, into the middle portion, known as the **jejunum**. The jejunum is where the majority of nutrient absorption takes place in the small intestine. As the food is forced through the small intestine, it moves into the final section, known as the **ileum**. Final absorption occurs in the ileum. Food moves through the ileum and into the large intestine.

The **large intestine** has two primary functions: **absorption of water**, and **elimination of waste**. As feces moves through the large intestine, water is absorbed. If too much water is absorbed, constipation may result. If not enough water is absorbed, diarrhea may result. The large intestine has four sections: the **ascending colon**, the **transverse colon**, the **descending colon**, and the **sigmoid colon**. As the feces leaves the sigmoid colon, it enters the rectum, where it is ready to be eliminated from the body.

Stages of Digestion

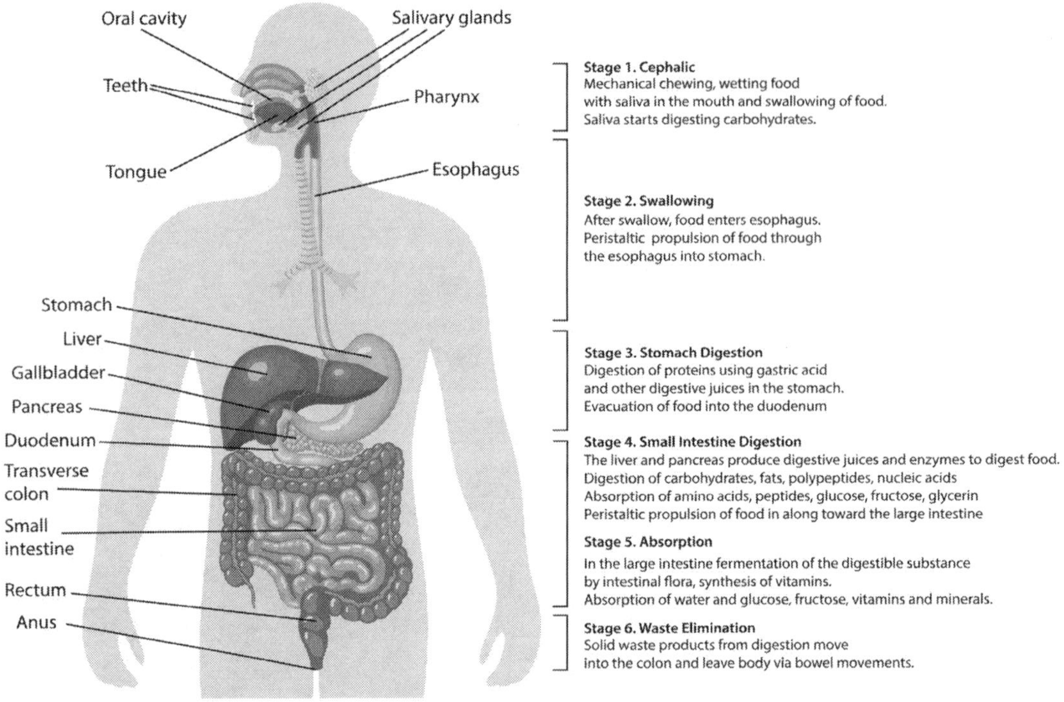

Mesentery

The mesentery is a fan-shaped extension of the peritoneum that **suspends the small and large intestines** from the posterior abdominal wall, holding them in place. The point of attachment where the mesentery attaches to the posterior abdominal wall is known as the **mesenteric root**. The mesentery additionally allows a **conduit** for blood vessels, nerves, and lymphatic channels to pass in the abdomen.

Several blood vessels use the mesentery as a conduit. Arteries found in the mesentery include the superior mesenteric artery and inferior mesenteric artery. Veins found in the mesentery include the superior mesenteric vein and inferior mesenteric vein.

In a person with Crohn's disease, the mesentery often presents with an increased amount of fat. This fat is thicker than the fat of a person without Crohn's disease, and this may lead to future treatments for Crohn's disease that specifically target the mesentery. In addition, these fat cells produce a type of protein known as **C-reactive protein**, which is normally produced by the liver. C-reactive protein(CRP) levels typically increase when there is some sort of inflammation in the body. High levels of CRP in the blood may indicate infection, inflammation, and other conditions such as heart disease or cancer.

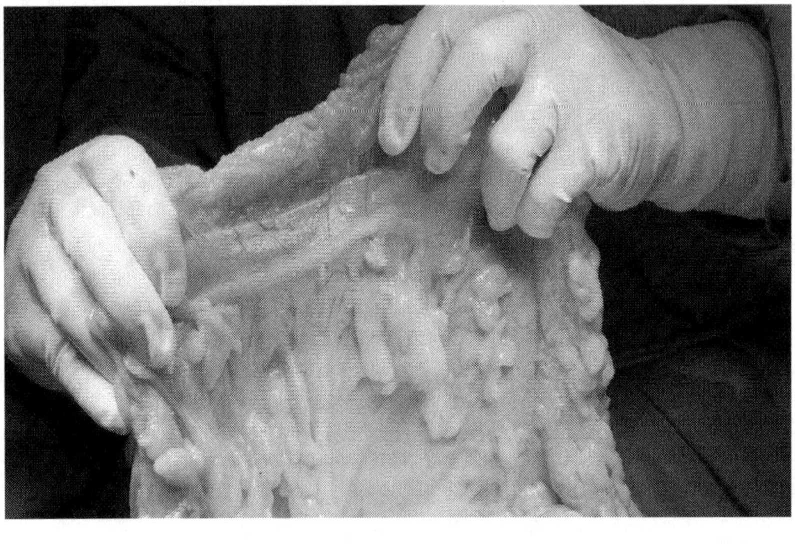

Sphincters

In the Digestive System, there are **ring-like bands of muscle** between digestive organs, known as **sphincters**. Sphincters function to allow food to enter into an organ, or to keep food from moving backwards.

There are four primary sphincters in the Digestive System:

The **esophageal sphincter** is located between the **pharynx** and the **esophagus**. It opens and allows food to move down into the esophagus. Another name for this sphincter is the upper esophageal sphincter.

The **cardiac sphincter** is located between the **esophagus** and the **stomach.** It is named after the region of the stomach it connects to, which is known as the cardia. When food enters the stomach, the cardiac sphincter closes, preventing food and stomach acid from ascending into the esophagus. Another name for this sphincter is the lower esophageal sphincter.

The **pyloric sphincter** is located between the **stomach** and the **small intestine.** It is named after the region of the stomach it connects to, which is known as the pylorus. When food enters the stomach, the pyloric sphincter closes, preventing food from leaving the stomach before digestion has taken place. When food has been properly digested, the pyloric sphincter opens, and food leaves the stomach and enters the small intestine.

The **ileocecal sphincter** is located between the **small intestine** and the **large intestine.** It is named after the parts of the two organs that come together, the ileum(small intestine) and cecum(large intestine).

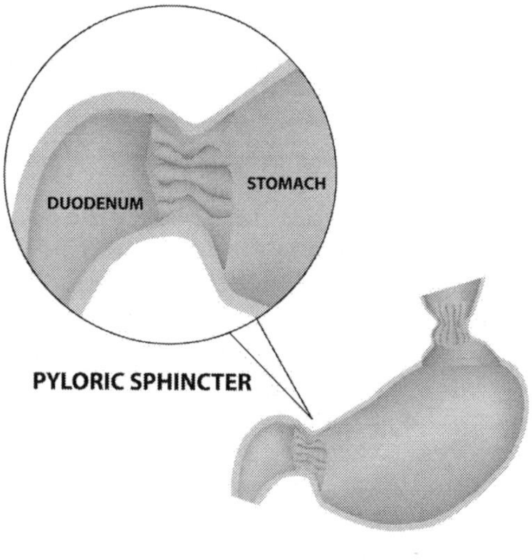

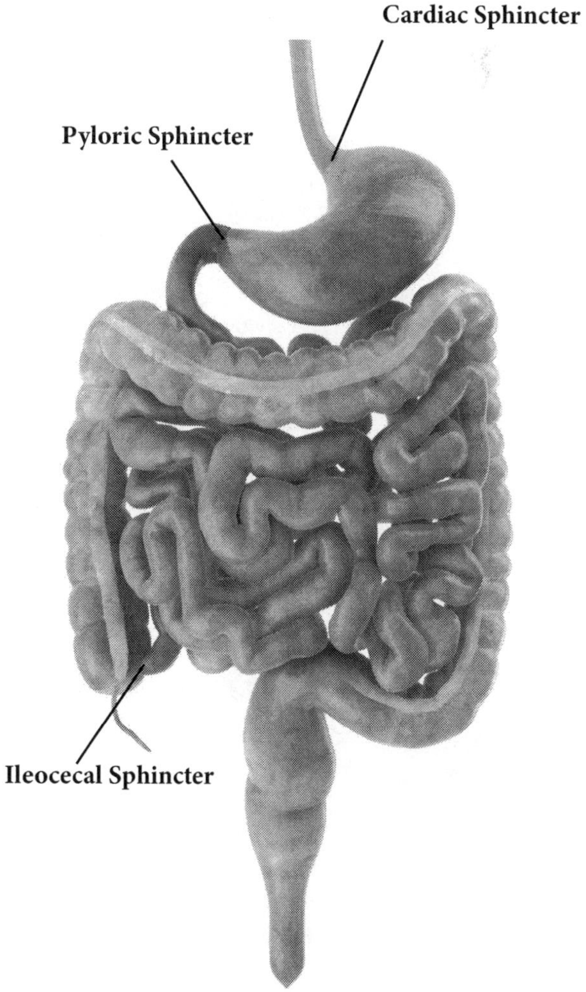

Endocrine System

The Endocrine System is responsible for coordinating specific activities of cells and tissues by releasing **hormones** into the body. Endocrine glands differ from exocrine glands in two specific ways: endocrine glands create and secrete hormones, while exocrine glands create and secrete things like sweat, saliva, and oil. Endocrine glands secrete hormones directly into the **blood stream**, while exocrine glands secrete their substances onto a **surface**(such as the surface of the mouth or skin). Endocrine glands have many different functions that help regulate body function and homeostasis.

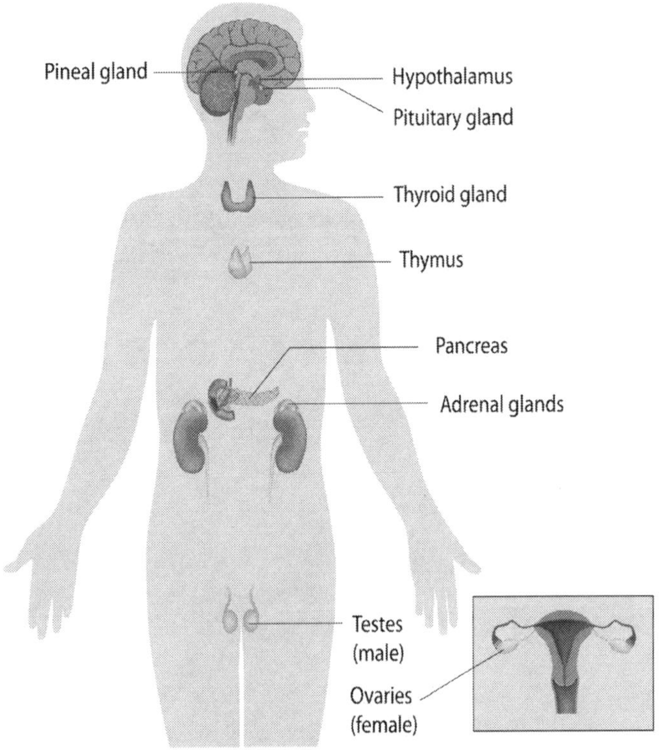

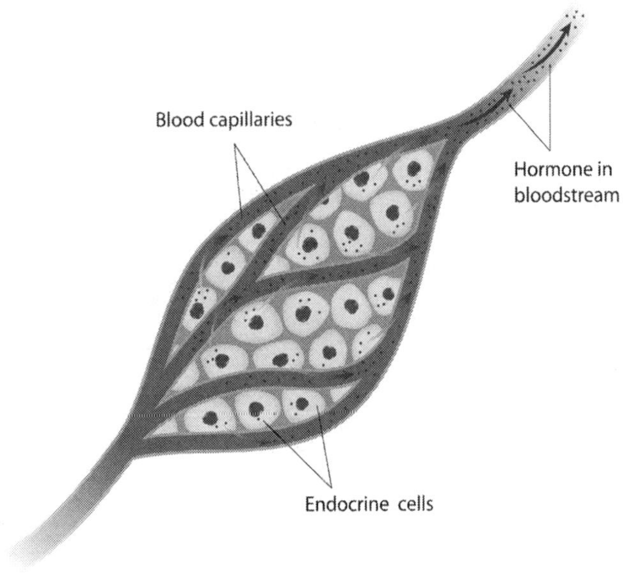

Hormone secretion into the blood stream

DID YOU KNOW?

While most hormones are made by these endocrine glands, other organs can also produce hormones! The placenta produces estrogen and progesterone, and the stomach produces ghrelin, the hormone that stimulates appetite!

Adrenal Glands

The adrenal glands, located **atop the kidneys**, secrete **epinephrine and norepinephrine**. These hormones help to elevate blood pressure, heart rate, and blood sugar. They are considered stress hormones, and are secreted when the body is under stress, or in the sympathetic nervous response.

Hypothalamus

The hypothalamus produces **dopamine**, an important hormone that increases blood pressure and heart rate. It is considered the **reward center hormone**. If you win at a game or contest, your hypothalamus may release dopamine, which gives a sensation of excitement.

Ovaries and Testes

The ovaries are the female gonads. They create **estrogen and progesterone**, two hormones important to female development and bone growth.

The testes are the male gonads. The testes secrete **testosterone**, the primary male hormone, responsible for increasing bone and muscle mass.

Pancreatic Islets

Pancreatic Islets are the parts of the pancreas that create **glucagon**, which **increases blood sugar levels**, and **insulin**, which **decreases blood sugar levels.** Glucagon is created by **alpha cells**, and insulin is created by **beta cells.**

Pineal Gland

The pineal gland is responsible for the production of **melatonin**, the hormone that regulates the body's wake/sleep cycle, also known as the **circadian rhythm.**

Pituitary Gland

The pituitary gland, which many consider the "master gland", secretes **growth hormone**, which regulates the amount of growth a person may experience. It also secretes **prolactin**, which stimulates milk production, and **follicle-stimulating hormone**, which influences production of female egg cells and male sperm cells.

Thyroid

The thyroid is a gland in the neck that produces **calcitonin**, which decreases the levels of calcium in the blood stream. preventing weakening of the bones and kidney stones.

Integumentary System

The Integumentary System is the body's first line of defense against pathogens and trauma. Its primary function is to protect the body. It also secretes substances, may absorb certain substances, and even eliminates waste.

Skin

The skin, which is the body's **largest organ**, is the main structure of the Integumentary System. The skin **protects the body** by creating a thick barrier that prevents pathogens from entering, and helps to cushion the body from blunt trauma.

Aiding the skin in protection are the **nails.** Finger and toe nails are made of **keratin**, the same cells that create thick layers in the skin called calluses. The nails prevent damage to the distal phalanges.

Hair also aids in protection, but in a different way. Hair is used to regulate temperature. When body temperature drops, smooth muscle that attaches to each hair, known as **arrector pili**, contract, forcing the hair to stand up. This creates an insulating layer, which is meant to trap warmth underneath the hair, much like a blanket. This does little for humans, but is utilized by animals to retain heat in cold environments.

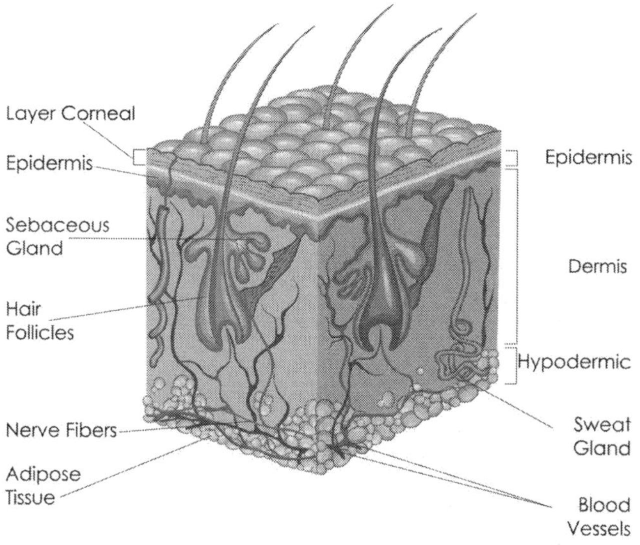

Glands

Inside the skin are glands, which also aid in protection. **Sudoriferous glands** emerge from deep in the skin to the surface directly through tubes. Sudoriferous glands create and secrete **sweat.** Sweat is mostly made of water, but may also contain salt and waste products such as ammonia. Sweat is used to lower body temperature by evaporating off the surface of the skin. The evaporation cools the skin, which helps lower the internal body temperature.

Sebaceous glands are glands that connect to hair, and produce **oil(sebum).** Oil helps to protect the body from pathogens and debris in the air. Blockage of a sebaceous gland, however, may lead to a bacterial infection, and acne.

Sensory Receptors

Inside the skin, there are many types of receptors that detect certain sensations, relaying the information to the brain. Sensory receptors aren't exclusive to the skin, but there are an abundance of them in the skin.

Nociceptors are a type of sensory receptor that detects the sensation of **pain.** While unpleasant, pain is actually vital in protection of the body. The term "noci-" is Latin for "hurt".

Meissner's Corpuscles are sensory receptors that are very superficial in the skin, and detect **light pressure.**

Pacinian Corpuscles are sensory receptors that are very deep in the skin, and detect **deep pressure.**

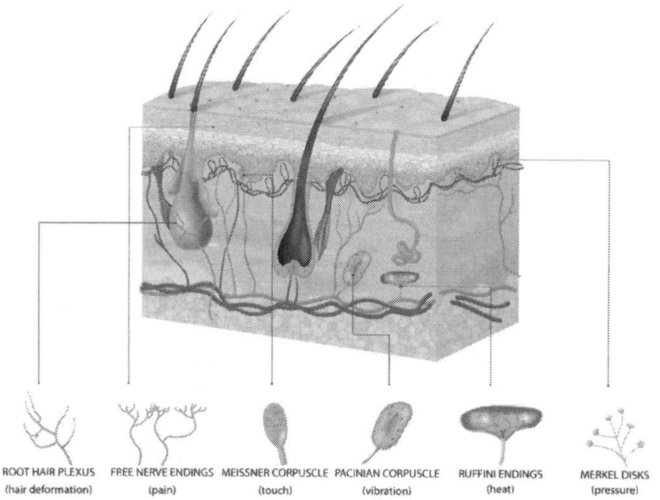

Easy to Remember: Nociceptors detect pain. Remember the old saying "No pain, No gain".

Easy to Remember: Pacinian Corpuscles detect deep pressure. Match up "Paci" of Pacinian with "Paci" of Pacific Ocean. The Pacific Ocean is deep!

Lymphatic System

The Lymphatic System is vital in the body's **defense against pathogens** and disease. Not only are leukocytes abundant in lymph, but antibodies are created in the Lymphatic System. The Lymphatic System contains lymph, lymph nodes, lymph vessels, and lymph organs.

Lymph, the primary structure of the Lymphatic System, is a **fluid** composed of water, protein, leukocytes, urea, salts, and glucose. Lymph allows transport of all of these substances through the body, ultimately dumping into the blood stream. Lymph is made of **interstitial fluid**, fluid found between cells.

Lymph travels throughout the body through **lymph vessels.** Lymph vessels are similar to blood vessels, but only flow in one direction, **towards the heart**. Lymph vessels absorb foreign bodies and nutrients from tissues, bringing them into the lymph to be transported to the blood stream or lymph nodes. The **largest lymph vessel** in the body is located in the trunk. It is known as the **Thoracic Duct**. The Thoracic Duct drains lymph into the **left subclavian vein**, where it joins with blood.

Lymph nodes are **large masses** of lymphatic tissue. They are responsible for production of **antibodies**, and help **filter and destroy** any foreign objects that enter the lymph. During an infection, lymph nodes may become tender and swollen.

The **thymus**, located in the chest, is responsible for production of **T-lymphocytes**, or T-cells. T-cells are vital in regulation of the body's immune system. If a person contracts HIV, the virus destroys the T-cells, which essentially disables the immune system.

The **spleen** is an organ of the Lymphatic System responsible for **destroying** dead or dying **red blood cells** from the blood stream, in addition to destroying pathogens and debris.

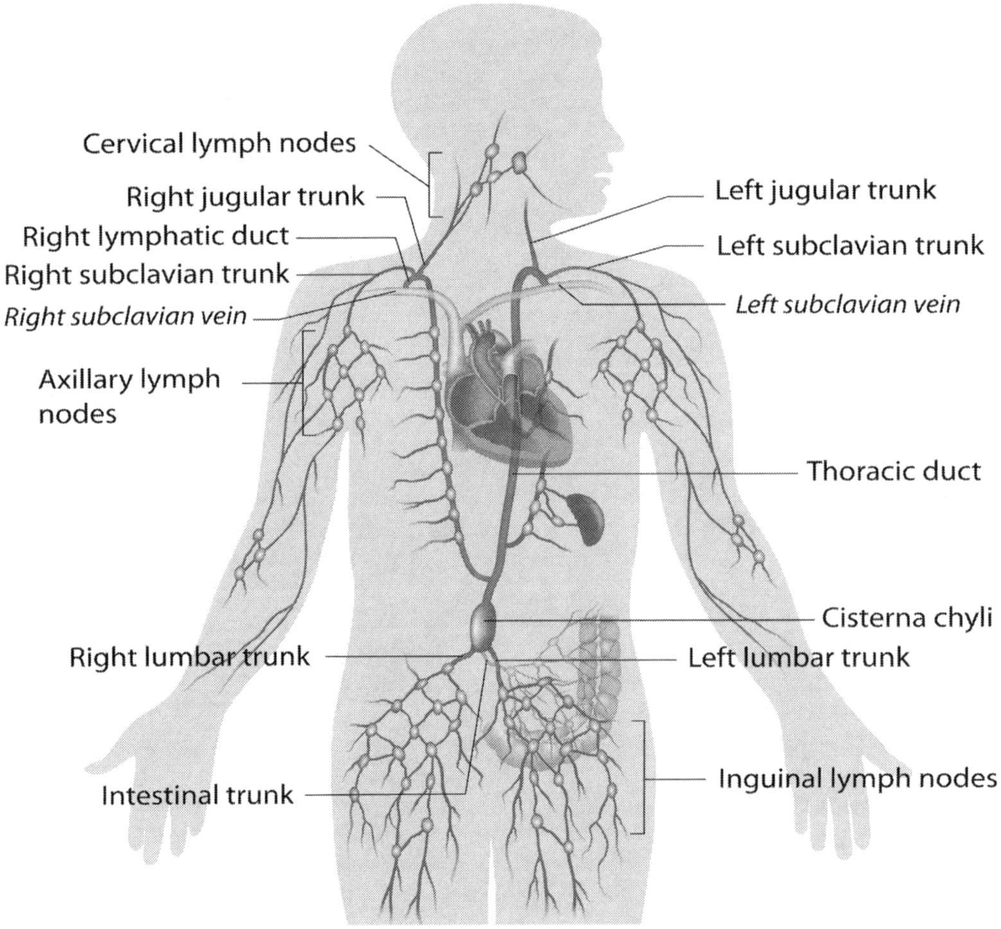

DID YOU KNOW?

The thoracic duct is the largest lymph vessel in the body!

Muscular System

Muscles have numerous actions in the body, primarily **producing body heat**, contracting to **allow movements**, and **constricting organs and blood vessels.**

Muscle Structure

Skeletal muscles are broken down into the following components:

- **Sarcomeres** are the functional units of skeletal muscle. When they shorten, the muscle contracts.
- **Actin** is part of a sarcomere, known as the **thin filament**. Actin is what myosin attaches to during a muscle contraction. Actin anchors to the **Z-Line** in a sarcomere.
- **Myosin** is part of a sarcomere, known as the **thick filament.** Myosin resembles a golf club head, and attaches to actin during a muscle contraction. The entire span of the thick filaments in one sarcomere is known as the **A-Band.**
- **Tropomyosin** is a protein that covers the attachment sites where myosin attaches to actin during a contraction. **Calcium ions** are responsible for removing the tropomyosin from the actin, allowing the myosin to attach to the actin and initiate a contraction.

Muscle contractions begin with **action potentials** sent from the brain. Action potentials terminate at the **neuromuscular junction**, releasing **acetylcholine(aCh)** into the synapse. This results in the aCh binding to certain receptors in the muscle fiber, which in turn allows sodium ions to enter the muscle fiber. The sodium ions come into contact with the sarcoplasmic reticulum, which causes a release of **calcium ions.** The calcium ions enter into the working unit of muscles, known as sarcomeres. A sarcomere contains thick filaments, known as myosin, and thin filaments, known as actin. When a muscle isn't in a state of contraction, the myosin and actin do not interact due to the presence of tropomyosin preventing myosin from attaching to actin. When the body wants to allow the muscle to contract, calcium ions bind to tropomyosin, causing them to reveal the attachment sites on the actin for the myosin. Once the tropomyosin is removed, the myosin attaches to the actin, pulling the Z-lines closer together. This causes the sarcomere to shorten. The shortening of all the sarcomeres in a muscle fiber result in the entire muscle contracting.

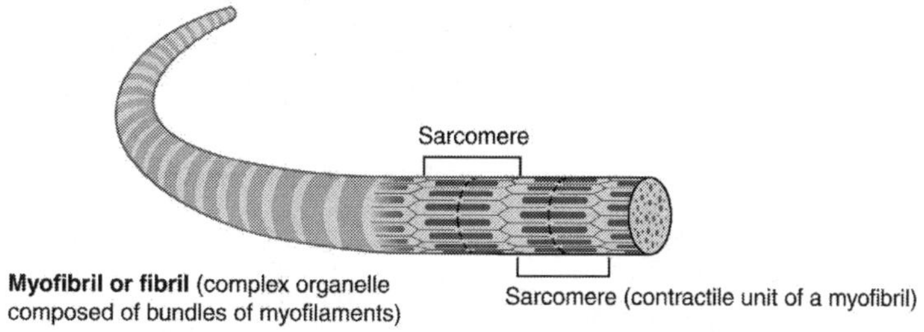

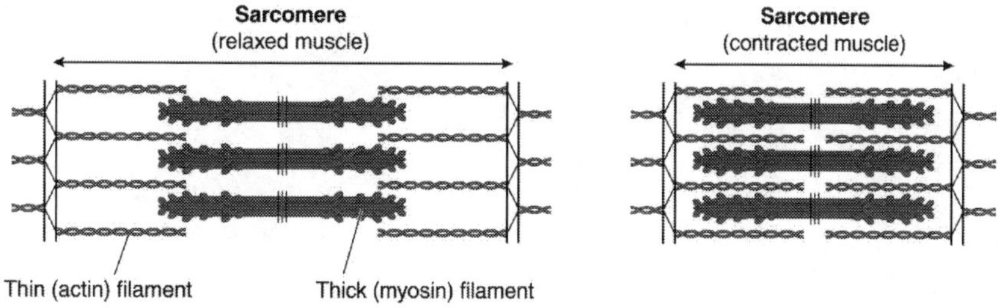

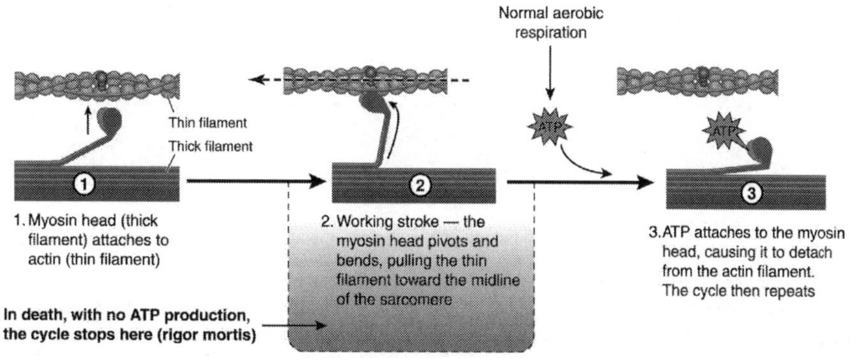

Muscle Contractions

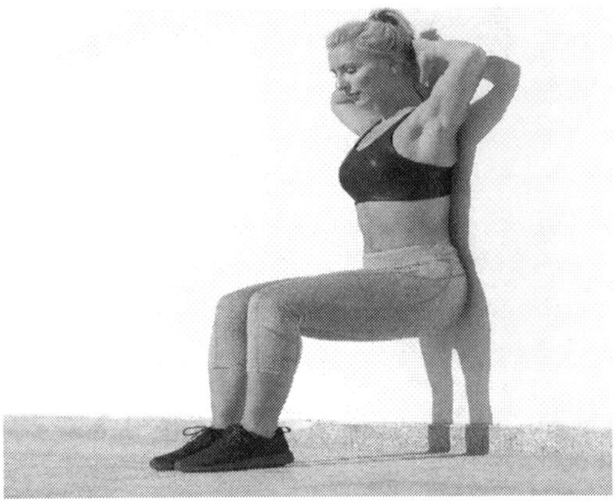

When there is **tension** in a muscle, it is **contracting**. A muscle can contract without causing movement, though. There are four types of muscle contractions.

Isometric Contraction

Iso means "**same**" or "**equal**". Metric means "**length**". When an isometric contraction occurs, as the name implies, the **length** of the muscle **stays the same**, but **tension** in the muscle **changes**. An example: imagine trying to lift something that is too heavy for you to lift. The muscles required to lift the object increase in tension, but because the muscles aren't strong enough, the length of the muscles doesn't change.

Isotonic Contraction

Iso means "**same**" or "**equal**". Tonic means "**tension**". When an isotonic contraction occurs, as the name implies, the **tension** in the muscle **stays the same**, but the muscle **length changes**. There are two separate types of isotonic contractions:

Concentric Contraction

When a concentric contraction occurs, several things take place. The tension in the muscle **initially increases** until the amount of tension required to perform the action is reached, then the tension **remains constant**. While the tension remains constant, the muscle **length decreases**. An example is performing a biceps curl.

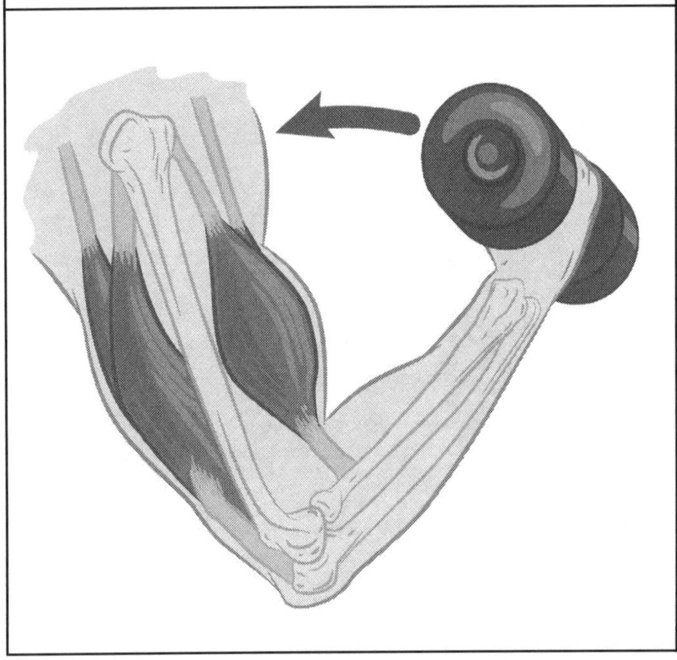

Eccentric Contraction

When an eccentric contraction occurs, several things take place. The tension in the muscle **initially decreases** until the amount of tension required to perform the action is reached, then the tension **remains constant**. While the tension remains constant, the muscle length **increases**. An example is extending the elbow and lowering the weight down after the biceps curl in a concentric contraction.

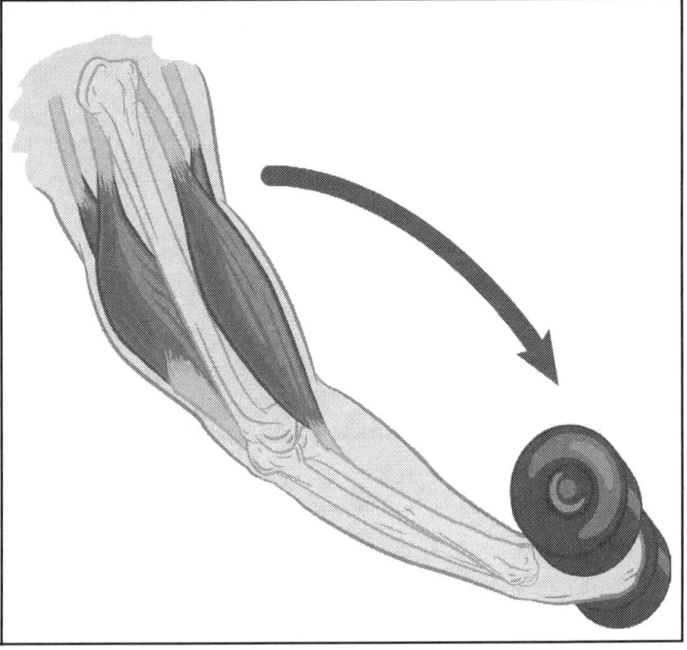

Proprioceptors

Proprioceptors are structures in the body that are responsible for detection of the body's **position in space**. Proprioceptors allow the location of the parts of the body, the body's weight, and center of gravity to be known even on a subconscious level. Proprioceptors can be found in several locations in the body, such as the skin, muscles, tendons, and ears. The two main types of proprioceptors in the muscles are **muscle spindles**, and **Golgi tendon organs**.

Muscle Spindles

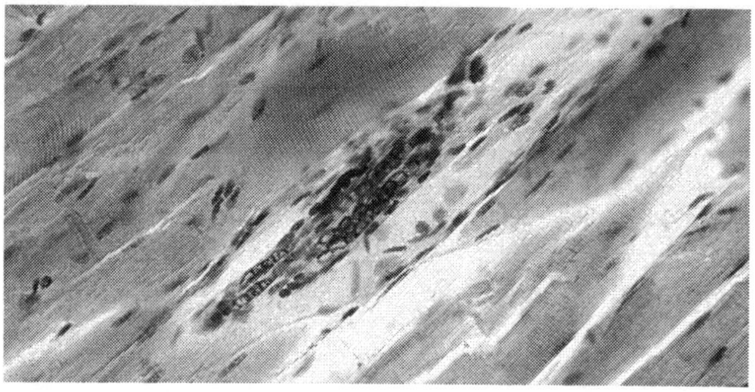

Muscle spindles, also known as **stretch receptors**, are able to detect when a muscle is stretching or elongating. When muscle spindles detect the muscle is stretching too far, they send a sensory impulse to the spinal cord, which responds by sending a motor impulse to the muscle that stimulates the muscle to **produce tension**. This counteracts the stretch and prevents damage to the muscle.

Golgi Tendon Organs

Golgi tendon organs are able to **detect the amount of tension** in a muscle. They are located at the origin and insertion of muscle fibers and tendons, also known as the **musculotendinous junction**. Golgi tendon organs detect when the muscle is producing tension, and if the tension is too great, Golgi tendon organs will **prevent the muscle from producing additional force**. This is done to prevent injury to muscles. An example is during weight lifting, when performing repetitions at the end of a set. The muscle may become more difficult to contract when lifting the weight due to the Golgi tendon organ preventing further force from being exerted by the muscle.

Muscle Shapes

Muscles have several different shapes. These include:

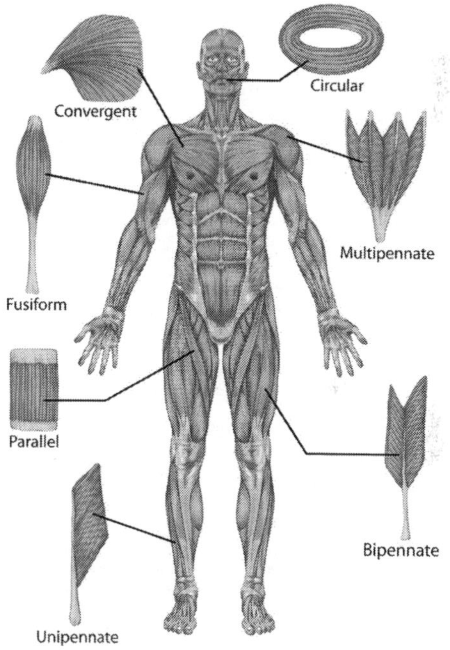

Circular: Circular muscles are arranged in a **circular** manner. Examples include orbicularis oris and orbicularis oculi.

Convergent: Convergent muscles are **spread out** on one end and **merge together** at another end. An example is pectoralis major.

Fusiform: Fusiform muscles are **thin** at the **attachment sites** and **wider in the middle**. An example is biceps brachii.

Parallel: Parallel muscles have muscle fibers that all run in the **same direction**. Examples include sartorius and coracobrachialis.

Pennate: Pennate muscles have an appearance resembling a **feather**. These muscles can be **unipennate**(one feather), **bipennate**(two feathers), or **multipennate**(multiple feathers). Examples include flexor pollicis longus(unipennate), rectus femoris(bipennate), and deltoid(multipennate).

Muscle Actions

Muscles perform numerous actions on the body, depending on which muscle is contracting. To see examples of all of these actions, refer to page 214. Muscle actions include the following:

Flexion: Decreasing the angle of a joint.
Extension: Increasing the angle of a joint.
Adduction: Moving a structure **towards the midline**.
Abduction: Moving a structure **away from the midline**.
Protraction: Moving a structure **anteriorly**.
Retraction: Moving a structure **posteriorly**.
Inversion: Turning the sole of the foot **in towards the midline**.
Eversion: Turning the sole of the foot **out away from the midline**.
Elevation: Moving a structure **superiorly**.
Depression: Moving a structure **inferiorly**.
Supination: **Rotating the palm** so it is facing **upwards**.
Pronation: **Rotating the palm** so it is facing **downwards**.
Rotation: **Turning a structure** around its **long axis**.
Circumduction: **Turning a structure** around the **circumference** of a joint.
Opposition: Moving structures in **opposite directions**.
Lateral Deviation: Moving a structure from **side-to-side**.
Plantarflexion: Pointing toes **down**.
Dorsiflexion: Pointing toes **up**.

When a muscle performs an action, other muscles associate with the muscle in different ways.

A **prime mover/agonist** is the muscle that primarily performs a specific action. An example: when plantarflexion is performed, the **strongest muscle** performing it is the gastrocnemius. That means gastrocnemius is the prime mover/agonist.

A **synergist** is the muscle that **assists the prime mover/agonist** in performing the action. Synergists are not as strong as prime movers. An example: when plantarflexion is performed, soleus contracts to allow more strength, assisting gastrocnemius in performing the action. That means soleus is the synergist.

An **antagonist** is a muscle that performs the **opposite action** of the prime mover/agonist. Every muscle has an antagonist. An example: gastrocnemius contracts, performing plantarflexion. To return the foot to the starting position, gastrocnemius relaxes, and tibialis anterior contracts, which performs dorsiflexion. This makes tibialis anterior the antagonist to gastrocnemius.

A **fixator** is a muscle that **stabilizes an area** or joint while an action is being performed. Stabilizing the joint prevents things like injury and allows optimal movement to occur. An example: supraspinatus stabilizes the head of the humerus in the glenoid fossa, keeping the joint together during the numerous movements the glenohumeral joint performs.

Easy to Remember: Just think of it like this: Batman is the Agonist, the main character, Robin is the Synergist, the helper, and The Joker is the Antagonist, who does the opposite of Batman!

Aerobic and Anaerobic Metabolism

Aerobic metabolism is the process in which cells utilize **oxygen** to **produce energy** to function properly. Oxygen is introduced into cells and enters into mitochondria. Mitochondria uses oxygen and glucose to create **adenosine triphosphate**, also known as **ATP**. ATP is a molecule that allows the transport of important nutrients, such as protein, inside the cell. ATP also stores energy for future use in the cell, and allows important bodily functions to occur, such as nerve impulse transmission and muscle contractions.

Anaerobic metabolism is the process in which ATP is produced **without** the presence of **oxygen**. This is performed when the lungs are unable to provide the cells with enough oxygen during high intensity exercise, such as running. The mitochondria produce ATP using only **glucose**, which in turn produces **lactic acid** as a waste product.

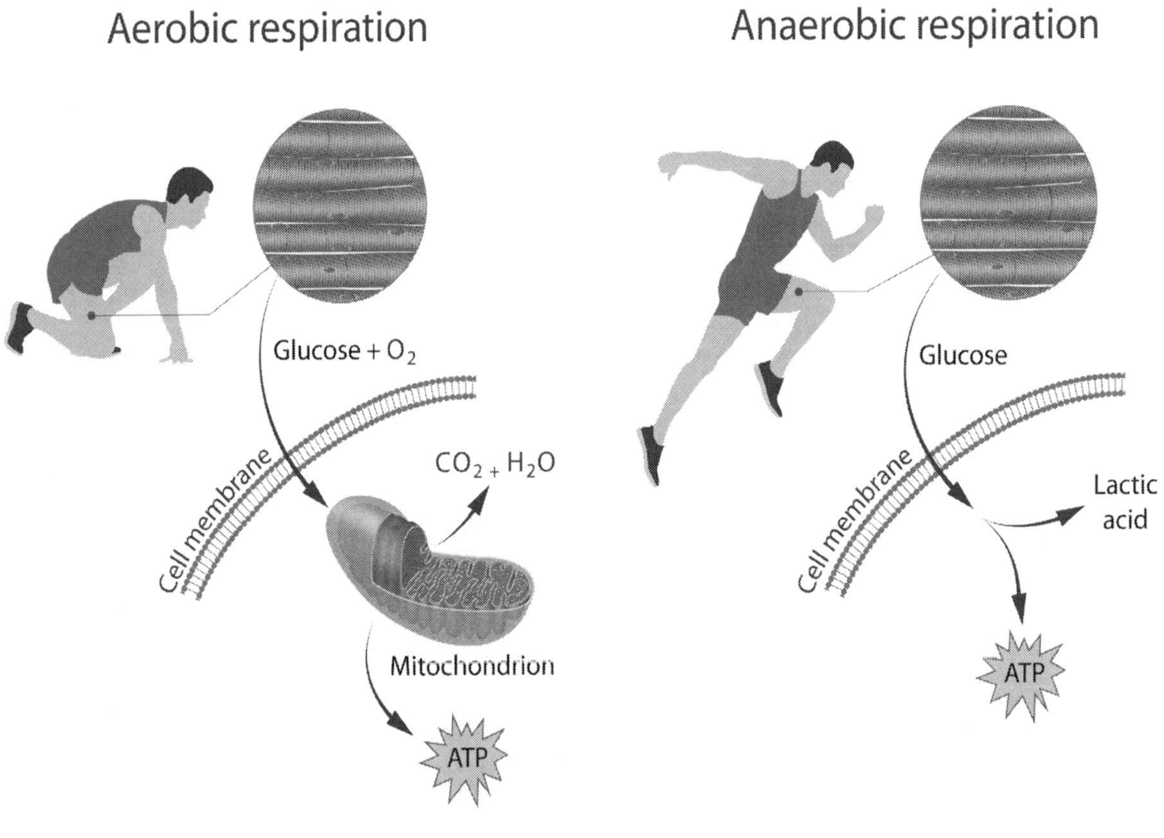

Muscles

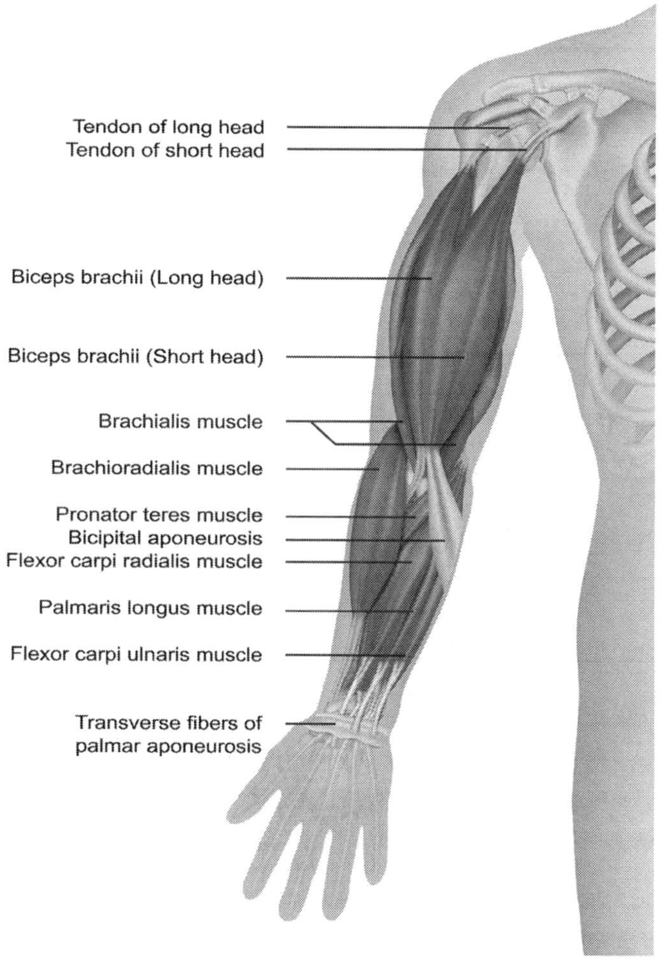

Anterior Right Upper Limb

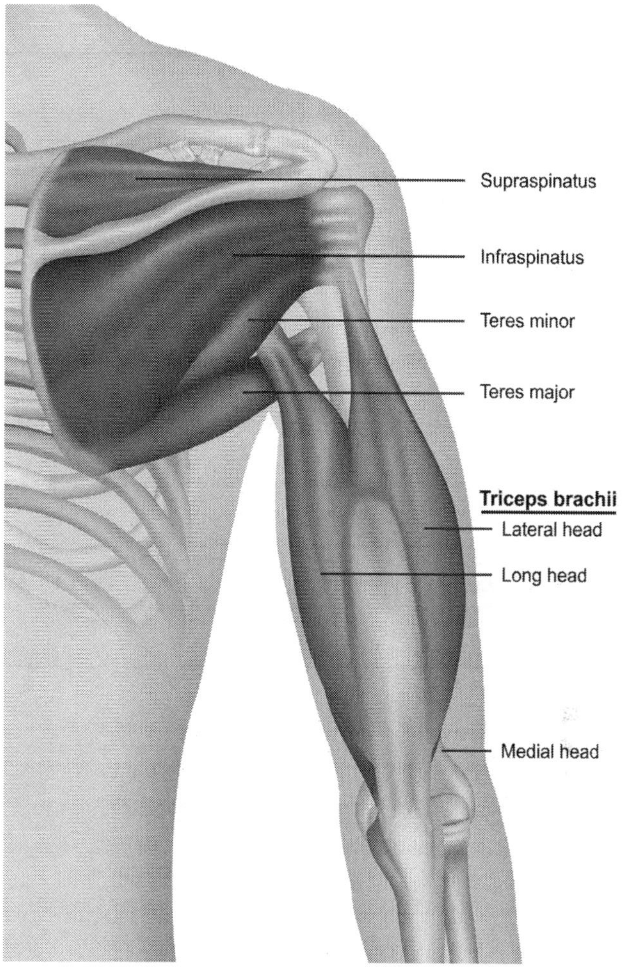

Posterior Right Upper Limb

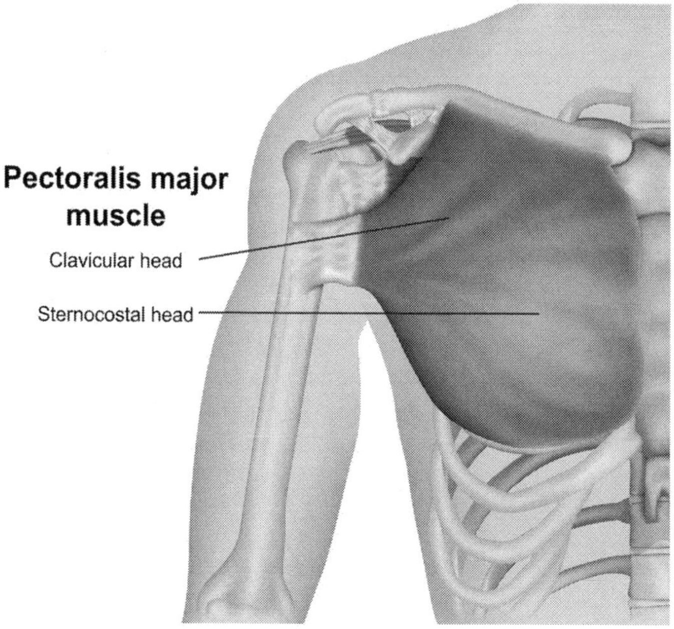

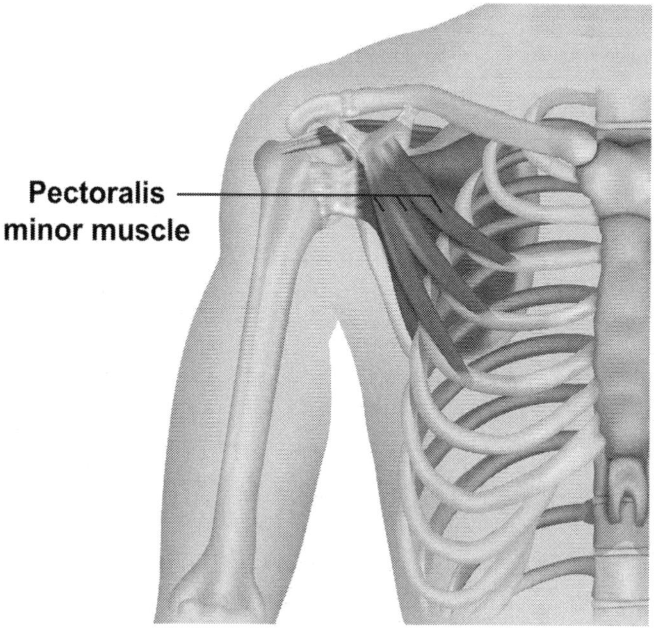

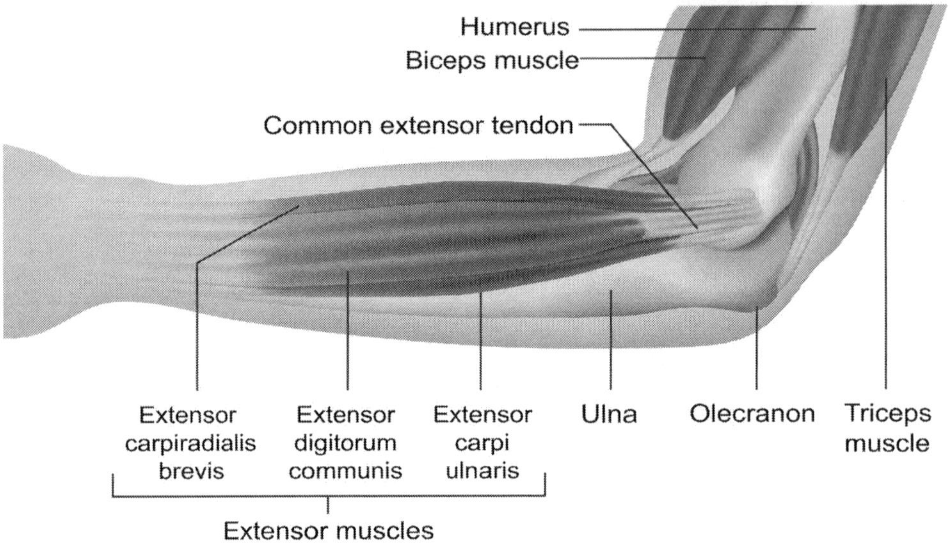
Humerus
Biceps muscle
Common extensor tendon
Extensor carpiradialis brevis
Extensor digitorum communis
Extensor carpi ulnaris
Extensor muscles
Ulna
Olecranon
Triceps muscle

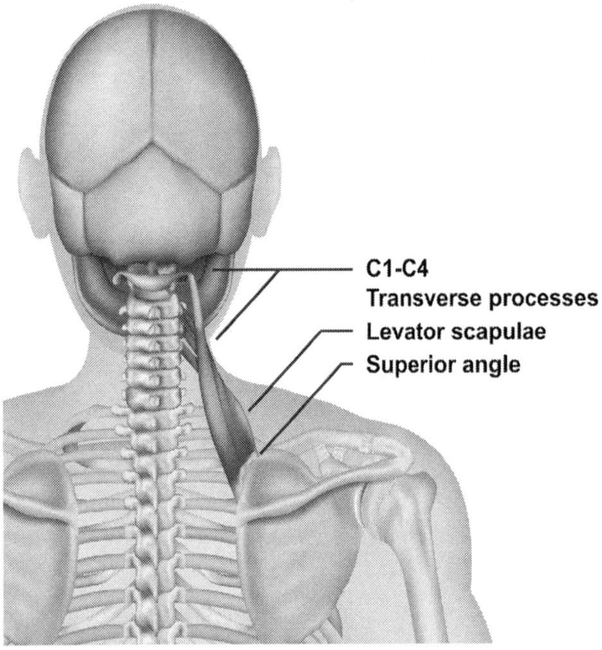
C1-C4
Transverse processes
Levator scapulae
Superior angle

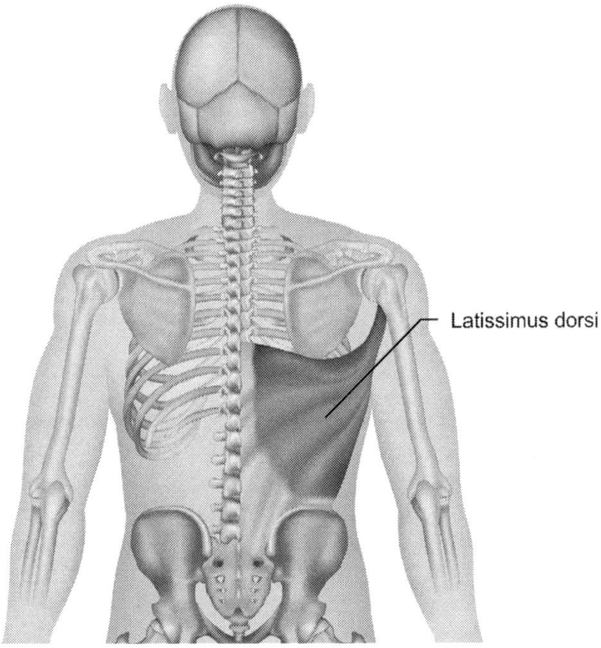
Latissimus dorsi

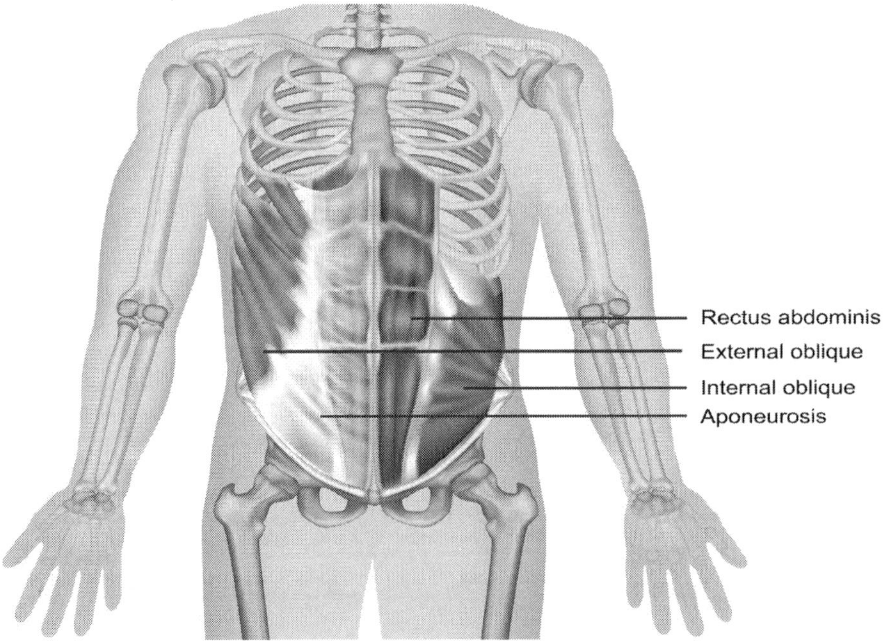
Rectus abdominis
External oblique
Internal oblique
Aponeurosis

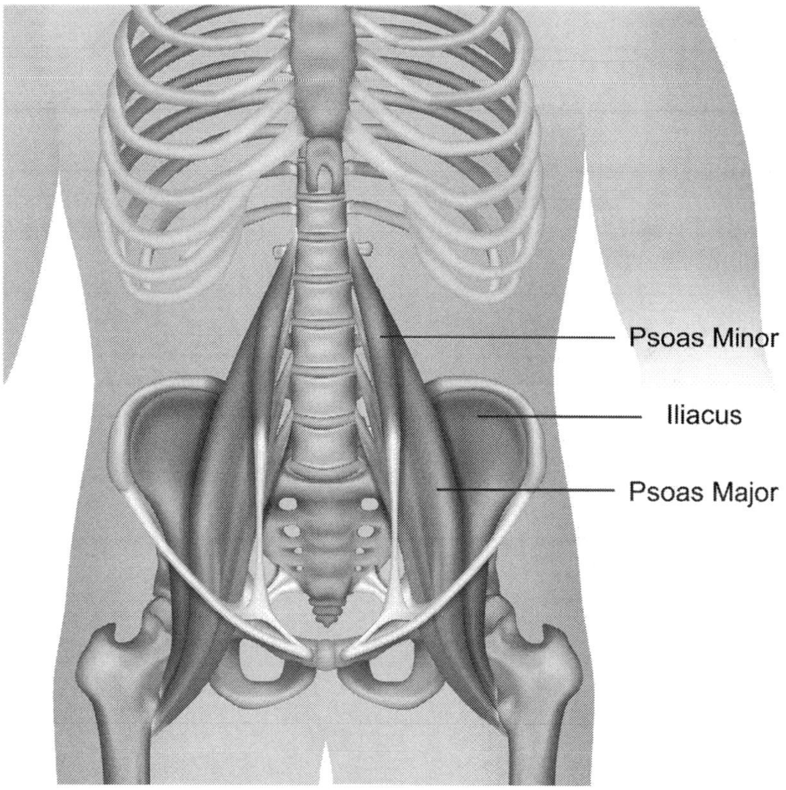
Psoas Minor
Iliacus
Psoas Major

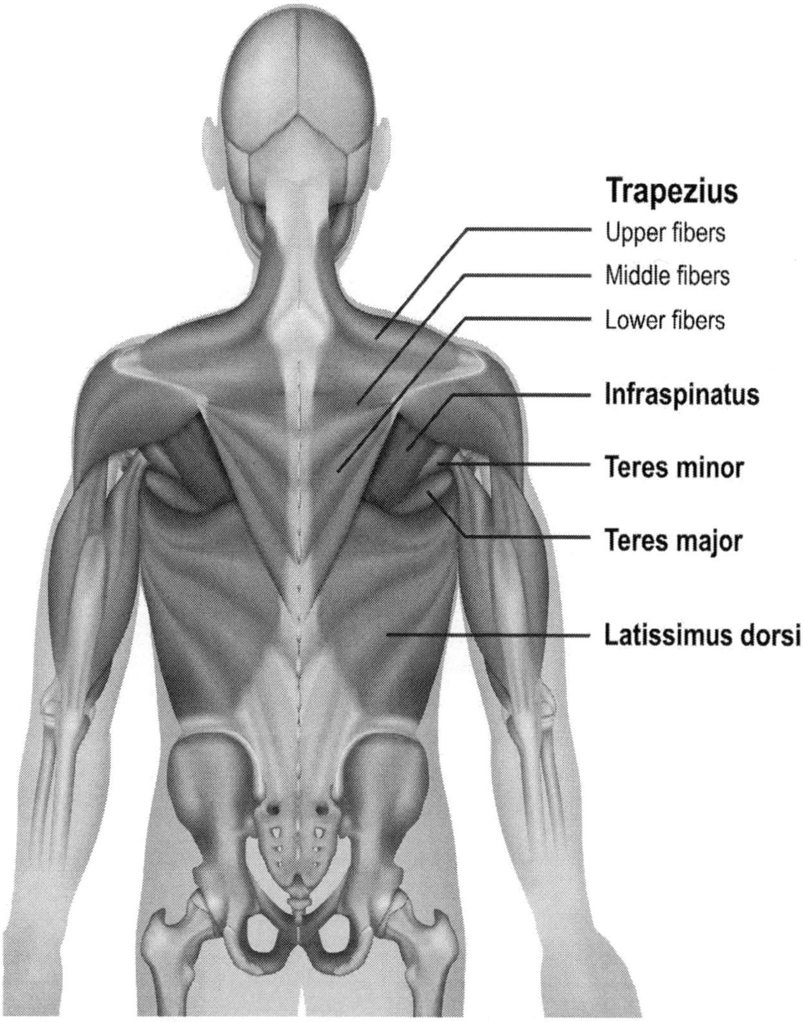
Trapezius
Upper fibers
Middle fibers
Lower fibers
Infraspinatus
Teres minor
Teres major
Latissimus dorsi

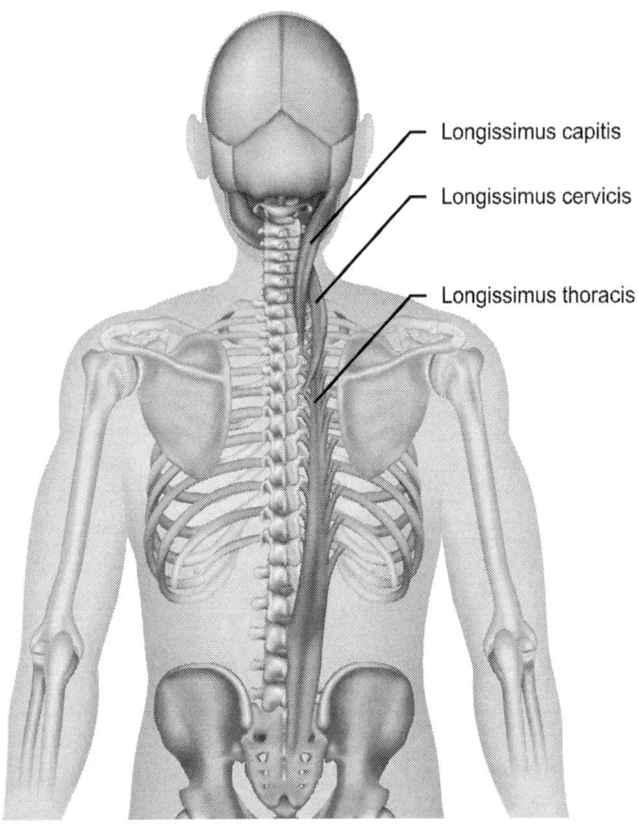
Longissimus capitis
Longissimus cervicis
Longissimus thoracis

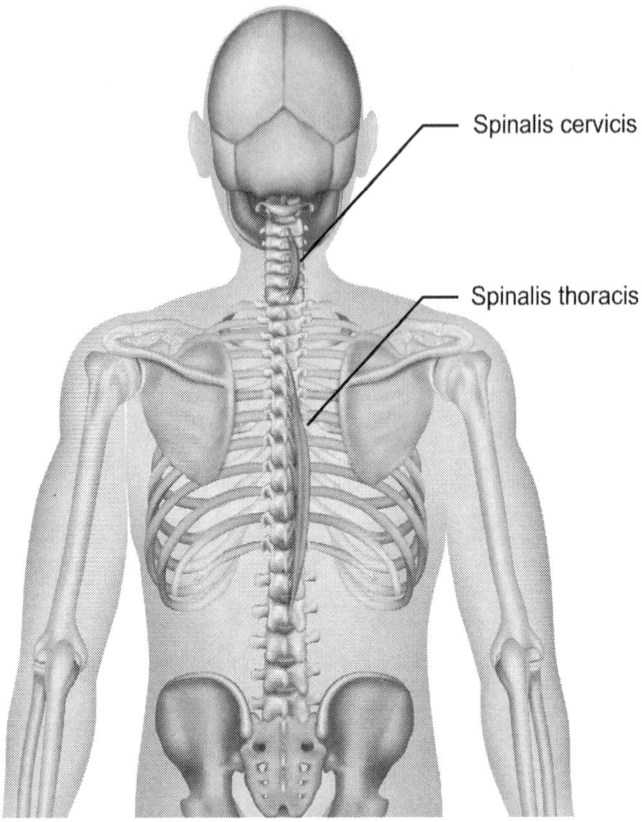
Spinalis cervicis
Spinalis thoracis

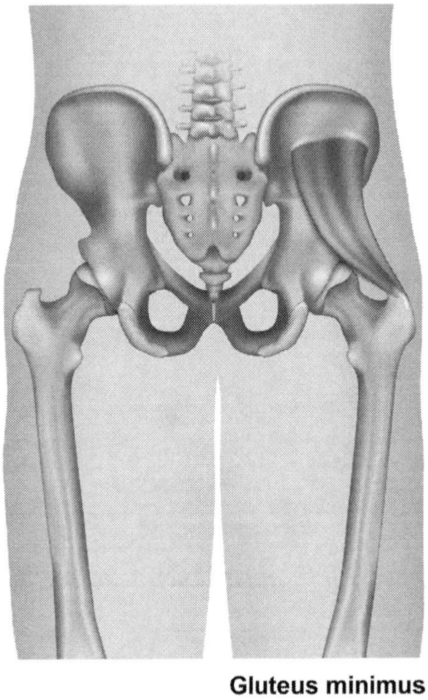
Gluteus minimus

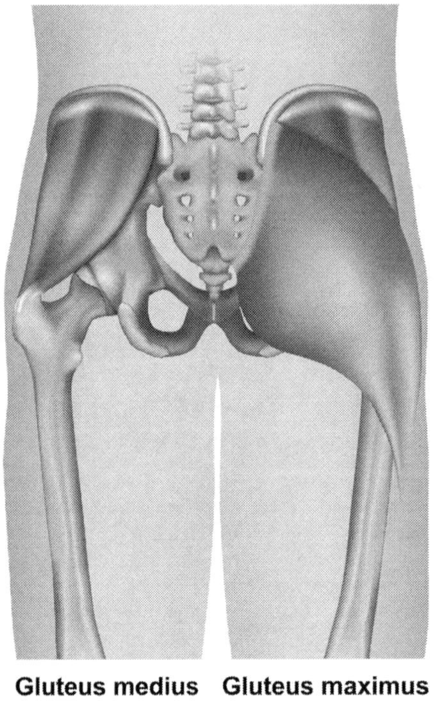
Gluteus medius
Gluteus maximus

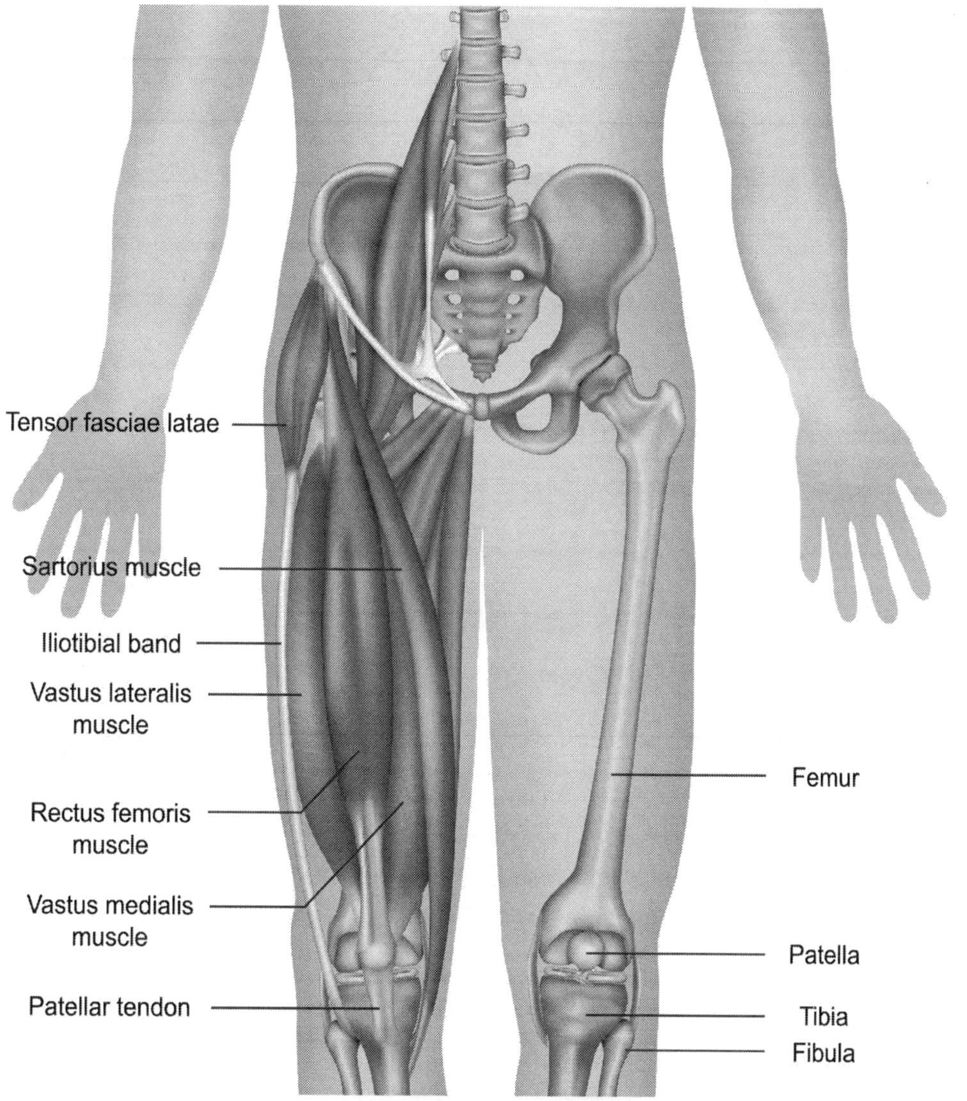
Tensor fasciae latae
Sartorius muscle
Iliotibial band
Vastus lateralis muscle
Rectus femoris muscle
Vastus medialis muscle
Patellar tendon
Femur
Patella
Tibia
Fibula

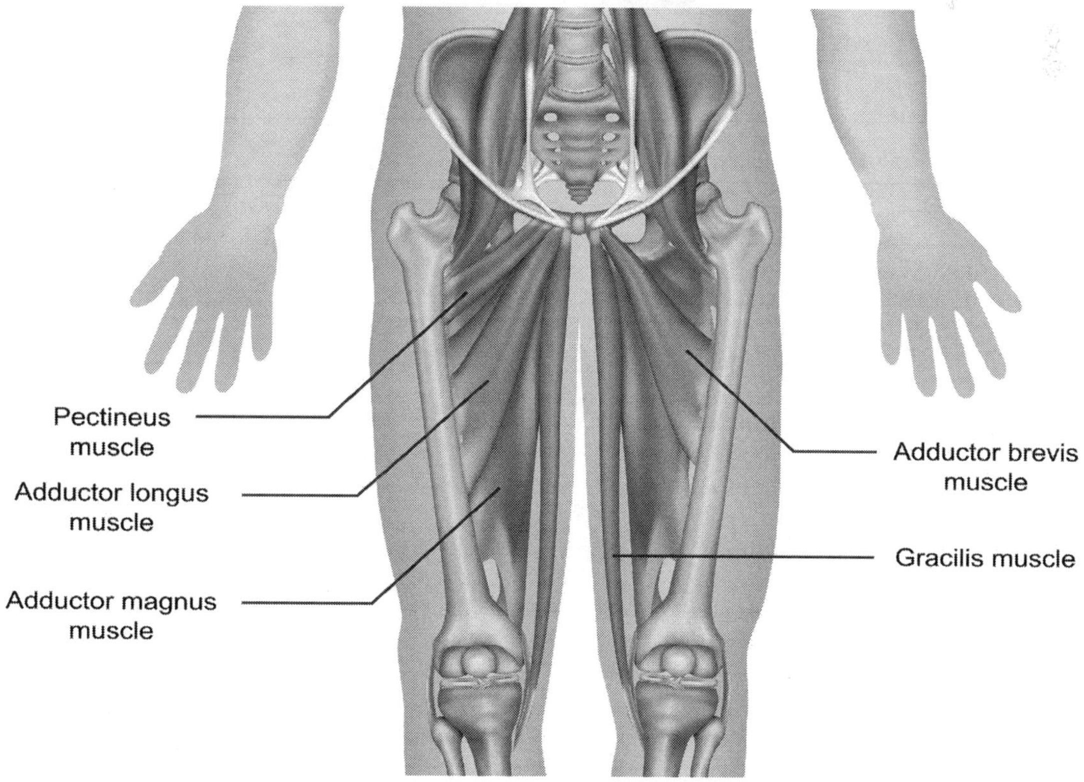
Pectineus muscle
Adductor longus muscle
Adductor magnus muscle
Adductor brevis muscle
Gracilis muscle

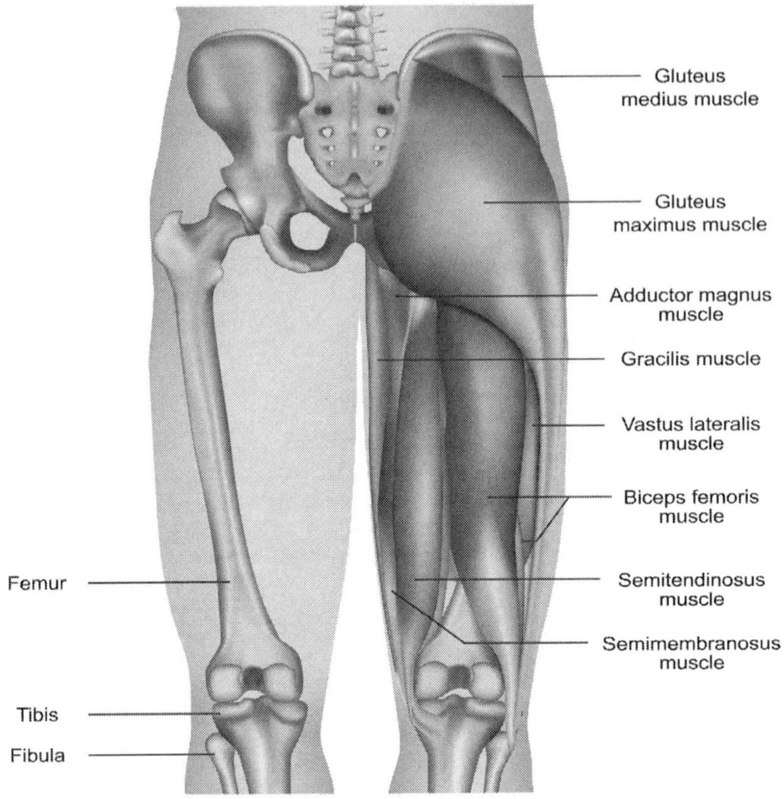
Gluteus
medius muscle
Gluteus
maximus muscle
Adductor magnus
muscle
Gracilis muscle
Vastus lateralis
muscle
Biceps femoris
muscle
Femur
Semitendinosus
muscle
Semimembranosus
muscle
Tibis
Fibula

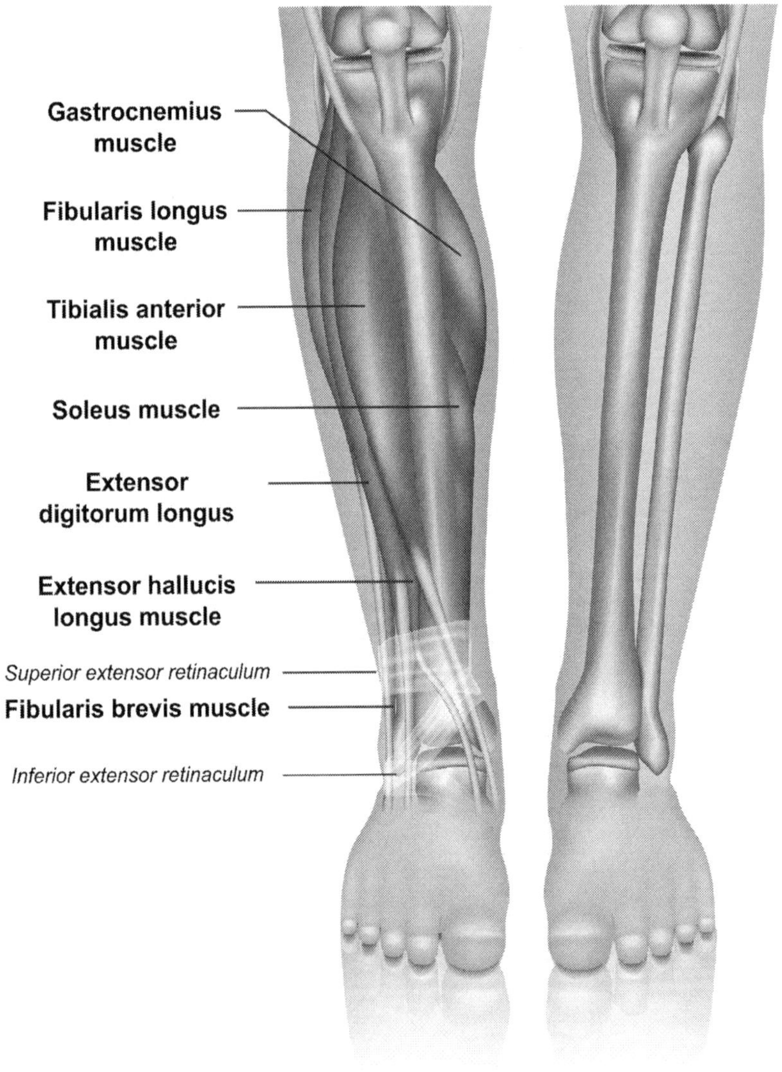
Gastrocnemius
muscle
Fibularis longus
muscle
Tibialis anterior
muscle
Soleus muscle
Extensor
digitorum longus
Extensor hallucis
longus muscle
Superior extensor retinaculum
Fibularis brevis muscle
Inferior extensor retinaculum

Nervous System

Nerves are structures in the Nervous System, made of nervous tissue. Nerves have many functions, from regulating vital functions within the body, to controlling muscles.

There are two divisions of the Nervous System: the **Central Nervous System**, and the **Peripheral Nervous System.** The Central Nervous System consists of the **brain and spinal cord**. The Central Nervous System is under involuntary control, responsible for interpretation of sensations and mental activity.

Central Nervous System

The brain consists of three parts: the **cerebrum**, which is the largest part of the brain and split into left and right hemispheres, the **cerebellum**, located at the back and bottom of the brain, and the **brain stem**, which connects the brain to the spinal cord.

Each side of the **cerebrum** is divided into **lobes**, named after the bones atop them: **frontal lobe**(processes motivation, aggression, mood), **temporal lobe**(processes memory, hearing, and smell), **parietal lobe**(processes most sensory information), and **occipital lobe**(processes vision).

The **cerebellum** is responsible for regulation of **muscle tone**, **balance**, **coordination**, and control of **general body movements.**

The **brain stem**, which consists of(in descending order) the **midbrain**, the **pons**, and the **medulla oblongata**, controls the **vital functions** of the body, such as breathing, heart rate, coughing, sneezing, vomiting, and blood vessel diameter.

Median section of the brain

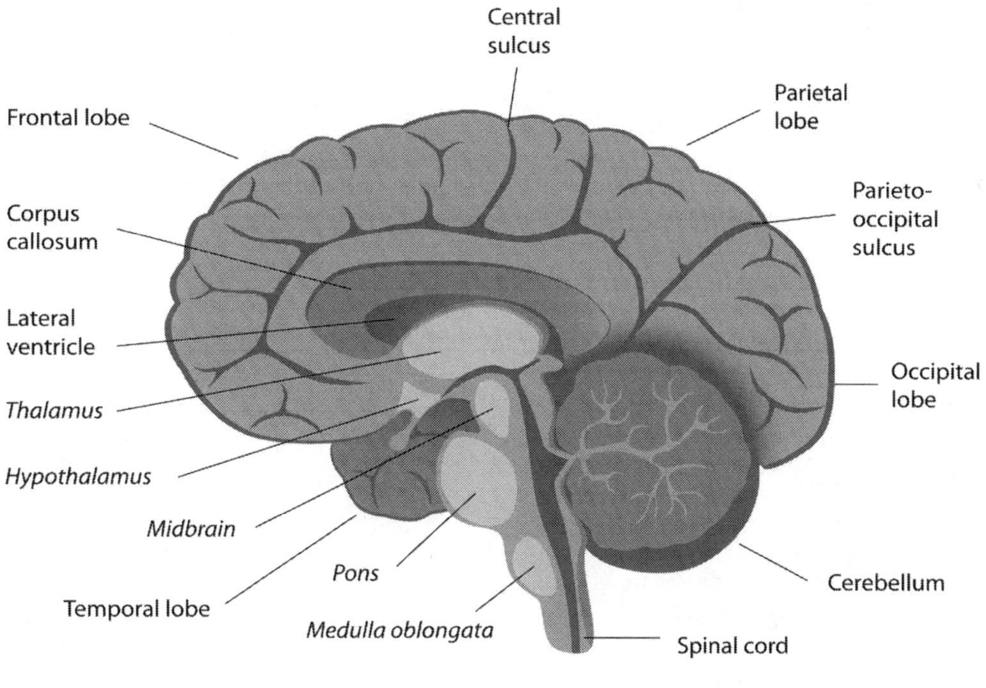

Meninges

Surrounding the brain and spinal cord are three layers of connective tissue known as the **meninges**. The deepest layer that comes into contact with the brain is known as the pia mater. The intermediate layer is known as the arachnoid. The most superficial layer, which comes into contact with the bones of the cranium, is known as the dura mater.

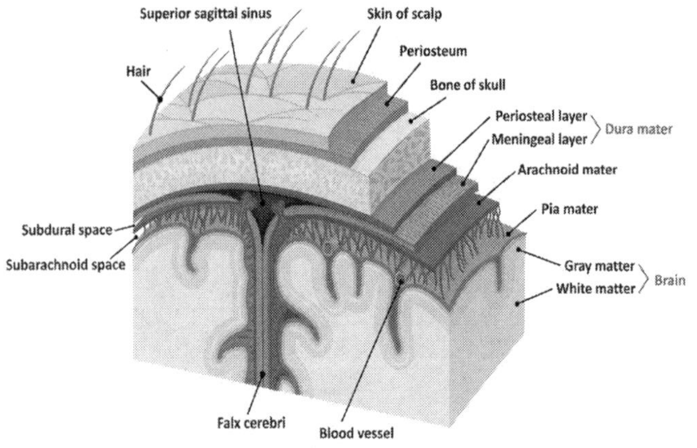

Pia Mater

The **pia mater**(tender mother), the **deepest layer**, is responsible for helping to protect the brain and spinal cord by containing cerebrospinal fluid. This fluid provides a cushion for the brain and spinal cord to help prevent injury. The pia mater is very delicate, and covers the brain completely by extending into the folds.

Arachnoid

The **arachnoid**, which is the **intermediate layer** of the meninges, is separated from the pia mater by subarachnoid space. The subarachnoid space contains cerebrospinal fluid, which helps to cushion and protect the brain and spinal cord. The arachnoid resembles cob webs or spider webs, which is where it gets its name. It is made of fibrous material that fluid is easily able to pass through. Unlike the pia mater, the arachnoid does not extend into the folds of the brain. The arachnoid is wrapped loosely around the brain.

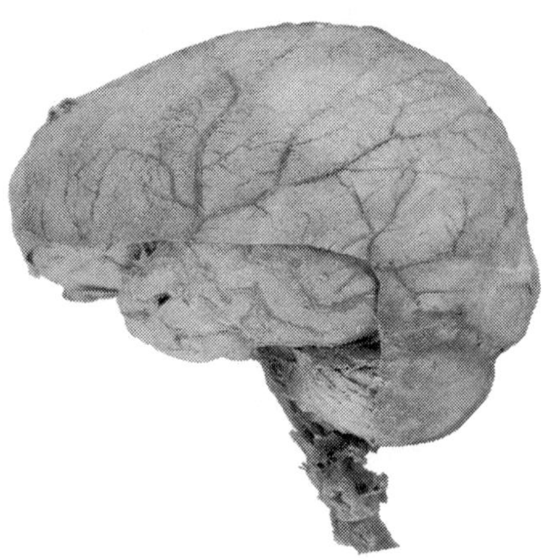

Brain covered with dura mater

Dura Mater

The **dura mater**(tough mother) is the **most superficial and strongest layer** of the meninges. The dura mater is responsible for protecting the brain by providing a thick padding around it. The dura mater is made of fibrous tissue, giving it the ability to properly protect the brain and spinal cord. It contains large blood vessels than branch off into capillaries that go into the pia mater.

Peripheral Nervous System

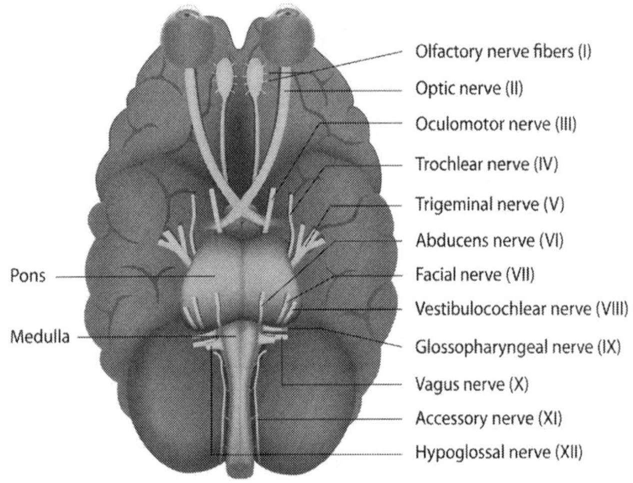

The Peripheral Nervous System consists of the body's **nerves**. There are two divisions of the Peripheral Nervous System: **Cranial Nerves** and **Spinal Nerves**. Cranial Nerves emerge from the brain, and help to regulate the functions of the head and face. There are **twelve pairs of Cranial Nerves**, each numbered in Roman Numerals:

- Olfactory(I)
- Optic(II)
- Oculomotor(III)
- Trochlear(IV)
- Trigeminal(V)
- Abducens(VI)
- Facial(VII)
- Vestibulocochlear(VIII)
- Glossopharyngeal(IX)
- Vagus(X)
- Accessory(XI)
- Hypoglossal(XII)

Spinal Nerves are much more numerous than Cranial Nerves. There are **31 pairs of Spinal Nerves**. The Spinal Nerves emerge from the spinal cord, and are responsible for controlling skeletal muscle.

A bundle of Spinal Nerves that emerge from the spinal cord is known as a **plexus**. There are three plexi in the body: **Cervical Plexus, Brachial Plexus, Lumbosacral Plexus**. The Cervical Plexus emerges from the spinal cord in the range of **C1-C4**. The primary nerve of the Cervical Plexus is known as the **Phrenic Nerve**. The Phrenic Nerve descends inferiorly from the cervical vertebrae and innervates(provides nervous stimulation to) the **diaphragm**.

Brachial Plexus

The Brachial Plexus emerges from the spinal cord at **C5-T1**. The nerves of the Brachial Plexus move distally, controlling the muscles of the **upper limb**. There are five primary nerves of the Brachial Plexus:

Radial
Musculocutaneous
Axillary
Median
Ulnar

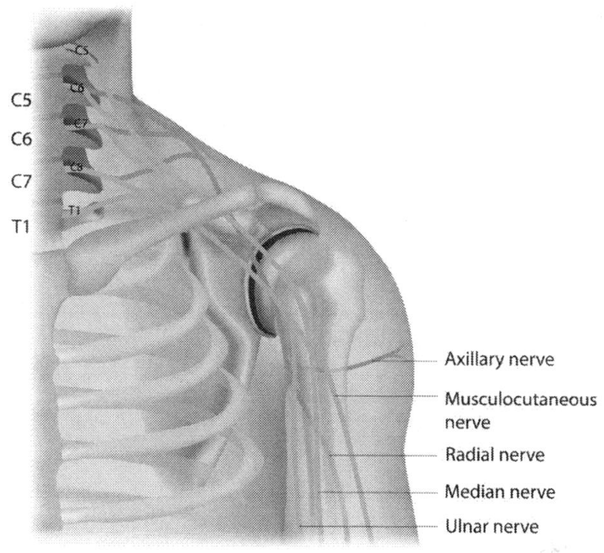

The **Radial Nerve** is located on the posterior arm and forearm, and innervates the triceps brachii, anconeus, brachioradialis, and wrist extensors.

The **Musculocutaneous Nerve** is located in the anterior arm, and innervates the biceps brachii, brachialis, and coracobrachialis.

The **Axillary Nerve** is primarily located in the armpit, and innervates the teres minor and deltoid.

The **Median Nerve** is located in the anterior arm, forearm, and hand, and innervates the wrist flexors, and most muscles on the lateral side of the hand.

The **Ulnar Nerve** is located on the anterior arm, medial forearm, and medial hand, and innervates the wrist flexors and most muscles on the medial side of the hand.

Lumbosacral Plexus

The Lumbosacral Plexus emerges from the **entire span** of the lumbar and sacral vertebrae. The major nerves of the Lumbosacral Plexus include:

- Sciatic
- Femoral
- Obturator
- Tibial
- Common Peroneal
- Deep Peroneal
- Superficial Peroneal

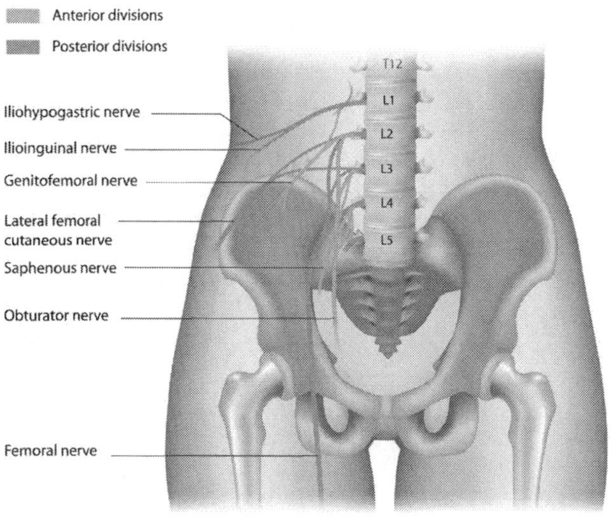

The **Sciatic Nerve** is a large nerve located on the posterior thigh. The Sciatic Nerve is actually both the Tibial Nerve and the Common Peroneal Nerve bundled together. Once the Sciatic Nerve reaches the back of the knee, it branches off into two separate nerves. The Sciatic Nerve innervates the Hamstring muscle group.

The **Femoral Nerve** is located on the anterior thigh, and innervates the quadriceps muscle group, iliacus, sartorius, and pectineus.

The **Obturator Nerve** is located on the medial portion of the thigh, and innervates the adductor muscle group.

The **Tibial Nerve**, after branching off the Sciatic nerve, runs down the posterior leg, and innervates the gastrocnemius, soleus, tibialis posterior, and plantaris.

The **Common Peroneal Nerve**, after branching off the Sciatic Nerve, actually branches off into two other nerves of its own: The Deep Peroneal and Superficial Peroneal Nerves.

The **Deep Peroneal Nerve** is located on the anterior leg, and innervates the tibialis anterior.

The **Superficial Peroneal Nerve** is located on the lateral portion of the leg, along the fibula, and innervates the peroneus longus.

Autonomic Nervous System

The autonomic nervous system helps to **regulate homeostasis** by release of hormones, controlling heart rate, breathing rate, and other bodily functions. There are two divisions of the autonomic nervous system: the **Sympathetic Nervous System**, and the **Parasympathetic Nervous System**.

Sympathetic Response

The Sympathetic Nervous System is also known as "**fight-or-flight**". When the body is in a state of **stress**, the Sympathetic Nervous System helps the body respond by releasing **norepinephrine** into the blood stream, which **increases heart rate and blood sugar**. The digestive organs will also shut down, and blood will be pulled from these organs and supplied to the muscles for use.

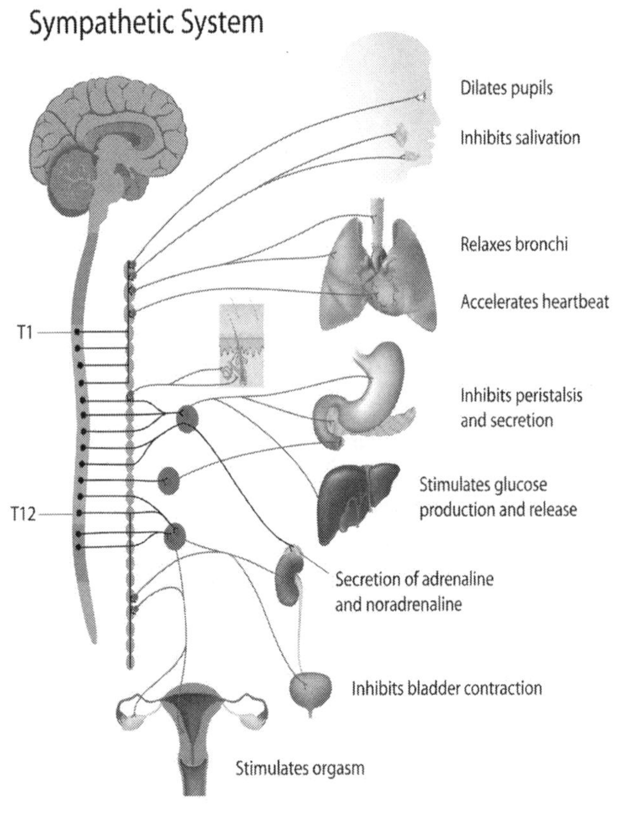

Parasympathetic Response

The Parasympathetic Nervous System is also known as "**rest-and-digest**". When the body is in a state of **relaxation**, the Parasympathetic Nervous System helps the body to calm itself. It decreases the body's heart rate, and increases blood flow to the digestive organs to **increase peristalsis.** The Parasympathetic Nervous System, decreasing heart rate, and peristalsis are all controlled by the **Vagus Nerve.**

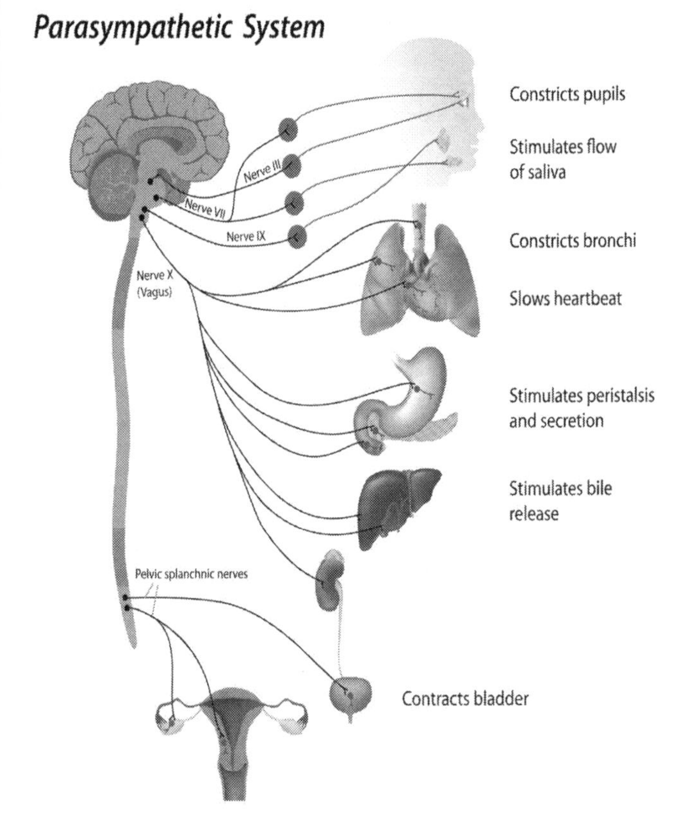

Reproductive System

The Reproductive System is responsible for **reproduction**, or the creation of offspring. Many organs and structures in the Reproductive System are shared with other body systems, such as the urethra, testes, and ovaries. There are two subcategories: the **Male Reproductive System** and **Female Reproductive System**. Each vary in structures and function.

Male Reproductive System

The Male Reproductive System is responsible for the production of **spermatozoa**(sperm) and male hormones, such as testosterone. Major structures of the Male Reproductive System include the penis, testes, scrotum, and ducts that carry sperm.

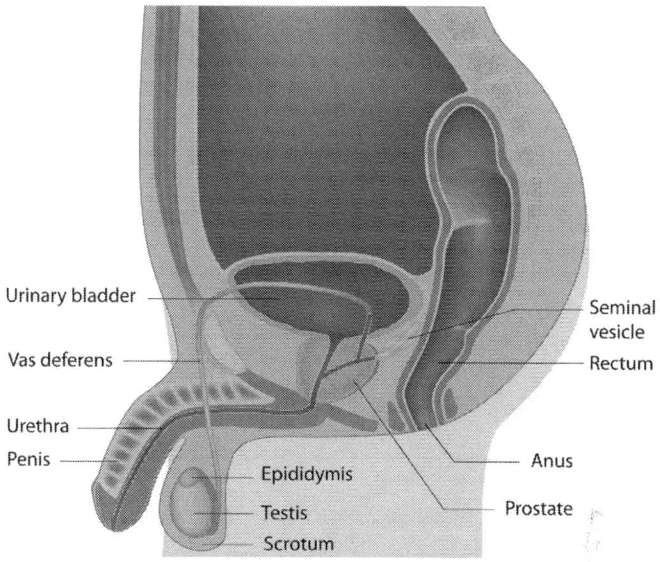

The **penis** is the primary organ of the Male Reproductive System, responsible for **sexual intercourse**, which allows passage of sperm outside the body through the urethra. The penis also allows urine to leave the body. During sexual arousal, nerves cause blood vessels in the penis to dilate, which then causes the penis to fill with blood. This results in an erection.

The **testes** are responsible for the production of **testosterone**. They are also responsible for **spermatogenesis**, or sperm production. After the testes produce sperm, it is stored in a tube located atop each testicle, known as the **epididymis**. Upon ejaculation, the sperm leaves the epididymis and enters the vas deferens.

The **vas deferens** are tubes that connect the **epididymis to the urethra**. During ejaculation, smooth muscle in the walls of the vas deferens contract rhythmically(known as peristalsis), forcing sperm into the urethra. The sperm mixes with secretions from structures such as the prostate, which creates semen.

Female Reproductive System

The Female Reproductive System is responsible for the production of **egg cells**, estrogen, progesterone, and **fetal development**. Major structures of the Female Reproductive System include the vagina, ovaries, fallopian tubes, uterus, and cervix.

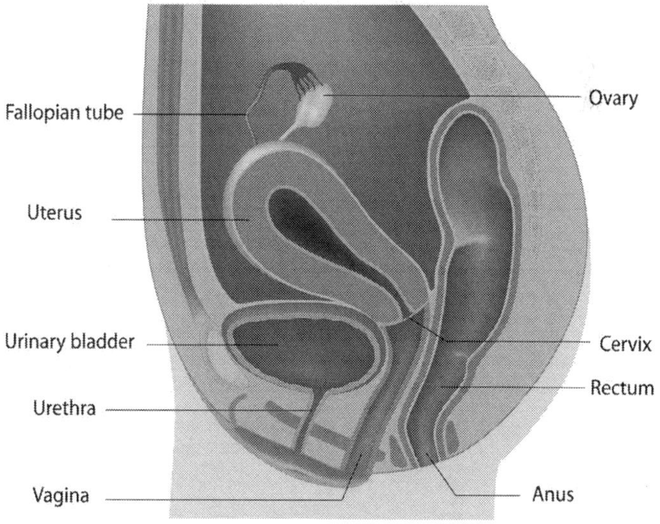

The **vagina** is the **passageway** located between the cervix and the opening to the outside of the body. The vagina is often confused with the outer, visible portion, known as the vulva. The vagina allows a passageway for the penis during sexual intercourse.

The **ovaries** are responsible for the production of **estrogen and progesterone**. The ovaries are also the structures that produce and release **egg cells**(oocytes) in women. Eggs are typically released once a month from one ovary.

The **fallopian tubes** allow **passage of oocytes** from the ovaries to the uterus. Fertilization most commonly occurs in the fallopian tubes.

The **uterus** is an inverted pear-shaped organ responsible for the **development of a fetus**. Upon fertilization, the embryo attaches to the wall of the uterus. The placenta develops, which connects to the embryo, providing it with blood flow and nutrients to help it grow. During childbirth, the placenta detaches from the uterus and exits through the cervix and vagina.

The **cervix** is a narrow, circular passage that connects the **vagina to the uterus**. During pregnancy, the cervix is closed by a thick layer of mucous. During childbirth, the cervix dilates widely, which allows a passage for the child to pass through.

Respiratory System

The Respiratory System has one essential function: to **bring oxygen into the body**, and **eliminate wastes such as carbon dioxide** from the body. The main organs of the Respiratory System are the **lungs**. The left lung has two lobes and is smaller than the right lung, which has three lobes. This is due to the presence of the heart on the left side of the chest.

Conduction of air is controlled by the **nose**. Air enters the body through the nose, and is filtered by **hair and mucous**. The nose also warms the air as it enters the body.

The **larynx**, also known as the voice box, is a short tube located inferior to the pharynx. As air passes over the vocal cords in the larynx, the **vocal cords vibrate**, which **produces sound** used with the tongue to create speech.

Sitting atop the larynx is a flap of tissue known as the **epiglottis**. Upon swallowing, the epiglottis lies on top of the larynx, blocking any food or fluid from entering the larynx, which **prevents choking**.

Connecting to the larynx inferiorly is a tube of cartilage known as the **trachea**, or the wind pipe. The trachea is the primary passageway for air to enter into the lungs.

Once air enters the lungs, it goes into each lung through **bronchial tubes**, which branch off of the trachea. These tubes branch into smaller tubes called bronchioles. Bronchial tubes **secrete mucous**, which helps to trap any dirt or debris that have made it into the lungs.

At the end of the bronchioles are tiny **air sacs**, known as **alveoli**. The alveoli resemble a cluster of grapes. Capillaries attach to the alveoli and move blood across the surface of the alveoli. This allows carbon dioxide to detach from the erythrocytes and exit the blood stream, and also allows oxygen to enter the blood stream and attach to erythrocytes. Alveoli are where **gas exchange** occurs in the Respiratory System.

Respiration is accomplished by contraction of the **diaphragm**, a large muscle connected to the rib cage that separates the chest from the abdomen. The diaphragm creates a vacuum inside the chest. When it contracts, it descends, pulling the chest down. This allows air to enter into the lungs. When the diaphragm relaxes, it ascends up into the chest, which forces air out of the lungs.

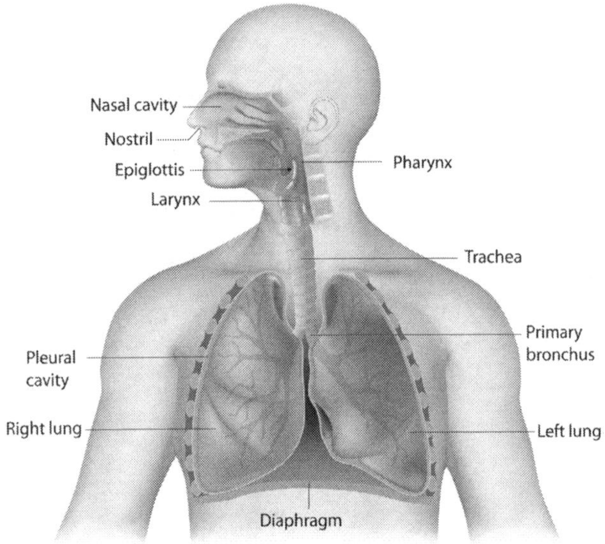

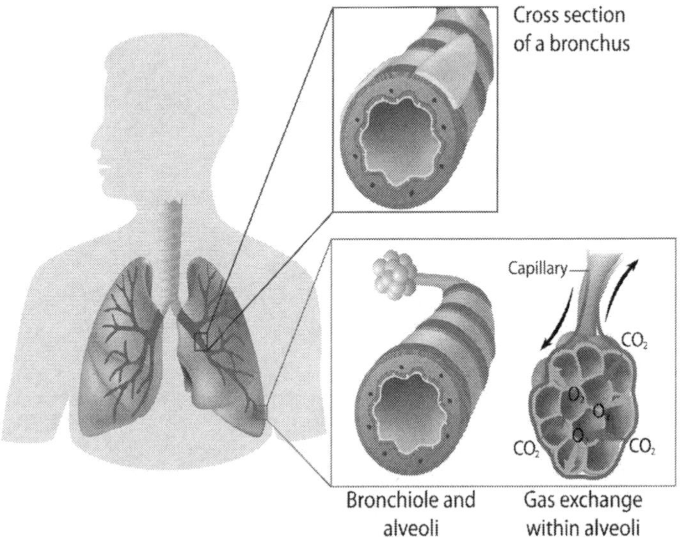

DID YOU KNOW?

There are four major structures that pass through the diaphragm: the aorta, the inferior vena cava, the thoracic duct, and the esophagus!

Skeletal System

The Skeletal System is a vital component of movement. Muscles attach to bones, and when a muscle contracts, it pulls on a bone(or bones), which performs an action. Bones also produce blood cells, provide stability for the body, and protect structures and organs in the body.

There are **206 bones** in the human body. Each bone can be classified as one of the following: Long bone, Short bone, Irregular bone, Flat bone, Sesamoid bone.

Long bones appear **longer than they are wide**. There are numerous long bones in the body, including, but not limited to, the clavicle, humerus, femur, metatarsals, and phalanges.

Short bones are **as long as they are wide**. Examples include the carpals and tarsals.

Irregular bones are bones that have generally **unusual shapes**. Examples include the mandible, vertebrae, and pubis.

Flat bones are named after how they look: **flat**. They are typically thin and flat. Examples include the scapula, ribs, and cranial bones.

Sesamoid bones are bones **embedded inside tendons**, and named after what they look like. They are rounded, and resemble **sesame seeds**. The primary examples are the patella and pisiform.

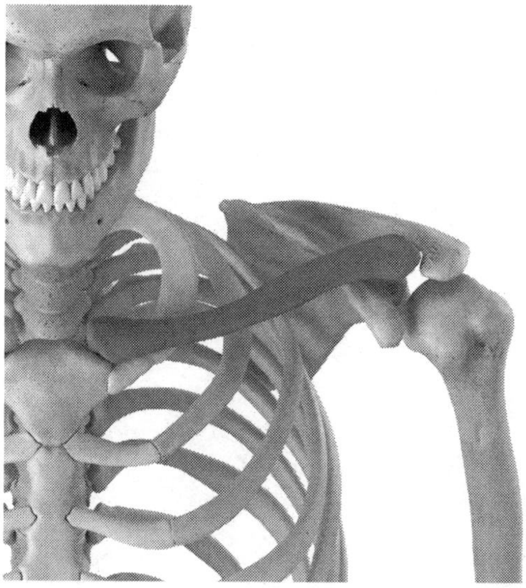

Long Bone(Clavicle)

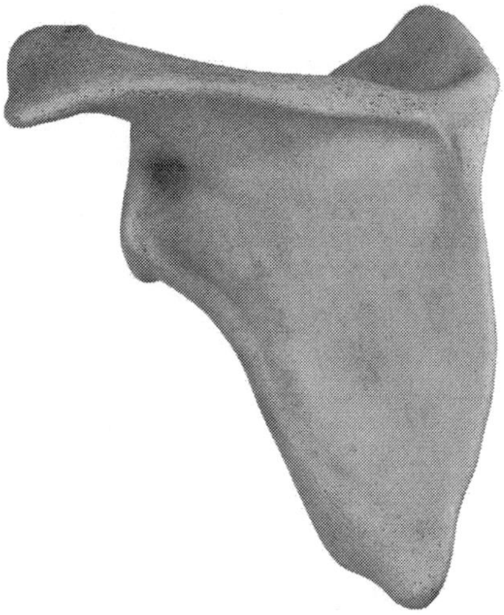

Flat Bone(Scapula)

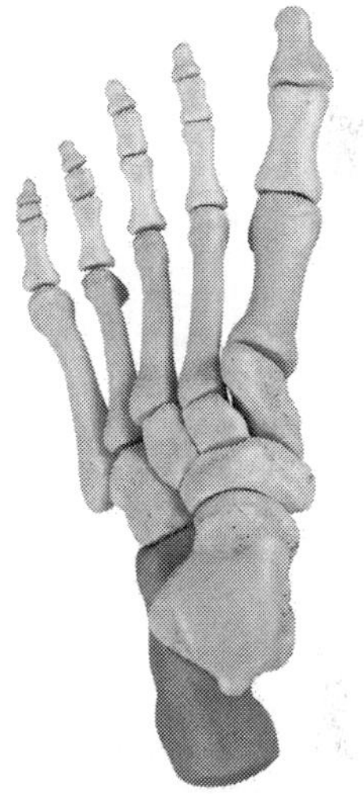

Short Bone(Calcaneus)

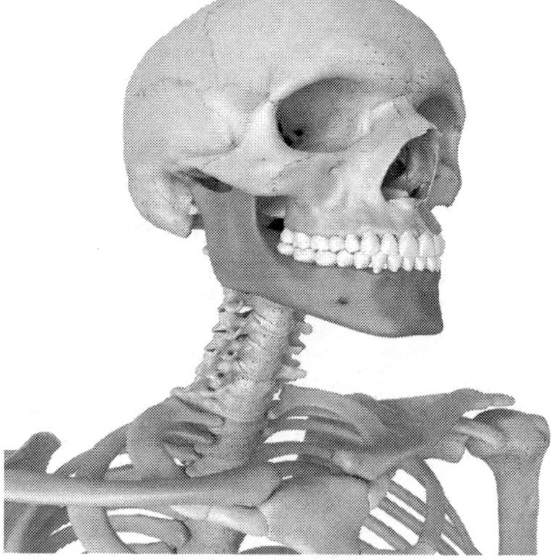

Irregular Bone(Mandible)

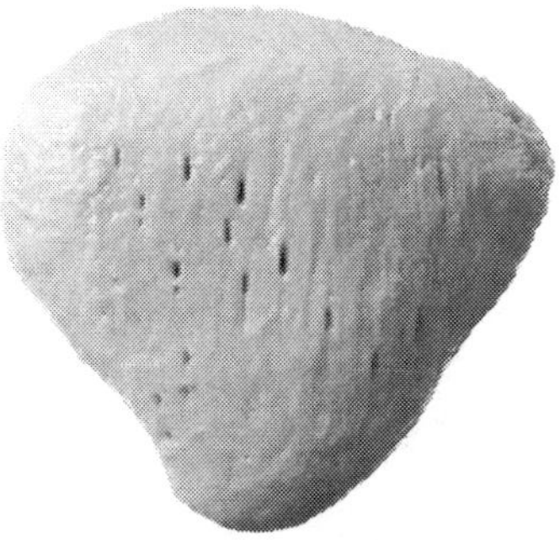

Sesamoid Bone(Patella)

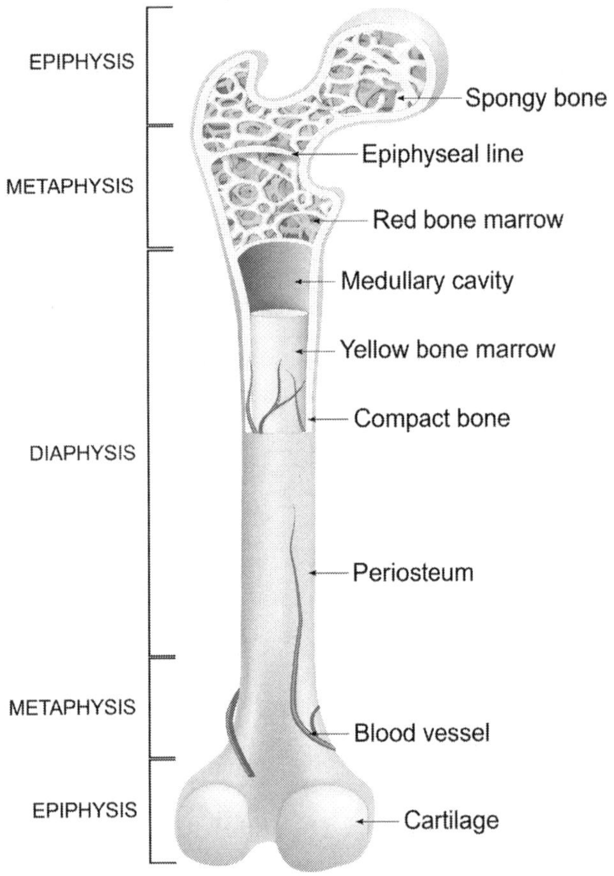

Long Bone Structure

Long bones consist of three main parts: the epiphyses, the metaphyses, and the diaphysis. The **epiphyses** can be found on the **ends of the long bone**, where the bone articulates with other bones. The epiphyses are **covered with cartilage** to prevent friction between the articulating bone surfaces. The epiphyses are primarily made of spongy bone, which allows certain bones to withstand extreme pressure without fracturing, such as the femur.

The **metaphyses** are the sections between the epiphyses and the diaphysis. Inside the metaphyses, there is a line of cartilage called the **epiphyseal plate/line**, and it is where **growth in the bone** takes place during childhood and adolescence. As a person grows, eventually the cartilage ossifies and becomes part of the bone, and growth in the bone no longer occurs.

The **diaphysis** is the **shaft of the bone**. Inside the shaft of the bone is the medullary cavity. The medullary cavity contains **red bone marrow** during childhood, which is the site of **red blood cell formation**. When the child ages, the red bone marrow is converted into yellow bone marrow, which is mainly just fat. The diaphysis is made of compact bone to provide as much strength as possible around the medullary cavity, while still giving enough space for the cavity itself to fill with marrow.

Joints

Where bones come together is known as an **articulation**. Another name for articulation is "joint". Joints are where **movements occur**. We don't flex muscles, we flex joints!

All joints are classified as one of the following: Synarthrotic, Amphiarthrotic, or Diarthrotic. **Synarthrotic joints** are joints with **little to no movement** in them, such as the sutures in the skull. **Amphiarthrotic joints** are joints that are **slightly movable**, such as the intervertebral joints. **Diarthrotic joints** are **freely movable** joints, and have no real movement restrictions, such as in the shoulder or hip.

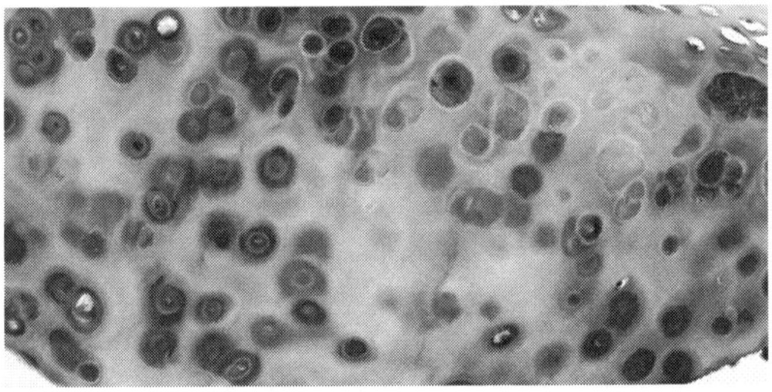

Hyaline cartilage

Joints have several structures that help create and support them. Between bones that articulate, on the epiphyses, there is **articular cartilage**. This type of cartilage is known as **hyaline cartilage**. It is a dense form of cartilage, very thick, and is a shock-absorber. Hyaline cartilage also **prevents friction** between the articulating bones, so bones don't rub against each other during movement.

Easy to Remember: To remember the joint classifications, just think of "SAD". This tells you the joint classifications in order from least movable joint to most movable joint. Synarthrosis, Amphiarthrosis, Diarthrosis.

Certain joints have a specific type of cartilage in them known as a **labrum**. The labrum, found in the glenohumeral joint and acetabulofemoral joint, is used to **deepen the joint**, providing a deeper socket for these ball-and-socket joints. This provides more **strength and stability** for the joint.

Bones are held together by **ligaments**. Ligaments are avascular, meaning they are not supplied with blood by blood vessels. Ligaments are strong, but do not stretch very far before injury can occur.

Four of the most important joints joined together by ligaments are located in the skull, between the cranial bones. These synarthrotic joints are called **sutures.** The **sagittal suture** runs along a sagittal plane on the top of the head, connecting the **two parietal bones.** The **coronal suture** runs on a coronal plane, connecting the **frontal bone** to the **parietal bones.** The **squamous suture** runs on a sagittal plane, but is located on the side of the skull, connecting the **parietal and temporal bones** together. Finally, the **lambdoid suture**, named for its resemblance to the Greek letter "lambda", connects the **occipital bone** to the **parietal bones.**

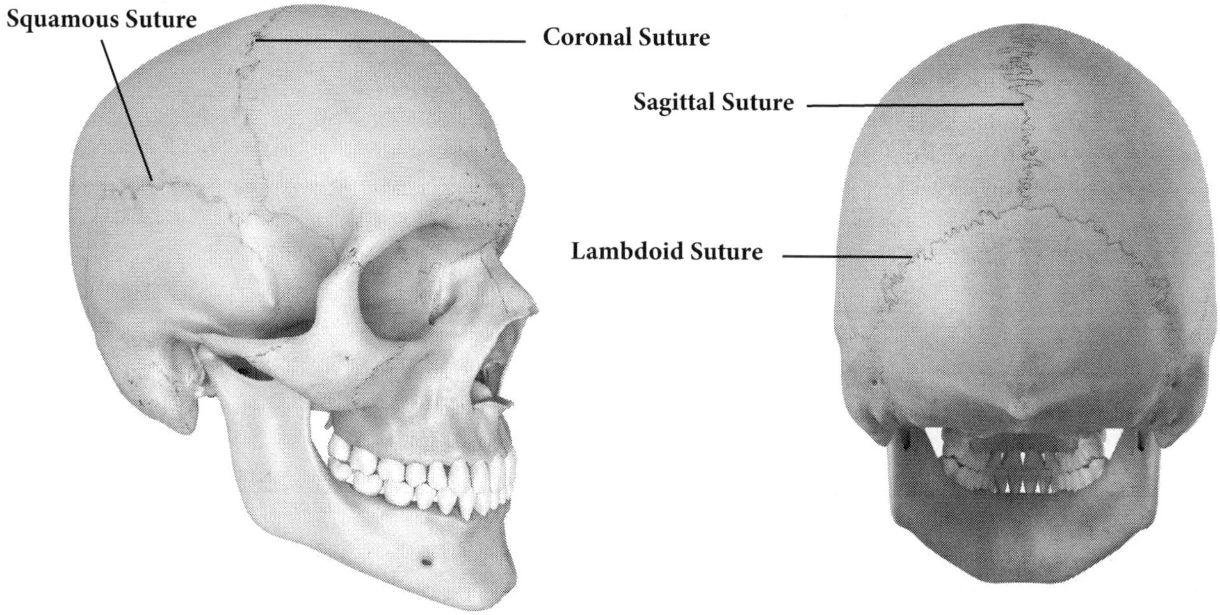

Muscles are held to bones via **tendons.** Tendons are similar to ligaments, but have a much more rich blood supply, and are able to stretch further before injury occurs.

Inside the joint itself, a membrane is present, known as the **synovial membrane.** The synovial membrane produces a fluid that helps to **lubricate the joint**, known as the **synovial fluid.** Lubrication of the joint is key in keeping the joint functioning optimally. Surrounding the entire joint is thick, dense connective tissue known as the **joint capsule.** The joint capsule keeps everything inside the joint, such as the synovial fluid, and provides even more strength and support for the joint.

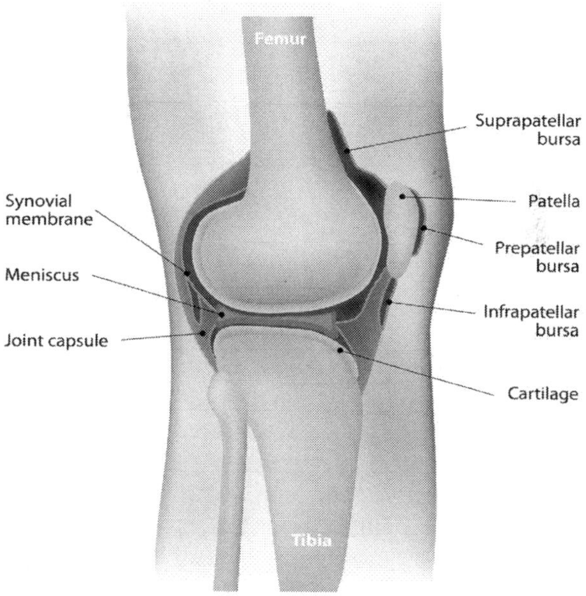

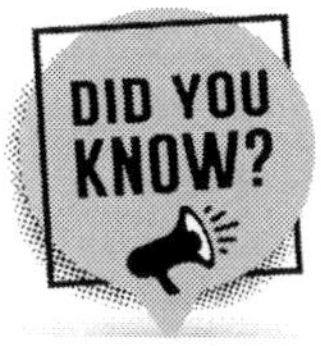

There are 360 joints in an average adult's body!

Types of Synovial Joints

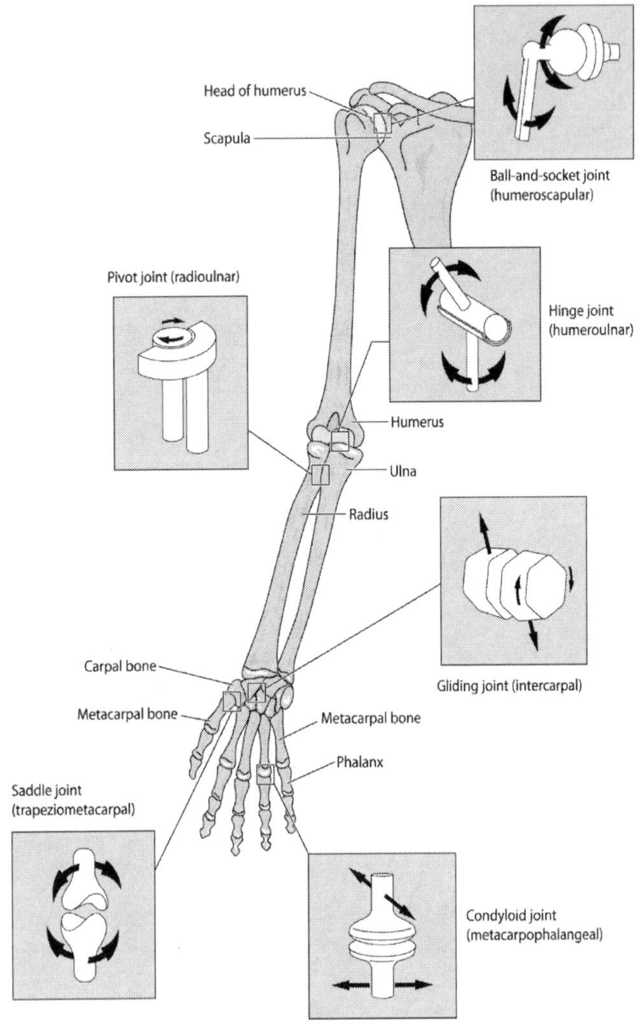

There are six different types of synovial joints.

Ball-and-Socket joints feature one bone with a **ball** at the epiphysis, and another bone with a **socket**. The ball fits in the socket, creating a ball-and-socket joint. Examples include the shoulder and hip joints. Ball-and-socket joints have the most amount of movement, able to move the joint in really any direction.

Hinge joints act much like the hinge on a door, only opening and closing. Hinge joints only allow movement in **one plane**, allowing only **flexion and extension**. Examples include the elbow and knee joints.

Pivot joints allow only one type of movement: **rotation**. All they do is allow structures to turn. An example is the atlanto-axial joint, which lets us shake our head "no". This is rotation.

Plane/gliding joints are produced when the articulating bones have **flat surfaces**, and there is a **disc of cartilage** between the bones. This allows the joint to move, or glide, in any direction, although with slight movement. Examples include the joints between the carpals and tarsals.

Saddle joints are only located in one part of the body: the **carpometacarpal joint of the thumb**. Saddle joints are named after the appearance of the articulating bones. The articulating surfaces are both shaped like saddles. The two bones that create the saddle joint are the **first metacarpal and the trapezium**.

Ellipsoid/condyloid joints are extremely similar to ball-and-socket joints. On one bone, there is a **condyle**, which resembles a ball, but isn't as pronounced. This condyle fits into an **elliptical cavity** on another bone, which is similar to a socket, but not as deep. This allows movements such as flexion, extension, adduction, abduction, and circumduction. An example is the radiocarpal joint.

Anatomical Laws

Davis's Law is an anatomical law described by Henry Davis, examining the **remodeling of soft tissue** due to outside factors. The law states that tissues such as muscle will **repair damage** done to the tissue to **strengthen the tissue** and prevent injury in the future. For example, if a person were to exercise and be sore the next day, the muscle will repair itself in a manner to increase muscle density and improve strength, leading to the person being stronger and not injuring the muscle the next time they exercise.

Hilton's Law is an anatomical law described by John Hilton, examining innervations of muscles and skin. The law states that **a nerve that innervates a muscle that crosses a joint** and acts on the joint **will also innervate the skin and joint atop the muscle.** An example, the tibial nerve innervates the gastrocnemius. The gastrocnemius crosses the popliteal region at the posterior knee, so the tibial nerve will also innervate the joint and skin at the back of the knee.

Wolff's Law is an anatomical law described by Julius Wolff, examining the **remodeling of bone tissue** due to outside factors. The law states that bone will **remodel itself to be more dense**, adding strength to the bone, **when the bone is placed under pressure.** For example, lifting a heavy object can place many pounds of pressure on the bones. The bones respond by remodeling to be able to support the increased demand on the bone, adding density and strength to the bone itself. If the bone is not placed under stress for a period of time, the bone will become less dense and weaken, which may lead to increased likelihood of fracture or the development of conditions such as osteoporosis.

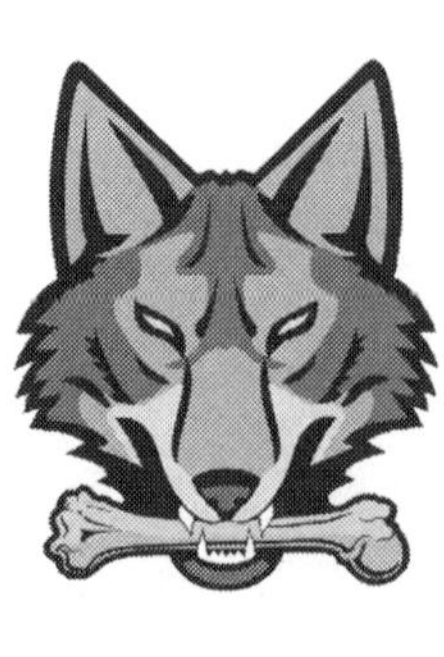

Easy to Remember:* *To remember Wolff's Law, just picture a wolf chewing on a bone that's so strong, it won't break!

Skeleton Divisions

There are two divisions of the skeleton: the Axial Skeleton and the Appendicular Skeleton.

The **Axial Skeleton** contains all of the bones that do not correspond to any appendages: the **skull**, **vertebral column**, and **thoracic cage**. These bones make up the trunk.

The **Appendicular Skeleton** contains all of the bones that correspond to the appendages: the **humerus**, **radius**, **ulna**, **carpals**, **metacarpals**, **phalanges**, **femur**, **tibia**, **fibula**, **tarsals**, **metatarsals**, **phalanges**, the **pectoral girdle**(clavicles and scapulae) and **pelvic girdle**(ilium, ischium, pubis, and sacrum).

Bones of the Axial Skeleton

Skull

The skull's primary function is to **protect the brain.** The bones that create the skull are:

Parietal
Frontal
Temporal
Occipital
Zygomatic
Maxilla
Mandible
Vomer
Ethmoid
Lacrimal
Sphenoid
Nasal

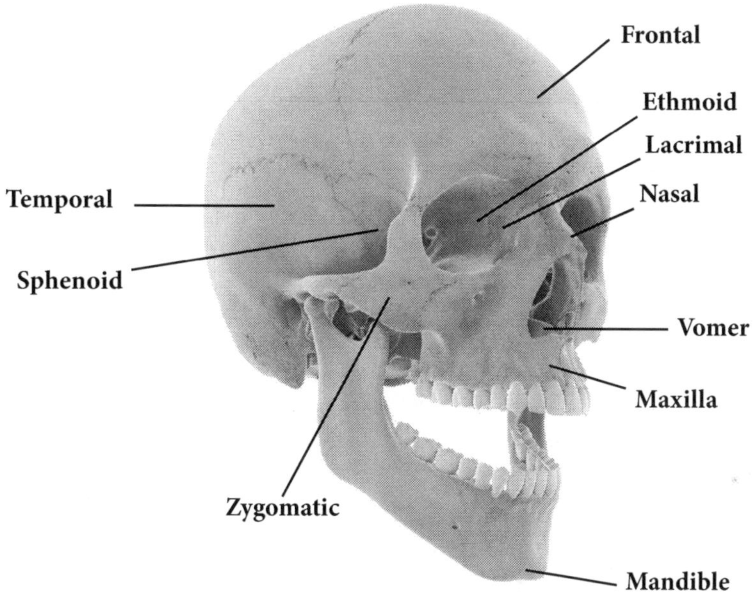

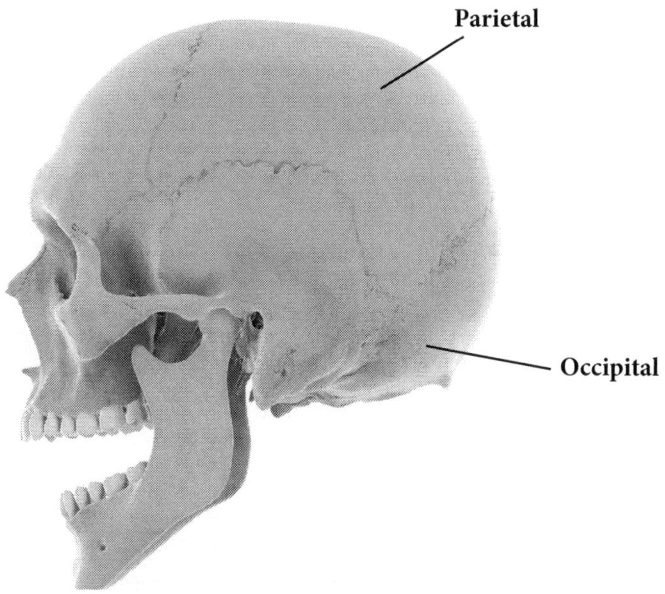

Vertebral Column

The vertebral column consists of **26 individual bones**. Its primary function is to **protect the spinal cord**, which runs through it. There are five regions of the vertebral column. They are:

Cervical(7 vertebrae)
Thoracic(12 vertebrae)
Lumbar(5 vertebrae)
Sacral(1 vertebrae*)
Coccygeal(1 vertebrae*)

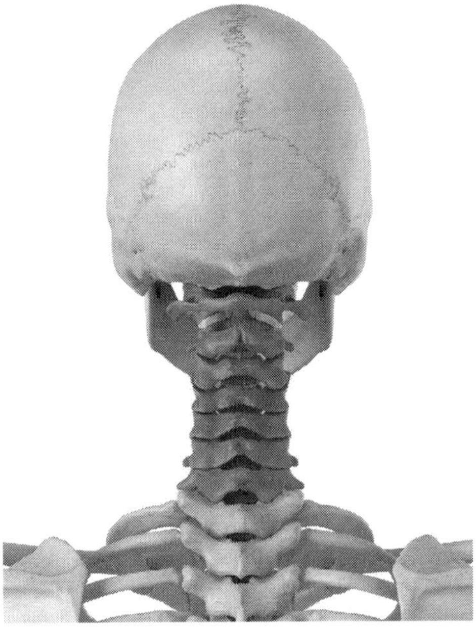

Cervical Vertebrae

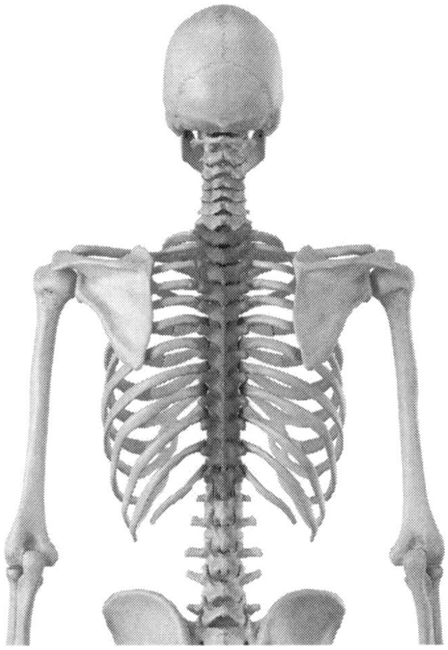

Thoracic Vertebrae

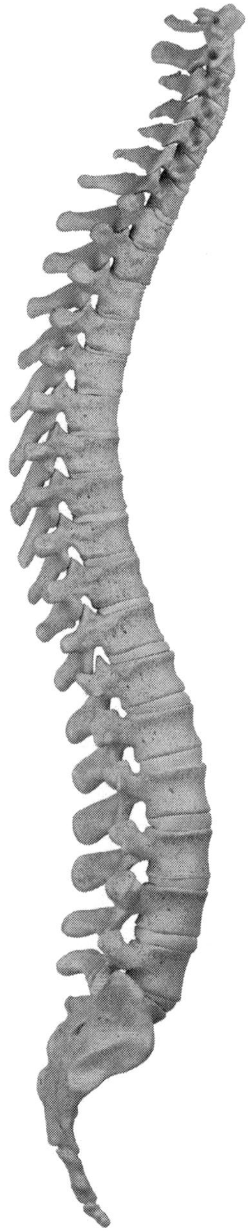

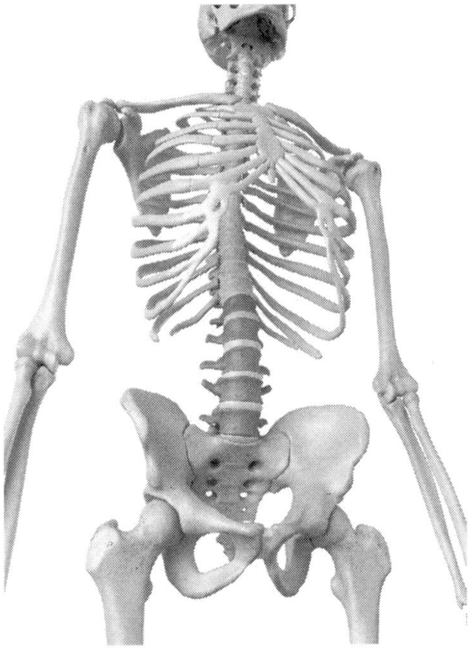

Lumbar Vertebrae

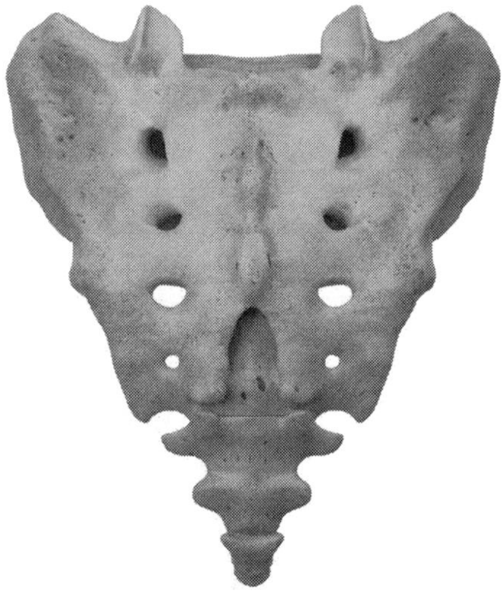

Sacrum and Coccyx

Easy to Remember: To remember how many vertebrae are in the cervical, thoracic, and lumbar regions, just think of breakfast, lunch, and dinner! Breakfast at 7(cervical), lunch at 12(thoracic), dinner at 5(lumbar)!

* The sacrum starts as five bones that fuse together to create one bone, and the coccyx starts as 3-5 bones that fuse together to create one bone.

Chest

The chest consists of the rib cage, and it contains **12 pairs** of bones. The primary function of the rib cage is to **protect vital organs** inside the thorax, and assist in breathing by giving the diaphragm a place to attach. The rib cage consists of:

True ribs(superior seven ribs, connect directly to the sternum via costal cartilage)
False ribs(inferior five pairs, do not directly connect to the sternum)
Floating ribs(ribs 11 and 12, protect the kidneys)

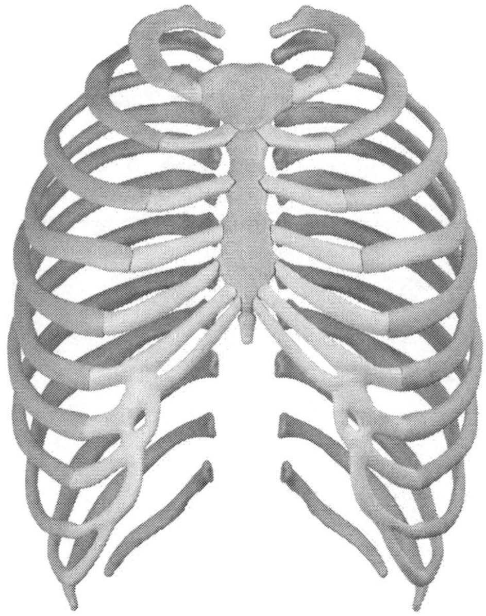

Bones of the Appendicular Skeleton

Pectoral Girdle

The pectoral girdle is responsible for holding the upper limbs to the body. The pectoral girdle consists of four bones:

Scapulae(2 bones)
Clavicles(2 bones)

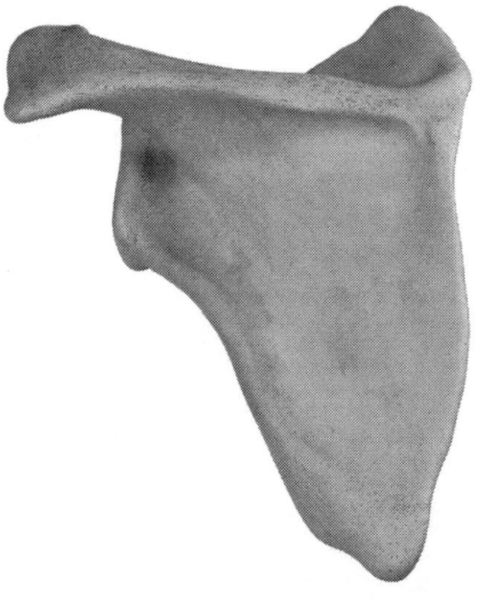

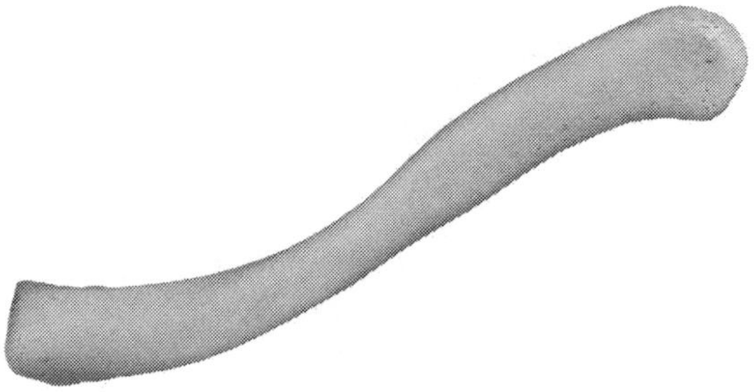

Pelvic Girdle

The pelvic girdle is primarily responsible for holding the lower limbs to the body. The pelvic girdle contains:

Ilium(2 bones)
Ischium(2 bones)
Pubis(2 bones)
Sacrum(1 bone)

DID YOU KNOW?

The iliofemoral ligament, which holds the head of the femur to the acetabulum, is the strongest ligament in the body!

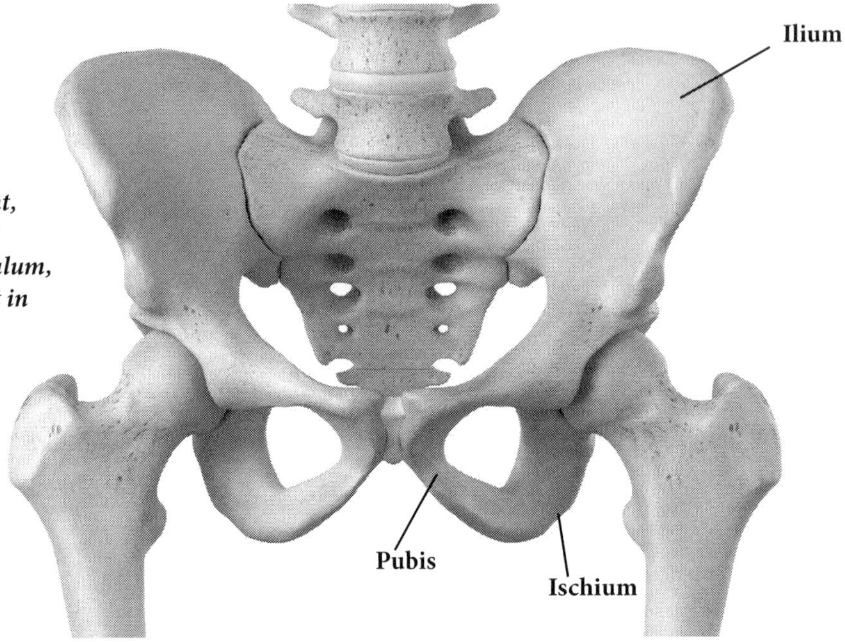

Arm

The arm contains one bone:

Humerus

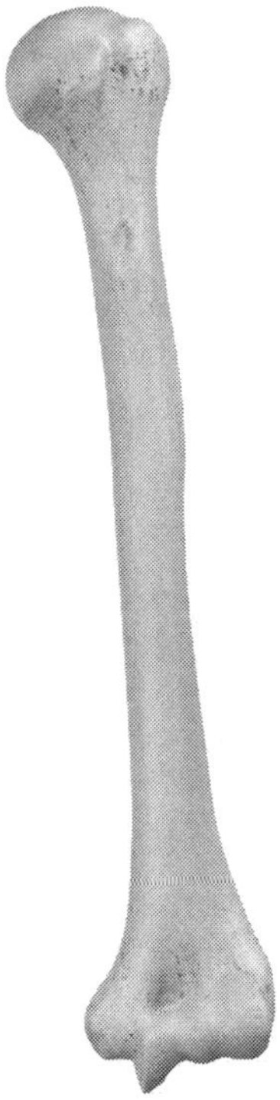

Forearm

The forearm contains two bones:

Radius

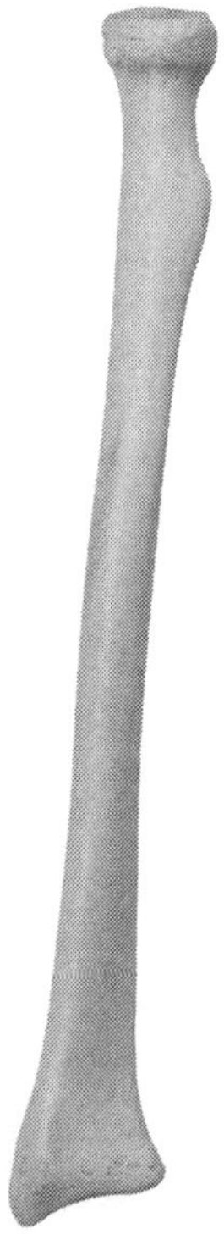

Ulna

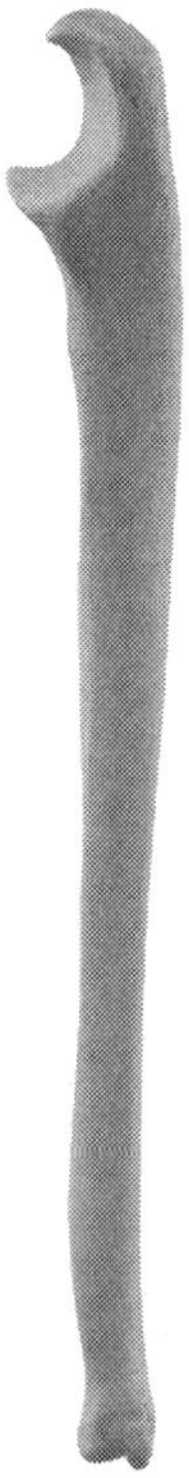

Wrist

The wrist is located distally to the forearm, and it contains the **carpal bones**. The carpal bones are divided into two separate lines, each containing four bones. The order begins on the lateral side and moves medially, then after the proximal line is finished, the order resumes on the lateral side of the distal line. The proximal line is listed first, then the distal line:

Proximal Line:
Scaphoid
Lunate
Triquetrum
Pisiform

Distal Line:
Trapezium
Trapezoid
Capitate
Hamate

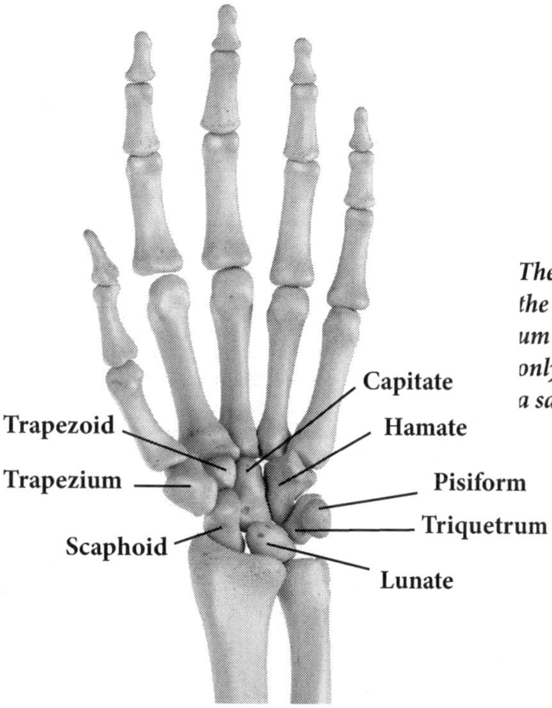

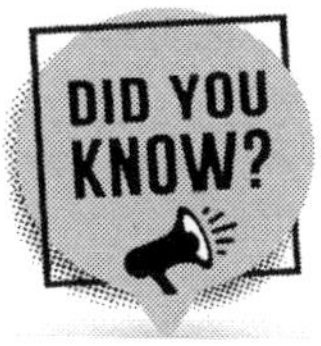

The carpometacarpal joint of the thumb, made by the trapezium and first metacarpal, is the only place in the body you find a saddle joint!

Easy to Remember: To remember the order of the carpals, think of this old saying: Some Lovers Try Positions That They Can't Handle(Scaphoid, Lunate, Triquetrum, Pisiform, Trapezium, Trapezoid, Capitate, Hamate)!

Hand

There are **19 bones** in each hand:

Metacarpals: 5 bones
Phalanges: 14 bones

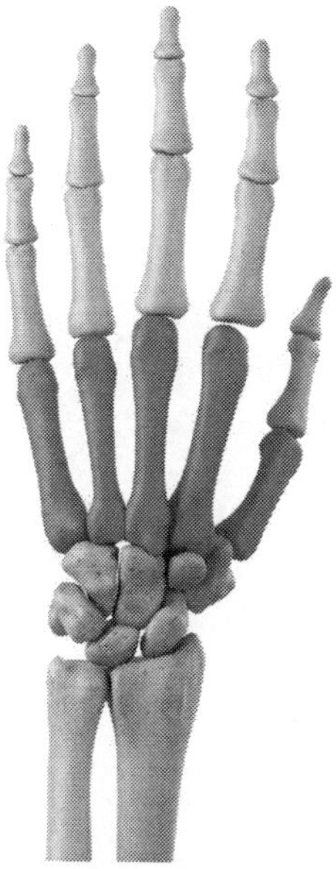
Metacarpals

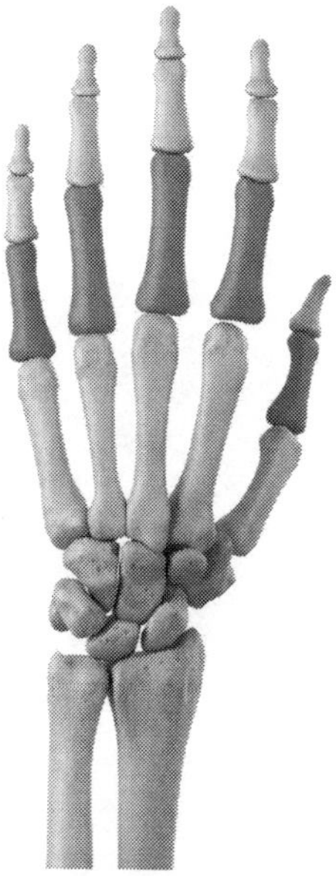
Proximal Phalanges

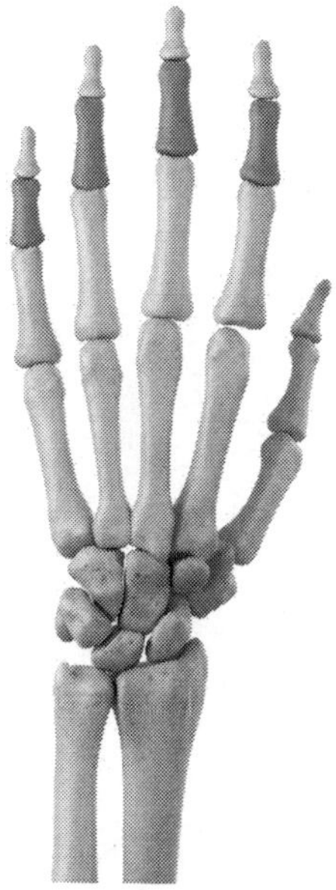
Intermediate Phalanges

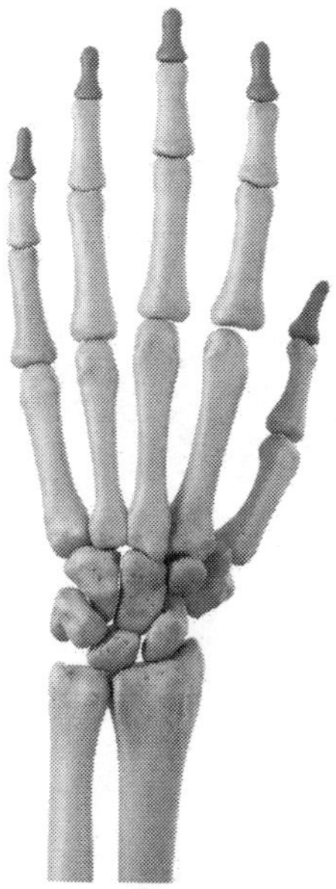
Distal Phalanges

Thigh

The thigh contains one bone:

Femur

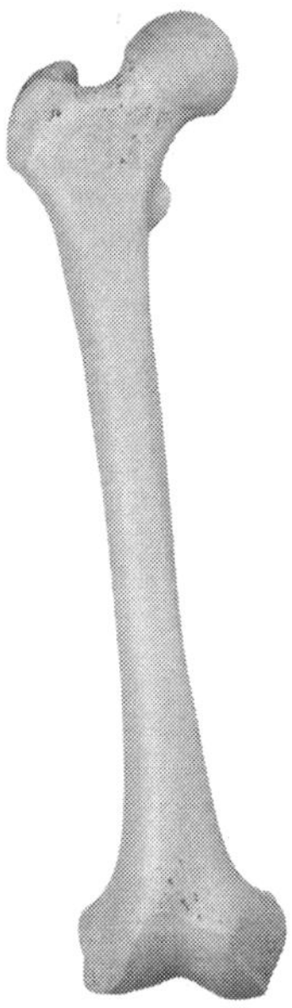

Leg

The leg contains two bones:

Fibula **Tibia**

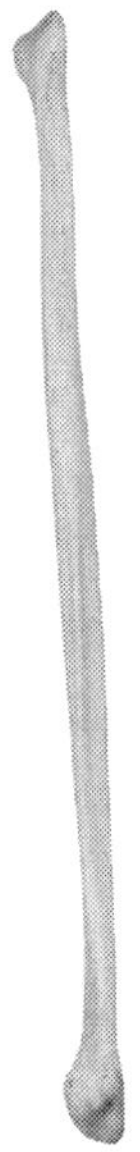

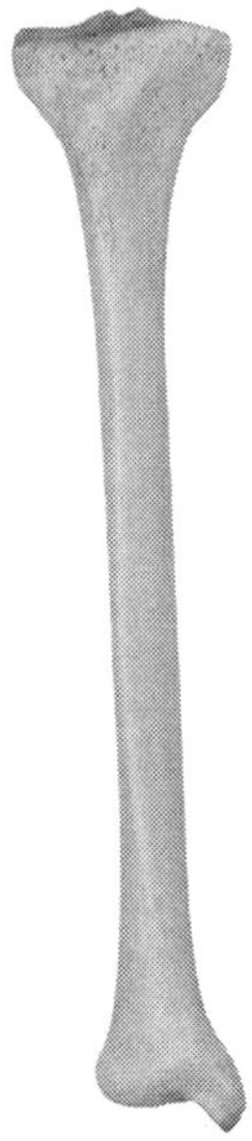

Ankle

The ankle is located distally to the leg, and contains the bones of the **tarsals**:

Calcaneus	Cuneiform I
Cuboid	Cuneiform II
Talus	Cuneiform III
Navicular	

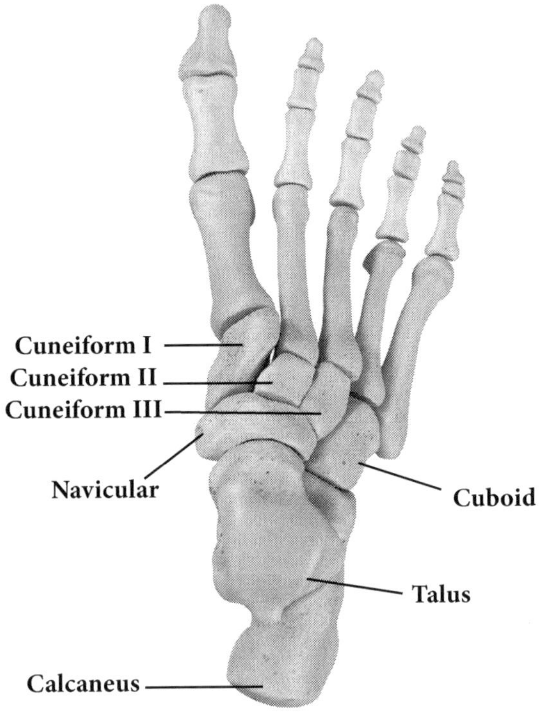

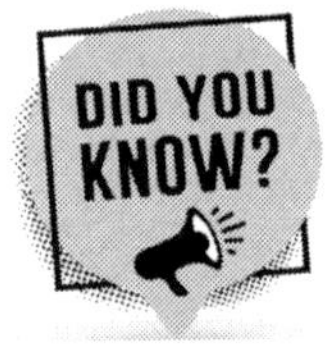

The femur is the longest and strongest bone in the body!

Foot

There are **19 bones** in each foot:
Metatarsals: 5 bones
Phalanges: 14 bones

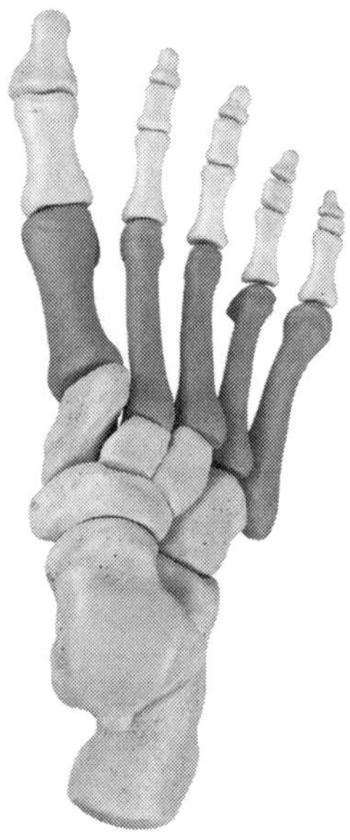

Metatarsals

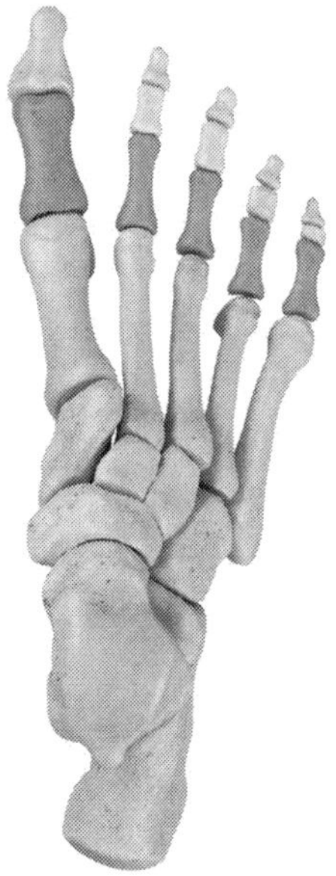

Proximal Phalanges

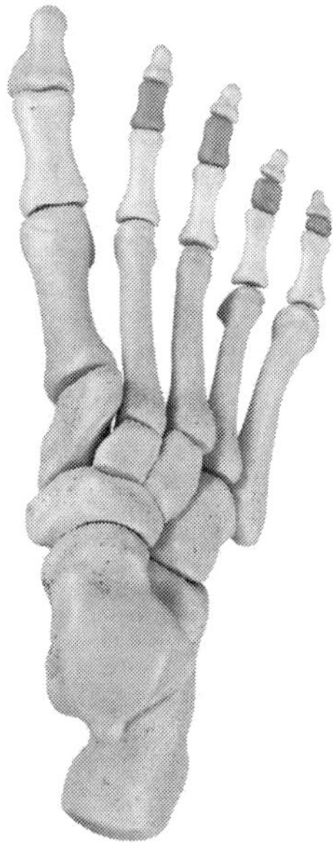

Intermediate Phalanges

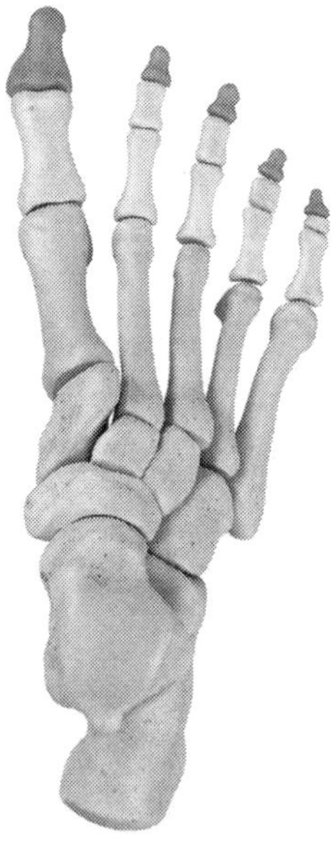

Distal Phalanges

Urinary System

The Urinary System is primarily responsible for **elimination of waste** from the body. It also assists in regulating the **pH level** of the body, and may also assist in reabsorption of substances back into the body. The four main structures of the Urinary System are(in descending order) the **kidneys, ureters, urinary bladder, and urethra.**

pH Scale

A **pH scale** is used to determine the **acidity or alkalinity** of a substance. If a substance reads between **7-14** on a pH scale, it is base, or **alkaline**. The higher the number, the more alkaline a substance is. An example, bleach is highly basic, and comes in at 12.6. Blood is slightly basic, and comes in at 7.4. On the other hand, if a substance comes in between **0-7** on a pH scale, it is **acidic**. The lower the number, the more acidic a substance is. An example, hydrochloric acid(the kind of acid in the stomach that helps digest food) comes in at 2.0, so it is highly acidic. Black coffee registers at about 5.0, so it is slightly acidic. The kidneys help regulate substances in the body that make the body's fluids either too acidic or too basic by filtration.

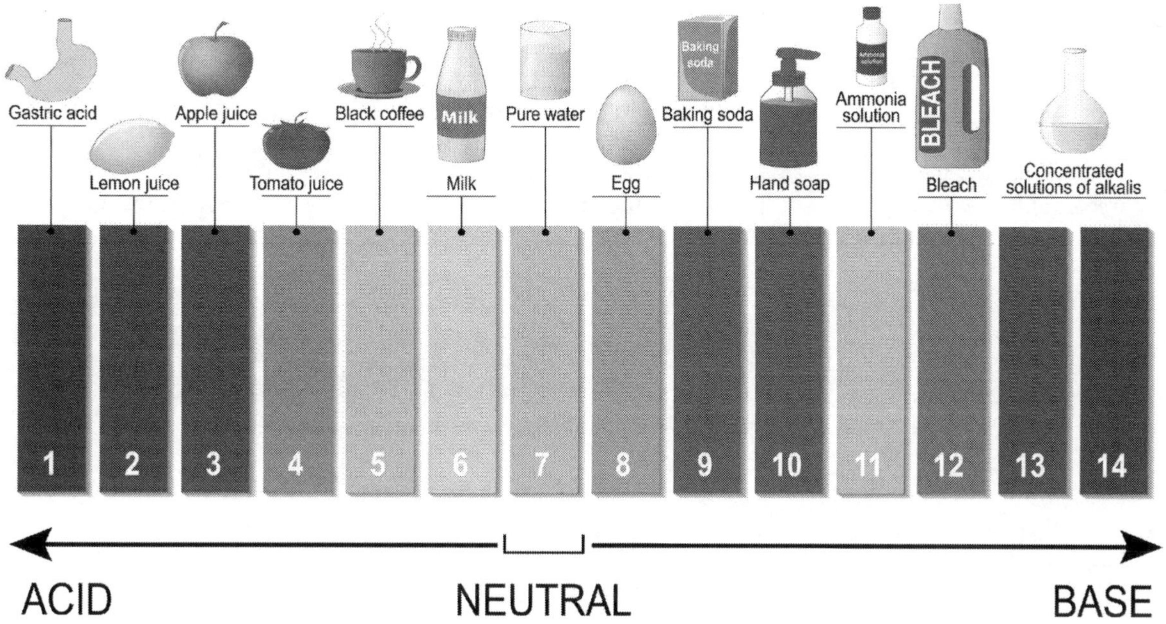

Flow of Urine

Blood enters the kidneys through the renal arteries. Inside the kidneys, blood is **filtered through the nephrons**, which extract waste products such as urea out of the blood. Inside each kidney, there are over one million nephrons. The waste products filtered out of the blood by the nephrons become **urine**. The nephrons also allow nutrients and water to be reabsorbed back into the blood stream.

Once urine has been created, it is sent from the kidneys to the urinary bladder through two small tubes known as ureters. The ureters only function as a **passageway for urine**.

Urine **collects in the urinary bladder**, until it is ready to be eliminated from the body. The urinary bladder expands as more urine is added to it. The urinary bladder can typically hold between 300-500 ml of fluid. Once urine is released from the urinary bladder, it passes through the urethra.

The urethra, much like the ureters, is a small tube that has one function: **transporting urine** from the urinary bladder **out of the body**.

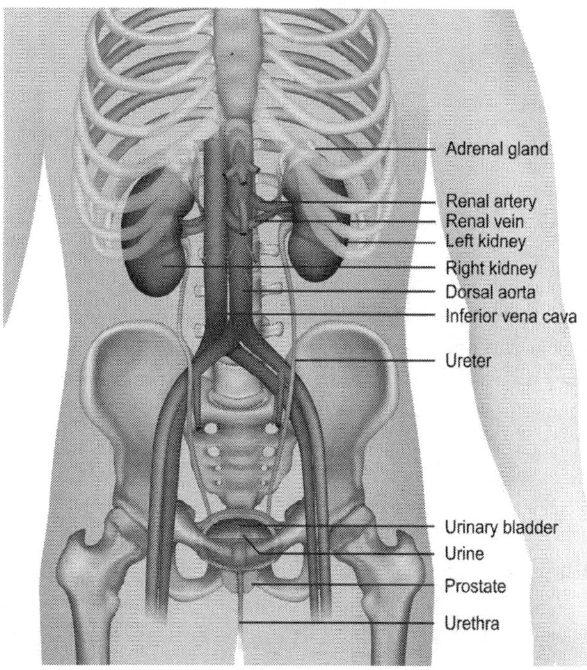

Sensory Organs

Sensory organs are organs that detect sensation, sending the information to the brain and/or spinal cord for processing, interpretation, and response. Sensory organs include the ear, eye, tongue, and skin.

Ear

The **ear** is responsible for detection of **sound**, producing **hearing**, and **balance**. The ear consists of the outer ear, middle ear, and inner ear.

The **outer ear** is known as the **auricle**. The auricle is mostly made of **elastic cartilage**. The **ear lobe** is made of flesh, allowing it to stretch and move, returning to its original size and shape, and contains an abundance of **blood vessels**. The function of the ear lobe is unknown, with some theorizing that they exist to keep the outer ear warm due to the presence of blood vessels.

Surrounding the outer ear is a **curved** structure known as the **helix**. A smaller version, further in the ear, is known as the **anti-helix**, and it opens into the ear canal.

Separating the outer ear and middle ear is the **tympanic membrane**. The tympanic membrane is also known as the **ear drum**. **Sound waves** cause the tympanic membrane to **vibrate**, which in turn vibrates the auditory ossicles in the middle ear.

The **middle ear** consists of the **tympanic cavity**. Inside the tympanic cavity are the **three auditory ossicles**. The auditory ossicles are three small bones that amplify and transmit sound further into the inner ear. These bones are the **malleus**, the **incus**, and the **stapes**, which is the **smallest bone** in the body.

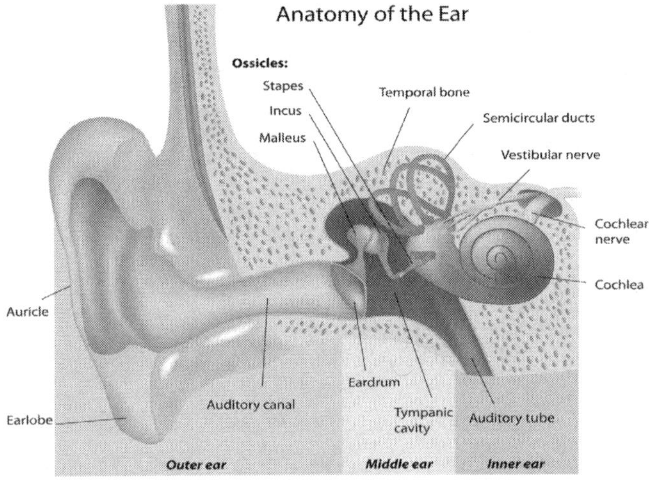

Also connecting to the middle ear is the **Eustachian tube**, a small tube that runs from the **middle ear** to the **pharynx**. The Eustachian tube allows **air pressure** and **fluid pressure** in the ear to be controlled. The Eustachian tubes open when a person yawns, swallows, or sneezes.

The **inner ear** contains the **bony labyrinth**. Inside the bony labyrinth are the semicircular canals and the cochlea. The **semicircular canals** are responsible for regulating **balance** and perception of **equilibrium**. This is achieved with the use of **fluid** in the canals that detect changes in motion.

The **cochlea** is a **spiral-shaped cavity**, named from the Greek word "kokhlias", which means "snail shell". The cochlea detects **vibration** from the middle ear, converting the vibrations into electrical signals that are sent to the brain stem for processing. This allows **hearing** to occur.

Eye

The eye is a round spherical organ responsible for **receiving** and **processing light** into an image that can be recognized by the brain.

Each eyeball is situated in the **orbital socket**, and is made of three layers: the outer layer, the middle layer, and the inner layer. The eye also contains two primary parts that fuse together: the anterior segment and posterior segment. The **anterior segment** of the eye consists of the iris, lens, aqueous humor, and cornea. The **posterior segment** consists of the sclera, retina, choroid, and vitreous humor.

The **outer layer** of the eye is known as the **sclera**, and is the tough, **white** portion of the eyeball. Light cannot penetrate the outer layer of the eye, instead focusing through the cornea into the eyeball.

The **middle layer** contains the **choroid**, and is where the majority of the eye's **blood vessels** are located. The middle layer also contains the **iris**. The iris is the **colored** portion of the eye, and is primarily made of **smooth muscle**. The iris contains an opening in its center known as the **pupil**. There are two sets of muscles in the iris, the dilator muscle and the contractor muscle.

When the **dilator muscle** contracts, the iris will pull the pupil open into **dilation**, allowing more light to enter the eye. This is useful in **low-light areas**. When the **contractor muscle** contracts, the iris will make the pupil **smaller**, known as **constriction.** This reduces the amount of light entering into the eye, useful in **high-light areas**.

Also contained in the **middle layer** is the **ciliary body**, responsible for controlling the overall shape of the **lens.** The ciliary body helps to **curve the lens**, allowing the lens to **focus** on objects that may be close or further away.

Aqueous humor is found in the space between the cornea and the lens. This fluid is clear and watery, helping to **maintain eye pressure** and provides **nourishment** to the cornea and lens, which are avascular and cannot receive nutrients from blood vessels directly.

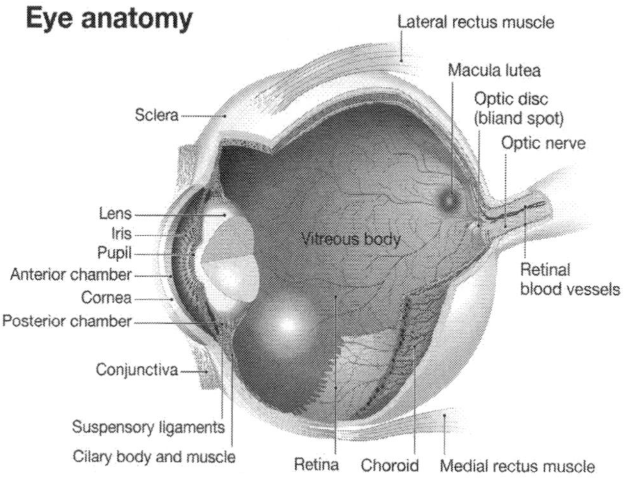

Vitreous humor is a thicker substance, often described as "**jelly-like**", found **behind the lens.** The primary function of the vitreous humor is to assist the eyeball in **maintaining its shape**. It also helps keep the retina fixed against the back wall of the eye.

The **inner layer** of the eye consists of the **retina.** The retina contains rods and cones. **Rods** are nerve cells that primarily function in **dim light**, and do not play a role in color vision. Rods do not allow high visual acuity. **Cones** function in **high light**, and **detect colors.** Cones produce high visual acuity. Rods and cones take the information from light and convert the information into electrical signals that leave the eye through the optic nerve.

Other structures contribute to proper functioning and overall health of the eye. Lining the eyelids and anterior portion of the sclera is a thin membrane known as the **conjunctiva**, which provides a layer of protection against dirt, debris, and pathogens. The **lacrimal glands** produce **tears**, which lubricate the eyes, helping to wash waste products and debris from the eye. The tears drain from the eye into the nasal passages.

Tongue

The **tongue** is a structure made of **skeletal muscle** surrounded by a mucous membrane that primarily acts to move food in the mouth, which assists in **mastication** by forcing food between the teeth when chewing. The tongue is covered in **papillae**, giving the tongue a rough texture. On the surface of each papillae are **taste buds**. Taste buds are sensory organs that react to chemicals in food, transforming the reactions into electrical signals that are sent to the brain. Taste buds allow a person to taste. The five main categories a person tastes in are sweet, salty, bitter, sour, and umami/savory.

Nose

The **nose** is the first organ of respiration, and is the location of olfaction. **Olfaction** is the sense of **smell.** Inside the nose, nerve endings detect **chemicals** in the air upon inhalation. These chemicals cause a reaction that is sent to the **olfactory bulb** in the brain, which processes the information to produce the sensation of smell.

Skin

The **skin**, aside from providing protection for the body, also acts to detect many **physical sensations**. Tactile sensations are primarily detected in the skin by various sensory receptors.

Merkel discs are primarily found in areas such as the **fingertips**, and are responsible for detection of **light sustained touch.** Merkel discs are located in the same level of the dermis as Meissner's corpuscles, at the base of the epidermis, and are therefore very superficial.

Ruffini corpuscles are primarily found in the deeper layers of the dermis, and are able to detect **tension** and **stretching of skin.** Ruffini corpuscles may also be found in connective tissues throughout the body, such as ligaments.

Thermoreceptors are found in the skin and detect either **warmth or cold**. Thermoreceptors are vital in helping to regulate homeostasis when temperature begins to negatively influence bodily function.

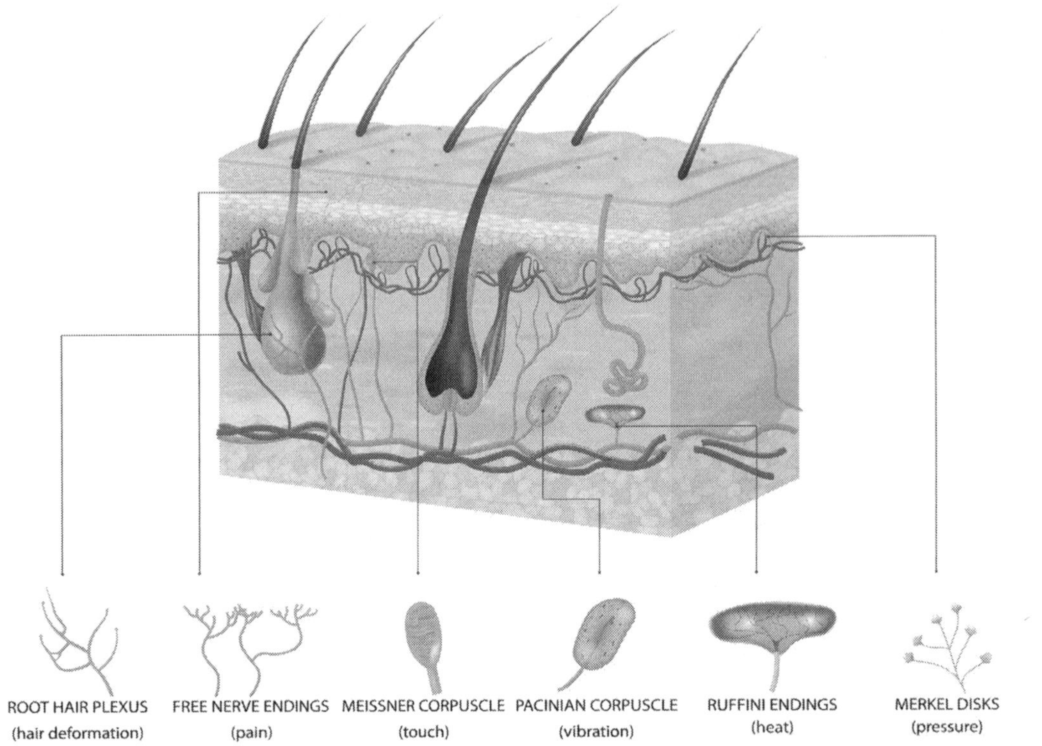

Sensation Processing

Nerve impulses are categorized as sensory or motor. **Sensory impulses** are detected by sensory receptors throughout the body (such as nociceptors, olfactory receptors, etc), and travel **to the brain and/or spinal cord** for processing. These impulses are called **afferent impulses**. In the case of reflexes, these impulses only reach the spinal cord, due to the immediacy of the required response. This is why reflexes are involuntary! Once the impulse reaches the brain and/or spinal cord, the brain and/or spinal cord interpret the sensation, and send a **motor impulse** back down the body to tell the body how to respond to the stimulus. These impulses are called **efferent impulses**.

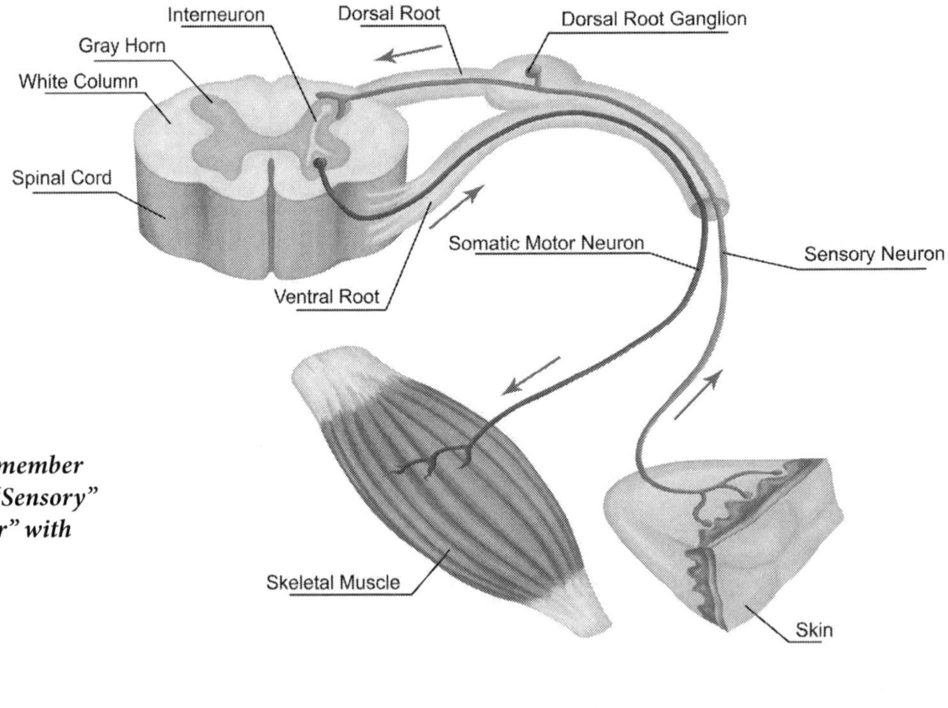

Easy to Remember: Just remember "SAME". You can pair up "Sensory" with "Afferent", and "Motor" with "Efferent"!

Human Growth, Development, and Milestones

Childhood

Childhood is the developmental stage **beginning after infancy**, ending when **puberty no longer takes effect** at the beginning of adulthood. Childhood is marked by physical growth in the bones at the metaphyses, which increases height. Bone in the head grows as well at an appropriate rate to match growth in the rest of the body. Once bones have reached peak growth, the cartilage that constitutes the metaphyses ossifies, and growth no longer occurs in the bones. Teeth first emerge usually during the first year of life. At around age six or seven, these baby teeth begin falling out, and are replaced with adult teeth.

Brain growth is extremely rapid during childhood, growing to nearly the size of an adult's brain by age seven. By age seven, a child should be able to rationally and logically think about daily life experiences.

Adolescence

Adolescence is marked by the **beginning of puberty** around age ten, which produces many changes in the body. Structurally, the child will see increased growth in height and muscle mass.

Physiological changes take effect, such as increased activity of sweat and oil glands, the development of pubic hair and armpit hair, the start of menstruation and the development of breasts in girls, the growth of the testes and increased production of testosterone in boys, and deepening of the voice.

Psychological changes begin during adolescence, in which the child begins exhibiting more abstract thoughts and feelings. This leads to the child establishing their own personal identity, which can evolve as thinking changes during this stage.

Adulthood

Adulthood has **no definitive physiological beginning.** Legally, in Western society, most are considered an adult at **age 18 or 21**. During adulthood, the bones stop growing, and each body system is functioning properly. As cells divide during this stage, errors in cell replication occurs, and this leads to degradation of the cell and causes aging.

Senescence

Senescence occurs **as a person ages**, and each body system begins to deteriorate and break down gradually. Senescence is typically marked with thinning and wrinkling of the skin, muscle atrophy, weakening of bones and joints, and the person may become more susceptible to infections due to a weakened immune system. Estrogen production declines, which leads to menopause in women. Testosterone production also declines in men, which may cause erectile dysfunction. Disorders may emerge as a person ages, such as dementia, and diseases such as cardiovascular issues may arise. Senescence ends with the person's death.

Death and Dying Stages

Death is the **end of life of a living organism**, in which all bodily functions cease. If a person has been diagnosed with a terminal disease, they may exhibit the **five stages of grief**. Established by **Elisabeth Kübler-Ross**, the five stages of grief theorize how people cope with death. The five stages are denial, anger, bargaining, depression, acceptance. The stage of **denial** is when the person refuses to believe the diagnosis, thinking it must be a mistake. **Anger** sets in when the person gives up denial, leaving the person to feel a sense of frustration and confusion over the situation. **Bargaining** begins as a way for the person to internally negotiate a lack of grief over the situation, usually by reforming their life or setting out on accomplishing goals that have not been met. During the next stage, a person may begin feeling **depressed** over the thought of dying, and lose interest in things or activities they would usually take joy in. Finally, the person may come to terms with their inevitable death, and decide not to fear or avoid it. This is the stage of **acceptance**.

Anatomy and Physiology Matching

______: Constant internal environment

______: Suture connecting the two parietal bones

______: Organ that creates bile and detoxifies blood

______: Tissue responsible for separating structures

______: "Rest-and-digest" response

______: Muscle contraction with constant tension and decreasing muscle length

______: Structure responsible for the creation of T-cells

______: Muscle contraction with constant tension and increasing muscle length

______: Region of vertebral column with five bones

______: Suture connecting the occipital bone and parietal bones

______: Sensory receptor that detects pain

______: Cell responsible for transporting oxygen and carbon dioxide

______: Tissue responsible for protection, secretion, and absorption

______: "Fight-or-flight" response

______: Glands responsible for production of estrogen and progesterone

______: Region of the vertebral column with seven bones

______: Body plane that splits the body into superior and inferior

______: Largest lymph vessel in the body

______: Body plane that splits the body into anterior and posterior

______: Organ that filters blood and creates urine

A: Erythrocytes
B: Thymus
C: Homeostasis
D: Kidneys
E: Liver
F: Cervical Vertebrae
G: Transverse Plane
H: Epithelial Tissue
I: Thoracic Duct
J: Ovaries
K: Sagittal Suture
L: Concentric Contraction
M: Parasympathetic Response
N: Lambdoid Suture
O: Nociceptor
P: Lumbar Vertebrae
Q: Eccentric Contraction
R: Frontal Plane
S: Sympathetic Response
T: Connective Tissue

Answer Key on Page 292

Anatomy and Physiology Crossword

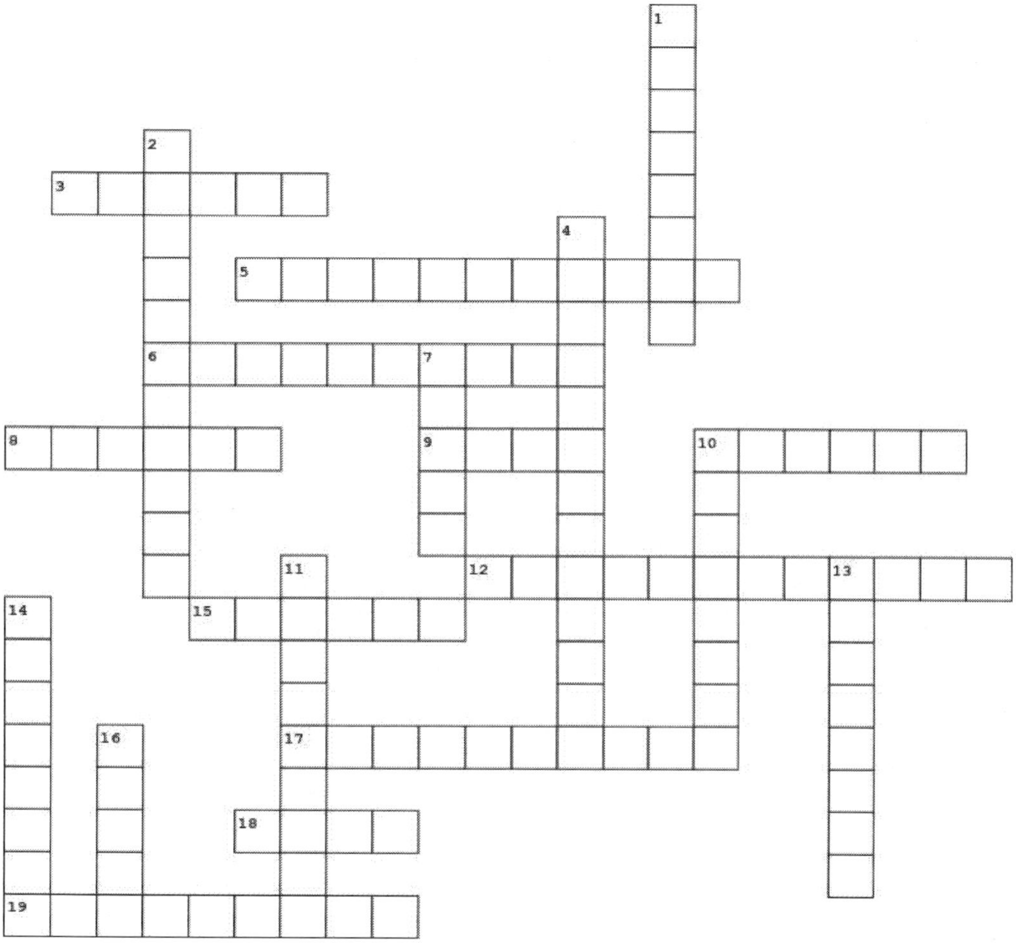

Across

3. Organ responsible for filtering old red blood cells from the blood stream
5. Existence and maintenance of a constant internal environment
6. Tissue responsible for protection, secretion, and absorption
8. Type of muscle responsible for performing peristalsis
9. Blood vessel responsible for bringing blood towards the heart
10. Gland responsible for producing and secreting melatonin, regulating the body's wake/sleep cycle
12. The largest lymph vessel in the body
15. Body cavity created by the cranium and vertebral column responsible for protecting the brain and spinal cord
17. Tissue covering the entrance to the larynx that functions to prevent choking
18. Substance created by the liver that helps emulsify fats
19. Organelles responsible for breaking down protein and waste products inside the cell

Down

1. Region of the vertebral column that contains twelve bones
2. Strongest ligament in the body
4. Type of joint located at the shoulder and hip
7. Organ located in the right hypochondriac region of the abdomen
10. Organ responsible for the production of insulin and glucagon
11. Bone that articulates with the metacarpal of the thumb to create the saddle joint
13. First segment of the small intestine
14. Body plane that splits the body into left and right sides
16. Nerve that controls and regulates the parasympathetic response

Answer Key on Page 293

Muscle Identification

Identify the numbered muscles. Write your answers on a separate piece of paper to allow yourself the ability to take this assignment multiple times!

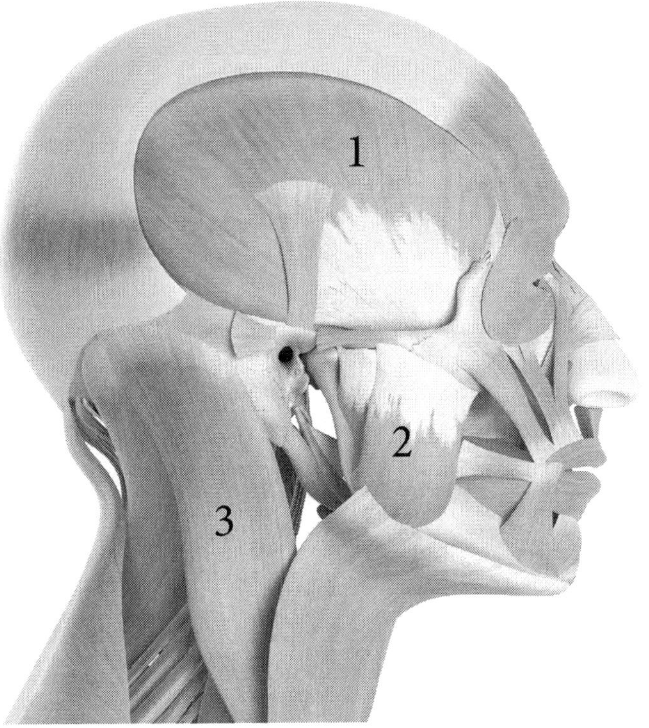

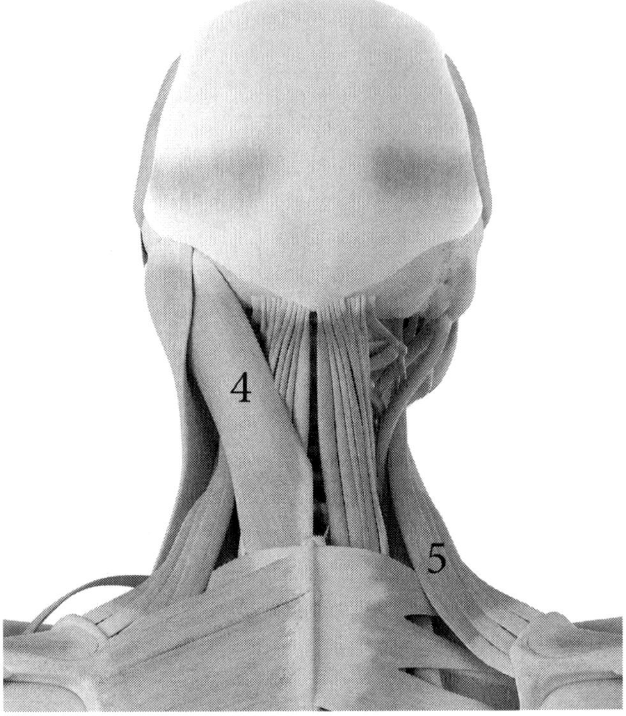

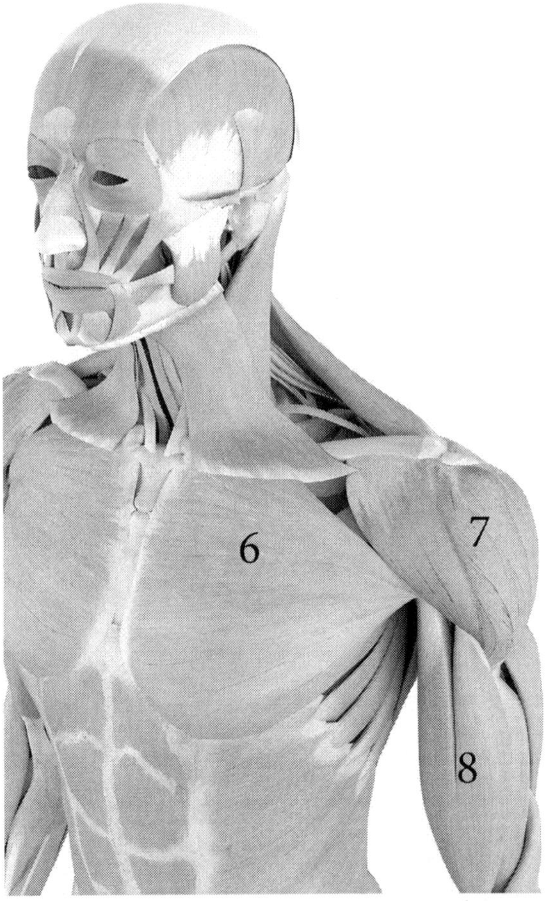

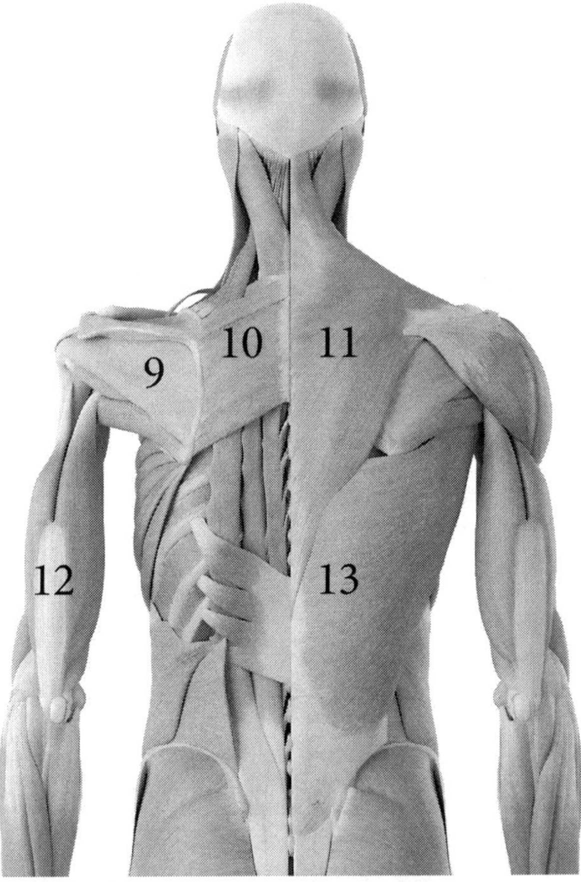

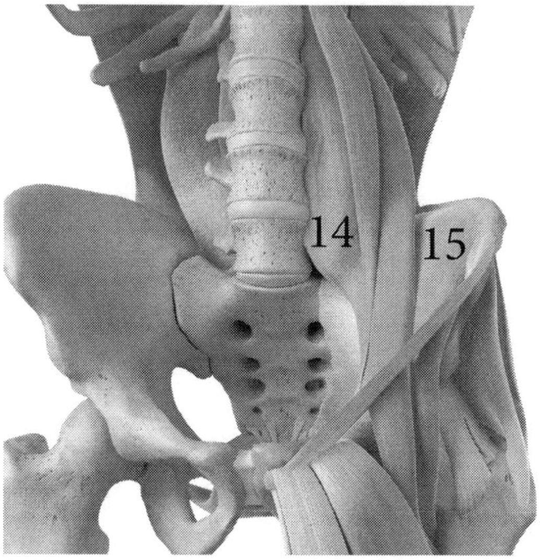

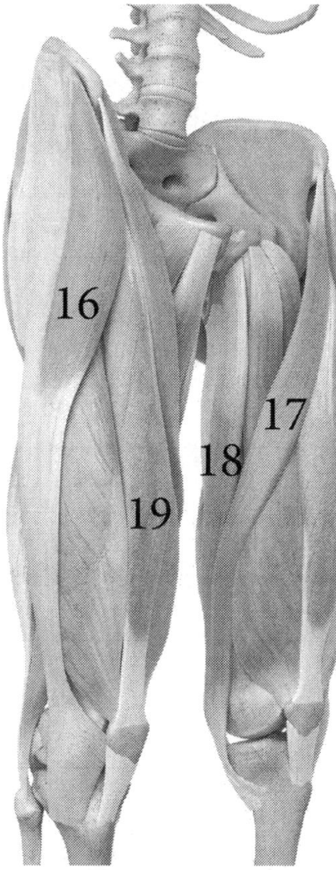

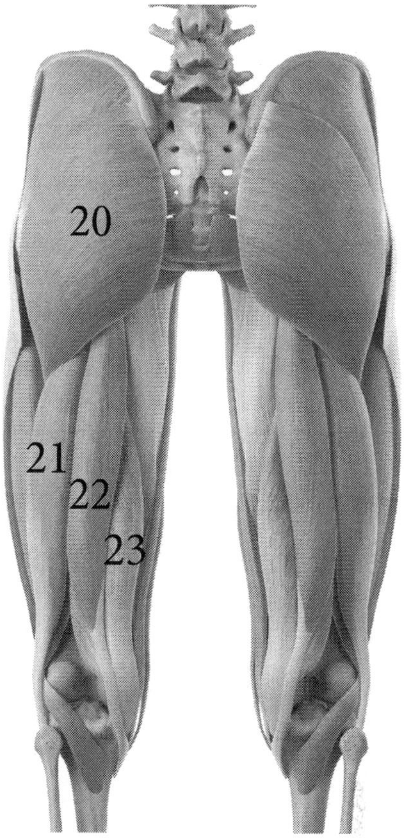

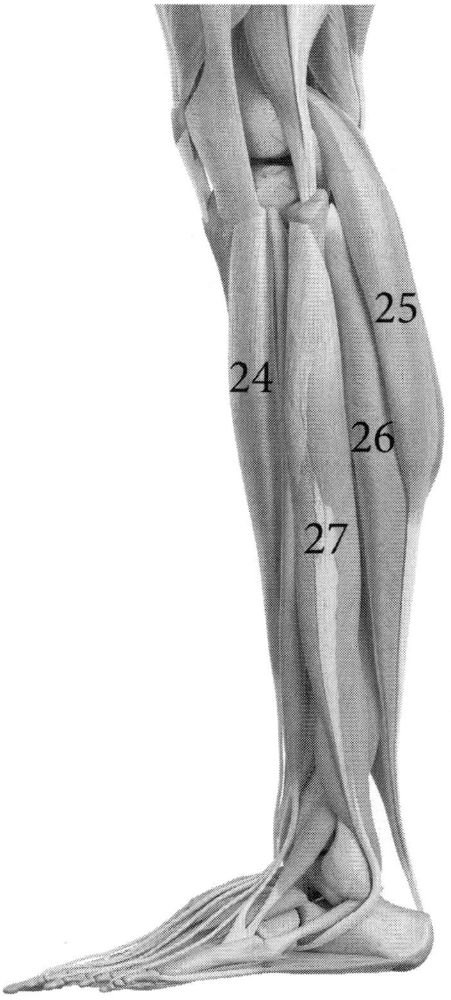

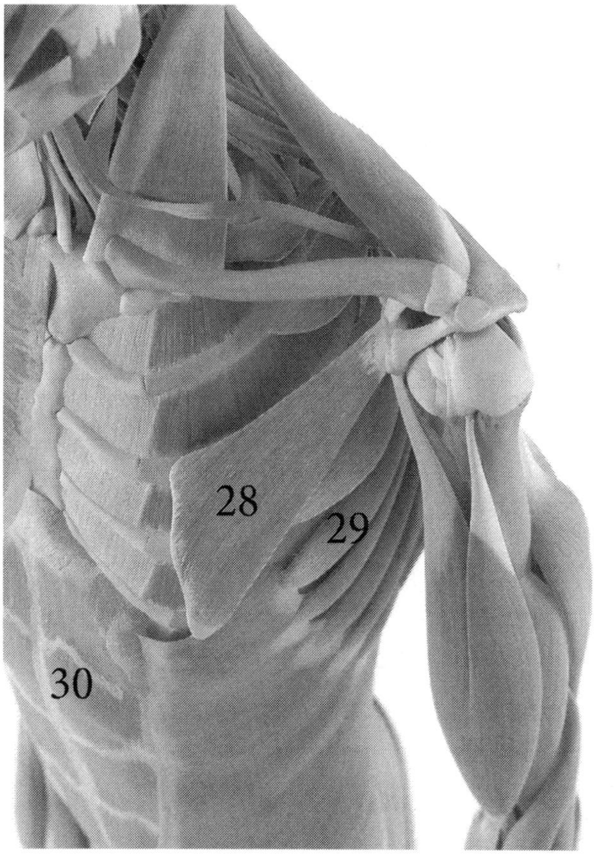

Answer Key on Page 294

Bone Identification

Identify the bones. Write your answers on a separate piece of paper to allow yourself the ability to take this assignment multiple times!

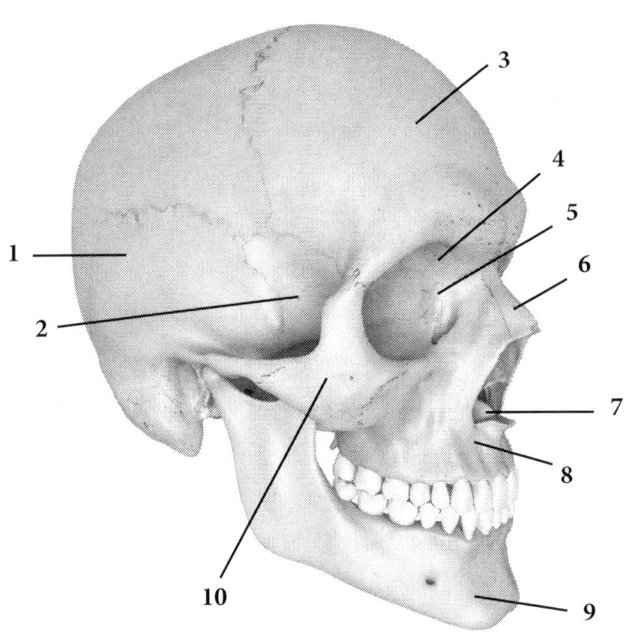

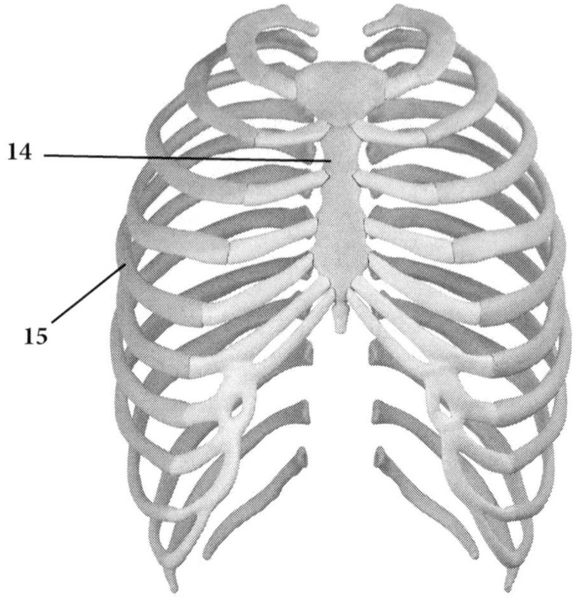

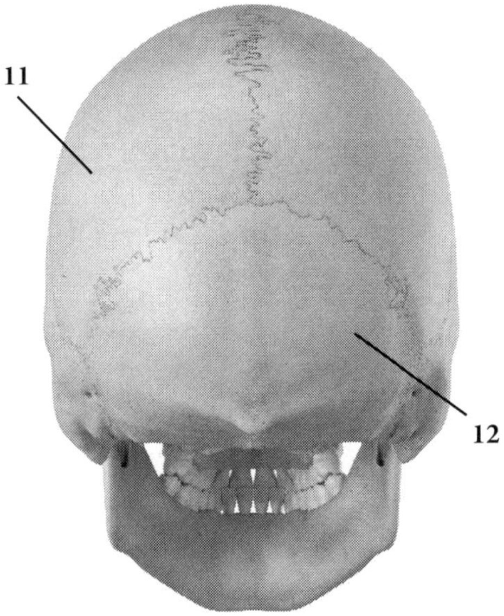

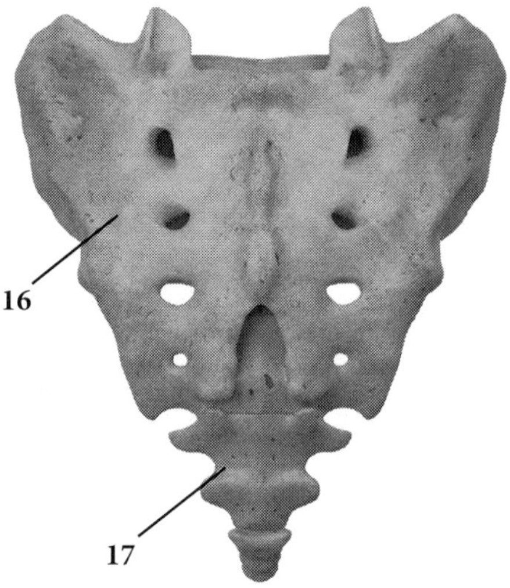

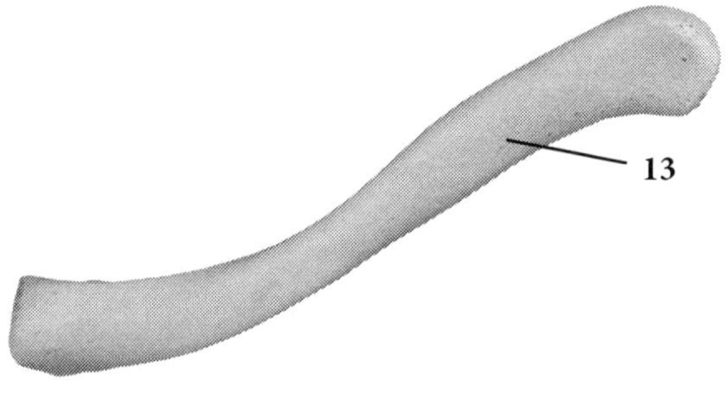

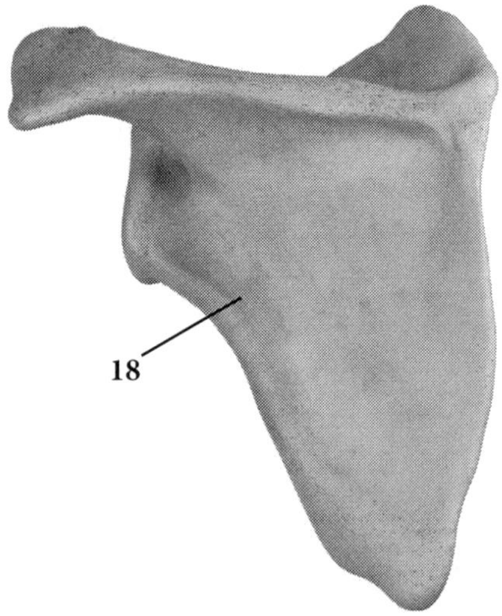

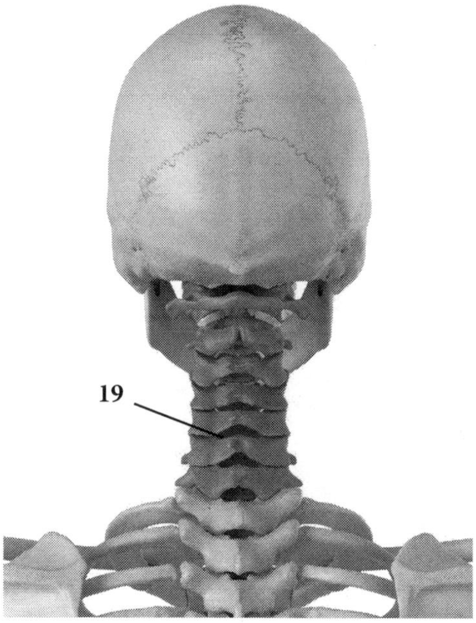
19

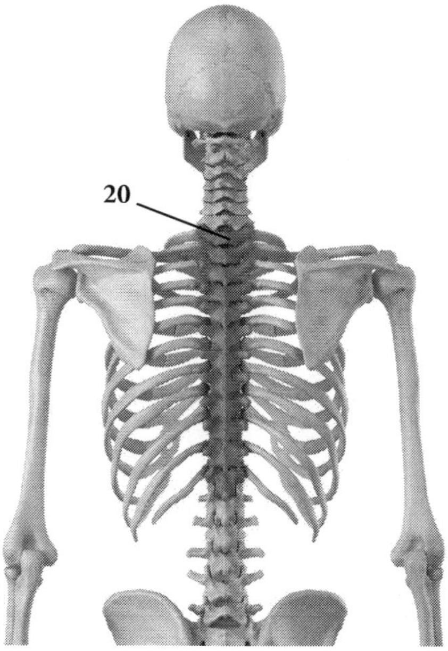
20

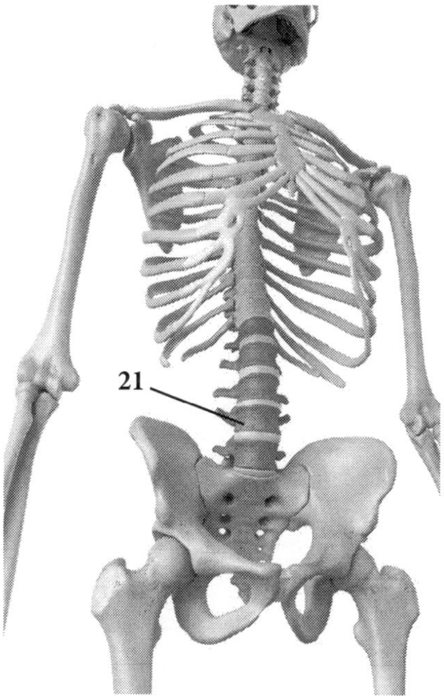
21

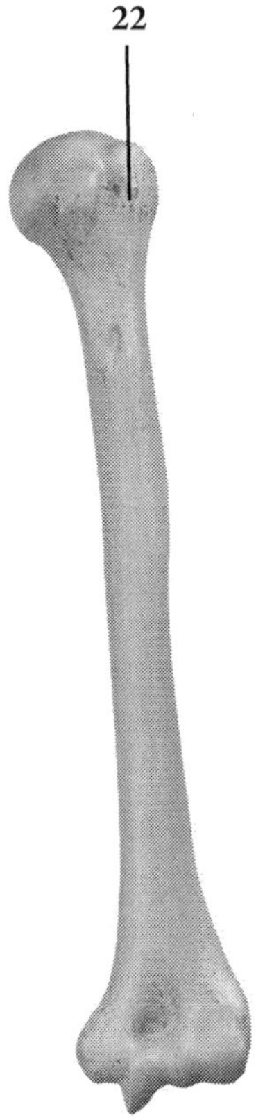
22

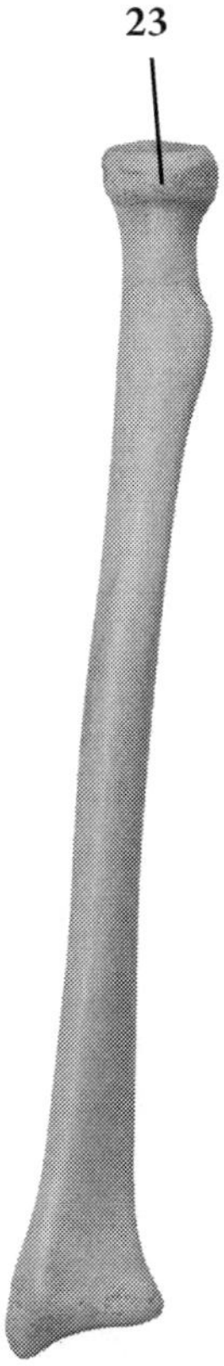
23

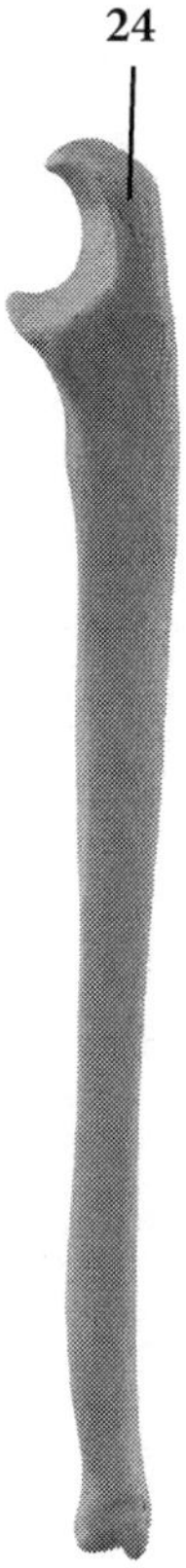
24

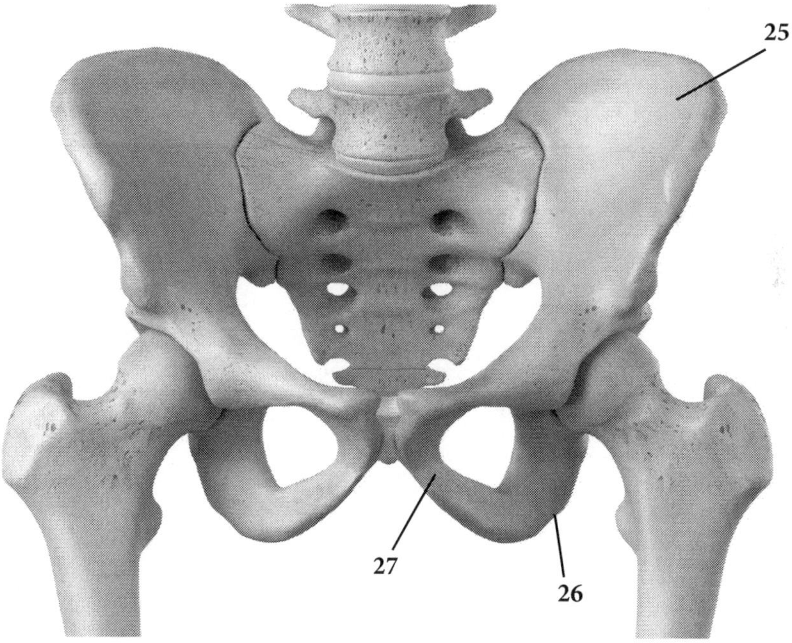
25
27
26

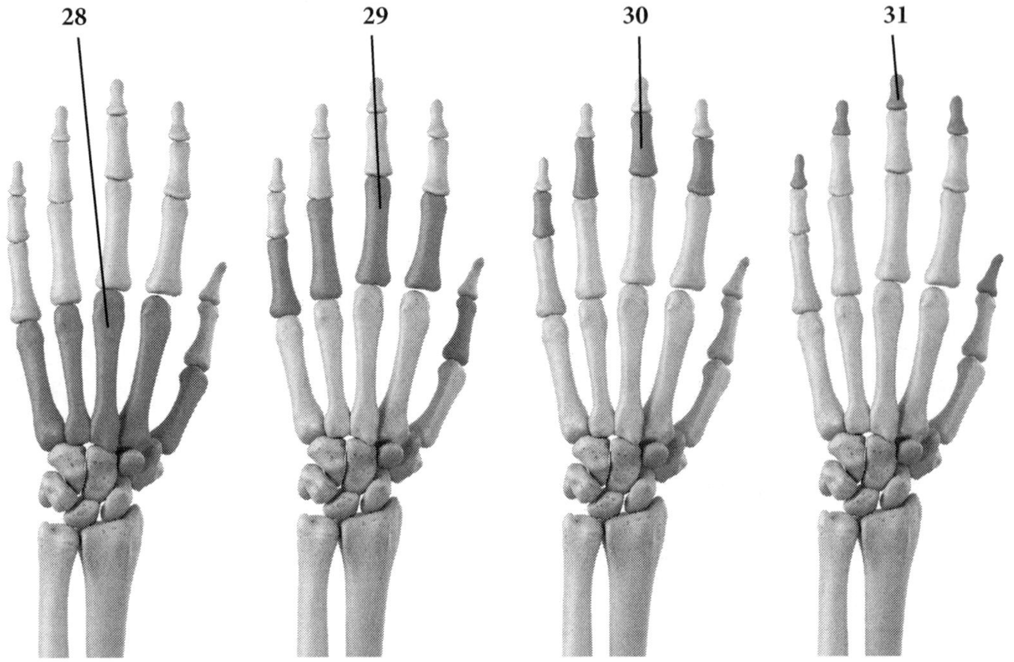
28
29
30
31

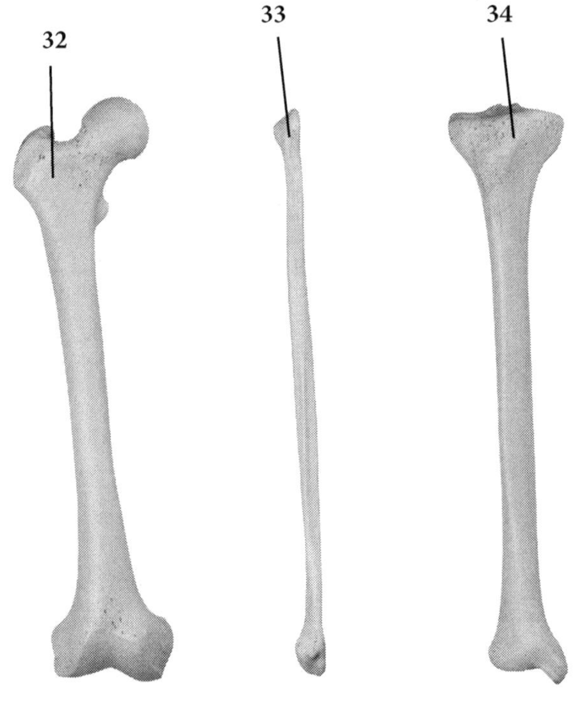
32
33
34

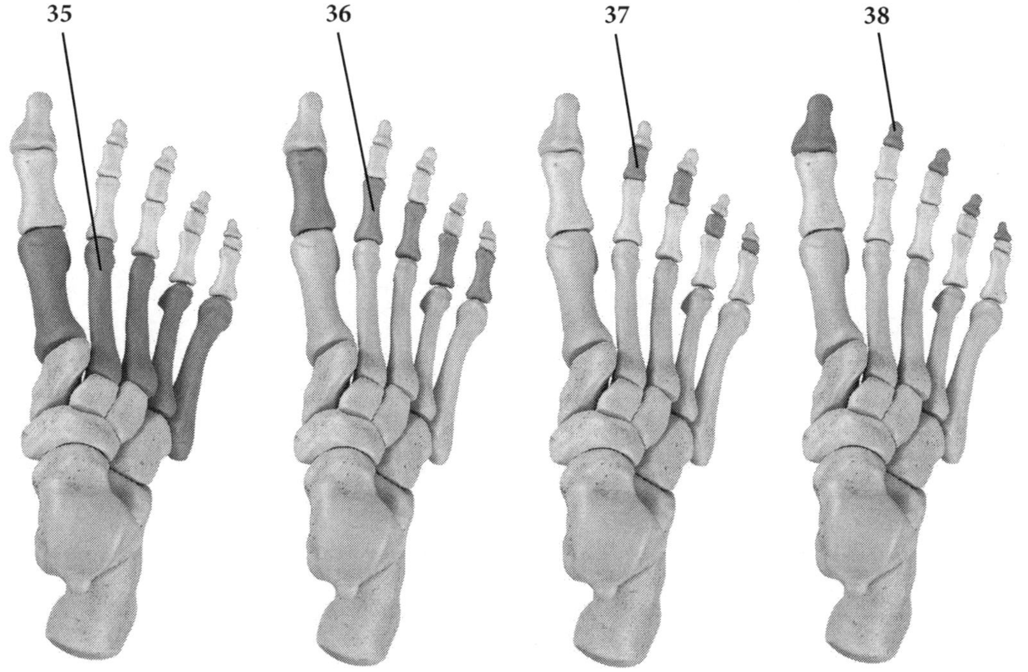

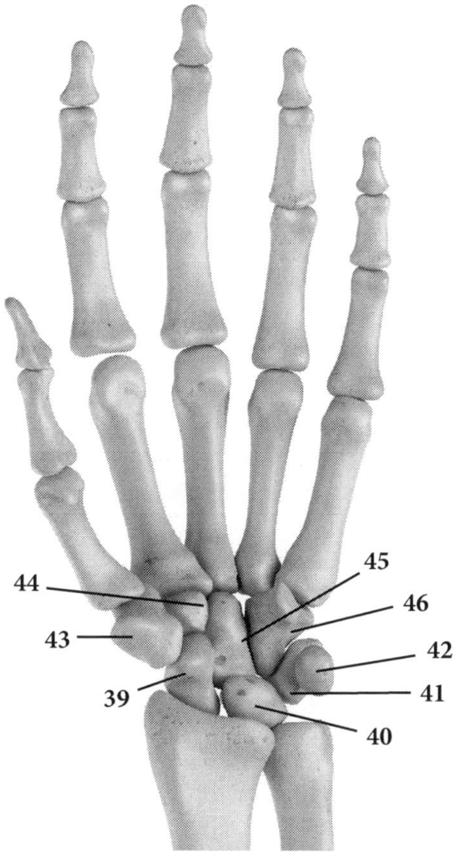

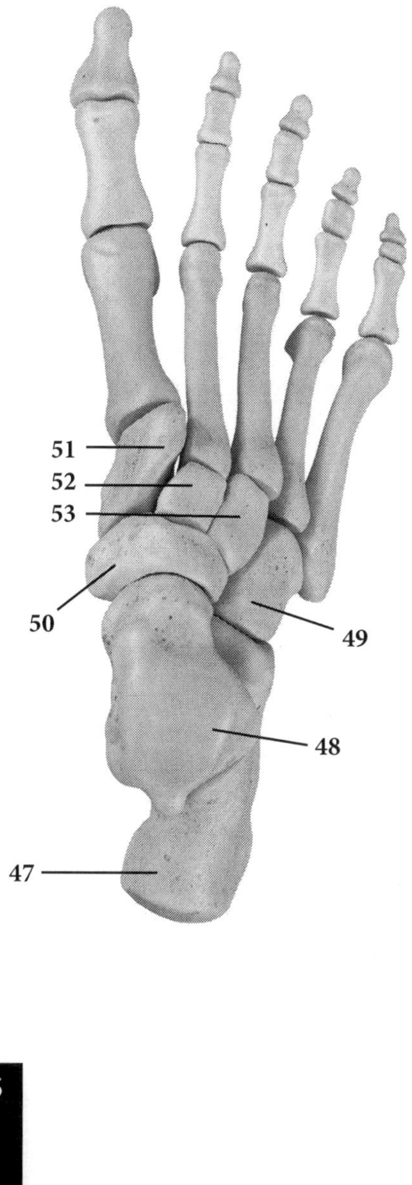

Answer Key on Page 295

Anatomy and Physiology Practice Test

1. The largest veins in the body, responsible for returning deoxygenated blood to the heart
A. Aorta
B. Pulmonary arteries
C. Pulmonary veins
D. Vena cavae

2. Which of the following describes the process of mitosis
A. The division of one mother cell into two daughter cells
B. The destruction of a pathogen or foreign agent performed by leukocytes
C. Production of adenosine triphosphate to provide energy to the body
D. Introduction of electrolytes into muscle tissue to produce contraction

3. Increased epinephrine, blood sugar, and heart rate are all key markers of
A. Parasympathetic response
B. Homeostatic mechanisms
C. Sympathetic response
D. Skeletal muscle heat production

4. Which developmental stage is marked by the beginning of puberty around age ten, producing structural changes in a child's body such as increased height and muscle mass
A. Childhood
B. Adolescence
C. Adulthood
D. Senescence

5. Substance released by sarcoplasmic reticulum upon contact with sodium ions, which binds to tropomyosin and reveals attachment sites on actin for myosin, allowing a muscle to contract
A. Calcium
B. Magnesium
C. Potassium
D. Vitamin A

6. Joints that have little to no movement
A. Biarthrotic
B. Synarthrotic
C. Diarthrotic
D. Amphiarthrotic

7. Which of the following best describes vitreous humor
A. Thick substance found behind the lens of the eye
B. Thick substance found within the tongue
C. Thin substance found in the auditory ossicles
D. Substance found between the cornea and lens

8. The dorsal body cavity
A. Surrounds the heart and lungs
B. Houses internal reproductive organs
C. Protects the digestive organs in the abdomen
D. Protects the brain and spinal cord

9. Stimulation of the parasympathetic nervous response has what action on the digestive tract
A. Decreases absorption
B. Shuts down peristalsis
C. Increases lymph circulation
D. Increases peristalsis

10. Contraction of cardiac muscle in the right ventricle sends blood
A. To the aorta
B. To the body
C. To the lungs
D. To the right atrium

Answer Key on Page 295

Pathology

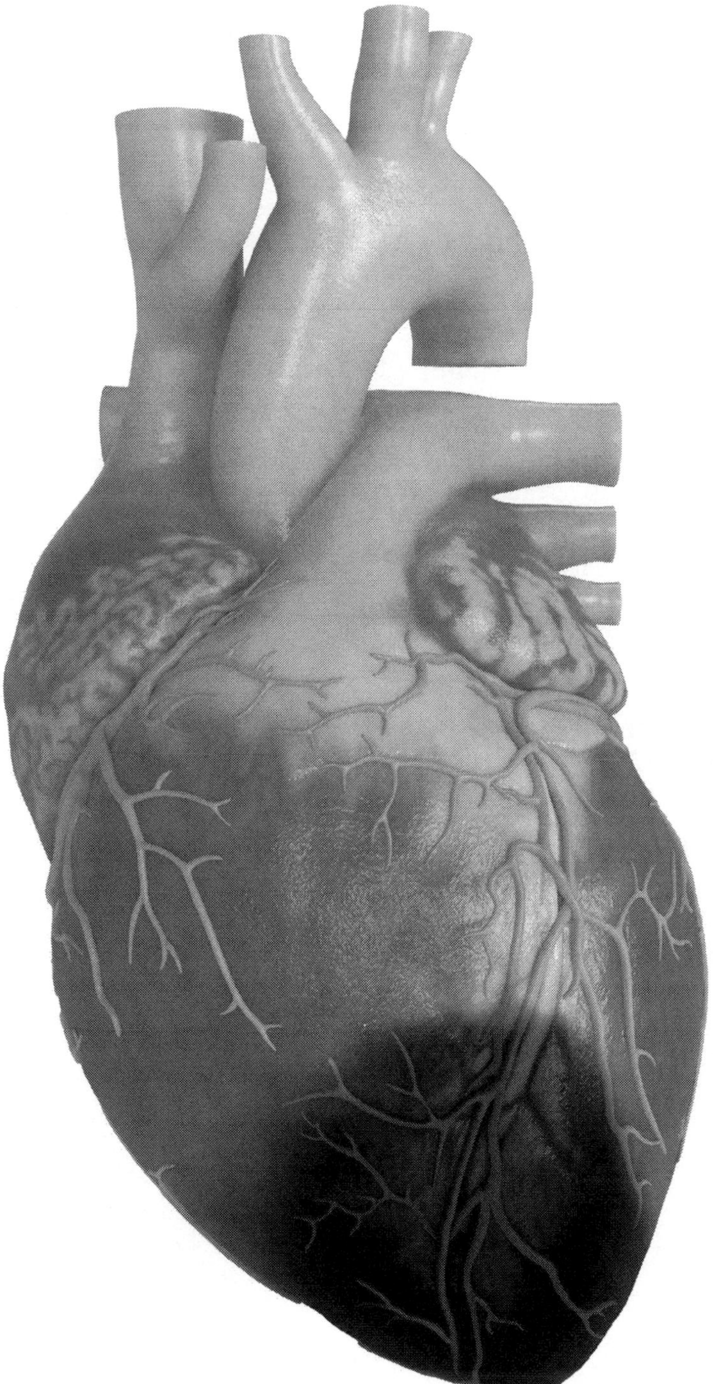

Disease

A disease is a condition affecting certain functions or structures in the human body, which can usually be associated with **signs or symptoms**. Diseases most commonly affect a specific location in the body, and aren't the result of physical trauma. Diseases range in severity from mild to severe, and in length from acute to chronic. These factors are determined by the type of disease, and the ability to treat the disease.

An **acute** disease or disorder has a **sudden onset**, which lasts for a **short period of time**. Acute conditions can be seen often with infections or trauma, and as the body's immune system fights off the infection, the acute condition dissipates. However, if the condition is severe enough, it may result in death. It is in this way that acute conditions are typically more dangerous in the short term than chronic conditions.

Chronic diseases or disorders are present for **long periods**, usually over three months. Examples of chronic diseases include asthma and hepatitis C. Chronic diseases may have periods of exacerbation and remission. The period where the disease is not actively showing signs or symptoms is the remission period, while the period where the disease is affecting a person's health is the exacerbation period. Other forms of chronic diseases, such as cancer or diabetes, are always present, and can make a person continuously ill.

Acquired Diseases

An acquired disease is a disease a person has obtained at some point **after birth**. Commonly thought of as some sort of infection, it actually just means the disease has appeared after birth. If a person has a disease that was not congenital, then it is referred to as an acquired disease.

Autoimmune Diseases

Autoimmune diseases are the result of the body's **immune system attacking cells and structures in the body that it cannot differentiate** from pathogens that have entered the body. Autoimmune diseases can attack different parts of the body with differing levels of severity.

In a person with an autoimmune disease, the body releases proteins known as **autoantibodies**. Autoantibodies are the cells that cannot tell the difference between normal tissue and foreign substances. Autoantibodies may attack only one specific structure, such as Graves' disease where the thyroid is the only structure attacked, or they may attack structures throughout the entire body, such as in lupus.

Autoimmune diseases may be hereditary, such as multiple sclerosis. If one person in a family has an autoimmune disorder, it may increase the likelihood of another family member having it as well.

Congenital Diseases

A congenital disease is a disease that is **present at birth**. These diseases may be inherited, or may be the result of certain environmental factors. Common examples of congenital diseases include heart defects, cleft lip, Down syndrome, HIV infection, and spina bifida. Causes for these diseases vary, but many are likely due to lack of maternal nutrition intake, alcohol use, drug use, and the fetus not receiving adequate nutrients.

Deficiency Diseases

Deficiency diseases are the result of the body **not receiving adequate nutrients**, vitamins, and/or minerals in the diet. Examples of nutrients include iron, vitamin C, zinc, calcium, and iodine. When a person does not receive these nutrients in adequate amounts, it can cause organs and structures in the body to function improperly, or not at all. For example, if a person lacks sufficient vitamin C in the diet, they may develop scurvy. If a person does not consume enough calcium, they may develop osteoporosis. Other examples of diseases caused by a nutrient deficiency include anemia, goiter, and rickets.

Hereditary Diseases

A hereditary disease, also known as a genetic disease, is the result of some sort of **abnormality in a person's genome**. These abnormalities vary in severity, and in turn, may cause differing levels of difficulty in normal function.

Genetic disorders are commonly passed down from the parents, but some genetic disorders may be the result of mutations in the genes due to environmental factors. Other times, the mutation in the gene may be completely random. There are differing types of gene inheritance that contribute to the development of hereditary diseases.

Single gene inheritances are the result of mutations occurring in **one single gene**. This leaves the majority of the body operating normally, but can change one specific aspect of the body. An example is cystic fibrosis, where the mutated gene causes the respiratory passages to produce an extremely excessive amount of mucous.

Multifactoral gene inheritances are the result of a **mutation in multiple genes**, in association with environmental factors. The gene may be present that can cause the disease, but it may lie dormant unless it is activated by environmental factors. Examples include cancers, hypertension, and cardiovascular disease. If the person avoids the environmental factors, they see less of a chance of developing the disease associated with the mutated gene.

Abnormal chromosomes are often caused by problems during cell division, known as **nondisjunction**, which can damage the chromosomes in the cell's DNA. An example of an abnormal chromosome disease is Down syndrome. This is caused by having an extra copy of chromosome 21. This gives the person 47 total chromosomes, instead of the standard 46.

Idiopathic Diseases

An idiopathic disease is a disease that has an **unknown origin or cause**. These diseases show no obvious sign of origin, and spontaneously appear. There may be theories about why a disease occurs, but the exact reason is unknown. Examples of idiopathic diseases include ankylosing spondylitis, chronic fatigue syndrome, and fibromyalgia.

Infectious Diseases

An infection is an **invasion of a microorganism** inside the body in some way, which can be localized and less serious, to systemic and life-threatening. These microorganisms are usually not inside the body, and therefore, the body does not have a knowledge of how to exactly combat the infection when first exposed. When there is an infection, the body develops antibodies, and these are used to destroy the invading microorganism.

There are four primary types of infections: bacterial, viral, parasitic, and fungal.

Psychological Diseases

Psychological diseases, often referred to as **mental disorders**, are often associated with problems a person may experience with their mood or thoughts. Causes are hard to pin-point, and may vary from person to person. These mental disorders can have an extremely adverse affect on the overall well-being of the person. Treatment via medications and psychotherapy may be available.

Mental disorders commonly seen in children include autism, ADHD(Attention Deficit/Hyperactivity Disorder), attachment disorder, and stuttering. Disorders commonly seen in adults may include addiction, depression, bipolar disorder, eating disorders, PTSD, and panic disorder.

Personality disorders are disorders that may influence how a person acts or responds to certain situations. Examples of personality disorders include Antisocial Personality Disorder, Dissociative Identity Disorder, and Obsessive-Compulsive Personality Disorder.

Immunity

Immunity refers to the ability of the body to **protect itself from disease and pathogens**. Immunity is the responsibility of the **immune system**, which destroys foreign objects that enter the body that may produce infection or disease. The process through which these substances are destroyed is known as the **immune response**.

The **humoral immune system** is the part of the immune system that takes place in the body's **fluids**, known as the **humors**. This results in the production of **antibodies** when a foreign substance is observed in the body. Antibodies react by neutralizing the pathogen, or allowing the pathogen to be destroyed easier by other cells.

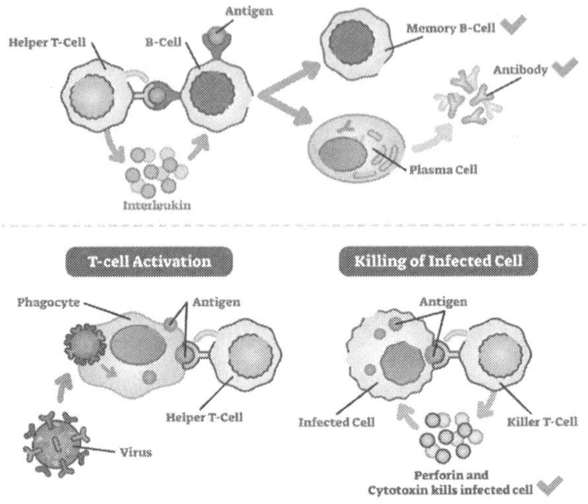

The **cell-mediated immune system** involves **T-lymphocytes**, also known as **T-cells**. These cells vary in type, depending on the kind of pathogen involved. The T-lymphocytes are responsible for destroying the pathogen, and do not utilize antibodies. Types of T-cells include effector, helper, cytotoxic, natural killer, memory, and regulatory, each responsible for a different aspect of immune support.

When a pathogen is detected in the body, a **B-cell** or **T-cell** will bind to the pathogen, and release **cytokines**. Cytokines are proteins responsible for allowing communication between cells. Cytokines will send a message to the immune system, which will then bring more B-cells or T-cells into the area to combat the pathogen.

Phagocytes

Phagocytes, which are certain types of **white blood cells**, are responsible for "**eating**" pathogens or debris in a process known as **phagocytosis**. Debris can include foreign objects or substances that have entered the body, or dead or dying cells that need to be removed from the body. An example is the fading of tattoos. Over time, tattoo ink is broken down by the body's phagocytes, because the body senses it is a foreign substance that should not be present. When enough ink is broken down by phagocytes, the tattoo fades. Laser tattoo removal works by breaking the ink into smaller pieces, which the phagocytes can then absorb and eliminate from the body easier.

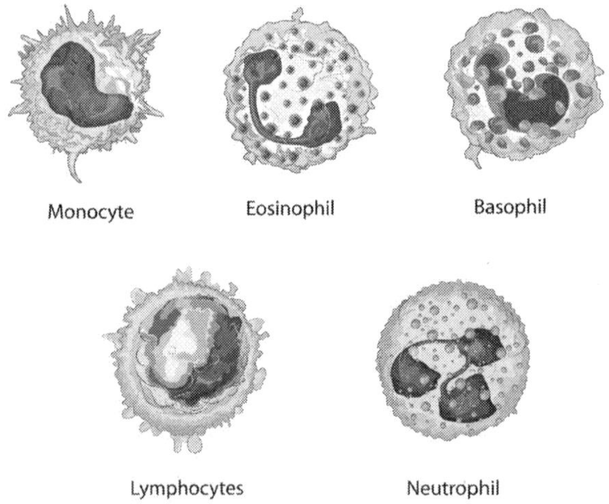

Examples of phagocytes include neutrophils, monocytes, macrophages, and dendritic cells. **Neutrophils** are typically the first phagocyte into the area. Neutrophils release enzymes that **destroy bacteria**, and perform phagocytosis. **Monocytes** move from the blood into the area, where they are then known as **macrophages**.

Much like neutrophils, they perform phagocytosis to eliminate the debris or infection. **Dendritic cells** are located on **surfaces** of the body such as the skin and gastrointestinal tract. Dendritic cells act by performing phagocytosis on a pathogen to retrieve its specific **antigen**. Once this information has been obtained, it is **passed on to T-cells** via cytokines produced by the dendritic cells.

Phagocytosis

Phagocytosis is the process of a cell "**eating**" an object or substance, a process known as **endocytosis.** The phagocyte envelops the debris or pathogen in a vesicle known as a **phagosome.** A phagosome is produced when the cell wraps the cell membrane around the structure and the cell membrane fuses together. The phagosome is introduced into the cell, holding the substance, where the substance is broken down by granules that produce toxic or acidic matter to dissolve the substances. Once the substance has been destroyed, the waste is removed from the cell in a process that is essentially the opposite of bringing the substance into the cell. The phagosome fuses back with the cell membrane, and the waste product is expelled into the extracellular fluid. This process is known as **exocytosis.**

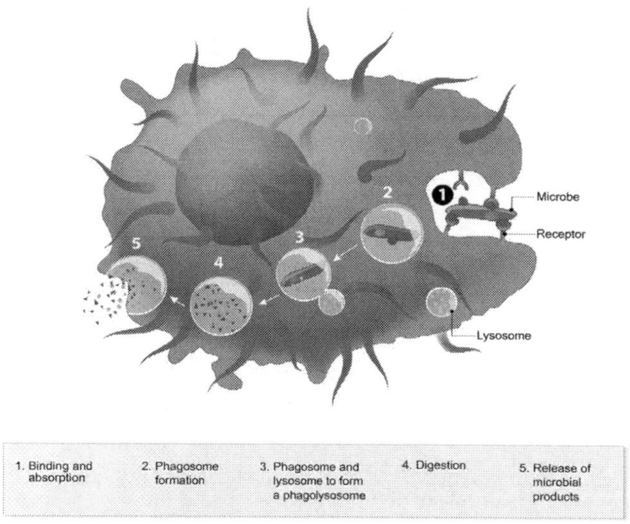

Antibodies

An **antibody**, also known as **immunoglobulin**, is a protein produced by **plasma cells** to neutralize pathogens in the body such as viruses and certain bacteria. Antibodies are **Y shaped.** The tips of the antibodies that produce the Y shape contain what's known as a **paratope**, which binds together with the **epitope**, the substance found in antigens that the body's immune system recognizes. **Antigens** are molecules the pathogen contains that the antibodies recognize and attach to, similar to a key fitting into a lock.

Antibodies are **produced and secreted by B-cells**, in two different forms. The first form is **soluble** and moves freely throughout the body. These types of B-cells are known as **plasma cells.** The second is a **membrane-bound form,** and it attaches to the surface of B-cells. These types are known as **B-cell receptors.** B-cell receptors bind to the surface of B-cells and are able to quickly identify pathogens seen before in the body. This allows the B-cells to produce sufficient antibodies to attack the pathogen with a faster response time.

Antibodies vary depending on the type of pathogen detected. For each different pathogen, a different type of antibody is produced. The amount of pathogens exposed to the body determines the amount of different antibodies being produced. If a person has been exposed to the pathogen before, **memory cells** may be produced, which **store information** on how the immune system is to destroy the pathogen. It is when this happens that a person is considered **immune** to a certain disease.

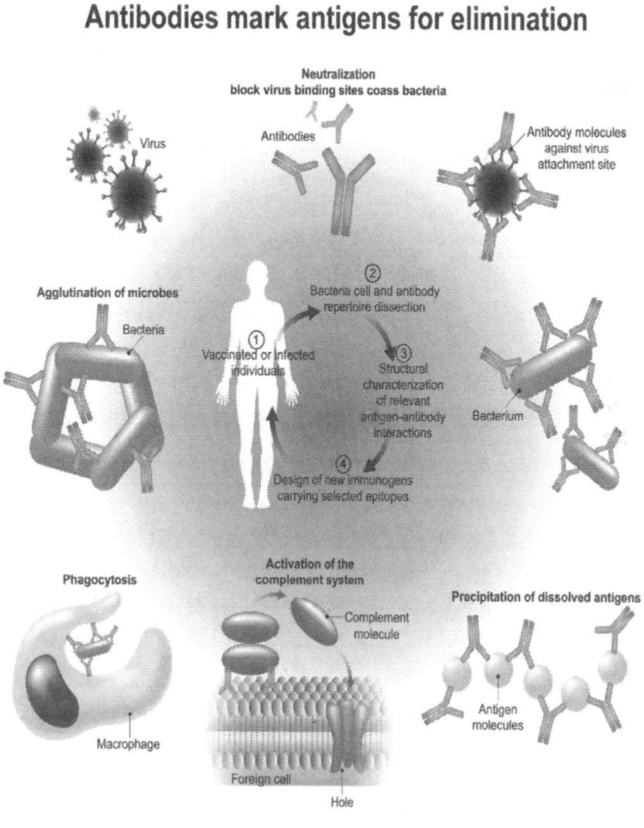

Tissue Repair

When a part of the body is injured or damaged, the damaged tissue must go through repair to allow proper functioning of the structure once again. The amount of repair correlates to the amount of tissue damage that has occurred. Some tissue may not be able to be repaired effectively, and may require scar tissue to complete the repair.

Inflammation

Upon damage to tissue, the tissue will experience **inflammation**. Inflammation starts with **dilation of capillaries** in the area of the trauma. Damaged tissues **release histamines** into the area, which stimulates the capillaries to dilate. When the capillaries dilate, the walls of the capillaries become thinner and **more permeable**. This allows **leukocytes and plasma** from the blood to enter the extracellular fluid in the damaged area, which is what produces inflammation. Because there is an increase in blood in the area, the inflamed area will feel **warmer** to the touch, and have a **reddish appearance**. The leukocytes release chemicals into the area, such as bradykinin, which causes **pain** by stimulating the nerve endings in the area. The four markers of inflammation are **pain**, **swelling**, **redness**, and **heat**.

As more leukocytes enter the area, they destroy any tissue that is damaged and any foreign objects or organisms that are present. Once the area is clear of damaged tissue and other organisms, the inflammation resolves. The capillary walls constrict, and the excess fluid in the area is removed through **lymphatic ducts**. As the blood and fluid is removed from the area, the swelling, redness, and heat subside.

Healing

Most tissue in the body can regenerate and create more tissue to replace any damaged tissue. Some tissue, such as nerve tissue and brain tissue, usually cannot. If a large portion of the body has experienced damage, the tissue may need to be removed to prevent the area from becoming gangrenous.

If a person has suffered a wound, and the **damaged areas are close together**, the body will heal itself through a process known as **primary intention**. Examples of wounds that are healed via primary intention are small cuts, scratches, and surgical incisions. These wounds allow for **blood clots** to form that hold the tissues together and stop bleeding. Beneath the clot, which is known as a **scab**, new tissue is formed, and the two sides of the wound join together. Once the new tissue is formed, the scab sloughs off, revealing the new tissue.

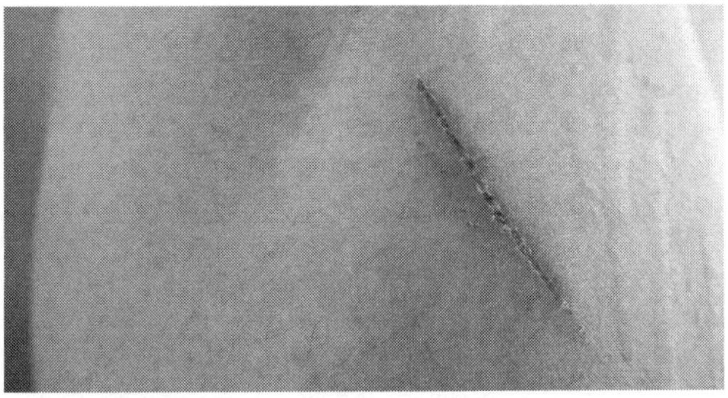

If a person suffers a wound that requires healing via **secondary intention**, the edges of the wound **cannot be approximated.** The edges are uneven, do not properly align, and may be far apart. This type of healing requires **granulated tissue** to form at the base and sides of the wound. As the healing progresses, the granulated tissue fills in the area missing tissue. This type of healing often takes far longer than primary intention healing, and will leave the area with scar tissue to help fill the damaged area. An example of secondary intention healing is seen with decubitus ulcers.

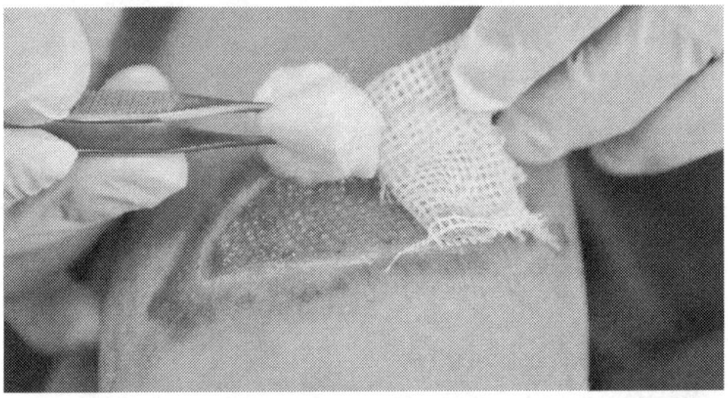

When a person experiences a wound that requires medical intervention, **delayed primary closure** may be utilized. With delayed primary closure, the **wound is left open** to ensure it is properly cleaned and free of bacteria or other pathogens before being closed. This is also known as **tertiary intention healing**. Once it is determined that there is no infection present, the wound is then surgically closed. An example of wounds that often require tertiary intention healing is animal bites.

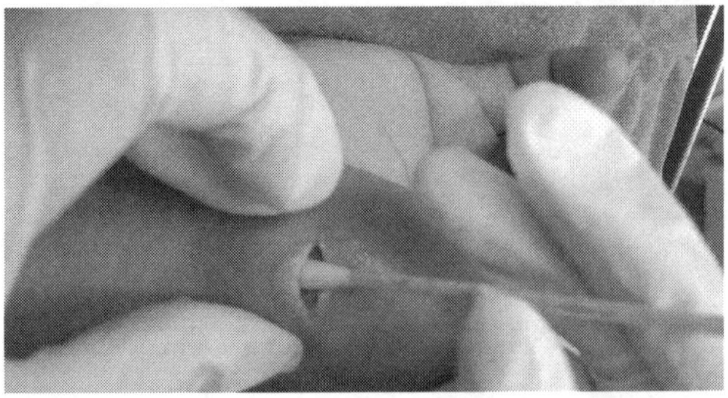

Bone Healing

Damage to bones, such as fractures, requires the use of **osteoclasts and osteoblasts** to help repair the structure. These cells continuously maintain the bone matrix, but if the bone is injured, they are the primary cells responsible for healing. After a bone is fractured, **osteoclasts** will begin **breaking down** the damaged bone tissue. This leaves the bone with a clean surface in which to build new bone tissue. It is similar to demolishing a building and erecting another building in its place. The rubble from the demolished building needs to be removed before another building can be constructed.

After the damaged surface has been cleared by the osteoclasts, **osteoblasts begin forming new bone matrix** to replace the matrix that has been lost. The material produced by osteoblasts is known as **callus**, and it binds the two sides of the fracture together, similar to scar tissue in the skin. The bone will absorb the callus, and the callus is then replaced by bone tissue. These cells are known as **osteocytes**. The bone is then remodeled into essentially its original shape, and osteoblasts stop producing osteocytes to replace the damaged bone.

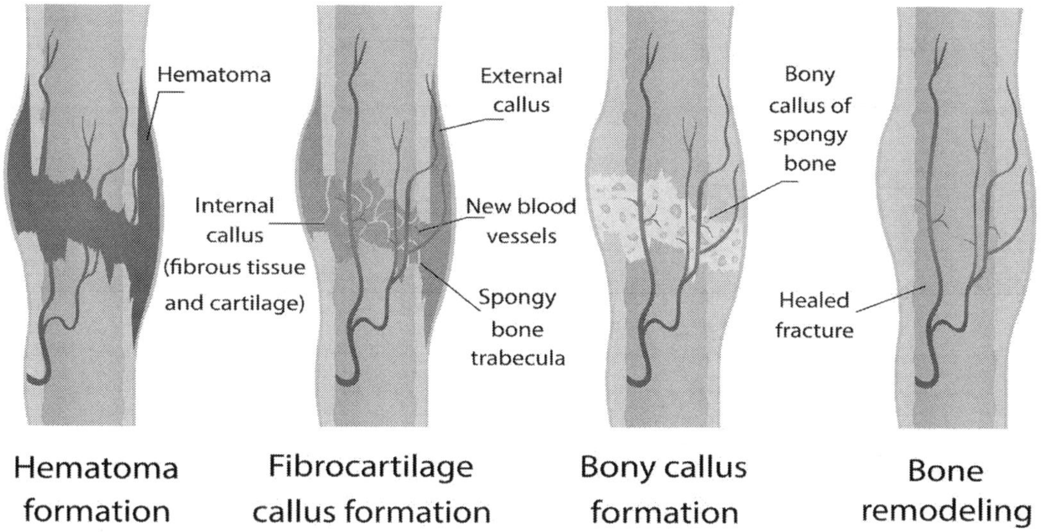

Scar

A scar, also known as **cicatrix**, is a fibrous tissue formed to help a wound heal. Scar tissue acts as a bandage, holding the damaged tissue together when it cannot be effectively replaced on its own. Scarring depends on the size, location, and depth of the wound suffered. Other factors that may play a role in scar development is a person's age, genes, and overall health of the person and the part of the body involved.

Different types of scars include acne scars, keloid scars, contracture scars, and hypertrophic scars.

Acne Scars

Acne scars may occur in a person with severe acne. These scars can leave **deep pits** in the skin, usually the result of a follicle wall being broken by an excessive accumulation of oil, bacteria, or fluid.

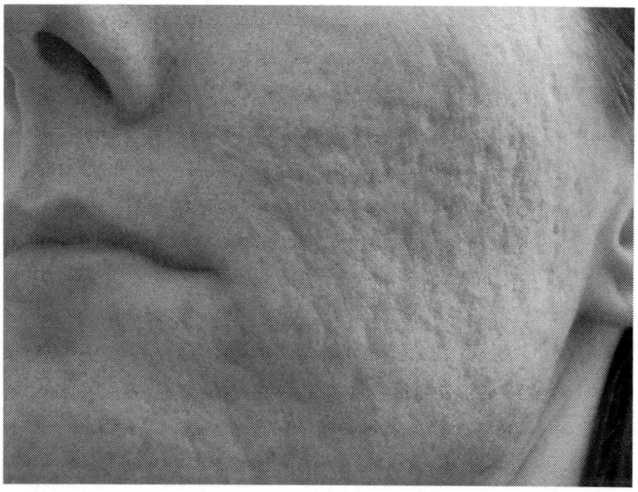

Contracture Scars

Contracture scars are usually seen in people who have suffered **burns**. These scars are spread out, and may extend deeper into the skin and affect muscles and nerves. The larger the burn, the more likely it is contracture scars may affect the ability to move certain parts of the body, depending on the location. If a person develops a contracture scar early in life, the scar may become mixed with healthy tissue.

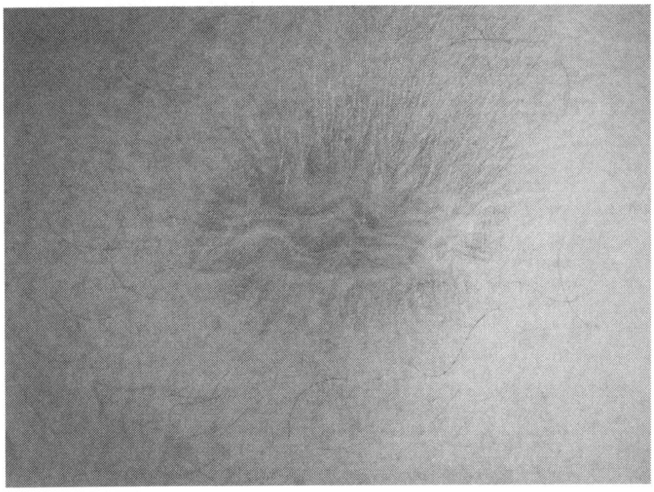

Hypertrophic Scars

Hypertrophic scars are similar to keloid scars, but they do not extend past the area of damage. These scars often **appear red**, and may be **tender or painful**. Hypertrophic scars are the result of a **collagen imbalance** at the site of injury, which does not allow the scar to form properly. **Excessive tension** on the area may also lead to the development of hypertrophic scars.

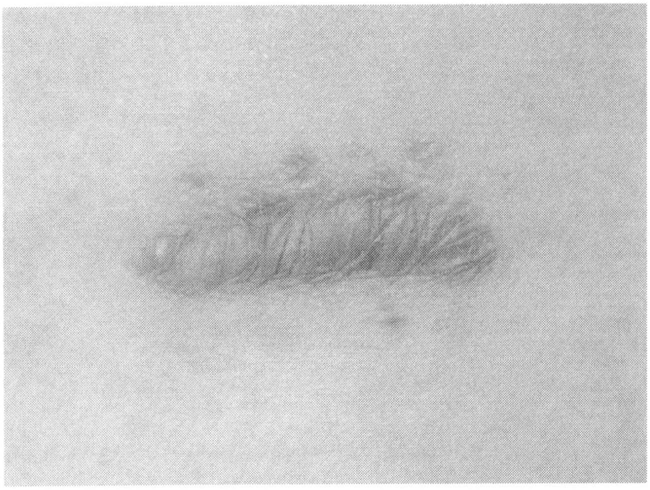

Keloid Scars

Keloid scars are more commonly seen in people with darker skin tone. These scars are the result of over-healing in the area. Keloid scars are often **raised off the skin**, extending beyond the area of damage. If large enough, these may be uncomfortable, cause pain, or reduce movement.

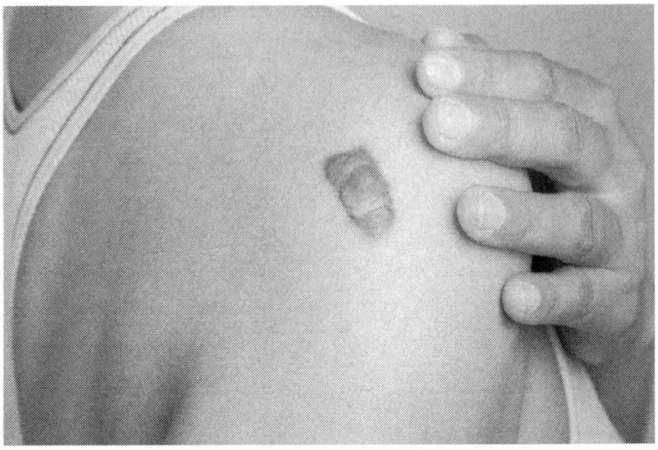

Striae

Striae, also known as **stretch marks**, are scars that form in the skin when the body experiences a **rapid growth**, such as during pregnancy, puberty, or during activities such as weight lifting. These scars generally have a different color than the surrounding skin. As the area grows, the skin is stretched and pulled apart. In response, the skin develops fibrous tissue to hold the expanding area together, which produces scarring.

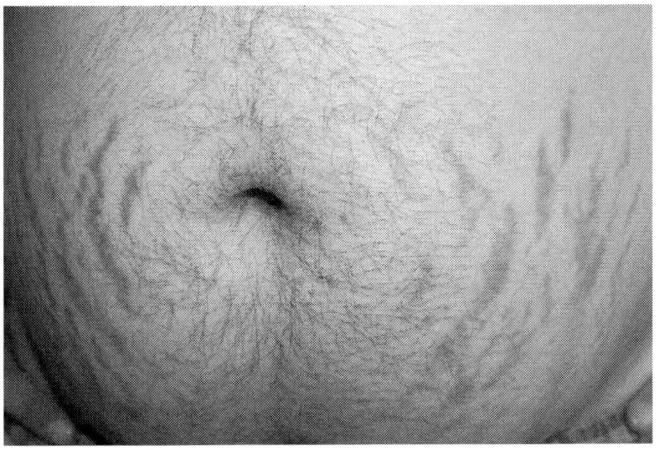

Cardiovascular Pathologies

Anemia

(an-: without; -emia: blood)

Anemia is a disease of the blood, resulting in a **lack of oxygen** and an **over-abundance of carbon dioxide** in the blood. There are many different types of anemia, ranging from **iron-deficient anemia** to **sickle cell anemia**. Anemia is the most common blood condition in the United States, with an estimated 3.5-4 million people afflicted with it.

Iron-deficient anemia is the most common form of anemia. The cells in the blood that are responsible for carrying oxygen and carbon dioxide throughout the body are the erythrocytes, or red blood cells. In the cytoplasm of erythrocytes, there is a protein present known as hemoglobin, which is made of iron. The hemoglobin attracts oxygen and carbon dioxide, allowing these molecules to attach to the erythrocytes.

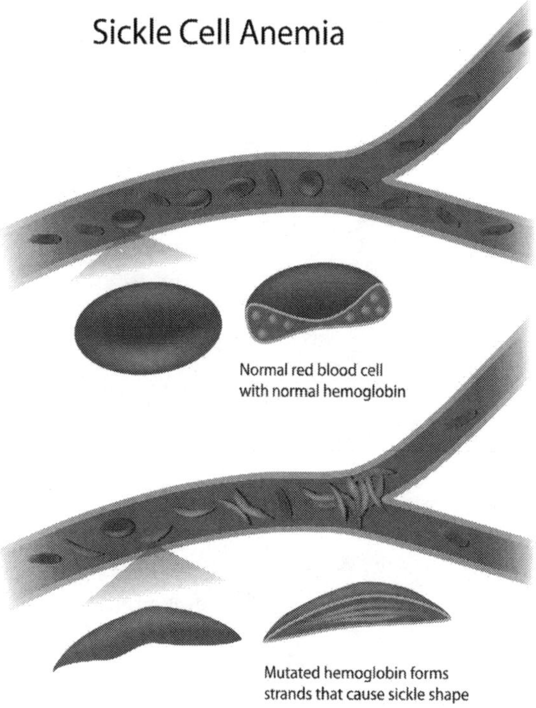

Causes

In iron-deficient anemia, the primary cause is a lack of iron being consumed. Less iron being consumed results in **less hemoglobin** in the erythrocytes, which in turn causes a lack of oxygen and carbon dioxide attaching to the red blood cells.

Sickle cell anemia is an inherited form of anemia, in which the erythrocytes have a sickle shape, as opposed to a normal erythrocyte, which is circular. This shape can cause the erythrocytes to become stuck in blood vessels, and reduce adequate blood flow to tissues.

Symptoms

People with anemia may feel sluggish, tired, have an increased heart rate, may show paleness in the skin, shortness of breath, and experience dizziness, all due to a lack of sufficient oxygen reaching tissues.

Sickle cell anemia may also result in the further development of infections due to damage caused to the spleen, pain in the thorax and abdomen(known as crises) due to blockage of blood vessels in these locations, and a lack of nutrients to the body, which can stunt growth.

People whose diet lacks proper amounts of iron or vitamin B-12 may develop anemia. Pregnancy, and a lack of folic acid, may result in anemia in pregnant women. Sickle cell anemia is primarily seen in African-Americans, resulting from a genetic defect.

Treatments

Treatments for anemia vary depending on the type, but may include increasing iron intake, bone marrow transplants, or blood transfusions. Pregnant women may require an increased intake of folic acid. People with sickle cell anemia face less treatment options. The only potential cure is through a bone marrow transplant. Often times, the only treatment is trying to minimize the number of crises a person may experience. Antibiotics and pain relievers may help in preventing infections in younger patients and reducing pain experienced during crises.

Aneurysm

(Greek "aneurysma": a widening)

An aneurysm is a condition of the arteries, resulting in a **bulge in the wall of an artery**. There are several different forms and causes of aneurysms. Different types of aneurysms include Aortic(bulge in the wall of the aorta), Cerebral(bulge in an artery supplying blood to the brain), and Ventricular(bulge in the wall of the heart).

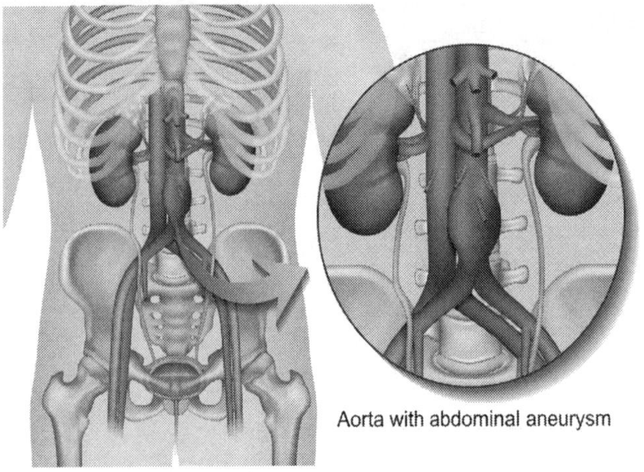

Aorta with abdominal aneurysm

Causes

Aneurysms are the result of a **part of an arterial wall becoming weakened**, which forces the wall out, creating a pouch or bubble. Most commonly, aneurysms are the result of hypertension putting too much pressure or strain on the artery. Ventricular aneurysms are most commonly caused by myocardial infarction, which can weaken the heart muscle.

When the arterial wall stretches due to weakness, it makes it much easier for the artery to rupture. Because the artery carries oxygen-rich blood, this makes aneurysms very dangerous, as any rupture will severely cut off blood flow to the structure supplied with blood by the artery.

Symptoms

Unfortunately, aneurysms that have not ruptured are asymptomatic. In fact, aneurysms themselves, unless very large, cause no symptoms at all. When an aneurysm ruptures, however, a person may experience severe chest or back pain, low blood pressure, severe headache, tachycardia, and lightheadedness.

People may develop aneurysms for many different reasons, including obesity, hypertension, diabetes, advanced age, and alcoholism. Some people develop aneurysms for no apparent reason at all.

Treatments

Common locations for aneurysms include the abdominal aorta and the brain. Aneurysms may be treated surgically before rupture to prevent major medical emergencies in the future. Beta blockers are commonly used as medications before surgery is required.

Angina Pectoris

(Latin "angere": to strangle; pectoris: chest)

Angina pectoris is **pain in the chest**, which results from **ischemia in heart tissue**.

Causes

The primary cause of angina pectoris is **blockages in arteries** that provide the myocardium with blood. When these arteries become restricted, the heart muscle is unable to get enough oxygen-rich blood. Lack of oxygen in tissue results in ischemia. During times of physical exertion, chest pain may develop as a result of the lack of oxygen entering the heart tissue. During times of rest, however, the heart does not have to work as hard, and the pain is non-existent. People who develop angina pectoris usually have increased emotional stress, and are chronic cigarette smokers. Because the arteries are narrowed, atherosclerosis may also be a contributing factor in the development of chest pain.

Symptoms

Symptoms of angina pectoris include acute instances of pain(less than five minutes), pain that dissipates with medication and/or rest, and pain that only appears when the heart is required to work harder, such as during physical activity.

Treatments

Treatment includes rest and medication, such as nitroglycerin, which relaxes the coronary arteries, and increases the volume of blood entering the myocardium.

Arrhythmia

(a-: without; rhythm: rhythm)

Arrhythmia is a condition of the heart, which results in the **heart's natural rhythm being altered**. There are several different forms of arrhythmia. Some of the most common forms of arrhythmia are Atrial Fibrillation, Bradycardia, and Tachycardia.

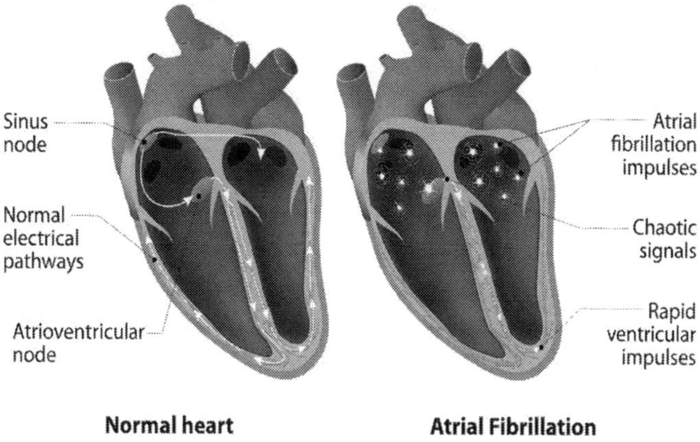

Causes

Atrial fibrillation, the most common form of arrhythmia, results when the atria, the heart's upper chambers, contract irregularly, which sends blood into the ventricles at uncoordinated times. This is caused by an electrical signal from the SA Node not firing correctly, which disrupts the timing of the atria contracting. This can affect the ability of the heart to consistently deliver oxygenated blood to the body.

Bradycardia*(brady-: slow; -cardia: heart)* results in the heart rate being reduced to a rate of contraction that is considered too slow to deliver substantial oxygen to the body.

Tachycardia*(tachy-: rapid; -cardia: heart)* results in the heart rate being increased to a rate of contraction that is considered too rapid. In tachycardia, the ventricles of the heart are contracting too rapidly, which may cause a lack of oxygen-rich blood from reaching the body, as the quick contractions do not allow the ventricles to properly fill with blood before being pumped out to the rest of the body. Older adults, those over age 60, are more likely to develop arrhythmia than younger adults and children. Heart diseases are a main contributing factor towards older adults developing arrhythmia. Other diseases may also play a role in the development of arrhythmia, so people who have had myocardial infarction may be more prone to developing the disease. Diabetes, sleep apnea, and hypertension all have contributed to the development of arrhythmia.

Symptoms

There are many different symptoms seen with arrhythmia. Symptoms include dizziness, fatigue, shortness of breath, pain in the chest, lightheadedness, and fainting. In severe cases, arrhythmia may result in cardiac arrest.

Treatments

Treatments vary, depending on the type of arrhythmia a person suffers from. Medical devices such as pacemakers may be implanted into the body to help regulate and control heart rhythm(IE, if a person's heart rate drops too low, the pacemaker will stimulate the heart muscle and cause it to contract, increasing heart rate back to safe levels). Alternative methods to controlling arrhythmia, such as massage therapy and yoga, may be applied in some cases.

Arteriosclerosis/Atherosclerosis

(arterio: artery; scler-: hard; -osis: condition);
(athero: fatty plaque; scler-: hard; -osis: condition)

Arteriosclerosis is a **hardening of the walls of arteries**, a condition that progresses slowly over time. Atherosclerosis is a **build-up of fatty plaque** inside the arteries. These two conditions are commonly caused by one another, and are often interchangeable.

Causes

Arteriosclerosis has many different contributing factors, including hypertension, high cholesterol, and smoking. Each of these can damage an artery. The body's response to this damage is to increase the thickness of the artery to prevent further damage. When this occurs, the artery becomes much harder and unable to move and stretch normally. This may also lead to increased deposits of plaque in the arteries, a condition known as atherosclerosis. This increased plaque, along with the hardening of the artery, may restrict blood flow and lead to conditions such as angina pectoris and myocardial infarction.

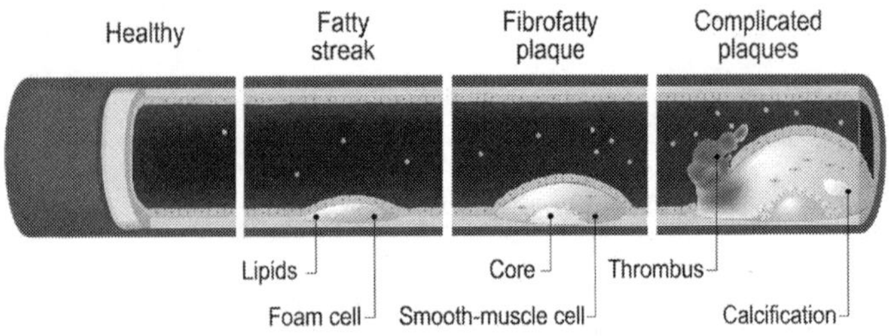

Symptoms

Symptoms include angina pectoris, shortness of breath, fatigue, and pain in any area of the body that may have any sort of restriction in the arteries.

Treatments

Medications are effective treatments for arteriosclerosis/atherosclerosis, including beta-blockers, statins, calcium channel blockers, and diuretics. If an increased plaque buildup is severe, an angioplasty may be performed, or a stent may be placed inside the artery to increase blood flow. Plaque may be surgically removed, or a bypass surgery may be performed to increase circulation into areas that may be experiencing ischemia.

Deep Vein Thrombosis

(thromb/o: clot; -osis; condition)

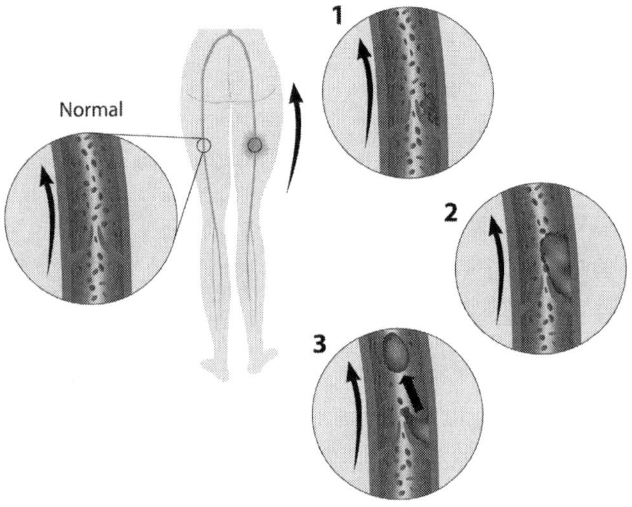

1. Clot formation, 2. Clot growth, 3. Clot dislodging

Deep Vein Thrombosis(DVT) is a condition in which **blood clots(thrombi) form in the veins** deep in the body, typically the **legs**. These blood clots can **block blood flow** in the veins, which can lead to several serious issues.

Causes

There are various causes for DVT. Primary causes are injury to a vein, surgery, impaired or limited mobility, and certain medications. An injury to a vein can result in blood clots, especially if there is significant damage to the vein. Surgery, which can result in cutting through veins, can also lead to blood clots. Post-surgery, if a patient is immobilized for extended periods, circulation starts to decrease in efficiency, which can lead to blood pooling in the veins of the legs. This pooling of blood can result in clots. It is this same reason people who have paralysis may develop blood clots as well.

Symptoms

Although symptoms may not be present in someone with DVT, others do show symptoms, which include a warm sensation in the affected area, pain in the affected area that can increase in intensity, and discoloration in the affected area. Most commonly, DVT affects the lower limb, so this is where a person will most likely experience these symptoms.

Treatments

The primary treatment for DVT is medication. Certain medications can help reduce the chance of developing DVT in the future, or even remove the blood clot from the body. Intravenous anticoagulants such as heparin help to thin the blood. Other anticoagulants, such as warfarin, work extremely well in conjunction with injectable anticoagulants.

If the blood clot is severe, the patient might be given a thrombolytic, a type of medication that destroys blood clots. These are typically only given in serious cases of blood clots, such as those that result in pulmonary embolism. Compression socks, which compress the leg up to the knee, can help reduce the amount of swelling a patient might experience with DVT.

Heart Murmur

(murmur: to mutter)

A heart murmur is a condition of the heart, which results in blood **flowing backwards in the heart**. A "murmur" refers to the sound of blood flowing through the heart. There are two types of heart murmurs: Innocent and Abnormal. Innocent heart murmurs are seen in children and infants, usually the result of congenital heart disease. Abnormal heart murmurs are much more serious, most likely due to the development of heart disease or valve malfunction.

Causes

Heart murmurs may not require any medical attention, depending on the cause. Other times, medical attention may be needed. Most commonly, heart murmurs are the result of a **bicuspid/mitral valve prolapse**, where the valve is pulled backwards into the left atrium. This allows blood to flow backwards in the heart, which may reduce the ability of the heart to pump enough oxygen-rich blood to the body.

People who have developed endocarditis or Rheumatic fever often develop heart murmurs due to damage to the valves in the heart.

Symptoms

While most heart murmurs aren't serious, abnormal heart murmurs may present with symptoms such as cyanosis on the fingers, chest pain, dizziness, shortness of breath, and fainting.

Treatments

Heart murmurs may require the person to take anticoagulants to prevent the formation of blood clots, may be treated for hypertension if it is resulting in heart murmurs, or may need surgery to repair or replace the malfunctioning valve.

Hypertension

(hyper-: above; -tension: tension)

Hypertension is a condition of the Cardiovascular System, resulting in **elevated blood pressure**. There are numerous factors that may contribute to the development of hypertension. For an average healthy adult, systolic blood pressure(pressure felt in arteries when the heart beats) is around 120 mmHg, and diastolic pressure(pressure felt in arteries when the heart is at rest) is around 80 mmHg. To be diagnosed with hypertension, a person's systolic pressure would be 140 mmHg and diastolic pressure would be 90 mmHg.

Causes

Hypertension may have no underlying cause, or may be the result of factors such as dysfunction of the adrenal glands or thyroid, dietary issues such as obesity or high sodium intake, kidney disease, and alcohol consumption. Hypertension is most commonly associated with people who smoke, drink excessive amounts of alcohol, are overweight, are older in age, consume excessive salt, and more.

Symptoms

Unfortunately, hypertension is largely asymptomatic. Only in extreme cases, where the heart's blood pressure spikes extremely high, will someone experience symptoms, such as dizziness and headaches. Most symptoms people associate with hypertension are actually side effects of medications.

Treatments

Untreated, hypertension may lead to numerous serious medical conditions, such as myocardial infarction, stroke, atherosclerosis, and aneurysm. Luckily, hypertension is very easy to detect, and very treatable. Often times, treatment is as simple as making lifestyle or dietary changes, such as consuming less sodium and increasing exercise. Other times, hypertension may require the use of medications such as beta blockers, statins, and diuretics.

Migraine Headaches

Migraine Headaches are a type of headache that affect the brain, which results in most side effects experienced.

Migraines have been referred to as "**vascular headaches**", due to the involvement of **blood vessels**. In migraines, when the brain is stimulated by a trigger, neurons rapidly send impulses which affects the blood vessels surrounding the meninges, three layers of connective tissue that surround and protect the brain. At first, the blood vessels constrict, which does not result in pain. A short time after constricting, the blood vessels will dilate, which places immense pressure on the meninges, which results in severe pain.

Causes

Migraines have numerous causes, which may be from exposure to substances like tyramine(a naturally occurring chemical found in foods such as aged cheese, alcoholic beverages, and cured meats), caffeine, stress, or even hormonal imbalance during stages such as menstruation. Migraines may even be considered hereditary.

Symptoms

Symptoms include nausea, fatigue, extreme pain, loss of sight, blurred vision, sensitivity to sound, and pain on one side of the head. Not everyone that experiences a migraine experiences all of the symptoms detailed, as each migraine is different.

Treatments

If a migraine is in the beginning stages, taking pain medication such as aspirin or ibuprofen can help reduce the symptoms of mild migraines. Other medications, called triptans, can help to constrict blood vessels, which can help reduce the effects of migraines.

Preventative drugs may be taken to reduce the chances of developing a migraine in the future. These medications include beta blockers, non-steroidal anti-inflammatory drugs, and even antidepressants.

Myocardial Infarction

(myo-: muscle; -cardia: heart; infarct: obstruction of blood flow)

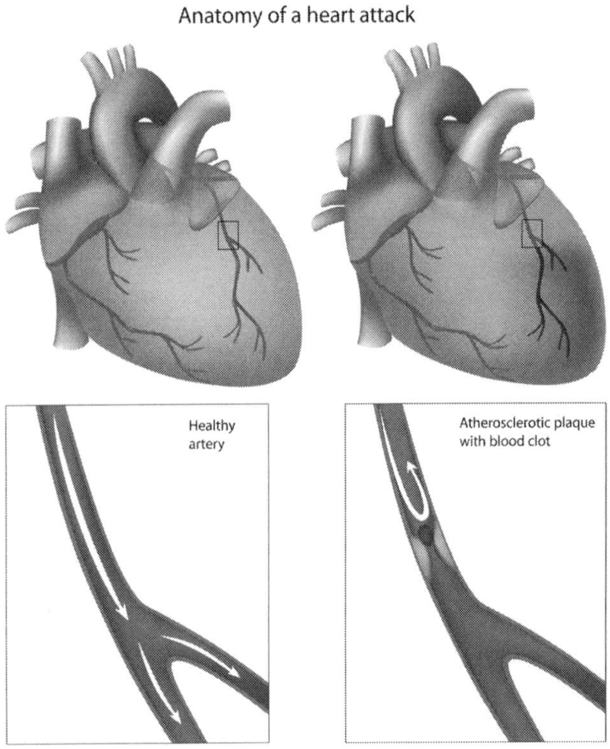

A Myocardial Infarction, or **heart attack**, is a condition that affects the heart muscle, reducing blood flow throughout the body.

An infarction is an **obstruction of blood flow** to a specific part of the body. In this case, blood flow to the heart is obstructed. The two arteries that supply blood to the heart muscle are known as the **coronary arteries**. When an abundance of substances such as **plaque build up** inside these arteries, it restricts blood flow to the heart muscle. When blood flow is restricted, the tissue does not receive adequate oxygen, which results in **necrosis of the affected tissue**. When too much cardiac muscle dies, the body experiences a myocardial infarction, or heart attack.

Causes

Myocardial infarctions may be the result of atherosclerosis, a condition which causes the artery walls to harden and thicken due to a build-up of plaque in the arteries. Hypertension, smoking, and obesity may also contribute to the development of atherosclerosis.

Symptoms

Symptoms of myocardial infarction may be acute, or build up over a period of days leading up to the myocardial infarction. In the preceding days, a person may experience malaise, fatigue, and discomfort in the chest. Acute stages of myocardial infarction include intense chest pain, pain in the neck and left arm, and increased heart rate.

Treatments

A person who has suffered from a myocardial infarction may have a coronary bypass surgery performed, an angioplasty or stent placed in the affected artery, or may not need any surgery and only require medications such as aspirin, beta blockers, and statins.

Phlebitis

(phleb-: vein; -itis: inflammation)

Phlebitis is a condition of the Cardiovascular System, affecting the **veins**, causing them to become **inflamed**. **Blood clots** may form in these veins.

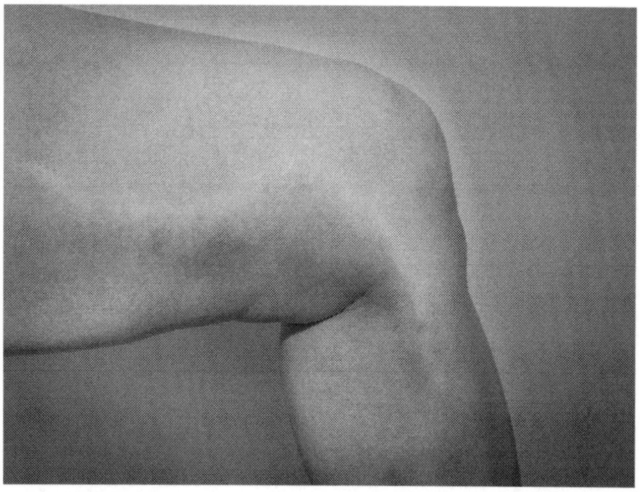

Causes

Phlebitis may have numerous causes, including **trauma to a vein**, and **immobility**. Trauma to a vein results in what is known as superficial phlebitis, usually the result of IV catheters being placed into a vein via needles.

Deep vein thrombosis is another type of phlebitis, taking place deeper in the body. Deep vein thrombosis(DVT) is most commonly caused by immobility of a limb. The body's veins move and stretch with the rest of the body during movement. If the veins are immobilized, they will become irritated, due to blood pooling in the veins. The blood pooling may result in blood clot formation. If a blood clot dislodges from its location and flows freely in the blood stream, it is known as an embolus, which could become lodged in other blood vessels throughout the body, cutting off blood flow and resulting in ischemia. Depending on the part of the body this takes place, it could even lead to possible death.

Symptoms

Symptoms of superficial phlebitis include tenderness and swelling around the injured vein, often with the affected vein presenting with a red line in the skin following the vein. The vein may feel hard to the touch due to inflammation.

Deep vein thrombosis may present with pain in the entire affected limb(usually the leg), along with swelling. If infection results, people may have fever.

Treatments

Treatments of phlebitis include anticoagulants for deep vein thrombosis such as heparin, ibuprofen, and antibiotics for superficial phlebitis.

Deep vein thrombosis requires immediate medical attention, as it may result in embolism, which could potentially be fatal.

Raynaud's Syndrome

Raynaud's Syndrome is a condition that results in **constriction of the blood vessels in the fingers and toes**, **reducing circulation** to these areas. This constriction is known as "vasospasm". Primary Raynaud's Syndrome occurs independently, while Secondary Raynaud's Syndrome is typically associated with other conditions.

Causes

The primary contributors to Raynaud's Syndrome are **cold temperatures**, **stress**, and **cigarette smoking**. Raynaud's Syndrome is typically not a debilitating disease. During a flare-up, the skin typically turns pale, the person may experience numbness or pain,

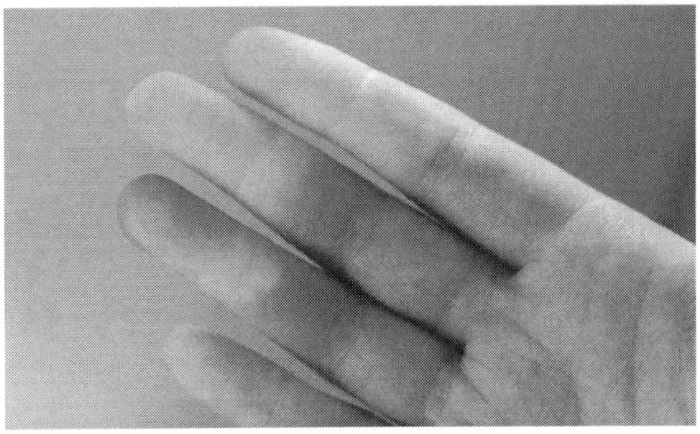

and the affected areas become very cold.

Secondary Raynaud's Syndrome may be associated with conditions such as lupus or scleroderma, and develops later in life than Primary Raynaud's Syndrome.

Symptoms

Symptoms of Raynaud's Syndrome include discoloration of the skin in affected areas, cold fingers and/or toes, numbness, and stinging pain upon warming of the area.

Treatments

Treatments for Raynaud's Syndrome include exercise, reducing stress, not smoking, and avoiding cold temperatures whenever possible. Secondary Raynaud's Syndrome may require medications such as statins to help regulate blood pressure and cholesterol.

Varicose Veins

(varicose: abnormally swollen)

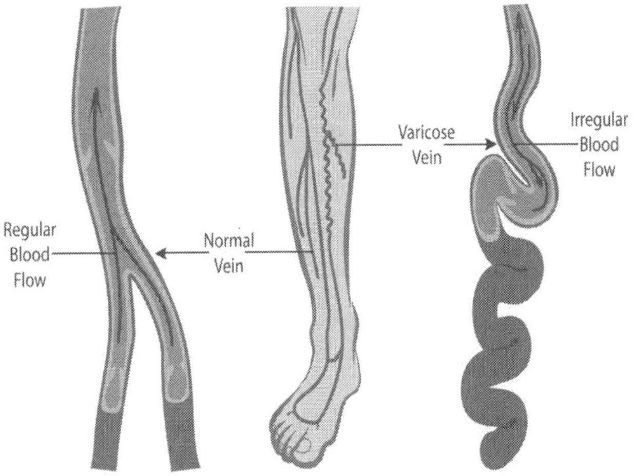

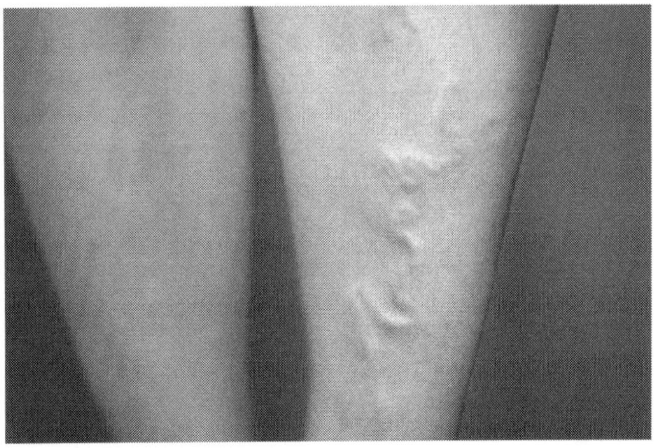

Varicose veins are the **abnormal swelling of veins** in the body, most commonly seen in the **legs**, but may be present in any vein. There are many different types, ranging from regular varicose veins, to spider veins, and even hemorrhoids.

Causes

Inside the veins, there are valves that push deoxygenated blood back up to the heart. Typically, as a person ages, the valves stop working as efficiently, which allows **blood to pool backwards** in the veins. This added pressure causes irritation and swelling of the veins. Blood pooling in the veins may also lead to complications such as the development of blood clots.

Because veins are much more superficial than arteries, when a vein becomes swollen, it is often visible. Varicose veins often present with a purple color, may look cord-like, and may even cause pain and discomfort. Causes of varicose veins include sitting or standing for prolonged periods, age, and even pregnancy.

Symptoms

Often times, varicose veins occur with no symptoms other than visual symptoms, such as discoloration of veins. If a varicose vein becomes painful, a person may experience burning, itching, edema, and cramping in the legs around the site of the varicose vein.

Treatments

Treatment is often unnecessary, outside of self-care. Self-care may include wearing compression socks, exercise, diet, and ele vating the legs to help circulation. If treatment is required, there are a number of different things that can be done, such as sclerotherapy, laser therapy, and removing the varicose vein from the body.

Digestive Pathologies

Appendecitis

(append: appendix; -itis: inflammation)

Appendicitis is inflammation of the appendix, a small tube extending off the ascending colon. The exact function of the appendix is unknown, but it is entirely possible to live without the appendix. When the appendix becomes inflamed, it risks rupturing and dumping infectious substances into the abdomen. This can possibly lead to peritonitis, which may be life-threatening. Appendicitis is always considered a medical emergency and must be treated immediately.

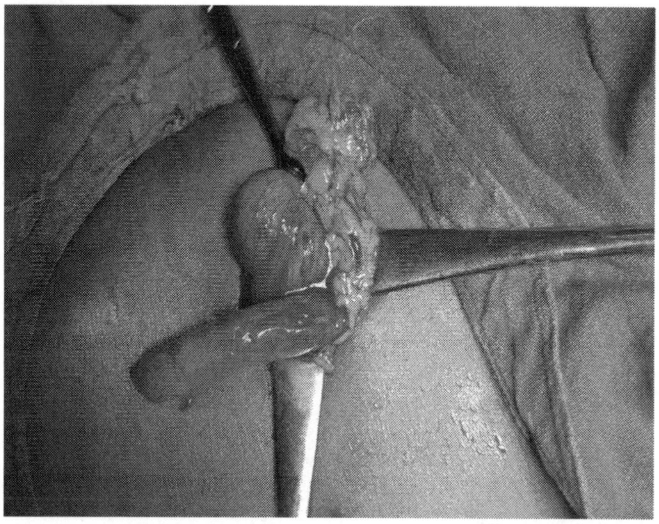

Causes

The most common cause of appendicitis is blockage of the appendix by fecal matter. This blockage keeps infectious material in the appendix, which may then become abscessed. A tumor may also block the appendix.

Symptoms

Symptoms of appendicitis include pain in the upper portion of the abdomen that moves down into the lower right abdomen which becomes extremely sharp, nausea and/or vomiting, low-grade fever, and loss of appetite. Painful urination, cramping, constipation, or diarrhea may also accompany appendicitis.

Treatments

Most commonly, appendicitis is treated by complete removal of the appendix, known as an appendectomy(surgical removal of the appendix). This ensures the appendix will not rupture and introduce infectious substances into the abdomen.

Cholecystitis

(chole-: bile; cyst-: bladder; -itis: inflammation)

Cholecystitis is **inflammation of the gallbladder.** If untreated, cholecystitis may lead to extremely serious conditions such as rupture of the gallbladder.

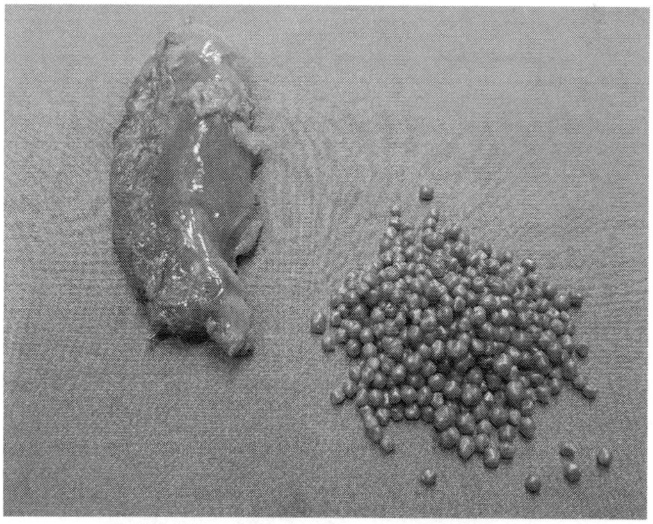

Gallbladder removal with presence of gallstones

Causes

Most commonly, cholecystitis is the result of **formation of gallstones.** Gallstones can block the cystic duct, which connects the gallbladder to the bile duct on its way to the duodenum, causing inflammation of the gallbladder as bile backs up in the organ.

There is no consensus on what causes gallstones to form. Some theories state gallstones form because the bile contains too much cholesterol, too much bilirubin, or the gallbladder doesn't properly empty bile into the duodenum.

Symptoms

Symptoms of cholecystitis include severe abdominal pain in the upper right quadrant near the liver, nausea, vomiting, fever, and pain in the right shoulder/back. These symptoms often occur after ingesting large meals.

Treatments

A diagnosis of cholecystitis almost always results in a hospital stay. Treatments may include antibiotics to fight off any associated infection, pain medication to reduce discomfort, and fasting to let the gallbladder rest and reduce inflammation.

Cholecystitis often recurs, and therefore most people who are diagnosed with cholecystitis require surgery to completely remove the gallbladder. The liver is then connected directly to the duodenum, allowing bile to enter into the small intestine.

Cirrhosis

(Greek "kirrhos": yellowish; -osis: condition)

Cirrhosis is **scarring of the liver**, due to other conditions such as **hepatitis**. Each time the liver is damaged, it repairs itself. During this repair process, **scar tissue** is formed. As the liver is damaged over time, more scar tissue forms, which makes liver function difficult. Cirrhosis gives the liver a **cobble-stone**, **yellow-orange appearance**.

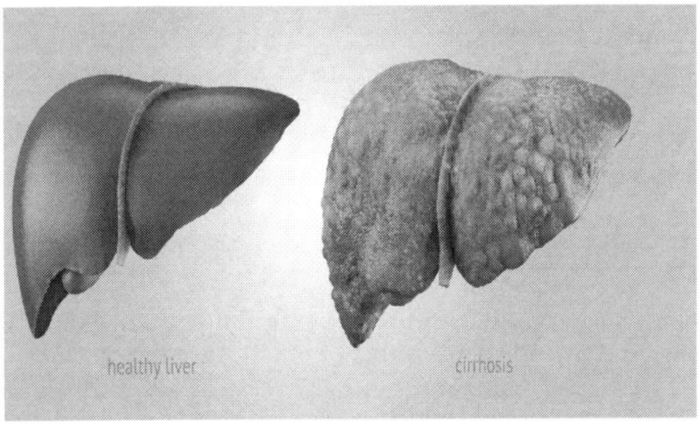

Causes

Most commonly, cirrhosis is the result of chronic hepatitis and alcohol abuse. Every time there is a flare-up of chronic hepatitis(HBV and HCV), it damages the liver, resulting in scar formation. Nonalcoholic fatty liver disease may also contribute to the development of cirrhosis.

Symptoms

Cirrhosis often does not present with symptoms until the damage caused is excessive. Symptoms may include nausea, weight loss, jaundice, bleeding and bruising easily, fatigue, edema in the legs, and an accumulation of fluid in the abdomen.

Treatments

Early stages of cirrhosis are treated by addressing the underlying cause, not the scarring itself, as the scarring is irreversible. A patient with early stages of cirrhosis may seek treatment for alcohol dependency to reduce the intake of alcohol, look into weight loss to reduce nonalcoholic fatty liver disease, and medications to help control HBV and HCV, which can substantially damage the liver.

Crohn's Disease

Crohn's Disease is an **inflammatory bowel disease**, which causes **inflammation of the digestive tract**. Crohn's has periods of exacerbation and remission, where the disease is actively causing inflammation, then periods where it is not. Crohn's disease typically appears in younger people, people who are of East European Jewish descent, people who have relatives with the disease, and people who smoke cigarettes.

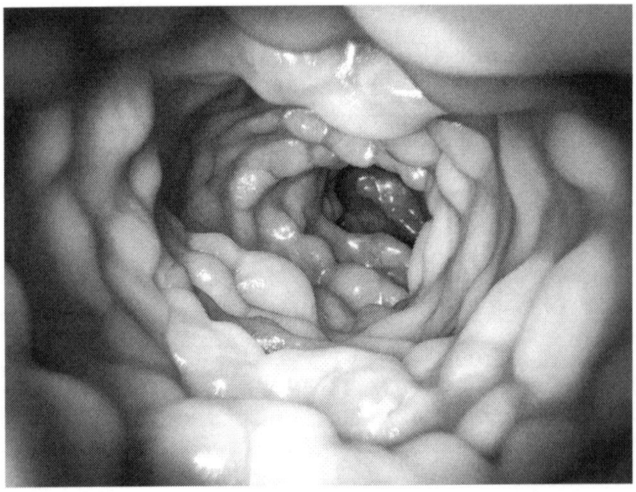

Damage to the digestive tract, including ulcerations and scarring, may result. Depending on the location of ulceration and scarring, abscesses and constipation may result.

Causes

The leading theories are heredity and an immune system that does not function properly are the main causes of Crohn's.

Symptoms

In acute stages of Crohn's, symptoms may include diarrhea, abdominal pain, cramping, fatigue, fever, and bloody stool. Depending on the severity of these symptoms, a person may need to visit a doctor.

Treatments

A variety of medications may be prescribed for a patient with Crohn's, including anti-inflammatory drugs such as corticosteroids to reduce inflammation in the digestive tract, immunosuppresors to help regulate the effects of the immune system on the digestive tract, and antibiotics to reduce any abscesses that may result. Pain relievers may also be prescribed.

In serious cases, surgery may be required. During Crohn's, scarring in the ileum or large intestine may result. In this surgery, the damaged portion of the digestive tract may be removed. This does not cure Crohn's, but can make it easier to manage.

Changes in diet, especially in acute stages, may be beneficial.

Diverticulitis

(diverticula: tubular sac branching off a cavity; -itis: inflammation)

Diverticulitis is a condition affecting the large intestine, but may also affect other structures such as the abdomen, or the entire Cardiovascular System. If a person is affected by diverticulosis, they have **small pouches** that develop in the large intestine. In certain cases, these pouches may become **inflamed and/or infected**, which then becomes diverticulitis.

Causes

Because diverticulitis puts strain on sections of the large intestine that are already weakened, ulcerations or open sores may result. These open sores may lead to infection, and leaking of feces into the abdomen, which results in peritonitis(inflammation of the peritoneum, a very serious condition that requires medical attention).

Symptoms

Symptoms of diverticulitis include fever, nausea, vomiting, pain in the lower left abdomen, and constipation. Tenderness in the abdomen may also be present.

Treatments

Diverticulitis may be treated in several different ways, depending on the severity. Pain medication may help with discomfort in less severe cases. In recurring diverticulitis, scarring may be present, which could lead to backing up of fecal content in the large intestine. Infections will require antibiotics.

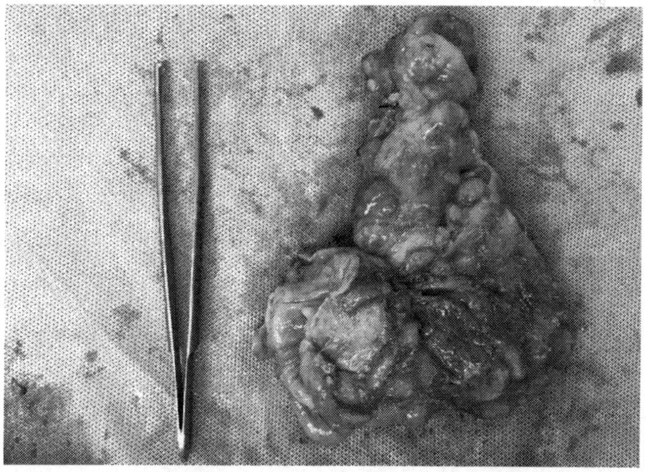
Removal of a segment of the large intestine affected by diverticulitis

If scarring is severe due to ulceration, surgery to remove the damaged part of the large intestine may be required.

Diverticulosis

(diverticula: tubular sac branching off a cavity; -osis: condition)

Diverticulosis is a condition affecting the large intestine, which presents with **pouches forming in the walls of the large intestine**, typically in the descending and/or sigmoid colons. It is a common condition seen in roughly half of people over the age of 65.

Causes

During peristalsis, the smooth muscle located in the walls of the large intestine contract, forcing food to move further through the organ and eventually out of the body. If the large intestine does not contain enough fecal matter, as in the case of a **low-fiber diet**, the contractions may result in weakening of the wall of the large intestine. As a result, small pouches may develop.

If a person develops diverticulosis, small pieces of feces, nuts, seeds, etc, may become stuck inside the pouches. If feces becomes trapped in a pouch, the large intestine will absorb all of the water from it, and it will become very solid and extremely hard

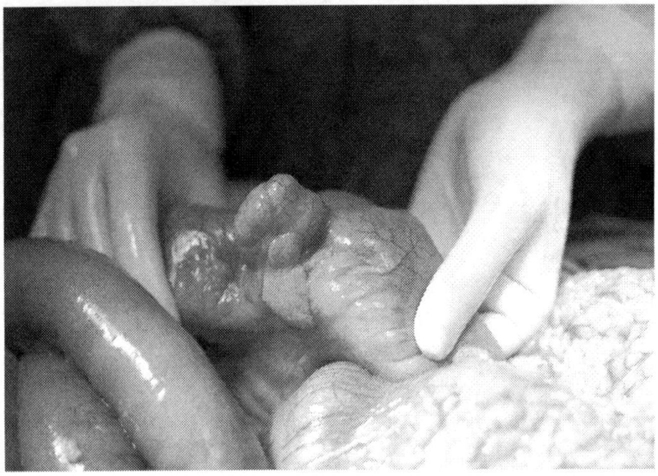

to remove. This may result in pain in the abdomen.

Symptoms

Typically, people with diverticulosis don't exhibit symptoms. When they do, however, symptoms may include diarrhea, abdominal cramping, or fever. These are typically the result of infection, which may lead to diverticulitis.

Treatments

Treatment primarily includes increasing intake of fiber via fruits and vegetables, and increasing fluid intake to make passing of stool easier to manage.

Gastritis

(gastr/o: stomach; -itis: inflammation)

Gastritis is **inflammation of the stomach**, specifically the **lining of the stomach**. Gastritis may occur suddenly or slowly over time.

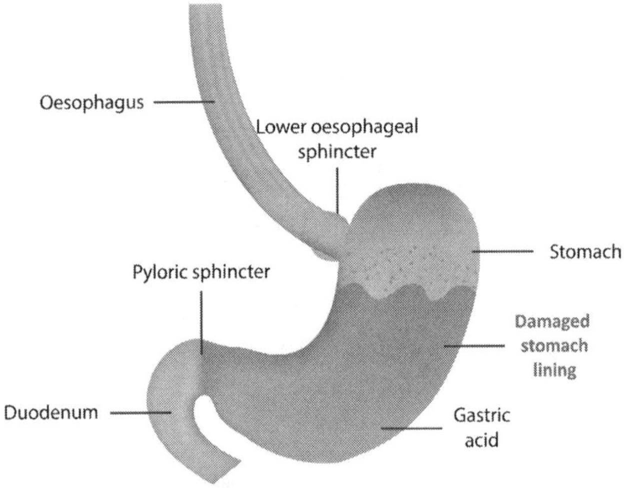

Causes

Some primary causes of gastritis include **infection by H. pylori bacterium**, excessive use of **alcohol**, use of **anti-inflammatory drugs, vomiting**, and **stress.** Gastritis should be treated, as it may lead to more serious conditions such as stomach cancer.

Symptoms

Some people with gastritis actually don't exhibit any symptoms. Those that do, however, may present with nausea, vomiting, loss of appetite, pain in the abdomen, and bloating in the abdomen.

Treatments

Treatment often consists of dietary changes, such as avoiding spicy food and dairy, taking antacids to reduce the amount of stomach acid present, and possibly even a round of antibiotics to combat infection by the H. pylori bacterium.

Gastroenteritis

(gastr/o: stomach; enter/o: small intestine; -itis: inflammation)

Gastroenteritis is **inflammation of the stomach and small intestine**, commonly known as the "**stomach flu**".

The primary cause of gastroenteritis is a **viral or bacterial infection**. These infections can be spread by coming into contact with someone who has it, or consuming contaminated food or water that contains the virus or bacterium. The main types of virus that cause gastroenteritis are **rotavirus and norovirus**. The main types of bacterium that cause gastroenteritis are **E. coli and salmonella**.

Symptoms

Symptoms of gastroenteritis include diarrhea, vomiting, fever, abdominal pain, and body chills.

Treatments

Most people recover from gastroenteritis without requiring any treatment. The primary goal of treatment for gastroenteritis is to prevent dehydration. Therefore, drinking plenty of fluids is advised. Over-the-counter medications that help with nausea and vomiting may also help.

Gastroesophageal Reflux Disease

(gastr/o: stomach; esophag/o: esophagus; reflux: flowing back)

Gastroesophageal Reflux Disease(GERD) is a condition in which **stomach acid**, or food from the stomach, comes **back up into the esophagus**, causing **irritation and burning** in the lining of the esophagus.

Causes

GERD is the result of acid flowing backwards into the esophagus. This is primarily caused by the lower gastroesophageal sphincter(also known as the cardiac sphincter) relaxing when it normally is contracted and tightened. This can happen abnormally, or be caused by the sphincter weakening over time.

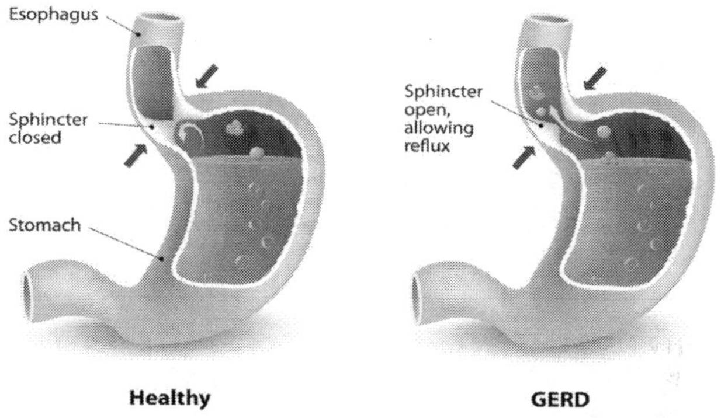

Symptoms

Symptoms include burning in the chest, pain in the chest, a dry cough, a sour taste in the mouth, and a sore throat. It is advisable to seek medical attention if chest pain is present, because symptoms are very similar to those seen in myocardial infarction.

Treatments

Over-the-counter medications, such as antacids, are the primary treatment for GERD. Other medications may be prescribed by a doctor if the GERD is not helped by antacids, such as H-2-receptor blockers, which reduce stomach acid production, and proton pump inhibitors, which completely block the production of stomach acid and give the lining of the esophagus time to heal.

Hepatitis

(hepat-: liver; -itis: inflammation)

Hepatitis is a condition that results in **inflammation of the liver.**

Causes

There are numerous causes of hepatitis, which affect numerous different organ systems. Most commonly, hepatitis is the result of a **viral infection**, but may also result from **toxic substances** entering into the body, such as **alcohol**. Short-term symptoms of hepatitis include jaundice(yellowing of the skin due to increased bilirubin in the blood stream), fever, and nausea. Long-term symptoms include cirrhosis(destruction of healthy liver cells), scarring of the liver, liver cancer, and liver failure.

There are five known hepatitis viruses: Hepatitis A, B, C, D, and E. Each varies in mode of contraction, and severity of symptoms.

Hepatitis A is the most common form, and is typically transmitted through ingestion of fecal matter(most commonly seen in parts of the world with low sanitation standards). People infected with Hepatitis A most frequently make a full recovery, and develop an immunity to the virus.

Hepatitis B is typically transmitted through exposure to body fluids such as blood. The virus produces symptoms for a period greater than Hepatitis A, but most people will develop an immunity to it after about four weeks. A small percentage of people who contract Hepatitis B will become chronically affected by it. Vaccines for Hepatitis B are available.

Hepatitis C, much like Hepatitis B, is contracted through exposure to body fluids such as blood. Hepatitis C is a chronic condition which damages the liver even further each time the person's symptoms are in the acute stage. Hepatitis C is one of the leading causes of liver failure.

Hepatitis D is an infection that only results in symptoms if the person is also infected with the Hepatitis B virus. When this occurs, major complications may arise. Because Hepatitis D is only activated by the Hepatitis B virus, the Hepatitis B vaccine may contribute to the prevention of Hepatitis D.

Hepatitis E, like Hepatitis A, is contracted through exposure to fecal matter. It is most commonly seen in developing countries, where sanitation standards may not be high. Hepatitis E, if severe, may lead to liver failure, despite being an acute infection.

Symptoms

Hepatitis often results in no symptoms. More severe cases of hepatitis may result in a person presenting with nausea, fatigue, mild fever, loss of appetite, abdominal tenderness, and jaundice, among others.

Treatments

Treatments vary, depending on severity. Immunizations are available for Hepatitis B, and medications may help reduce the symptoms.

Hernia

(hernia: a rupture)

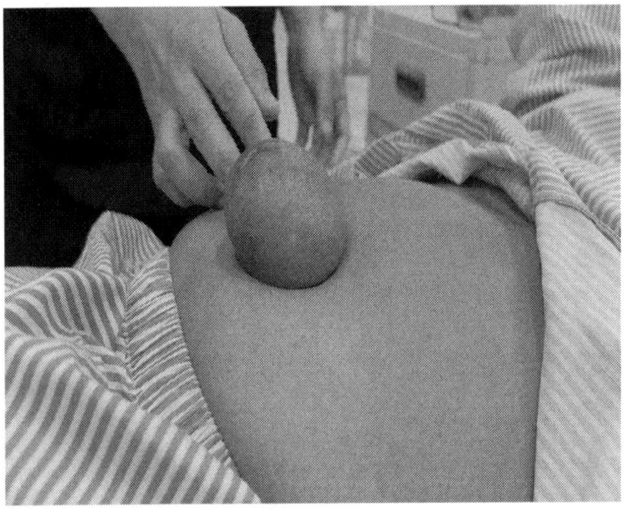

Umbilical hernia

A hernia is a rupture in a muscle or connective tissue, allowing an organ or other tissue to **protrude** through its normal location. There are many different types of herniae in the Digestive System, including **hiatal**, **umbilical**, and **inguinal**.

A hernia is caused by a weakness in the affected tissue, and/or straining of the tissue. When the tissue tears, the organ, usually the small intestine, protrudes through it. This can lead to many complications, such as organ strangulation, constipation, pain, or even trauma to other structures, such as the testes.

A hiatal hernia results from part of the stomach protruding upwards through the diaphragm, into the chest. Gastroesophageal Reflux Disease may result from this type of hernia, where stomach acids leak from the stomach backwards into the esophagus.

An umbilical hernia, most commonly seen in infants, is caused by the small intestine protruding through the abdominal wall and into the umbilicus. This condition usually resolves on its own.

An inguinal hernia, most commonly seen in men, is caused by the small intestine protruding through the wall of the abdomen, which typically descends into the scrotum. This may cause trauma to the testes. Sometimes, the small intestine may even drop farther down the body, into the thigh.

Symptoms

Symptoms vary depending on the type of hernia suffered. Examples include swelling beneath the skin in the abdomen or groin in an inguinal or umbilical hernia, and heart burn and pain in the upper abdomen in hiatal herniae.

Treatments

Treatments may include dietary changes in cases such as a hiatal hernia, weight loss, medication such as antacids, or even surgery to repair the hernia.

Jaundice

(jaund/o: yellow)

Jaundice, also known as **icterus**, is a condition that causes the skin to turn a **yellowish color**. Jaundice is the result of an increased amount of **bilirubin in the blood stream**(hyperbilirubinemia). Bilirubin is a byproduct of the breakdown of heme in the body, a normal process in which the body recycles blood cells. Bilirubin is filtered through the liver and in to the digestive tract, binding with bile, where it will then be eliminated from the body. Bilirubin is a yellow substance. When there is an abnormal amount of bilirubin in the blood, it can be absorbed into the skin and whites of the eyes, resulting in the yellow pigment.

Causes

Jaundice may result when there is damage to the liver. Examples include viral infections such as hepatitis(page) or alcoholism. Blockage of the gallbladder resulting from gallstones may contribute, as can certain medications taken over a prolonged period such as acetaminophen.

Neonatal jaundice occurs in infants, usually due to the breakdown of erythrocytes in the fetus at a higher level than normal. Neonatal jaundice is sometimes considered a serious condition, as excessive bilirubin is considered a neurotoxin and may damage the Nervous System. Usually, however, neonatal jaundice resolves itself within a day or two without any issues.

Symptoms

Jaundice is usually the result of another problem, and is considered a symptom of other conditions such as hepatitis. People with jaundice may exhibit yellowing of the skin and whites of the eyes, nausea, pale stools, dark urine, fever, chills, and diarrhea. When the primary cause of jaundice resolves, the jaundice should resolve with it.

Treatments

Treatment for jaundice usually revolves around treating the underlying cause, whether it be hepatitis, malaria, or gallstones.

Pancreatitis

(pancreat/o: pancreas; -itis: inflammation)

Pancreatitis is **inflammation of the pancreas**. Pancreatitis may be either acute or chronic, each presenting with differing levels of severity.

Causes

Pancreatitis results when **enzymes** produced by the pancreas, **insulin and glucagon, become active in the pancreas** before entering into the digestive tract or blood stream. This causes the pancreas to become irritated and inflamed. Things that may contribute to pancreatitis include blockage of the bile duct by gallstones, alcoholism, pancreatic cancer, infection, and cystic fibrosis.

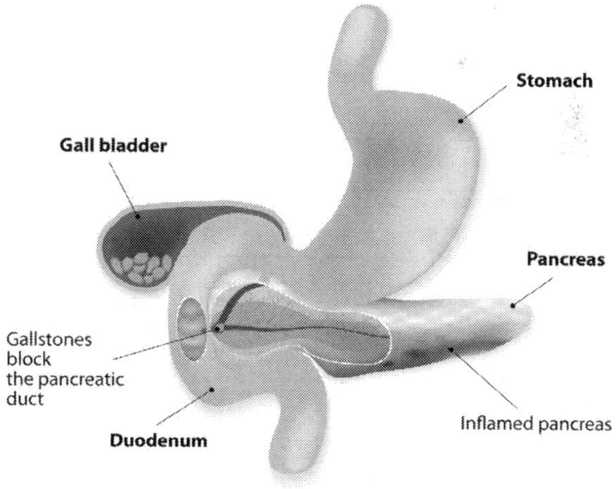

Symptoms

Acute pancreatitis presents with fever, nausea, vomiting, pain in the upper abdomen, abdominal tenderness, and pain radiating to the back. Chronic pancreatitis may also present with the same symptoms in the acute stage, but weight loss may also occur. Pancreatitis may lead to the development of other serious conditions such as diabetes, pancreatic cancer, and kidney failure.

Treatments

Upon admission to a hospital, a patient with pancreatitis will be prescribed pain medication. Fasting reduces the production of insulin and glucagon, and is therefore beneficial to decrease irritation. Other treatments that treat the underlying causes of pancreatitis can include removal of the gallbladder or gallstones, and treatment for alcohol dependency.

Peptic Ulcer

(peptic: digestion; ulcer: open sore)

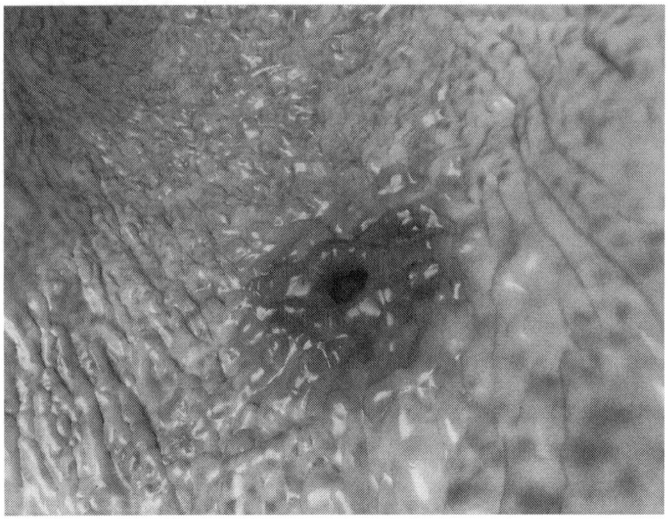

An ulcer in the digestive tract is typically referred to as a stomach or peptic ulcer. These ulcers are **open sores** in the **inner linings of the stomach**, which can cause pain in the stomach.

Causes

Peptic ulcers are usually caused by **stomach acid** such as pepsin **eating away** the inner lining of the stomach and/or small intestine. Mucous lines the stomach, but when acid levels in the stomach rise and mucous production fails to match the rise in acid levels, the acid will eat through the mucous and the stomach lining. Reasons for increases in stomach acid can vary between prolonged use of things like aspirin, or a bacterial infection(H. pylori being the primary type of infection causing peptic ulcers). Excessive prolonged alcohol consumption may also contribute to the development of ulcers.

Symptoms

Peptic ulcers may cause painful burning sensations in the stomach, heartburn, nausea, and bloating. In less common cases, a person may also experience vomiting and have bloody stool.

Treatments

Treatment for peptic ulcers largely revolves around the cause of the ulcers. If H. pylori is the suspected cause, antibiotics will be prescribed to fight off the infection. Antacid medications may also be prescribed to lower the acid content of the stomach back to normal levels, giving the stomach lining a chance to heal and recover mucous.

Pharyngitis

(pharyng/o: pharynx; -itis: inflammation)

Pharyngitis is **inflammation of the pharynx**, or the throat. A **sore throat** is considered pharyngitis.

Causes

Pharyngitis is usually the result of a **viral infection** from the **common cold or the flu. Bacterial infections** may also result in pharyngitis, such as **strep throat.** Non-exudative pharyngitis, the kind usually caused by a virus, does not produce increased mucous, while exudative pharyngitis, the kind usually caused by bacteria, does produce mucous. Both types of pharyngitis are contagious.

Symptoms

Pain in the throat is one of the main symptoms of pharyngitis. Speaking and swallowing food may be painful. A person may develop a fever, and the tonsils and lymph nodes in the neck may enlarge. Excessive mucous may be produced if it is caused by bacterial infection.

Treatments

Antiviral medications may prevent the condition from worsening. If the condition is caused by bacterial infection, antibiotics can help combat the infection and improve the condition.

Strep Throat

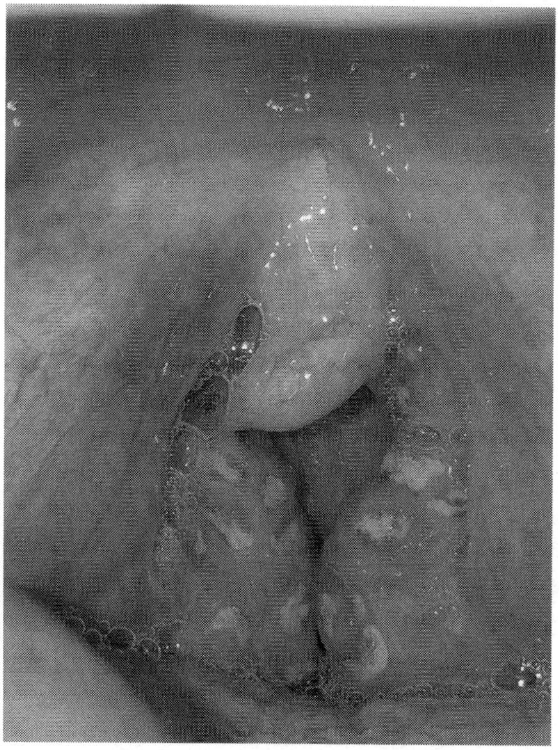

Strep throat is a **bacterial infection**, resulting in **sore throat**. Typically, a throat culture is performed in order to diagnose strep throat.

Causes

Strep throat is caused by an infection of the streptococcal bacteria, which is contagious. Children are most at risk of contracting strep throat, but it can occur in people of all ages.

Symptoms

In addition to sore throat, a person with strep throat may exhibit red spots on the roof of the mouth, white patches on the tonsils, swollen lymph nodes in the neck, pain upon swallowing, and fever, amongst others. If left untreated, strep throat may contribute to the development of rheumatic fever, which can cause damage to heart valves.

Treatments

Because strep throat is caused by bacteria, antibiotics are the primary treatment. Acetaminophen is useful in treating any pain that may be present due to the infection. After starting a course of antibiotics, a person should begin feeling better within a couple days. Taking all the medication prescribed is required to prevent the infection from returning and becoming resistant to the antibiotics.

Ulcerative Colitis

(ulcer: open sore; col/o: large intestine; -itis: inflammation)

Ulcerative colitis is an **inflammatory disease** of the digestive tract, specifically affecting the **inner walls** of the **large intestine** and **rectum**. Ulcerative colitis presents with chronic inflammation and **ulcers**, which can result in several symptoms. There are several different types of ulcerative colitis: Proctosigmoiditis(ulcers in the sigmoid colon and rectum), Ulcerative proctitis(ulcers in the rectum), Left-sided colitis(ulcers in the descending and sigmoid colons), and Pancolitis(ulcers throughout the entire large intestine). All forms of ulcerative colitis are chronic conditions, aside from acute severe ulcerative colitis, which is not common.

Causes

Direct causes of ulcerative colitis are unclear, but heredity may play a role. There is some belief that ulcerative colitis may be caused by an autoimmune disorder of some sort.

Symptoms

Symptoms of ulcerative colitis may include bloody diarrhea, weight loss, fever, fatigue, pain in the abdomen, difficulty defecating, and pain in the rectum. Symptoms are usually mild, and a patient may go long periods without developing symptoms.

Treatments

There are several treatments available for ulcerative colitis, but there is no cure. Treatments include application of corticosteroids to reduce inflammation, antibiotics to combat any infections that may be present, acetaminophen to reduce pain, and possibly immunosuppresants to prevent inflammation.

Endocrine Pathologies

Acromegaly

(acro-: extremity; -megaly: irregular enlargement)

Acromegaly is **abnormal growth during adulthood**, resulting from the release of **excessive amounts of growth hormone** by the **pituitary gland.** This can cause bones to keep growing, increasing a person's size and changing their appearance.

Acromegaly can result in numerous severe complications, such as cardiovascular issues, hypertension, sleep apnea, and arthritis.

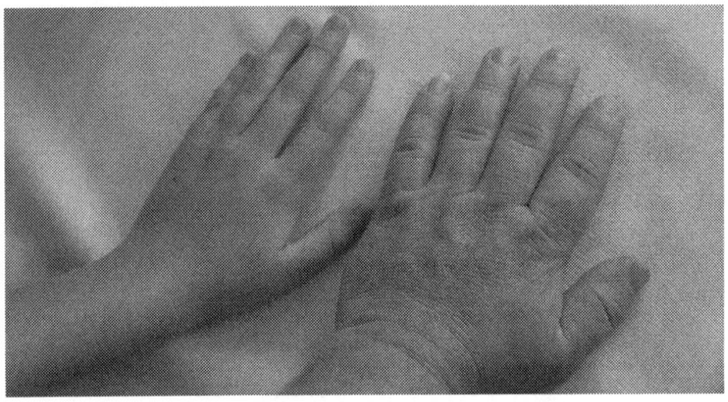

Enlarged features pictured on the right

Causes

Acromegaly is caused by increased amounts of growth hormone being produced by the pituitary gland. The most common reason for this to occur is a tumor growing on the pituitary gland. The tumor produces growth hormone and secretes it into the blood stream, increasing the growth hormone levels in the body. Rarely, a tumor elsewhere in the body, such as the adrenal glands, may produce growth hormone. This can also increase growth hormone levels in the body.

Symptoms

Symptoms of acromegaly generally take some time to appear as the disease slowly progresses. Enlarged hands and feet are an extremely common symptom. Enlargement of facial features, including the jaw and brow lines, can typically be seen in advanced stages. Skin can become thickened and the voice can deepen.

Treatments

If acromegaly is the result of a tumor, surgery may be performed to remove the tumor. Removing the tumor should stabilize the growth hormone levels in the body. After surgery, radiation therapy may be performed to destroy any remaining tumor cells in the body. This can help ensure the tumor does not return. Medications may help reduce the effects of growth hormone in the body.

Addison's Disease

Addison's Disease is an **autoimmune disorder affecting the adrenal glands**, which results in a lack of cortisol and/or aldosterone production.

Causes

Addison's Disease is caused by **damage to the adrenal cortex** by the body's **immune system**. Damage to these glands results in an inability to produce cortisol, which regulates stress levels in the body by helping control blood sugar, blood pressure, and metabolism, and aldosterone, which aids in reabsorption of water and sodium back into the blood stream.

Symptoms

Addison's Disease may result in fatigue, weight loss, low blood pressure, hair loss, hyperpigmentation of the skin, and nausea. It may become life-threatening if not treated. Acute adrenal failure, also known as Addisonian Crisis, may result in severe vomiting and diarrhea, dehydration, low blood pressure, and pain in the low back, abdomen, and/or legs.

Treatments

Treatment primarily consists of hormone replacements, which may be taken orally or injected.

Cushing's Disease

Cushing's Disease is a disease of the pituitary gland, which results in **hyper-production of adrenocorticotropic hormone(ACTH).**

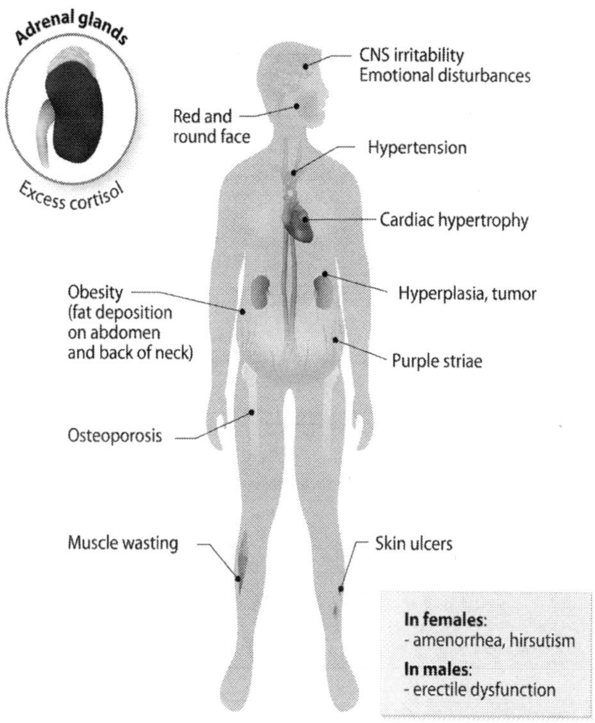

Causes

Cushing's Disease is the result of hyperplasia(excessive growth) of the pituitary gland, or development of a tumor. This causes too much ACTH to be released in the body, which stimulates hyper-production of cortisol.

Symptoms

Cushing's Disease may result in weight gain around the face and torso, weakening of bone, thinning of skin, fatigue, and acne, amongst other complications.

Treatments

Treatments for Cushing's Disease include surgery to remove a tumor, and hormone therapy to reduce the amount of cortisol being produced.

Diabetes Mellitus

(diabetes: to pass through; mellitus: sweet)

Diabetes Mellitus is a condition of the Endocrine System that affects **insulin function in the body**. There are three types of diabetes: Diabetes Type I, Diabetes Type II, and Gestational Diabetes.

Causes

Diabetes Type I is often known as **juvenile diabetes**, as it begins in childhood. In Type I, the body's immune system attacks the pancreas, the organ that produces insulin. This results in the body not producing enough insulin, which the body needs in order to convert glucose to energy.

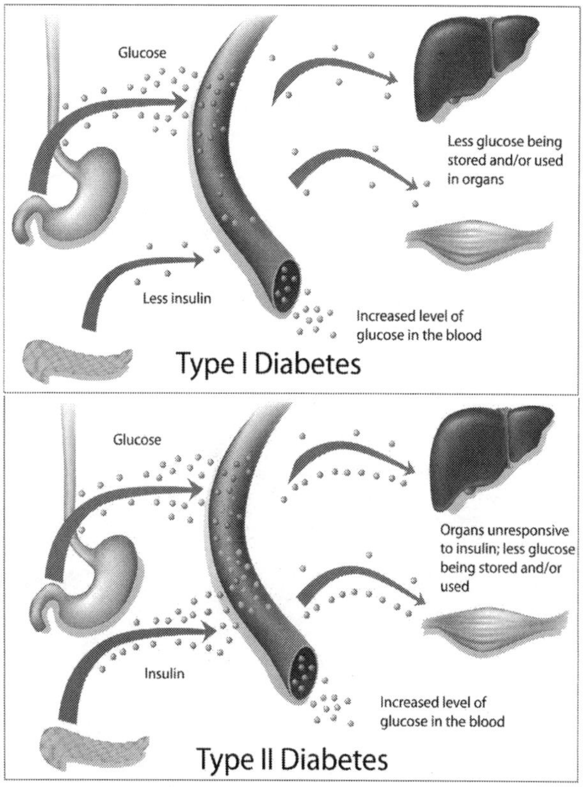

Diabetes Type II, the most common form of diabetes, is caused by the body having an **insulin resistance.** The insulin in the body is unable to break down glucose, which causes high levels of sugar in the blood stream. Obesity is a common cause of Diabetes Type II.

Gestational Diabetes is only present **during pregnancy**. Gestational Diabetes affects less than 10% of all pregnant women, and typically resolves after pregnancy ends.

Symptoms

Symptoms of diabetes include frequent urination, fatigue, weight loss, pain and/or numbness in the hands or feet, extreme thirst, and extreme hunger.

Treatments

Treatment for Diabetes Type I is primarily insulin injections. Treatment for Diabetes Type II includes medications, but exercise and dietary changes are most common. Treatment for Gestational Diabetes includes exercise, regulating weight gain during pregnancy, and insulin medication depending on the severity.

Goiter

(Latin "guttur": throat)

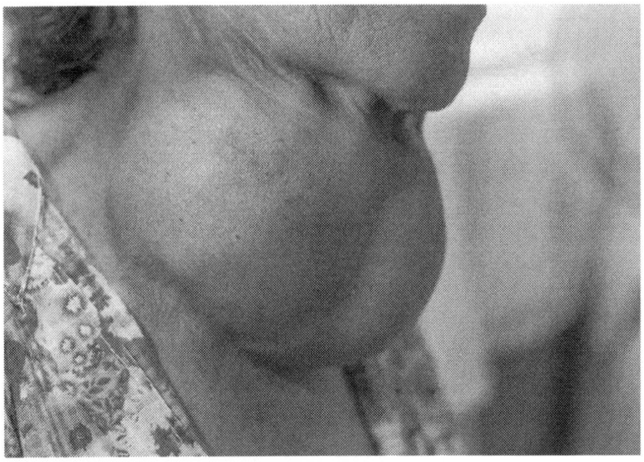

A goiter is an **enlargement of the thyroid gland**, located at the base of the neck.

Causes

The primary cause of a goiter is a **lack of iodine in the diet**. If a person does not consume enough iodine, the body is unable to produce sufficient thyroid hormones. Other conditions such as Graves' disease or Hashimoto's disease can affect the levels of thyroid hormone being produced. Too much thyroid hormone or too little thyroid hormone being produced can have negative effects on the thyroid and could produce a goiter.

Symptoms

Goiters produce a bulge in the throat, which may place pressure on other structures such as the esophagus or trachea, making it difficult to eat or breathe.

Treatments

Treatment of a goiter typically depends on the cause. If it is caused by low levels of thyroid hormones, thyroid hormone replacement medications may be prescribed. If the thyroid is producing too much thyroid hormone, medications may be prescribed to stabilize the levels of thyroid hormone in the body. Surgery to remove the thyroid may be an option if the goiter causes any difficulty in breathing or swallowing, or causes discomfort.

Increasing iodine consumption may be all it takes to reduce the goiter. Iodized salt may be added to the diet, along with other foods high in iodine such as seafood.

Graves' Disease

Graves' Disease is an **autoimmune disorder** in which the body's **immune system attacks the thyroid gland**, causing an **increase in thyroid hormone production(hyperthyroidism)**.

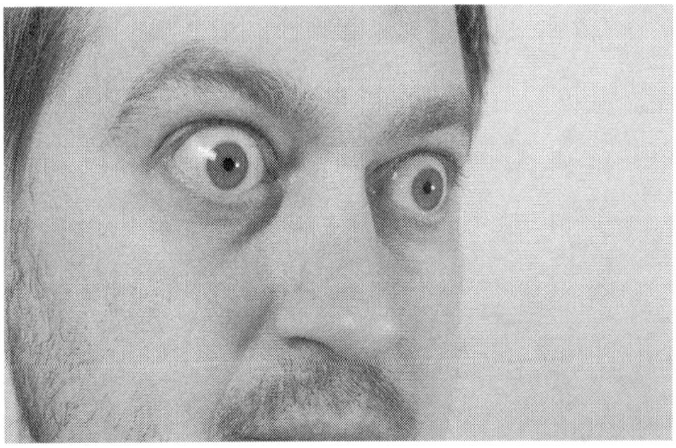

Causes

The exact cause of Graves' disease is unknown.

Symptoms

Graves' disease can affect numerous parts of the body, resulting in sensitivity to heat, weight loss, the development of a goiter(enlargement of the thyroid), bulging of the eyes, and irregular heart rhythm. Women are more likely to develop Graves' disease, as well as people under the age of 40.

Treatments

Treatment for Graves' disease include medications such as beta blockers and anti-thyroid medications. If medication isn't helpful, surgical removal of the thyroid may be an option.

Hyperthyroidism

(hyper-: excessive; thyroid: thyroid gland; -ism: condition)

Hyperthyroidism is an **increase in production of thyroxine**, a hormone secreted by the thyroid gland. Thyroxine is primarily responsible for **stimulating tissues to consume oxygen**. Excessive amounts of thyroxine can significantly increase the body's metabolism, which can have numerous effects.

Causes

Hyperthyroidism is often caused by other conditions such as Graves' disease. Tumors may grow in or on the thyroid, which can increase production of thyroxine.

Symptoms

Symptoms of hyperthyroidism are vast, and may be confused with other medical conditions. The main symptom of hyperthyroidism is sudden, rapid weight loss due to an increased metabolism. This may even cause an increase in appetite, despite the lost weight. Arrhythmia, specifically tachycardia, may also result. Heat sensitivity and sweating are other symptoms to be aware of.

Treatments

Treatments are often the same as those seen with Graves' disease, including a prescription of oral radioactive iodine. Other medications may help lower the amount of hormone being produced by the thyroid. If a person has tachycardia as a result of hyperthyroidism, beta blockers may also be prescribed. In cases where these treatments aren't helpful, surgical removal of the thyroid may be performed.

Integumentary Pathologies

Acne

Acne is an infection of the skin, resulting from numerous factors. Acne may result in whiteheads, blackheads, or even cysts if left untreated.

Causes

Acne is caused by an increased production of sebum on the skin, which results in blocked pores. These **blocked pores may become infected**, which may develop into pustules. There are several contributing factors that lead to the development of acne, including **testosterone production**, stress, hormonal imbalances, and poor personal hygiene.

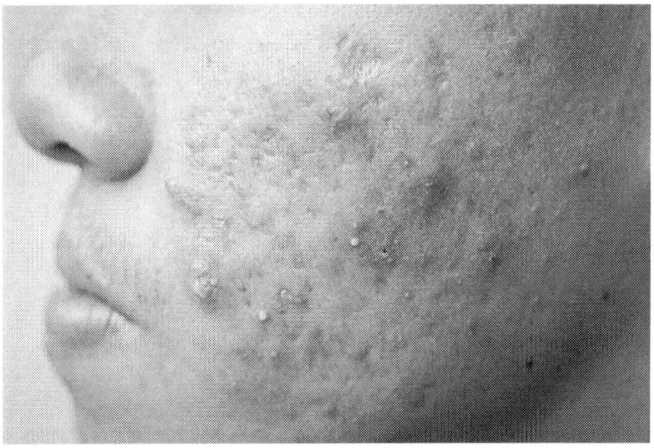

Symptoms

Acne may result in the development of whiteheads, blackheads, pimples, or even cystic lesions beneath the skin. These are often painful to the touch and may present with infection and inflammation.

Treatments

Treatment includes over-the-counter skin care products for mild acne, or in the case of severe acne, medications such as birth control pills to regulate hormone levels in women, and antibiotics to eliminate bacterial growth. Other treatments include light therapy and chemical peels.

Athlete's Foot

(tinea: fungus; pedis: foot)

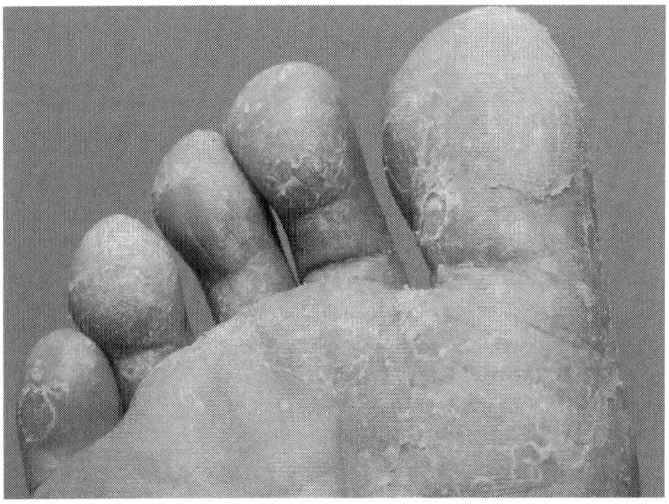

Athlete's Foot(also known as Tinea Pedis) is a **fungal infection of the foot**. Despite the name, anyone may develop athlete's foot, not just athletes. Athlete's foot, like other fungal infections such as ringworm and jock itch, is highly contagious.

Causes

Athlete's foot is caused by exposure to fungus on the foot. When a person wears tight-fitting shoes, it provides an environment for the fungus to thrive: a warm, humid, dark space. The fungus spreads, growing between the toes, then expanding across the foot. The infection causes the skin to become dry and scaly, which may result in breaking of the skin and bacterial infection.

Symptoms

Symptoms of athlete's foot are typically the development of a red, scaly rash between the toes, which may spread proximally. Blisters and ulcers may be present in the area. Itching of the affected area is common.

Treatments

Treatment of athlete's foot primarily consists of over-the-counter medications, in addition to self-care, such as ensuring the foot and footwear are dry as much as possible, wearing shower shoes in public bathing areas, etc.

Boil

A boil is a **bacterial infection of a hair follicle**, also known as a **furuncle**. A group of these infections together in one localized area is known as a carbuncle.

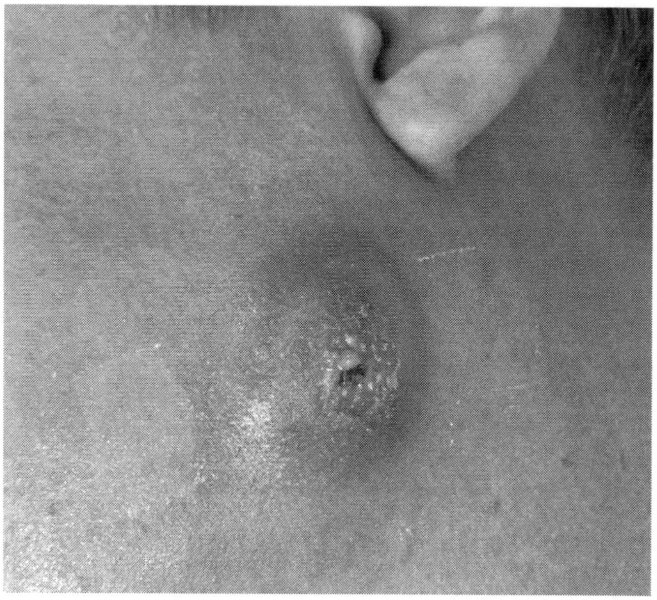

Causes

A boil typically results from small cuts in the skin(caused by things like shaving), allowing staphylococci bacterium to enter the body and reproduce. Boils can be red, inflamed, and painful to the touch. The lump initially produced by the infection begins to soften over a few days, and becomes much more painful. Pus develops on the affected area.

Symptoms

A boil may result in pain around the boil, the development of a fever, and swelling of lymph nodes. More boils may develop around the site of the original boil.

Treatments

Boils are treated by lancing(draining) the area and applying antibacterial soap and water, or in more severe cases, prescription of antibiotics to combat the bacterial infection.

Burns

Burns are a skin condition in which the skin is damaged due to exposure to **heat**, **chemicals**, or other means. This may result in inflammation, blister formation, or necrosis, depending on the severity of the burn.

Burns of the skin can be categorized as first, second, third, or fourth degree, with first being the least severe.

A **first degree burn** only affects the **epidermis**. It may lead to pain and inflammation of the skin, but nothing more. A common first degree burn is a sun burn. The pain and inflammation subsides in a day or two, and the skin returns to normal.

A **second degree burn** is more severe. In a second degree burn, the burn moves through the epidermis and **into the dermis**. Because the burn goes deeper into the skin, it causes more damage, which can be seen by **blistering**. Blisters form to help repair the damage done by the burn. Second degree burns may result in scarring if they are too severe.

Third degree burns move even deeper into the skin, reaching the **subcutaneous layer of the skin**. Third degree burns often cause **severe tissue damage and necrosis**. Skin grafts may be needed to help repair an area damaged by a third degree burn.

While first, second, and third degree burns are most common, a **fourth degree burn** moves completely **through all layers of the skin**, and goes deeper into tissues beneath the skin such as tendons, ligaments, muscles, and bones.

Causes

Burns may be caused by many different factors, including heat(thermal burns), chemicals, electricity, radiation(such as sunburns), friction(rug burns), and even extreme cold temperatures.

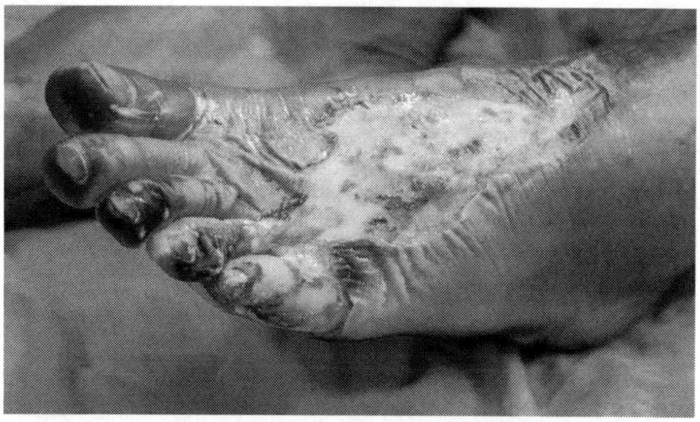

Tissue damage resulting from scalding

Symptoms

Burn symptoms vary based on severity. First degree burns often present with inflammation and pain. Second degree burns present with pain, blistering, and discoloration of the skin as the body repairs the damaged tissue. Third degree burns may present with blackened, charred tissue, with the skin having a waxy appearance. Because tissue is destroyed in third and fourth degree burns, loss of sensation may occur resulting from nerves being destroyed.

Treatments

Treatment for burns often depends on the severity of the burn. Application of aloe vera may help reduce the pain in first degree burns. Second degree burns may require bandages with topical antibiotic cream to prevent infection. Third degree burns may require surgery and skin grafts to repair the affected areas.

Cellulitis

(cell: cell; -itis: inflammation)

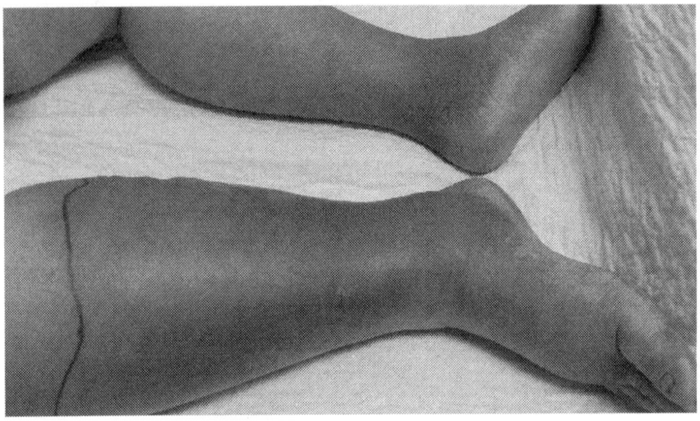

Cellulitis presenting with defined border of infection

Cellulitis is a **bacterial infection of the skin**, causing symptoms such as inflammation of the infected area, fever, pain, and blisters.

Causes

Cellulitis is caused by **staphylococci bacterium** entering the body through **exposure to wounds**, most commonly on the legs. The infection typically stays localized, but continues to spread to surrounding tissues as the bacteria grows. The infection can present with well-defined borders of infection. If the infection enters the blood stream, it may result in septicemia, a potentially life-threatening condition. Spider or insect bites may also introduce the bacterium into the body. Any insect bite should be cleaned thoroughly to prevent infection.

Symptoms

Cellulitis may present with many symptoms, including a red area of skin that spreads and increases in size over time, swelling, pain, fever, and blisters on the infected area.

Treatments

Treatment for cellulitis includes antibiotic medication, taken orally. Cellulitis is not typically contagious.

Contusion

A contusion, also known as a **bruise**, is **damage to blood vessels in the skin**, resulting in **bleeding**. The bleeding usually stops quickly due to thrombocytes clotting the blood, but blood remains in a localized area until it can be slowly removed by the body over time.

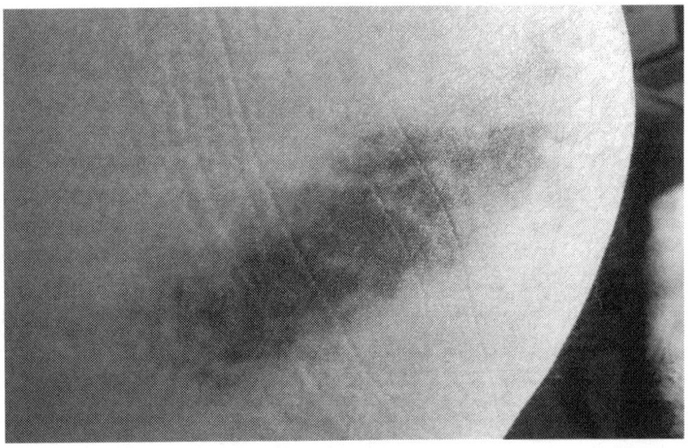

Causes

Contusions are caused by trauma to an area damaging and breaking open capillaries in the skin. The trauma is usually caused by a direct blow to the skin.

Symptoms

In the acute stage, pain may be present in the area, as there is trauma. Inflammation may occur as a result to tissue damage. After the contusion has stopped bleeding, the inflammation usually subsides. There may be a dull ache in the contusion as the tissue is being repaired internally.

Contusions leave discoloration in the skin until they are healed and the blood has been removed from the area. The closer to the time trauma occurs, the darker the bruise is. The contusion lightens over time as the blood is removed from the area.

Treatments

PRICE is the best method of treating a bruise: protect the area from further damage, rest the area, ice the area to reduce pain and inflammation, compress the area to further decrease inflammation, and elevate the area to promote effective blood flow and limit inflammation. Over-the-counter pain medication may be used if the area is painful.

Decubitus Ulcer

(decubitus: the act of lying down; ulcer: open sore)

A decubitus ulcer is a condition affecting the skin, resulting in the development of open sores.

Causes

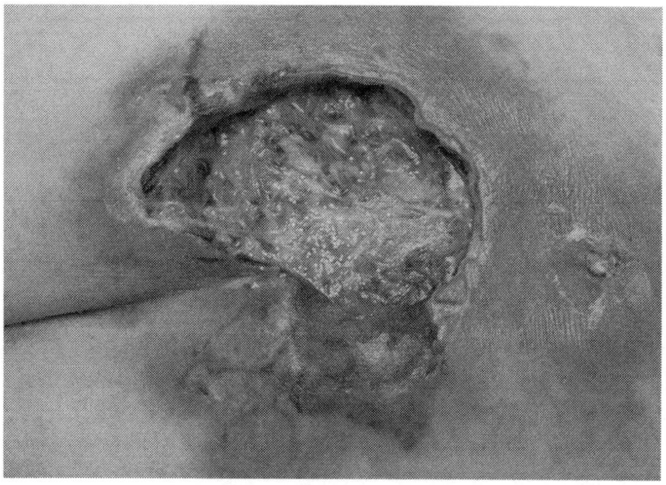

Decubitus ulcers are also known as **bed sores or pressure ulcers**. When the body is in a static position for an extended period of time, such as when lying down, the parts of the body coming in contact with the bed, floor, or chair experience **ischemia**, a reduction of blood flow to the tissues due to pressure. When ischemia is present for too long, the tissue experiences **necrosis** due to a lack of oxygen. The dead tissue becomes ulcerated, and bacterial infection may occur.

People who are prone to decubitus ulcers are the elderly, disabled people, and people confined to a bed or wheelchair.

Symptoms

Symptoms of decubitus ulcers include discoloration of the skin, tenderness in the affected area, temperature variation in the affected area, and swelling. In severe cases, infection may result after ulceration has occurred.

Treatments

Treatments for decubitus ulcers vary, depending on the severity of the ulceration. If an infection is present, antibiotics may be prescribed. If there is an abundance of necrotic tissue, cleaning of the area(debridement) may be performed. If there is ischemia, but no ulcer, massage and application of heat may help bring blood back into the area.

Dermatitis

(dermat/o: skin; -itis: inflammation)

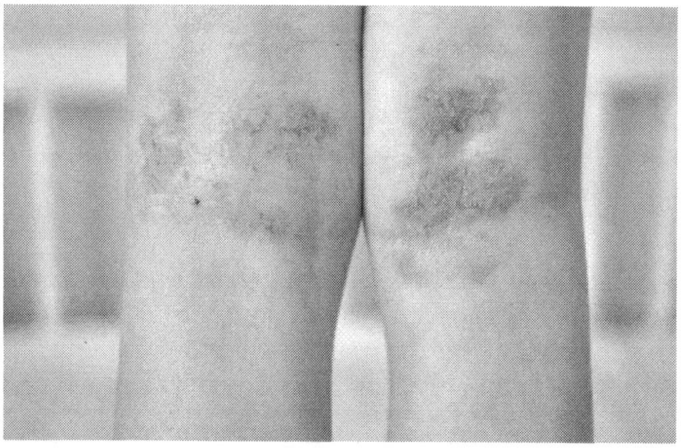

Dermatitis is **inflammation of the skin.** There are several types of dermatitis, including **contact dermatitis**, **atopic dermatitis**, and **seborrheic dermatitis.** Each has different causes, but each presents with some sort of inflammation of the skin.

Causes

Contact dermatitis results when the skin comes in to contact with some sort of irritant or allergen, causing the skin to become inflamed. Atopic dermatitis, also known as **eczema**, can be caused by numerous factors, including an improperly functioning immune system, bacteria, dry skin, and the environment. Eczema usually begins in infancy. Seborrheic dermatitis is typically the result of a fungus growing on the skin, usually in regions that are more oily than others such as the scalp.

Symptoms

Contact dermatitis presents with inflammation and possible blistering where the skin has come into contact with an irritant. This is usually an acute condition, and will improve after the irritant has been cleaned or removed from the body. Atopic dermatitis presents with red, itchy patches on the body, usually near joints that flex and extend. This can be a chronic condition, and the patches may go away and come back later depending on factors such as the weather. Seborrheic dermatitis can cause itchy patches around the face, cheeks, nose, back, and chest.

Treatments

Often times, application of an over-the-counter corticosteroid cream is all that's needed to alleviate dermatitis symptoms. If over-the-counter creams are ineffective, prescription strength corticosteroid creams may be administered, which usually take care of the dermatitis. Other treatments can even include exposure to sunlight.

Herpes Simplex

(herpein: to creep; simplex: simple)

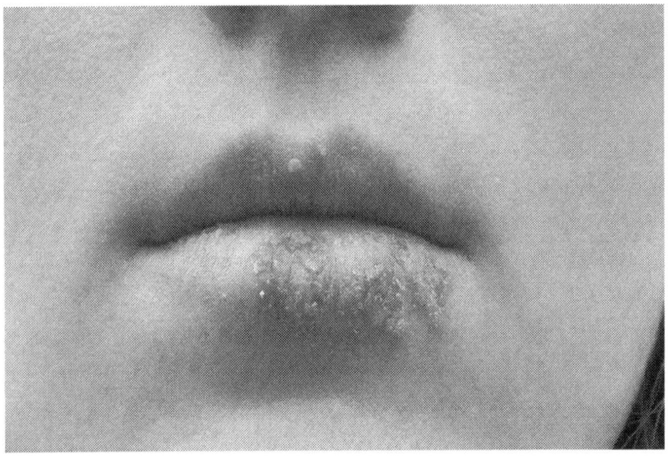

Herpes Simplex is a **viral infection of the skin**. There are two types of herpes simplex: **Herpes Simplex I**, which causes sores around the mouth, and **Herpes Simplex II**, which causes sores around the genitals.

Causes

Herpes simplex is highly contagious, passing between people via direct contact. During an acute outbreak, a sore may appear on the skin, most commonly the mouth, face, or genitals. This sore disappears after a short time. Despite not having any sores present, a person may still be able to transmit the virus to another asymptomatically.

Symptoms

Symptoms vary depending on the type of herpes simplex a person has. Herpes simplex I primarily presents with sores around the mouth, while herpes simplex II may cause painful urination. Both forms, however, may result in fever, headache, and swollen lymph nodes.

Treatments

While there is no cure for herpes simplex, medications may be prescribed to reduce the chance of spreading the infection to others.

Impetigo

(impetere: to attack)

Impetigo is a **bacterial infection of the skin**, most commonly seen in **children**. Impetigo is often confused with Hand, Foot, and Mouth Disease, which is a viral infection.

Causes

Impetigo is a highly contagious infection, caused by staphylococci or streptococci, which most commonly enter the body through already damaged skin, but may affect healthy skin as well. When the bacteria enters the skin, it produces sores that blister and leak a yellow, crust-like fluid. These sores typically develop around the mouth, nose, and ears.

Symptoms

Symptoms of impetigo include red sores that may pop and leave a yellowish crust, swollen lymph nodes, and fluid-filled blisters. The affected areas may also itch.

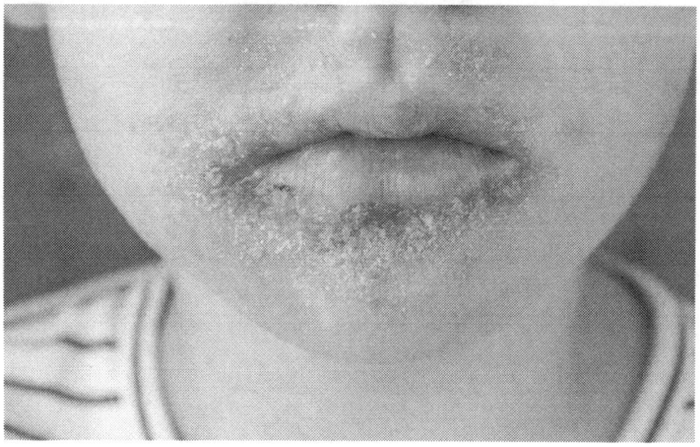

Treatments

Depending on the severity of the infection, impetigo may be treated with topical antibiotic cream for less severe cases, or with oral antibiotics for more severe cases. Recovery time is typically around one week with medication.

Lice

Lice, plural for a head louse, are small **parasites** that live on the **head** that **feed on human blood**. They primarily live on the scalp. Children are most likely to contract a lice infestation, also known as **pediculosis capitis**.

Causes

Lice are spread via direct contact. Lice do not jump or fly, and therefore must physically come into contact with a person to transfer to them. After lice have attached to a new host, they lay eggs on hair shafts. Once the eggs hatch, more lice are present.

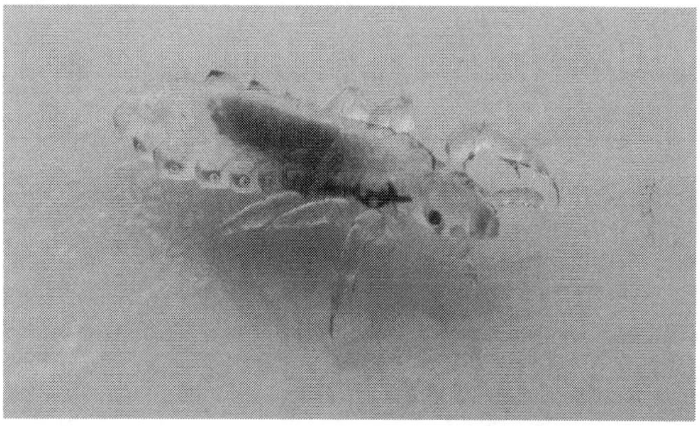

Symptoms

The main symptom of lice is itching, caused by an allergy to the saliva of the lice.

Treatments

Over-the-counter or prescription medications may be prescribed to help kill the lice. Shampoos specifically designed to eliminate lice are often used.

Onychomycosis

(onycho-: nails; myc-: fungus; -osis: condition)

Onychomycosis is a **fungal infection of the nails**, most commonly the result of an infection by the **dermatophyte fungi**.

Causes

Onychomycosis is caused by fungi entering a nail, typically more common in older people due to the natural drying and cracking of nails that happens with age. The fungus enters into these cracks and begins growing, infecting the nail. Athlete's foot may also spread in to the area and infect the nail.

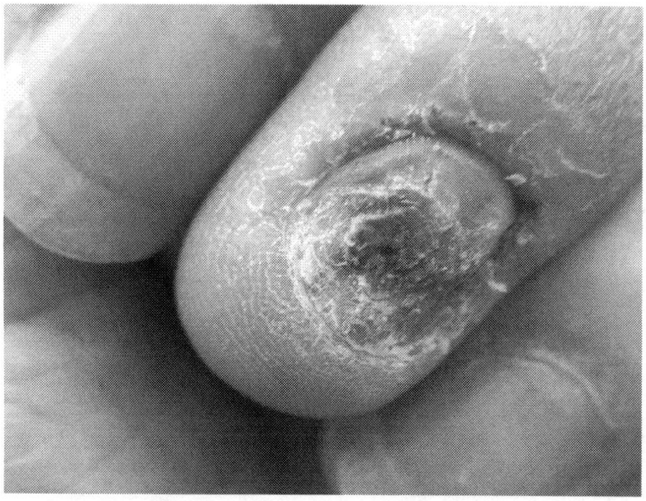

Symptoms

Symptoms of onychomycosis include thickening of the infected nail, change in the nail shape, discoloration of the nail turning it yellow or brown, and the nail becoming brittle.

Treatments

If symptoms are mild, treatment may not be necessary. When treatment is required, however, antifungal medications are the main form of treatment. Oral antifungals are used more often than topical creams, as they can work quicker. If the in fection is severe, the nail may need to be surgically removed to allow antifungal cream to be applied directly to the nail bed.

Psoriasis

(psora-: to itch; -iasis: condition)

Psoriasis is an **autoimmune disorder of the skin**, resulting in the **production of thick, dry, scaly patches**. Psoriasis has periods of exacerbation and remission, where the patches appear and then may resolve themselves.

Causes

The exact cause of psoriasis is unknown. Certain triggers, such as stress, may cause the body's immune system to attack the skin. Normally, skin cells have a life span of 3-4 weeks, and ultimately flake off the body. When the immune system attacks the skin, the body responds by increasing production of epithelial cells at an extremely rapid pace, which is much faster than the cells are being destroyed. This rapid pace of cell production is what produces the patches on the skin.

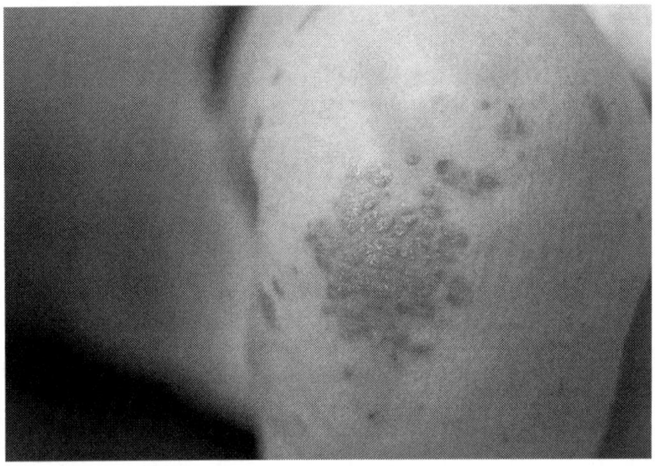

Symptoms

Symptoms of psoriasis differ based on each person, but may include red, patchy skin covered in thick, silvery scales, dry skin that may crack and bleed, thickened finger and toe nails, and itchy skin.

Treatments

There is no cure for psoriasis, but treatments are available to help manage the condition. Treatments include topical creams(which may contain steroids), exposure to sunlight, and application of aloe vera.

Ringworm

(dermato-: skin; phyt-: plant; -osis: condition)

Ringworm. also known as dermatophytosis, is a **fungal infection of the skin** similar to athlete's foot. Despite the name, it is not a parasitic infection. It results in a **ring-like area of infection**.

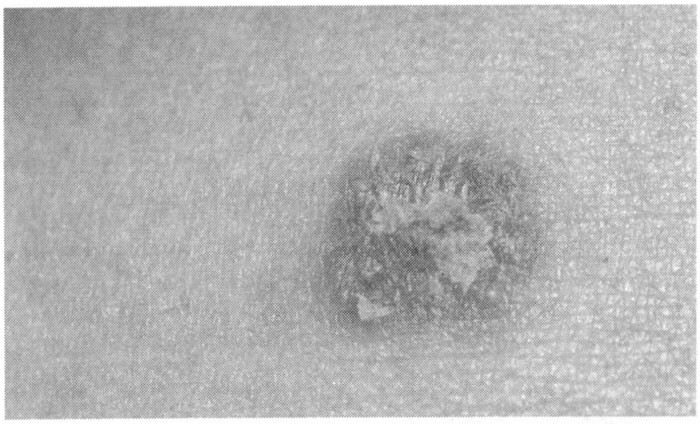

Causes

Fungus, like the kind found in ringworm, live on the dead cells of the body, such as the epidermis. When ringworm is contracted, it forms red blisters and a ring of infection begins to show, which then spreads as the infection grows through the skin.

Ringworm is contagious, and may be spread from person to person. It is especially common in athletes, whose bodies come in close contact with one another, such as wrestlers.

Symptoms

Ringworm typically presents with well-defined circular patches of infection on the skin, usually more red on the outer edges than inside. These patches can be itchy and develop blisters.

Treatments

Treatment includes good personal hygiene, and most commonly application of antifungal ointment to the affected area. More severe cases may require oral antifungal medication.

Scabies

Scabies is a **parasitic infection caused by a mite**, known as **Sacroptes scabiei.** This mite **burrows under the skin and lays eggs**, causing **intense itching**. The tunnels the mite creates are visible in the skin. Scratching due to a scabies infection may lead to an infection, and is not recommended.

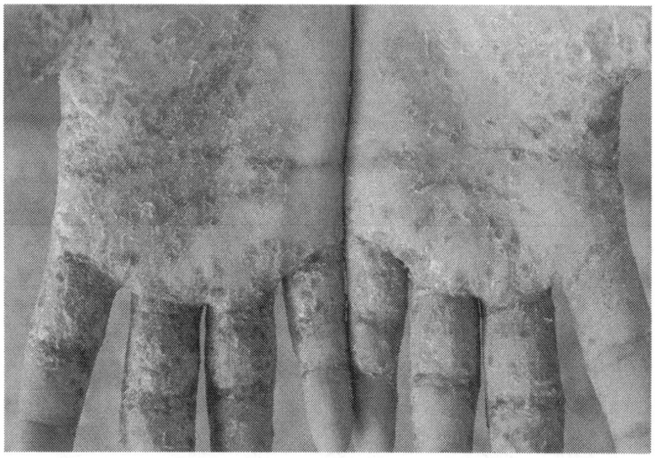

Causes

Scabies are extremely contagious, transmitting easily from one person to the next via physical contact, or sharing clothing or other linens.

Symptoms

The main symptoms of a scabies infection are severe itching and visible burrows in the skin where the mite has worked its way in to the body.

Treatments

Topical creams that are specifically designed to kill mites are prescribed to treat scabies. They kill the mites quickly, but itching may persist for some time after treatment begins.

Sebaceous Cyst

A sebaceous cyst is a condition affecting the skin, but may affect other tissues as well. These are typically the result of a **blockage in a sebaceous gland** that causes a backup of sebum, which is then **surrounded by a membrane** to keep it or an infection from harming the rest of the body.

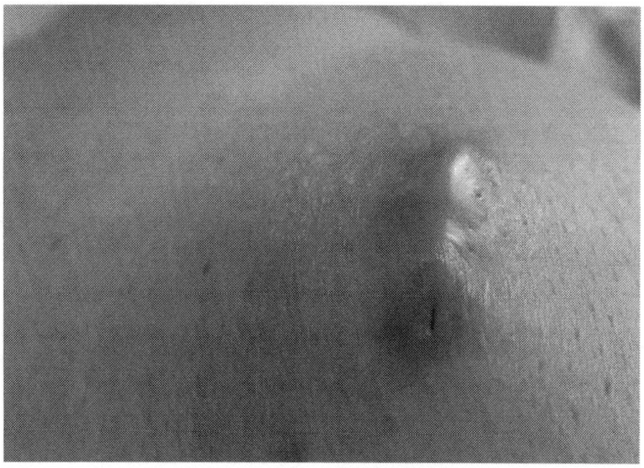

Causes

A sebaceous gland produces oil, and secretes oil onto the surface of the skin. If a blockage of a sebaceous gland occurs, oil cannot escape the gland, and bacteria may infect the area. If too much bacteria is present, the body may develop connective tissue that surrounds the infected sebaceous gland, trapping it inside.

Sebaceous cysts may be large or small. They may be painful to the touch, or may lead to localized infections known as abscesses. Cysts may need to be removed surgically. If the entire cyst membrane is not removed, there may be a chance of the cyst returning in the future.

Symptoms

Some cysts show no symptoms, but symptoms are more likely to appear the larger the cyst is. Small cysts usually do not cause pain, but large cysts may cause pain and discomfort in the surrounding area.

Treatments

Treatment, if necessary, includes moist compresses on the area to help drain the cyst, or possible surgery if there is a risk of infection. Surgical removal may be required if the cyst is large, causes pain, or may be cancerous.

Wart

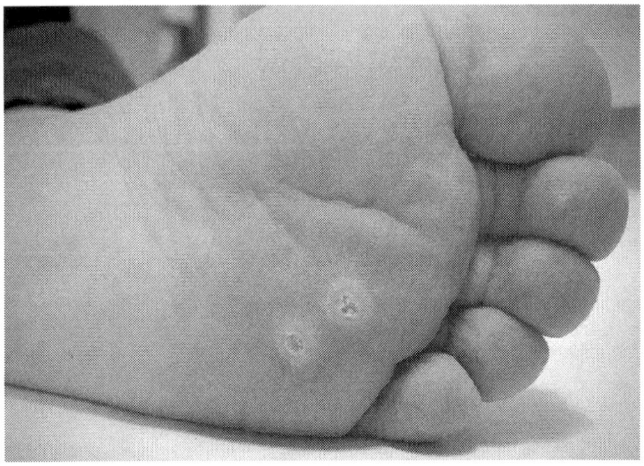

Warts, also known as verrucae, are small **benign growths on the skin** caused by the **human papilloma virus(HPV)**.

Causes

Warts are contagious, and may be spread by direct skin contact. The human papilloma virus stimulates the skin to produce more keratin, which causes a hard, thick overgrowth on a small localized area.

Warts may be located in numerous locations on the body, including the hands, feet(plantar warts), and genitals(genital warts).

Symptoms

Warts are typically rough, grainy bumps, which may be a range of colors, from the color of the person's skin to white, tan, or even pink. Often, warts may have black spots in them, which is nothing more than blood clots.

Depending on the location of the wart, such as plantar warts, the wart may be painful due to calluses forming over them, pushing them deeper into the skin.

Treatments

Warts often go into remission on their own, and treatment is not necessary. Treatment options include cryotherapy to freeze the wart, excising(cutting out) the wart, or electrosurgery to burn the wart.

Wounds

Wounds are the result of a **breakage in the skin**, which exposes underlying tissues. There are several different types of open wounds.

An **abrasion** is a **scraping off of layers of the skin**, such as a skinned knee from falling. An **avulsion** is when the skin or another structure, such as a finger or toe nail, is **pulled and ripped**. An **incision**, such as produced during surgery, is a **clean cut through tissue**. A **laceration** is a cut that produces **jagged edges**. A **puncture** is caused by an object **piercing the skin**, producing a hole.

Causes

Wounds can be caused by many different factors. Ischemia may cause wounds in cases such as decubitus ulcers. Infections may cause wounds to appear in the skin as well. Damage to blood vessels, like those seen in diabetes mellitus can result in wounds. Trauma is usually the main cause of wounds, however. These include abrasions, lacerations, incisions, and punctures.

Symptoms

Wounds in the acute stage often present with bleeding, pain, and redness in the area. These symptoms usually resolve with the healing process. If a wound is not properly treated, infection may occur, along with fever if the infection becomes systemic. A wound that becomes infected and results in necrosis is known as gangrene, caused by a severe lack of blood flow in the area.

Treatments

Wounds should be cleansed with soap and water, and a sterile bandage should be applied to stop bleeding. If a wound is caused by a bite from an animal or insect, medical attention may(and probably should) be recommended.

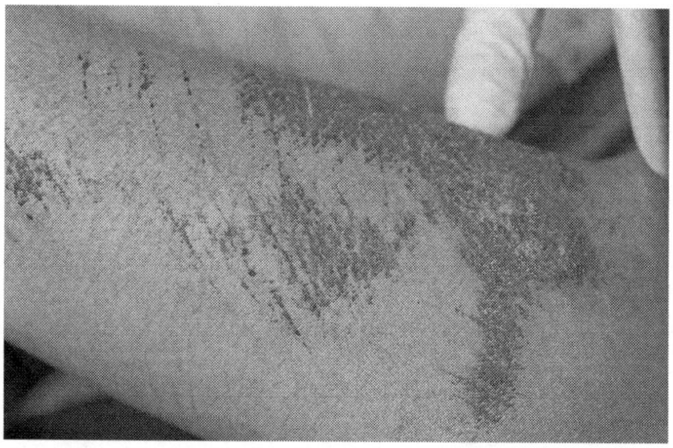

Abrasion

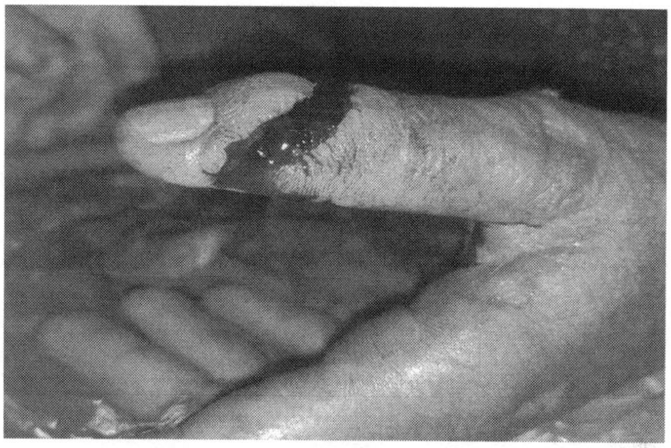

Avulsion

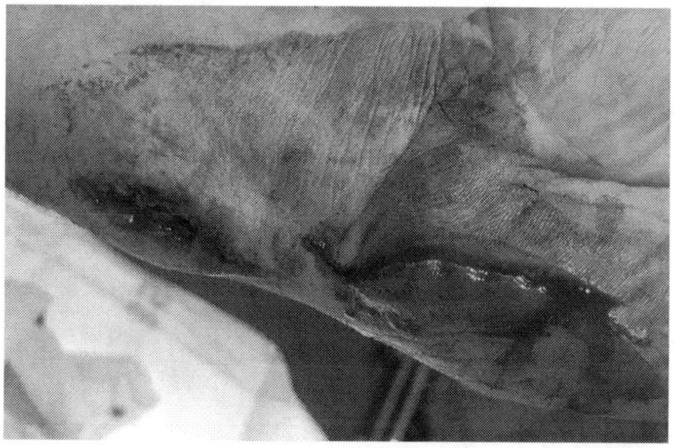

Laceration

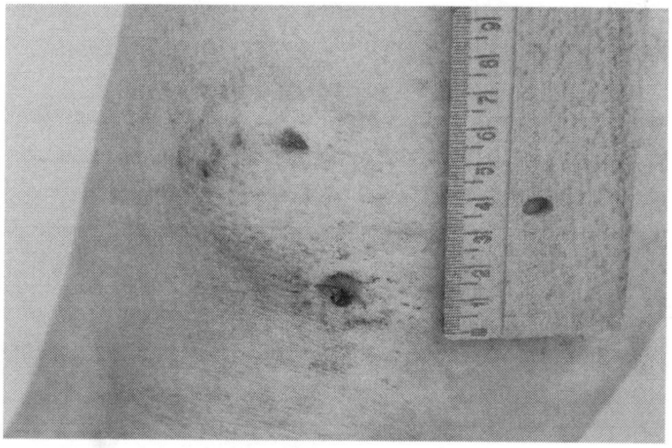

Puncture

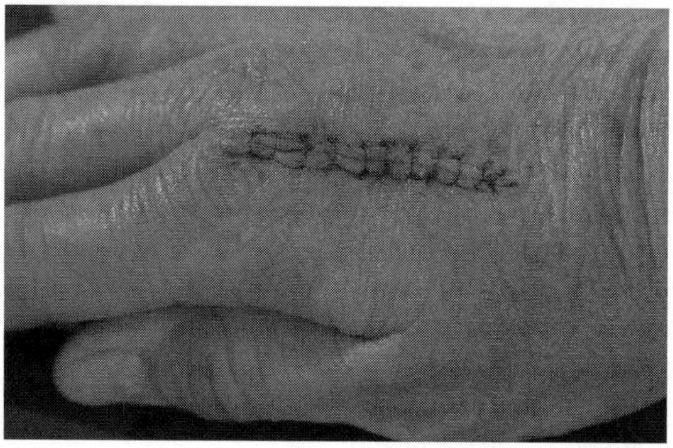

Suture

Lymphatic Pathologies

Acquired Immunodeficiency Syndrome

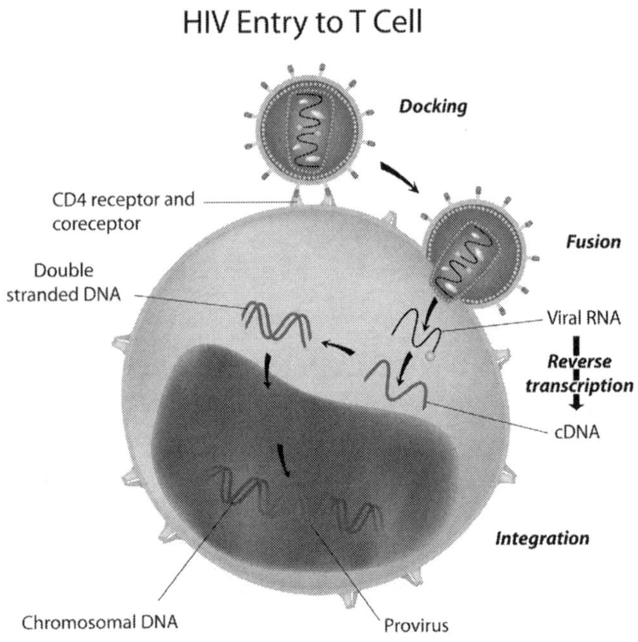

Acquired Immunodeficiency Syndrome, also known as **AIDS**, is a chronic condition caused by HIV, the human immunodeficiency virus. Once in the body, **HIV destroys the body's T-cells**, which function to regulate the response of the body's immune system to antigens. When HIV destroys too many of the body's T-cells, the immune system is considered compromised, and a person is then diagnosed with AIDS. While most people who are infected with HIV in the United States are properly treated and don't develop AIDS, a small portion of people do gets AIDS after HIV infection, typically around ten years after initial infection.

Causes

HIV is spread though unprotected sex, through needles that have been shared by an infected person, as a result of a mother passing HIV on to their unborn child, or even through blood transfusions if the blood has not been properly screened beforehand. HIV cannot be spread through skin contact, water contact, through the bites of insects such as mosquitoes, or breathing in the air of an infected person.

Symptoms

Close after the initial infection has occurred, a person may experience fever, fatigue, body aches, headache, and swollen lymph nodes. As the infection spreads, symptoms emerge such as diarrhea and weight loss in conjunction with previously mentioned symptoms.

Complications caused by infection by HIV include being more prone to infection of other conditions such as pneumonia. A type of cancer known as Kaposi's Sarcoma may develop. Severe wasting of the body may occur, in which a person loses at least ten percent of their total body weight.

Treatments

A person infected with HIV should be prescribed antiretroviral therapy to help prevent the virus from further replicating.

Allergy

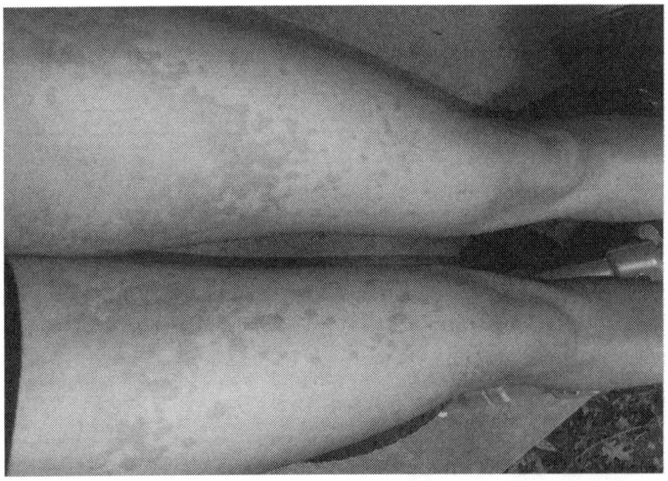

An allergy is a reaction of the body's immune system in response to substances that **normally do not affect people**. Common substances people may be allergic to include dust, pollen, mold, certain foods, pet dander, and medication.

Causes

Allergies occur when a substance enters the body that the body's immune system thinks is dangerous. The body produces **antibodies** for that specific substance. When the substance enters the body, the body releases the antibodies and other substances such as **histamines** to attack the substance. The release of histamines is what gives people allergy symptoms.

Symptoms

Allergies may be mild, or may be severe and result in serious conditions such as anaphylactic shock, which requires the use of an epinephrine shot to reverse the effects of the allergen. Less severe allergies may result in a runny nose, itchy eyes/skin, and hives.

Treatments

Typical treatments of allergens include the use of antihistamines, decongestants, and steroid nasal sprays. Avoiding the allergen is advised.

Lupus Erythematosus

(lupus: wolf; erythemat-: red skin; -osus: pertaining to)

Lupus Erythematosus is an **autoimmune disorder affecting the connective tissues of the entire body**, but can be physically seen in the skin by the formation of a **butterfly rash** that appears on the face during flare-ups. This rash is similar in shape to the markings found on the face of a wolf, which is where lupus gets its name.

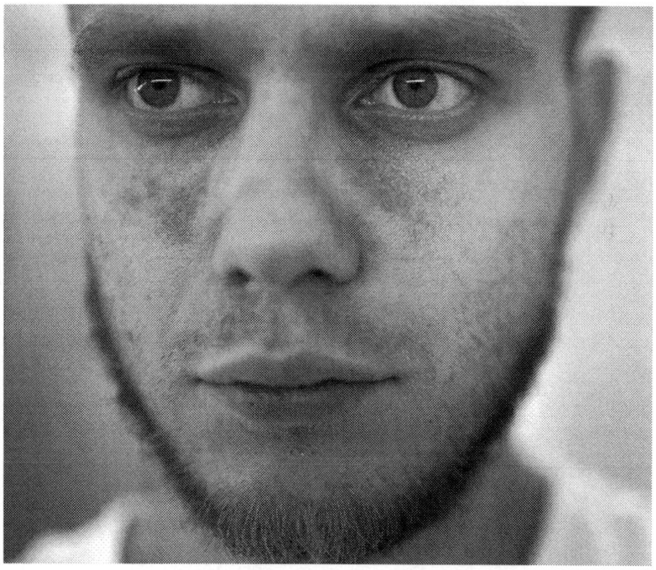

Causes

The exact cause of lupus is unknown. Some experts believe it is a genetic disorder that influences the immune system's function. Lupus may also be triggered by smoking, sunlight, infections, and medications.

Symptoms

Symptoms of lupus erythematosus include fever, the formation of a butterfly rash, joint pain, discomfort, fatigue, and sensitivity to sunlight. It may also contribute to the development of other medical conditions, such as Raynaud's Syndrome.

Treatments

There is no cure for lupus erythematosus, but treatment is available to help manage the condition. Non-steroidal anti-inflammatory drugs may help with systemic inflammation in non-severe cases. Topical corticosteroid creams may help alleviate rashes. Blood thinners may also be used in more severe cases.

Lymphedema

(lymph: lymph; -edema: swelling)

Lymphedema is a condition of the Lymphatic System that results in **increased interstitial fluid in a limb**, which causes **swelling.**

Causes

Causes of lymphedema vary. Most commonly, it results from damage to the lymph nodes and vessels during treatment for cancer(such as a mastectomy, where breast tissue and lymph channels may be completely removed). This results in lymph not draining properly. Other causes include obesity and advanced age.

Symptoms

Symptoms of lymphedema include swelling in the limbs, restricted range-of-motion, discomfort in the affected area, and thickening of the skin.

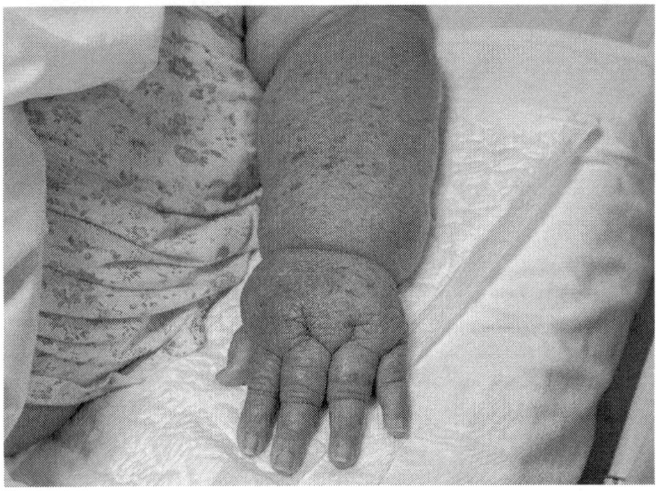

Treatments

While there is no cure for lymphedema, treatments may help reduce the amount of fluid in the area by stimulating lymph circulation. Massage therapy is highly effective at increasing lymph circulation. Compression clothing may help move lymph. Exercise is also extremely helpful in increasing lymph flow.

Pitting Edema

(edema: swelling)

Pitting edema is a form of lymphedema that produces **pits in the skin after pressure is applied and released**. Lymphedema does not leave pits, and the skin rebounds immediately due to the amount of fluid in the area.

Causes

Pitting edema may be non-serious, or may have severe underlying causes. A common cause of pitting edema is pregnancy, due to the body creating much more fluid than it normally has. This increases fluid retention. Other more serious causes include heart failure, liver failure, or most commonly amongst these, **renal failure**. If these organs are not functioning properly, fluid is not effectively drained from the body, which increases swelling.

Symptoms

Pitting edema results in pits left in the skin after applying pressure. Other symptoms may include swelling, pain, numbness, and cramping in the area. If the swelling is near a joint, movement of the joint may become difficult.

Treatments

For serious cases of pitting edema, it is recommended to visit a doctor to find the underlying cause. Once the cause is determined, a proper treatment plan may be developed. Typically, if a person is suffering from organ failure, diuretics may be prescribed to help drain excess fluid from the body. Keeping limbs such as the legs elevated may also help reduce swelling.

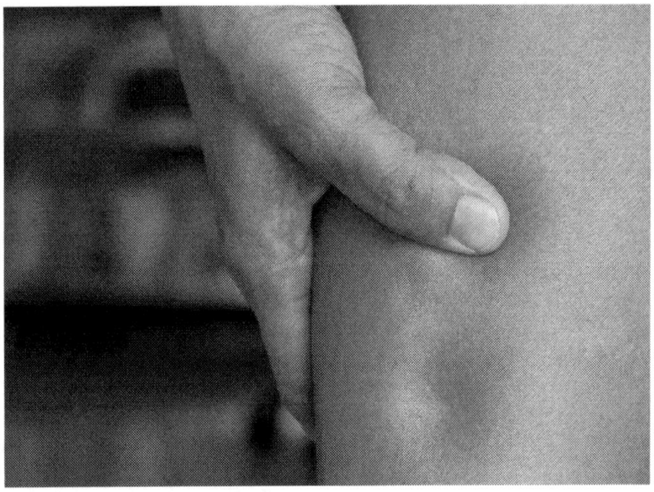

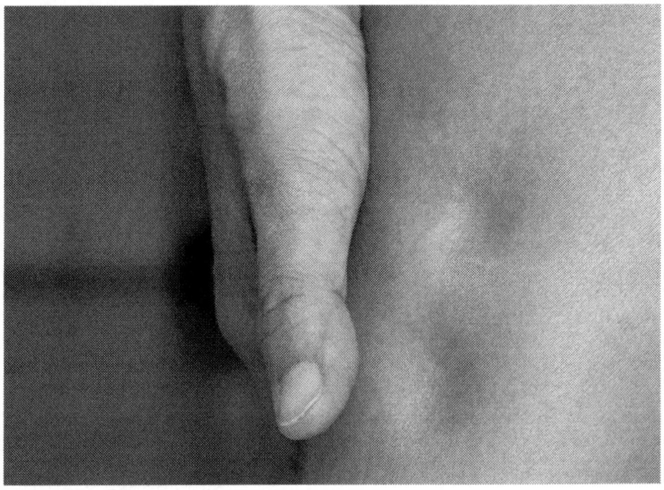

Muscular Pathologies

Adhesive Capsulitis

(capsul-: capsule; -itis: inflammation)

Adhesive capsulitis is a condition resulting in **restricted range-of-motion at the shoulder joint**. Another name for adhesive capsulitis is "**Frozen Shoulder**".

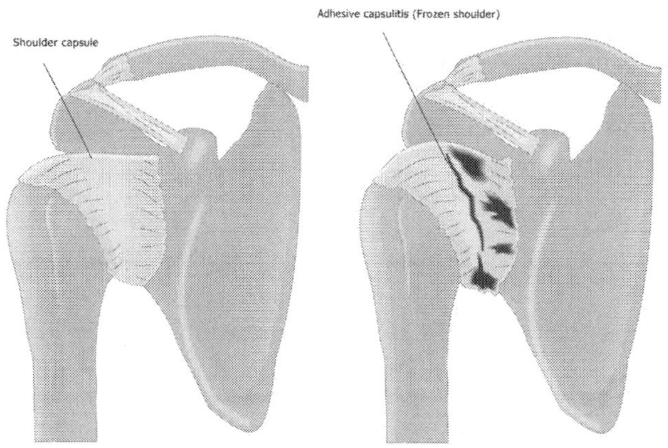

Causes

Surrounding the glenohumeral joint is connective tissue known as the joint capsule. This joint capsule holds everything in the joint in place, such as the bones themselves, synovial membrane, synovial fluid, etc. If there is irritation or over-use of the shoulder joint, **adhesions** may form between the **joint capsule and the head of the humerus.** These adhesions can decrease range-of-motion in the joint, and make movement in the joint uncomfortable.

The **subscapularis** muscle is often called the "Frozen Shoulder Muscle", due to its possible role in adhesive capsulitis. If the subscapularis is hypertonic, it may pull back on the humerus, which can restrict range-of-motion.

Symptoms

As adhesive capsulitis progresses, symptoms vary. In beginning stages, pain may be present, with a gradual decrease in the range-of-motion. As the condition advances, pain may subside, with a severely reduced range-of-motion.

Treatments

Treatments include stretching exercises and massage therapy to help break up the adhesions restricting range-of-motion, or to relax the subscapularis.

De Quervain's Tenosynovitis

(teno-: tendon; synov-: synovial; -itis: inflammation)

De Quervain's Tenosynovitis is a form of tenosynovitis that specifically **affects the thumb.**

Causes

De Quervain's Tenosynovitis is caused by **over-use of the thumb**, which contributes to straining of the tendons around the thumb and their protective sheaths. This may cause pain around the thumb, inflammation, and difficulty in moving the area.

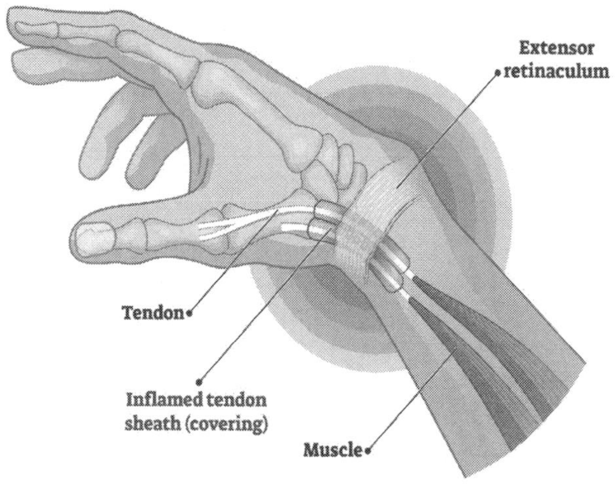

Symptoms

Symptoms include pain and inflammation at the base of the thumb, loss of sensation in the posterior thumb, and difficulty moving the thumb and/or wrist while performing certain actions. Pain may gradually increase and radiate to other areas, such as the posterior forearm.

Treatments

Treatments primarily consist of rest and ice to reduce pain and inflammation in the area. Any repetitive actions that are causing the inflammation should be stopped to allow irritation to subside.

Dupuytren's Contracture

Dupuytren's Contracture is a condition that results in **deformation of the hand**, due to tissues under the skin **hardening, thickening, and shortening.** These tissues pull the fingers into flexion, and don't allow the fingers to completely straighten.

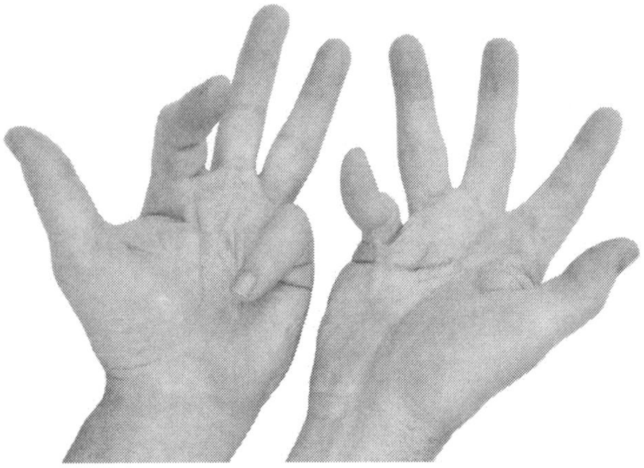

Causes

There are no known causes of Dupuytren's contracture. Men over the age of 50 are more likely to develop the condition, but exact reasons why are still not understood.

Symptoms

Deformity of the hand, specifically in the pinky finger, can occur. The skin on the palm of the hand can thicken, and the fascia under the skin thickens, pulling the pinky and ring finger towards the palm. This causes the affected fingers to lose the ability to fully extend, impairing function of the hand.

Treatments

Treatments include injecting enzymes into the cords to help soften them, a technique called needling in which needles are inserted in to the cords that help to break them, or surgery to partially or completely remove the cords from the hand. Each treatment has varying degrees of success, and the contracture may return.

Fibromyalgia

(fibro-: fibrous; my-: muscle; -algia: pain)

Fibromyalgia is a condition causing **pain throughout the body**, in conjunction with **fatigue**. Trouble with memory may also be present. Fibromyalgia may occur suddenly, or may worsen over time. Fibromyalgia typically affects women much more often than men. Diagnosis involves first ruling out other conditions that may be causing symptoms. If these other conditions are ruled out, then the duration of pain(over three months) and location of pain(using the **Widespread Pain Index**) are taken into account.

Causes

The exact cause of fibromyalgia is unknown. Many theories state the cause could range from hereditary to environmental factors, such as stress or trauma.

Symptoms

Symptoms of fibromyalgia primarily include widespread pain, usually a dull ache, in specific regions of the body for longer than three months, general fatigue, and issues with memory.

Treatments

Medications are important in the treatment of fibromyalgia. Pain relievers help to reduce the pain a person may be experiencing, while antidepressants can help treat depression that may result due to the fatigue a person can experience.

Golfer's Elbow

Golfer's Elbow is a form of **tendonitis** that affects and weakens the **flexors of the wrist**. Golfer's Elbow is also known as Medial Epicondylitis, **inflammation of the medial epicondyle**.

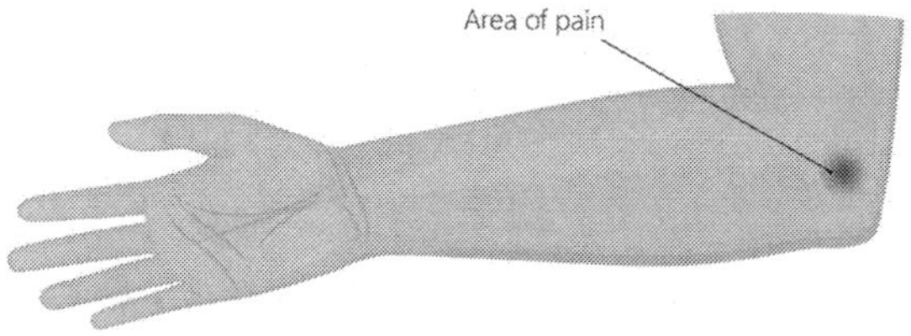

Causes

Golfer's Elbow is caused by repetitive motions such as elbow flexion, which put strain on the tendons connecting the flexors of the wrist to the humerus, at the medial epicondyle.

Symptoms

Golfer's Elbow may present with pain and inflammation at the medial epicondyle of the humerus, weakness in the elbow joint, and numbness in digits four and five.

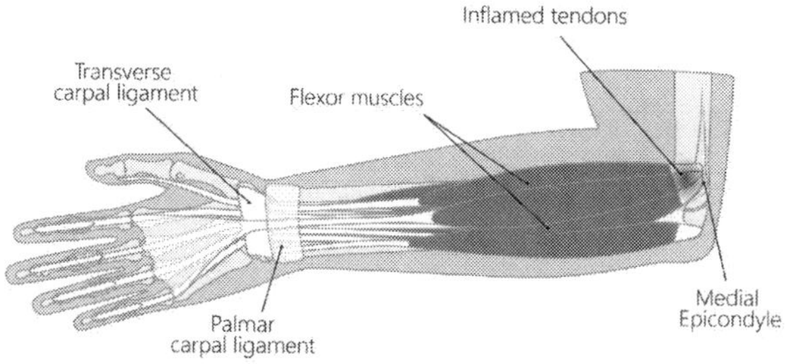

Treatments

Treatment typically involves rest, and ice on the medial epicondyle to reduce inflammation. Any repetitive actions that are causing the inflammation should be stopped to allow irritation to subside.

Muscle Cramps

Muscle cramps are **involuntary contractions of a muscle**, and are usually **painful.**

Causes

Dehydration and overuse of a muscle are prime causes of muscle cramps. However, a cramp may develop due to other factors, including a low supply of blood which reduces oxygen intake in the muscle, or compression of nerves. Loss of electrolytes, such as sodium or potassium, may also lead the muscle cramping.

Symptoms

Pain in the location of the cramp is the prime symptom of muscle cramps. A person may also be able to visibly see the muscle cramping under the skin.

Treatments

Cramps are typically not serious, and only require minimal treatment to fix. Stretching and utilizing **reciprocal inhibition** (contracting the opposing muscle of the muscle cramping) can help calm the cramping in the acute stage. Keeping hydrated and providing the body with nutrients such as potassium may help prevent muscle cramping.

Strain

A strain is an **injury to a tendon or muscle**, usually caused by over-exertion or over-use.

Causes

Activities such as exercise are a common cause of strains. Much like burns, there are three grades of strains: grade 1, grade 2, and grade 3. The less severe the strain, the lower the grade.

A **grade 1 strain** results in **slight tearing** of a tendon or muscle. An example could be a person's muscles being sore after exercise. The muscles have experienced slight tears during exercise, but will heal after a day or two.

A **grade 2 strain** results in more tearing of a muscle or tendon. Grade 2 strains may require surgery to repair, or may heal on their own with rest. There may be accompanying **bruising and inflammation** around the strain.

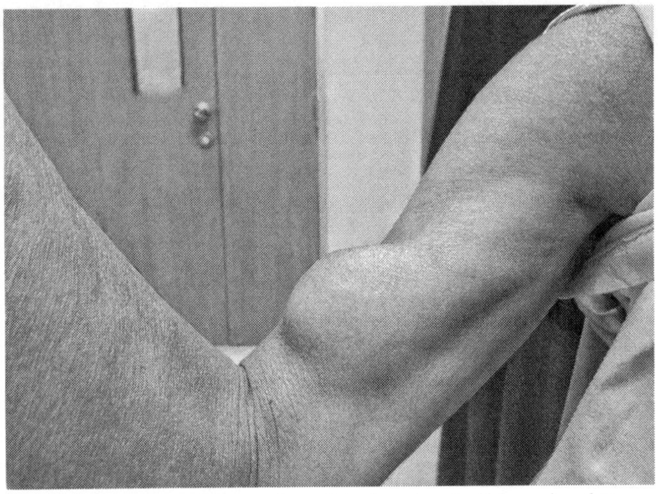
Grade 3 strain of the tendon of the long head of biceps brachii

A **grade 3 strain** results in **complete tearing of a muscle**, or more commonly, **a tendon**. Surgery is required to repair a grade 3 strain. The quadriceps and biceps brachii are two muscles prone to grade 3 strains more than others. Grade 3 strains will inhibit movement involved with the muscle involved, due to its inability to pull on the bone.

Symptoms

Strains may result in pain, inflammation, and an inability to move the injured muscle or tendon.

Treatments

Treatment varies depending on the severity of the strain. Grade 1 strains should be able to receive massage and heat therapy after 24-48 hours to increase circulation and promote healing. Grade 2 strains may need to rest longer before treatment. Grade 3 strains would require surgery to repair.

Easy to Remember: To remember the difference between a strain and sprain, look for the "t" in "strain"! "T" for "tendon"!

Tendonitis

(tendon-: tendon; -itis: inflammation)

Tendonitis is an injury that results in **inflammation of a tendon.**

Causes

Tendonitis is a mostly repetitive strain injury, caused by repeated use of one specific muscle, which can over-exert the tendon. When the tendon is over-exerted, it may tear slightly, which causes pain and inflammation.

There are several different types of tendonitis, including Golfer's Elbow(inflammation of the tendon at the medial epicondyle of the humerus), Tennis Elbow(inflammation of the tendon at the lateral epicondyle of the humerus), and Jumper's Knee(inflammation of the patellar tendon). All these conditions are caused by repetitive movements.

Symptoms

Symptoms may include pain upon moving a muscle connected to an affected tendon, and inflammation.

Treatments

Treatment for tendonitis is primarily rest and application of ice to reduce any inflammation. Repetitive actions causing the inflammation should be stopped until the irritation subsides.

Tennis Elbow

Tennis Elbow is a form of tendonitis that **affects and weakens the extensors of the wrist**. Tennis Elbow is also known as Lateral Epicondylitis, **inflammation of the lateral epicondyle.**

Causes

Tennis Elbow is caused by repetitive motions such as elbow extension, which put strain on the tendons connecting the extensors of the wrist to the humerus, at the lateral epicondyle.

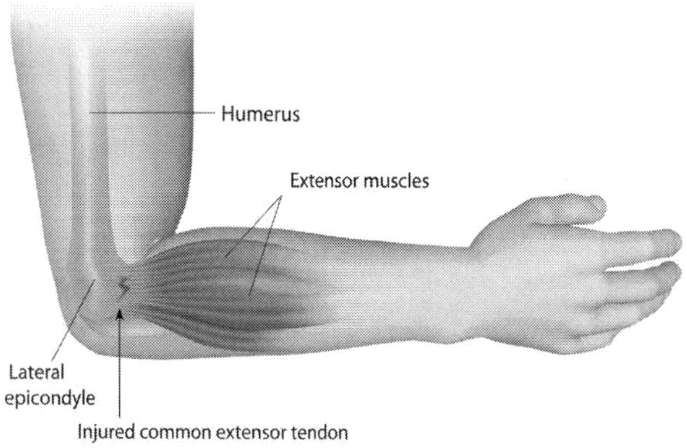

Symptoms

Tennis Elbow commonly presents with pain that radiates distally to the posterior forearm. Weakness may result, especially when performing actions that require grasping.

Treatments

Treatment typically involves rest, and ice on the lateral epicondyle to reduce inflammation. Any repetitive actions that are causing the inflammation should be stopped to allow irritation to subside.

Tenosynovitis

(teno-: tendon; synov-: synovial; -itis: inflammation)

Tenosynovitis is a **repetitive strain injury** that results in **inflammation of a tendon and its protective sheath.**

Causes

Tenosynovitis primarily affects the hands, wrists, and feet due to the length of the tendons in these areas. The longer the tendon is, the easier it becomes to strain. Because there may be inflammation, pain may be present, and it may be difficult to move the affected area.

A common type of tenosynovitis is known as De Quervain's Tenosynovitis, which causes inflammation around the thumb due to over-use.

Symptoms

Tenosynovitis may produce pain and inflammation in affected joints, making it painful to move these joints. The area of the inflamed tendon may also be red.

Treatments

Tenosynovitis is typically treated the same as any strain, with rest and ice to reduce pain. Less commonly, tenosynovitis may be the result of bacterial infection, which may produce a fever. If a fever is present, medications such as antibiotics and antipyretics may be prescribed to combat bacterial growth and fever.

Nervous Pathologies

Alzheimer's Disease

Alzheimer's Disease, the most common form of **dementia**, is an over-arching term for **memory loss**, **confusion**, and a **general loss of intellectual abilities.** Alzheimer's is a result of brain tissue gradually dying over time. Increased age is a risk factor of developing Alzheimer's, and becomes much more common after the age of 65 in those affected.

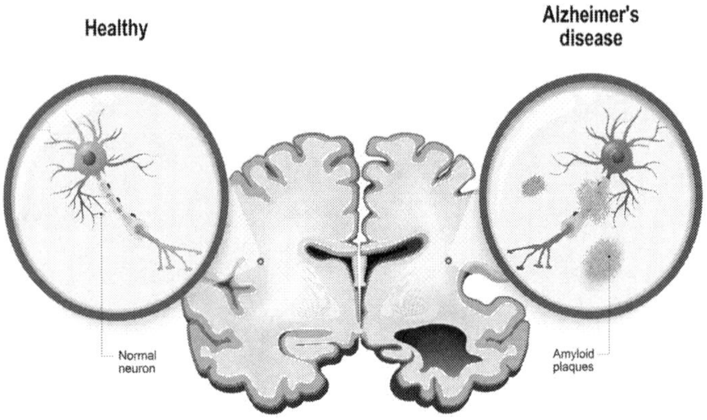

Causes

While the exact cause of Alzheimer's is unknown, environmental factors are the most likely culprit. Few people with Alzheimer's disease develop the disease due to genetic factors.

Two factors strongly contribute to the death of nervous tissue: plaque and tangles. Plaque is the formation of deposits of a protein known as beta-amyloid, which develops in the space between nerves, restricting communication between nerve cells. Tangles are the development of another protein known as tau inside the nerve cells, which can cut off the natural flow of nutrients through cells.

Symptoms

Symptoms begin with difficulty remembering information, such as locations of items or things just learned. As the condition progresses, more brain tissue is lost, and a person may have difficulty making decisions, identifying people or places, and become more irritable or aggressive. Later stages of Alzheimer's may see the loss of the ability to read, write, dance, sing, and other activities learned early in life.

Treatments

There is no cure for Alzheimer's, but there are treatments available that can help manage the condition. Medications may be prescribed that can help with memory loss and other cognitive symptoms. In later stages, other medications may be prescribed that can help with memory, speech, and the ability to perform simpler tasks.

Amyotrophic Lateral Sclerosis

(a-: without; my/o-: muscle; -trophic: nourishment)

Amyotrophic Lateral Sclerosis(ALS) is a **degenerative disorder** affecting **motor neurons**, which control muscles. The nerve degeneration causes **loss of voluntary muscle control**, and can eventually lead to death within five years of diagnosis due to **respiratory failure**. A small percentage of people diagnosed with ALS survive longer than five years.

Amyotrophic Lateral Sclerosis is also known as **Lou Gehrig's Disease**, named for the baseball player who was diagnosed with the condition in 1939.

Causes

The precise cause of ALS is unknown. Genetics seem to play a factor. Men are more likely to develop the condition than women, and it is much more common in people over the age of 50.

Symptoms

Symptoms of ALS begin subtly and may not be noticeable until they become more advanced. A person may experience muscle cramping and twitching, weakness in the muscles of the arms, legs, and neck, trouble chewing and swallowing, and slurred speech as the muscles responsible for vocalization are affected. As the disease progresses, muscle atrophy sets in and the person loses the ability to stand or walk.

Treatments

There is no cure for ALS, but treatment options may include medication to assist with muscle pain and cramping, physical therapy and speech therapy, and the use of ventilators as natural breathing support fails.

Bell's Palsy

(palsy: paralysis)

Bell's Palsy is a condition affecting the **facial nerve**, causing **paralysis on one side of the face.**

Causes

The exact cause of Bell's Palsy is unknown, but is likely the result of an attack to the facial nerve(cranial nerve VII) by the herpes simplex virus. The inflammation damages the nerve, causing the muscles of the side of the face controlled by the facial nerve to become paralyzed or severely weakened. The side of the face affected may also become numb. Bell's Palsy is mostly a temporary condition, and should resolve over the course of a month or two. In some cases, it can become permanent.

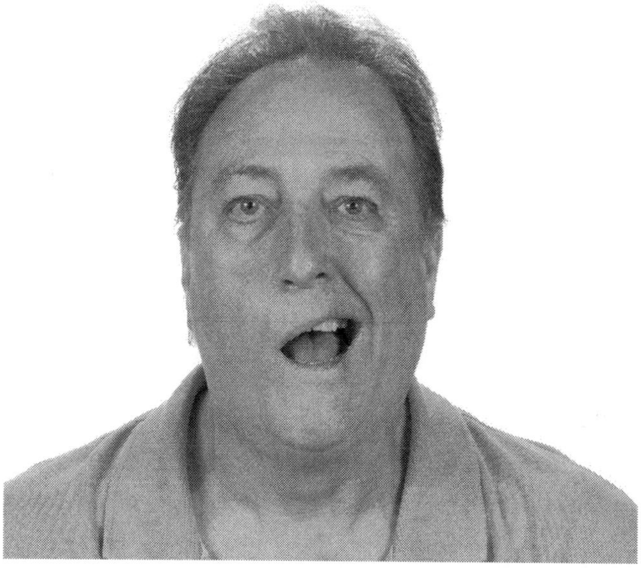

Symptoms

Symptoms, which are usually only present on one side of the face, include the inability to close the eye, difficulty chewing, twitching of muscles in the face, and watery eyes. These symptoms typically resolve within three weeks at the earliest, but may persist for several months, or even become permanent.

Treatments

A person with Bell's Palsy may take corticosteroids to help treat the muscle weakness. Self care, including facial exercises, are recommended.

Carpal Tunnel Syndrome

Carpal Tunnel Syndrome is a condition caused by **compression of the median nerve between the carpals and the transverse carpal ligament.**

Causes

Several factors may contribute to the development of carpal tunnel syndrome, although the most common cause is **repetitive movements.** These repetitive movements can cause straining of the tendons that run through the carpal canal, which can place pressure on the median nerve. If the transverse carpal ligament tightens, it can also place pressure on the median nerve. When pressure is placed on the median nerve, numbness, pain, or tingling sensations may be experienced in the thumb, index, ring, and lateral side of the ring finger.

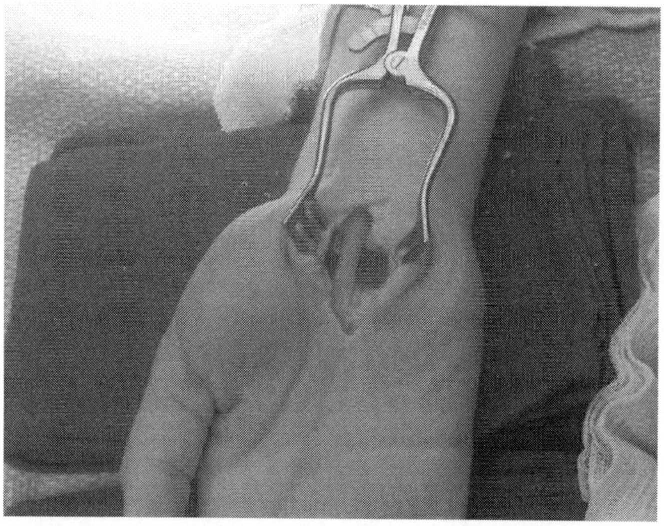

Carpal tunnel surgery, revealing the median nerve

Symptoms

Carpal tunnel syndrome often results in pain, numbness, and tingling sensations in the hand and wrist. Atrophy of the hand muscles may result due to lack of use.

Treatments

Several treatments are available for carpal tunnel syndrome. Self-care is recommended, including stretching the forearm and wrist flexors, massaging the transverse carpal ligament and hand muscles, and icing the area. Because carpal tunnel syndrome is often caused by repetitive actions, ceasing these actions is recommended. Non-steroidal anti-inflammatory medications may be prescribed. Surgery to remove the transverse carpal ligament may also be an option if the condition is severe.

Encephalitis

(encephal-: brain; -itis: inflammation)

Encephalitis is primarily a **viral infection** that results in **inflammation of the brain**.

Causes

Causes of encephalitis vary, but may include mosquito-borne viruses, such as West Nile, the Herpes Simplex virus, and the Rabies virus. Symptoms of encephalitis are usually mild, with the infected person suffering no more than flu-like symptoms, but severe cases may result in brain damage or death.

Symptoms

Symptoms of encephalitis vary depending on severity. Mild cases result in flu-like symptoms, such as fever, headache, general body ache, and fatigue. More severe cases may result in unconsciousness, seizures, weakness, and difficulty speaking or hearing.

Treatments

Most cases of encephalitis are mild, and treatment often consists of bed rest, and letting the virus work through its course. Antiviral medications may also be administered via an IV if the infection is more severe.

Meningitis

(mening-: meninges; -itis: inflammation)

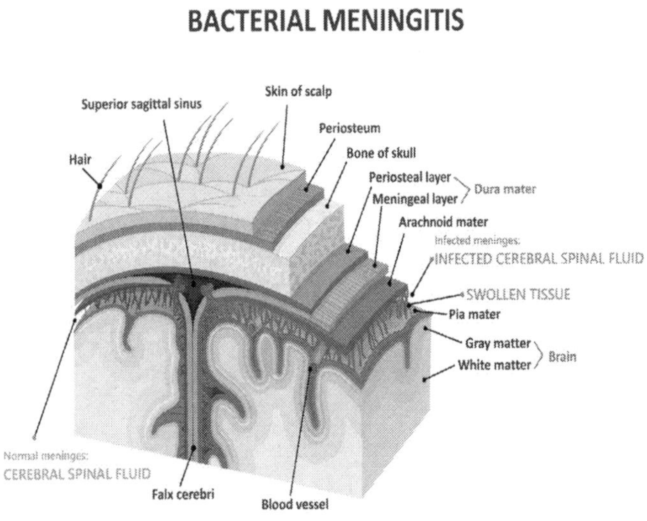

Meningitis is **inflammation of the meninges**, the protective connective tissue surrounding the brain and spinal cord. In the US, meningitis is most commonly caused by **viral infection**. However, certain **bacterial and fungal infections** may also cause meningitis. Bacterial meningitis is the most severe form of meningitis, usually preceded by a sinus or ear infection.

Causes

Being exposed to a pathogen, such as streptococci bacterium, or West Nile virus, are the causes of meningitis. Exposure to these may differ, and contracting them does not necessarily mean a person will develop meningitis. West Nile virus, which also may cause encephalitis, is often transmitted by mosquitoes. Rarely, meningitis may be caused by things that are not infectious, such as medications or allergies to certain chemicals.

Symptoms

Symptoms vary depending on the underlying cause. Viral meningitis may present with symptoms extremely similar to influenza, and will likely clear up on their own within a couple weeks. Fever, headache, nausea, vomiting, and an unusually stiff neck are symptoms to watch for. Meningitis is considered a medical emergency, and a person with suspected meningitis should be seen by a medical professional right away.

Treatments

Bacterial meningitis is treated with intravenous antibiotics to combat the infection, and a course of corticosteroids to prevent inflammation in the brain. Draining the infection from the sinuses may be helpful. Viral meningitis, however, is far less serious, and often clears up after a couple weeks. Treatment for viral meningitis is simply rest and increasing fluid intake. Pain relievers may also help if a person has general body aches or is suffering from mild fever.

Multiple Sclerosis

(scler-: hard; -osis: condition)

Multiple Sclerosis is an **autoimmune disorder**, affecting the **myelin sheaths** that protect the axons of the Nervous System.

Causes

The cause of Multiple Sclerosis is unknown, but may be hereditary, and even environmental factors have been linked to the development of the disease. The disease begins with the body's immune system attacking the myelin sheaths, the protective fatty layers surrounding axons. These sheaths help to insulate the axons and prevent damage to the axons. When the myelin sheath is attacked and destroyed, it exposes the axons, which can have many different effects. Impulses traveling along an axon may terminate at the site of myelin degeneration, which may cause loss of functions. Scar tissue may form over the axons, which leads to extreme pain.

Nerve affected by MS

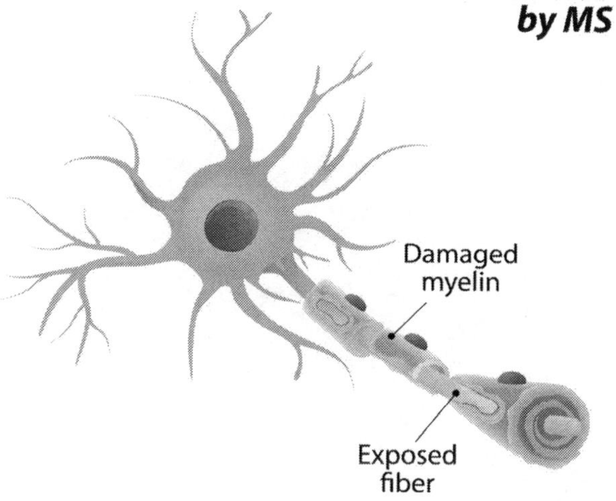

Symptoms

Symptoms of Multiple Sclerosis in acute stages include pain, weakness, fatigue, numbness(usually in the face), tingling sensation, blurry vision, and difficulty walking.

Treatments

There is no cure for Multiple Sclerosis. People may be prescribed disease-altering drugs that suppress the functions of the immune system. People may seek other means of managing Multiple Sclerosis and the accompanying pain and fatigue, including massage therapy, yoga, and meditation.

Paralysis

(paraleyin: disable)

Paralysis is a **loss of function** of a part of the body. This condition can affect a small area, or a large portion of the body.

Causes

Paralysis is caused by **damage to a nerve** that innervates a muscle or muscles. When a nerve is damaged, it can cause weakness(partial paralysis) in a muscle, making it extremely difficult to use, or even result in complete loss of function. The three main types of paralysis that result in complete loss of function are paraplegia, quadriplegia, and hemiplegia.

Paraplegia is paralysis affecting the **lower limbs**. This is typically caused by an injury to the spinal cord, but may also be caused by conditions such as spina bifida.

Quadriplegia(also known as tetraplegia) is paralysis affecting **all four limbs and the trunk**. This is typically caused by an injury to the spinal cord around the C4 vertebrae, which eliminates nerve supply to the limbs.

Hemiplegia is paralysis that affects **one side**(hemisphere) of the body. This is typically caused by a stroke, transient ischemic attack, or even multiple sclerosis.

Symptoms

Primarily, paralysis results in loss of sensation. Depending on which type of paralysis, different parts of the body may lose sensation. In the initial acute stage of paralysis, a person may experience weakness, extreme pain in the back, head, or neck, difficulty walking or standing, difficulty breathing, and loss of control over the bladder or bowels. In the acute stage, a person needs medical attention immediately.

Treatments

Treatment for paralysis may be helpful in cases of partial paralysis, where there is still some function. Physical and occupational therapy may also help the nervous tissue regenerate.

Parkinson's Disease

Parkinson's Disease is a motor disease that results in **trembling** due to a **loss of the neurotransmitter dopamine**.

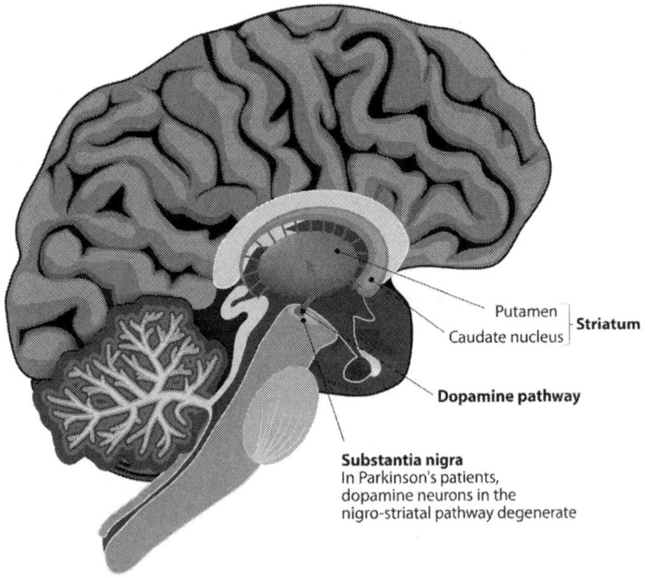

Causes

There is no known cause of Parkinson's Disease. Neurons in the brain that produce dopamine are gradually destroyed. Dopamine is the neurotransmitter that stabilizes the body during motor movements, especially fine movements like writing. When dopamine levels in the body drop, trembling and shaking increases. Over time, as dopamine levels drop, the trembling increases. As dopamine continues to drop, larger movements become affected, like walking and talking.

Symptoms

Symptoms of Parkinson's Disease include tremors, which usually begin in the hands and fingers and advance to larger body areas, difficulty writing, slower movement, difficulty in speech, and the loss of movements such as blinking.

Treatments

While there is no cure for Parkinson's Disease, treatments are available to help manage the condition, including dopamine replacement medications.

Sciatica

Sciatica is a condition causing pain radiating down the buttocks, posterior thigh, and leg.

Causes

Sciatica is most commonly caused by a **herniated disc in the lumbar vertebrae**, which puts compression on the nerves that comprise the **sciatic nerve**. Bone spurs may also place pressure on the nerves.

Piriformis Syndrome is often confused with sciatica. Piriformis syndrome is caused by tightness in the piriformis muscle, which may place substantial pressure on the sciatic nerve.

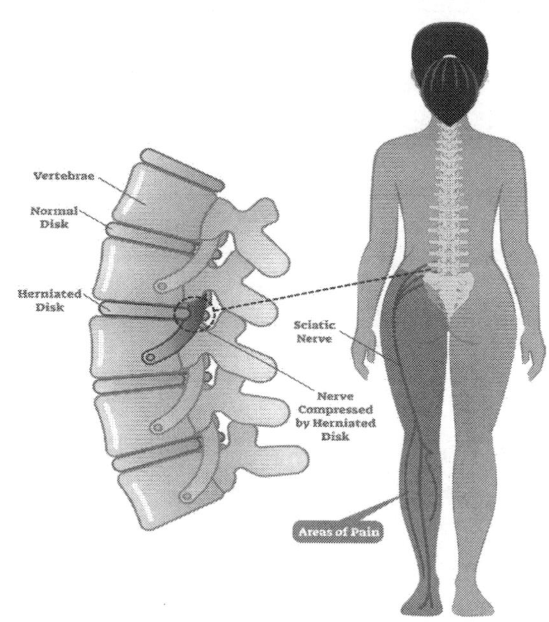

Symptoms

The primary symptom of sciatica is pain in the posterior leg, thigh, and glutes, usually only on one side of the body. There may also be numbness and tingling in the affected area.

Treatments

Treatment for sciatica may include physical therapy, anti-inflammatory medications, or surgery if the condition is severe enough.

Thoracic Outlet Syndrome

Thoracic Outlet Syndrome is a condition caused by **compression of nerves and blood vessels passing through the thoracic outlet.**

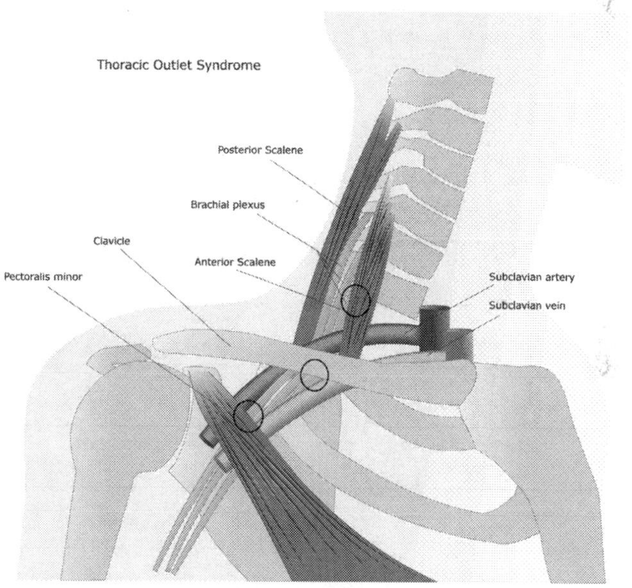

Causes

Thoracic outlet syndrome may be caused by tight muscles, including **pectoralis minor and scalenes**, obesity, and tumors in the neck, such as those seen in Non-Hodgkin's Lymphoma.

Symptoms

Pressure placed on the nerves and blood vessels may cause pain, numbness, and weakness in the upper limb. If a blood vessel is compressed, it may cause the hand to become a bluish color due to lack of circulation, cause pain and fatigue in the arm, and coldness in the hands and fingers. If a nerve is compressed, numbness in the limb and atrophy of the muscles innervated by the nerve may result.

Treatments

Treatments primarily consist of stretching of the tight muscles to release pressure on the nerves and blood vessels. In the case of a tumor, surgery to remove the tumor may be required.

Trigeminal Neuralgia

(neur-: nerve; -algia: pain)

Trigeminal Neuralgia is a chronic condition causing **extreme pain in the face**.

Causes

The **trigeminal nerve**(cranial nerve V) sends sensory information from the face to the brain. When a blood vessel comes into contact with the trigeminal nerve at the brain stem, it results in dysfunction of the trigeminal nerve. This dysfunction results in hyper-sensitivity of the face, making even light touch extremely painful.

Symptoms

Extreme pain in the face, which may last from days to weeks, is the primary symptom of trigeminal neuralgia. This pain is typically only felt in one side of the face, but may worsen over time.

Treatments

Treatments for trigeminal neuralgia include medications to reduce pain, botox injections, or possible surgery to reduce pressure on the trigeminal nerve caused by blood vessels.

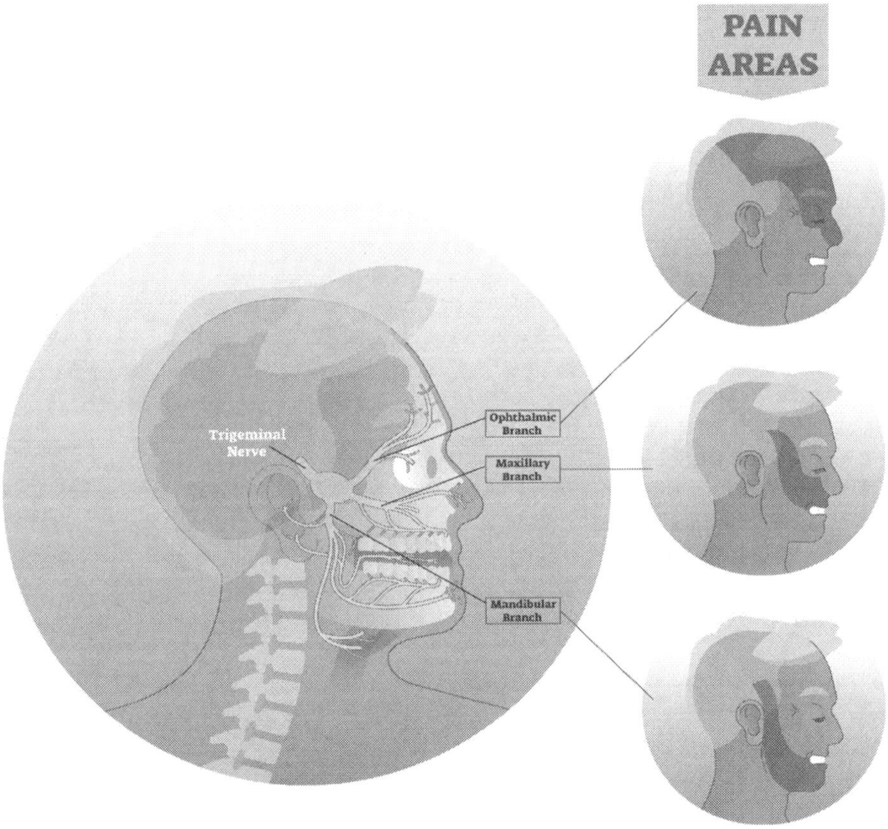

Reproductive Pathologies

Amenorrhea

(a-: without; men-: menstruation; -rrhea: discharge)

Amenorrhea is a **lack of menstruation** that takes place over **three menstrual cycles**. This most commonly occurs with pregnancy, although hormones and issues with reproductive organs may also contribute.

Causes

The main cause of amenorrhea is pregnancy. As a woman ages and experiences menopause, amenorrhea will also occur. Birth control may also stop menstruation, along with other medications such as antidepressants.

Problems with hormone production, such as if a woman has polycystic ovarian syndrome(PCOS), may also prevent menstruation. Stress may also lead to hormonal imbalance.

Symptoms

A lack of menstruation is the main symptom of amenorrhea. Other symptoms may include headaches, change in vision, production of acne, and loss of hair.

Treatments

Treatment depends on the root cause. If pregnancy is the cause, normal menstruation should return after pregnancy. Stopping birth control will return menstruation. Medications to treat hormonal imbalances may be prescribed. In cases such as PCOS, surgery may be performed to remove the cyst or cysts causing problems, or remove the ovary completely. Reducing stress may also help reestablish menstruation.

Chlamydia

Chlamydia is a **bacterial infection** of the Reproductive System, known as a sexually transmitted infection. It occurs most commonly in sexually active women, but anyone may contract it via **sexual or oral intercourse.**

Causes

Direct contact to the bacteria during vaginal, anal, or oral intercourse may result in contraction of chlamydia. Despite contracting the bacteria, a person may not know they have it, as symptoms do not always appear.

Symptoms

Discharge from the penis or vagina, painful urination, and pain in the abdomen are common symptoms of chlamydia, although as previously stated, symptoms don't always appear. If symptoms do occur, they usually appear a couple weeks after contracting the bacteria.

Treatments

If any symptom is seen, a person should see a doctor to get diagnosed. If diagnosed with chlamydia, antibiotics are prescribed to kill the bacteria, and the infection is usually resolved within a couple weeks after starting medication.

Dysmenorrhea

(dys-: difficult; men-: menstruation; -rrhea: discharge)

Dysmenorrhea, known as **menstrual cramps**, is pain experienced during menstruation, typically at the beginning of menstruation. The pain usually goes away after a few days. Pain may be experienced in the lower abdomen and lower back, and may be either dull or more intense and interfere with daily life.

Sometimes, dysmenorrhea may be the result of more serious problems, such as endometriosis.

Causes

During menstruation, the uterus sloughs off its inner lining by contracting. The release of substances such as prostaglandins, which are associated with pain and inflammation, cause the uterus to contract, and pain results.

Symptoms

Symptoms include a dull ache in the lower abdomen or back, potential nausea, and headaches.

Treatments

Usually, over-the-counter pain relievers such as ibuprofen are taken to assist with the management of pain. If dysmenorrhea is the result of another more serious condition, surgery to correct the issue may be performed, such as removing fibroids from the uterus.

Endometriosis

(endo-: inside; metri-: uterus; -osis: condition)

Endometriosis is an **abnormal growth of uterine lining**, known as the endometrium, **outside the uterus**. The lining often grows on the ovaries and fallopian tubes. The tissue still behaves like normal uterine lining, breaking down and bleeding during each menstrual period. The tissue stays inside the body, whereas during a normal menstrual period, the uterine lining is expelled from the body. Scar tissue and cysts may form, especially involving the ovaries, and pain may be present.

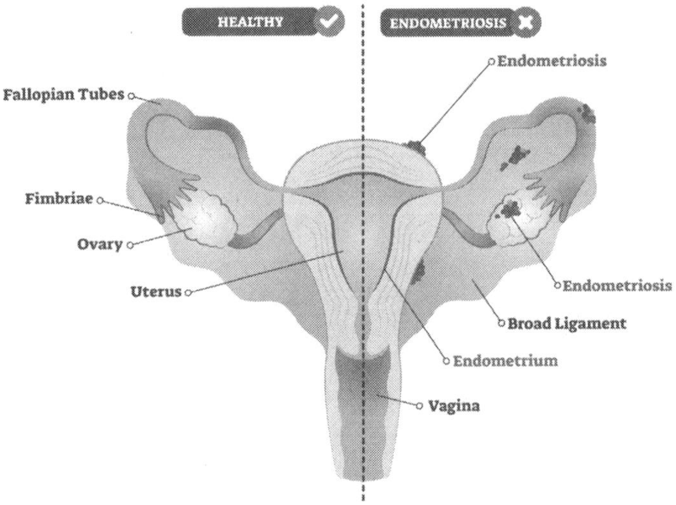

Causes

There is no exact cause that has been determined. Some theories include menstrual blood flowing backwards through the fallopian tubes and out to the pelvic cavity, possible complications from surgeries such as C Section, or even problems with the immune system that make it difficult to break down the growth of tissue.

Symptoms

Painful menstruation, sometimes severe, may occur. Excessive bleeding and infertility may also occur as a result due to blockage of the fallopian tubes by endometrial tissue.

Treatments

There are many treatments available. Pain medication may be prescribed to manage pain, while birth control may be administered to help regulate hormones responsible for building up uterine lining. Surgery is an option to remove endometrial tissue. If other treatments are not helpful, a hysterectomy may be performed to completely remove the uterus.

Genital Herpes

Genital Herpes is a **viral infection** of the genitals, caused by contact with the **Herpes Simplex 2 Virus.** Herpes Simplex 1 may also cause genital herpes, but is usually only transmitted during oral sex, and is much less common than Herpes Simplex 2. The virus is primarily transmitted sexually, and a person who has contracted it may not know they have it due to symptoms not being present immediately after infection.

Causes

Exposure to the herpes simplex virus through sexual contact is the cause of genital herpes.

Symptoms

Symptoms are often recurring, and a person may experience them several times a year. Symptoms include pain, itching, ulceration, skin that forms a crust that scabs, and the development of red bumps or white blisters that contain fluid.

Treatments

There is no cure for genital herpes. Antiviral medications may be prescribed to help slow the progression of symptoms.

Genital Warts

Genital Warts is the development of warts in the genital region. Genital warts is one of the most common sexually transmitted infections. Genital warts are caused by coming in to contact with the **human papilloma virus(HPV)**, the same virus that causes cervical cancer.

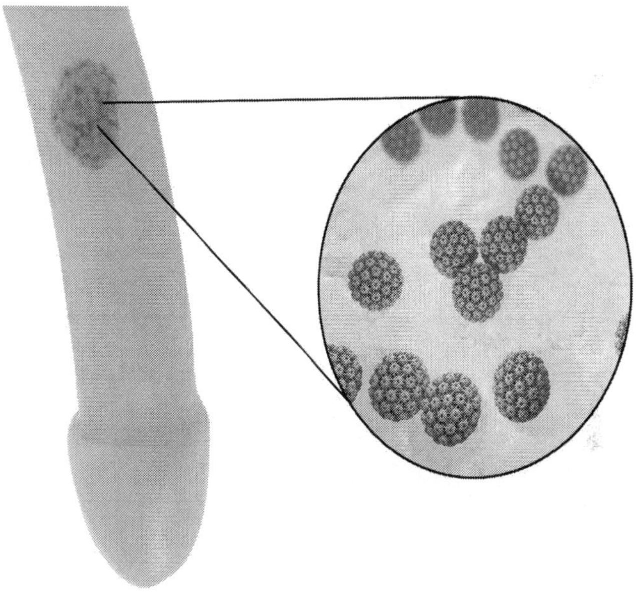

Causes

Genital warts is caused by the human papilloma virus. Not every strain of HPV causes genital warts, and the virus is generally destroyed by the body before warts can develop.

Symptoms

Warts form around the genitals. The warts may itch or cause discomfort. Like other warts, genital warts may go away on their own and return later.

Treatments

Most common treatment is application of topical creams that either boost the immune system to destroy the warts, or creams that destroy the wart tissue. Surgical removal may be performed if warts are larger or are unresponsive to topical creams.

Gonorrhea

(gono-: semen, seed; -rrhea: discharge)

Gonorrhea is a **bacterial infection** of the genital region. The infection results from sexual contact with the **Neisseria bacterium.** Although gonorrhea most commonly affects the genitals, it can also infect the mouth, throat, eyes, and rectum.

Causes

Sexual contact is the most common cause of bacteria transmission in gonorrhea.

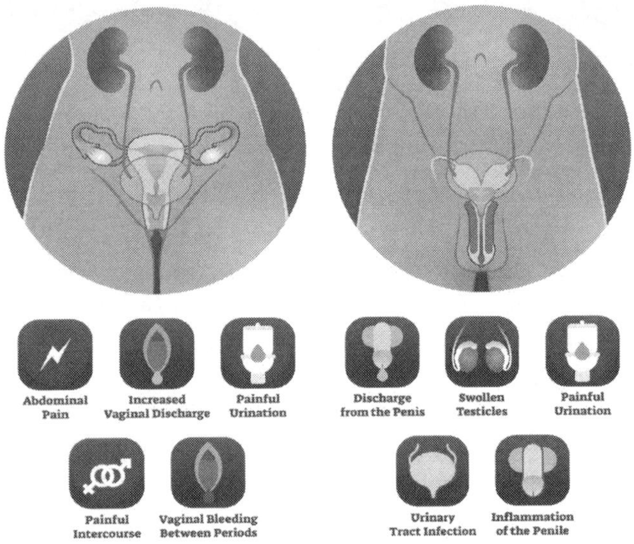

Symptoms

Commonly, symptoms of gonorrhea never appear, and a person may not know that they have been infected. When symptoms do appear, they include discharge from the penis or vagina, pain during urination, and bleeding from the vagina between menstrual periods in women.

Treatments

People with gonorrhea are treated with antibiotics to kill the bacteria. A course of antibiotics should be completed, even if symptoms have disappeared in the middle of the prescribed dose.

Mastitis

(mast-: breast; -itis: inflammation)

Mastitis is **inflammation of breast tissue**, the result of a **bacterial infection**. Mastitis most commonly occurs after pregnancy as a result of breast feeding. The breast may become red and tender. If not properly treated, an abscess may develop in the breast, which would need to be drained surgically.

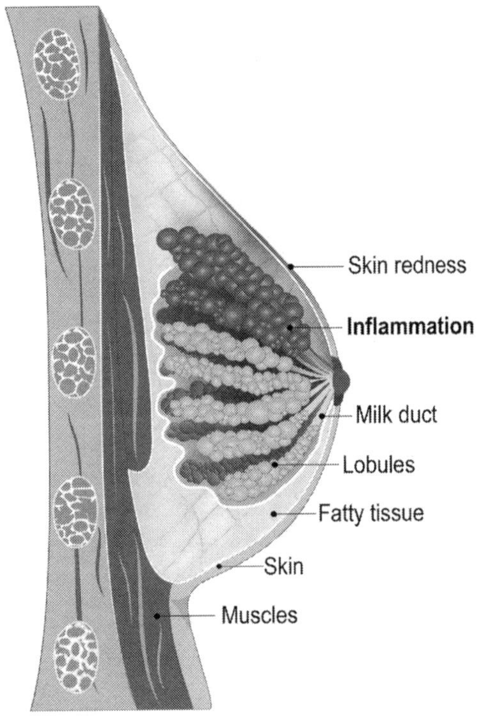

Causes

Bacteria is a common cause of mastitis, entering the breast while breast feeding. Not properly draining the breast after bacteria has entered the breast can provide a suitable environment for the bacteria to reproduce.

A blockage in a milk duct may also produce mastitis, causing bacteria to become trapped, leading to infection. Breasts should be sufficiently drained to prevent blockages.

Symptoms

Breasts may become red and swollen, a fever may present, and the breasts may be more tender than normal.

Treatments

Antibiotics are useful in treating mastitis caused by bacterial infection. Again, if an abscess is present, it may need to be surgically drained. Over-the-counter pain relievers may help with general aches associated with the breast inflammation.

Menopause

Menopause is the **permanent cessation of menstrual cycles**. As a woman ages, her body naturally produces less estrogen and progesterone, two hormones vital in regulating menstruation. The average age of a woman to reach menopause is 51, at which point the ovaries no longer release eggs, and menstruation stops. Osteoporosis is a common side effect of menopause.

Causes

Most commonly, menopause is a result of natural aging. Less commonly, it is associated with other medical procedures, such as hysterectomy(surgical removal of the uterus), problems arising from the ovaries, or even temporary menopause seen with chemotherapy or radiation treatments stemming from cancer.

Symptoms

There are numerous symptoms associated with menopause, depending on the stage of menopause a person is in. Hot flashes and changes in mood are common. Hair may become thin and brittle. A person may see increased weight gain, and experience problems sleeping.

Treatments

There are no treatments to prevent menopause from occurring. Treatments are available that may help with some symptoms as sociated with menopause. Hormone replacement therapy can help maintain estrogen levels in the body, which may assist with hot flashes and reduce the chances of developing osteoporosis.

Polycystic Ovarian Syndrome

(poly-: many; cyst-: bladder)

Polycystic Ovarian Syndrome(PCOS) is a disorder marked by the development of **small fluid-filled sacs** in an **ovary**, which may prevent eggs from being released, and cause problems with estrogen and progesterone release. It is more commonly seen in obese women.

Polycystic Ovarian Syndrome may lead to infertility, miscarriage, the development of gestational and/or Type 2 Diabetes, and hypertension during pregnancy.

Causes

The precise cause of Polycystic Ovarian Syndrome is unclear, but factors that may contribute include excessive amounts of insulin in the blood, which can lead to increased production of male specific hormones, and genetic factors.

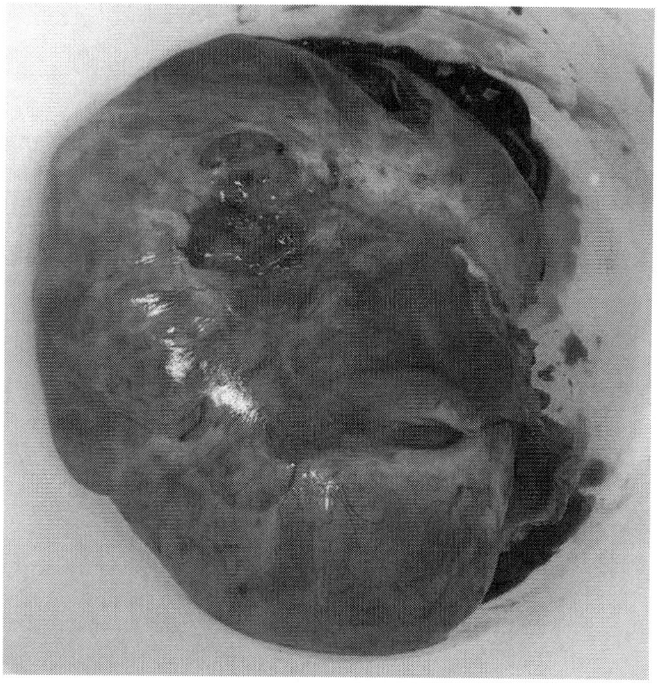

Symptoms

Common symptoms include a lack of regular menstrual cycle, cysts that develop in an ovary(which may affect both ovaries), increased amounts of facial hair, and increased acne due to excessive amounts of male hormones.

Treatments

Because Polycystic Ovarian Syndrome occurs more commonly in obese women, weight loss is recommended to combat the condition. Certain medications may be prescribed to help regulate estrogen and progesterone levels in the body, reducing the effects of male hormones.

To help with ovulation, medications such as Metformin may be prescribed. If the cysts in the ovary are too large, surgery to remove the ovary completely may be performed.

Preeclampsia

(pre-: before; -eclampsia: a convulsive state)

Preeclampsia is a potential complication of pregnancy, and is considered a serious condition that may potentially lead to death if left untreated. Preeclampsia may be a sign of damage to organs such as the kidneys and liver. It is marked by **high blood pressure** and **increased protein in the urine** where there hasn't been any before.

Because preeclampsia is a serious condition, it may lead to **early induced labor.**

Causes

Causes of preeclampsia often involve blood vessels in the placenta. If blood vessels aren't formed properly and are unable to effectively deliver blood to the fetus, it can result in preeclampsia. Other disorders, such as gestational hypertension, may result in preeclampsia.

Symptoms

Although preeclampsia may be asymptomatic, common symptoms include hypertension, an abnormally large amount of protein in the urine, nausea, headaches, and abdominal pain. The amount of urine being produced may decrease, as well as the levels of thrombocytes in the blood.

Treatments

Treatments before delivery are available, but the only way to completely rid the body of preeclampsia is to deliver the child. Severe complications may arise until then, including stroke and seizures. Medications include corticosteroids to improve thrombocyte levels in the blood, and antihypertensives to lower blood pressure.

Premenstrual Syndrome

Premenstrual Syndrome is the predictable occurrence of a series of symptoms around the time a woman leading up to menstruation.

Causes

Hormonal changes are thought to be a major contributing factor to the development of premenstrual syndrome. During menstruation, **hormone levels change dramatically**, and this can result in altered behavior and thought processes.

Symptoms

Symptoms are extremely varied, and no one person experiences exactly the same symptoms as another. Common symptoms include depression, mood swings, changes in appetite, fatigue, headache, bloating, feeling anxious, fluid retention, and tenderness in the breasts.

Treatments

Despite changes in lifestyle being the preferred treatment, a doctor may prescribe medications if symptoms are more severe. Diuretics help with excessive fluid accumulation, and antidepressants may help with hormone regulation associated with mood swings. Lifestyle changes may include increasing exercise and incorporating massage therapy or yoga to promote relaxation and reducing stress.

Prostatitis

(prostat-: prostate; -itis: inflammation)

Prostatitis is **inflammation of the prostate**, a small gland located beneath the bladder in males. Prostatitis commonly affects men over the age of 50, but can occur at any age.

The prostate produces fluids that mix with sperm to create semen, connecting with the urinary tract. **Bacteria** may enter into the prostate through the urine, resulting in acute prostatitis.

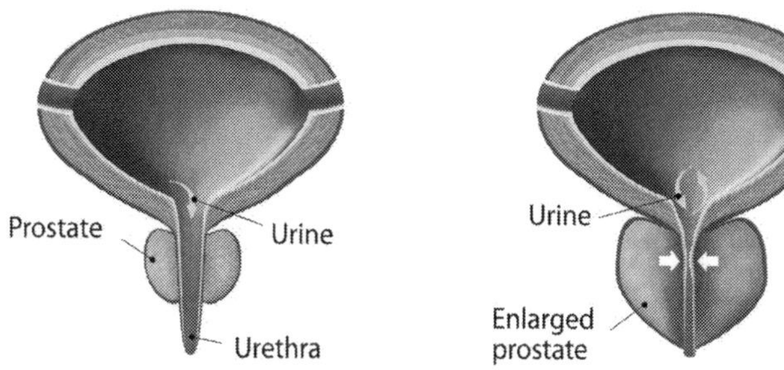

Causes

The most common cause of prostatitis is a bacterial infection. Damage to the nerves that control urination may also lead to the development of prostatitis.

Symptoms

Difficulty urinating is a common symptom of prostatitis. Painful urination may present, along with the need to frequently urinate at night. A person may experience pain in the abdomen and pelvis, and the urine may look cloudy.

Treatments

Most commonly, prostatitis is treated with antibiotics. Non-steroidal anti-inflammatory drugs may also help alleviate inflammation of the prostate, but will not fix the underlying cause.

Syphilis

Syphilis is a **bacterial infection of the genitals**, most commonly spread by **sexual intercourse**. Syphilis is easily treatable, but may lie dormant in the body for years before becoming activated. Advances stages of a syphilis infection can cause brain or heart damage, and can be fatal.

Causes

Direct sexual contact with a person infected by syphilis transmits the bacteria. Although less common, the bacteria may be transmitted during childbirth(known as congenital syphilis), or through direct contact to syphilis lesions during activities such as kissing.

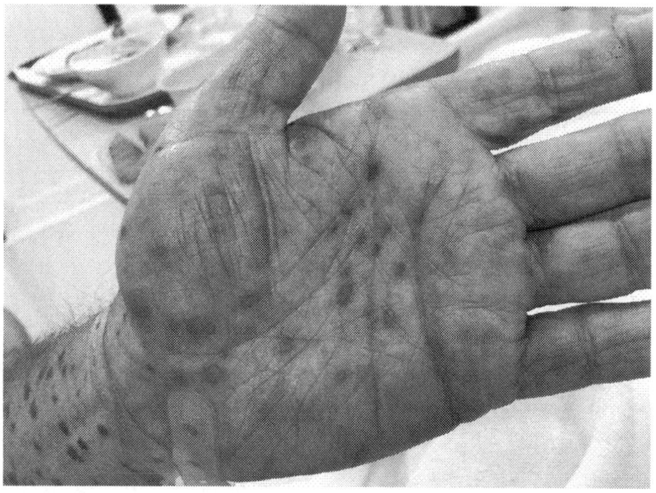

Symptoms

There are several different stages of a syphilis infection. The first stage is known as primary syphilis, and presents with a small sore that is usually painless on the area where infection occurred. Secondary syphilis presents with a widespread rash that usually starts on the torso, then spreads over the entire body. Latent syphilis occurs when there are no symptoms, but a person is still infected by the bacteria. Tertiary syphilis, which develops in the late stages of a syphilis infection, may cause damage to the brain, heart, liver, or eyes. The amount of damage caused could lead to stroke, dementia, and the development of aneurysms.

Treatments

Because syphilis is caused by bacteria, antibiotics are prescribed to destroy the infection. Early stage syphilis is easily treatable.

Respiratory Pathologies

Apnea

(a-: without; -pnea: breathing)

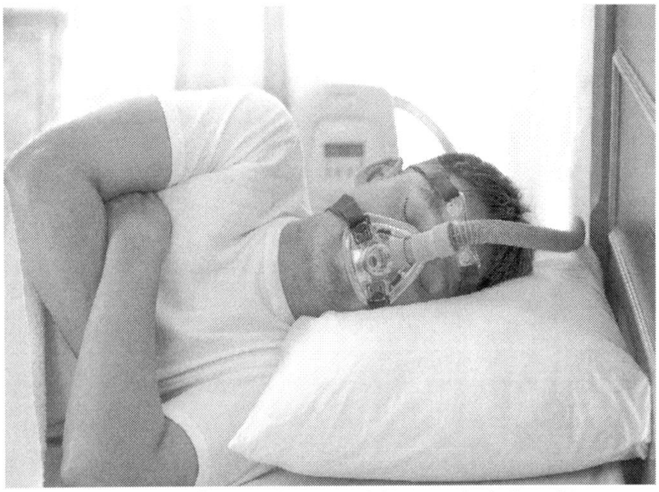
Patient utilizing a CPAP machine to assist in breathing

Apnea, commonly referred to as sleep apnea, is a **temporary cessation of breathing during sleep**. Apnea may be a serious condition, depending on the patient. There are three types of sleep apnea: central sleep apnea, obstructive sleep apnea, and complex sleep apnea syndrome.

People who are overweight have a much higher rate of occurrence than others. Advanced age and being male are also common demographics for the development of sleep apnea.

Causes

Central sleep apnea is the result of the brain not stimulating muscles responsible for breathing. A patient may experience shortness of breath due to lack of oxygen intake. This form of sleep apnea is not common.

Obstructive sleep apnea is the result of throat muscles relaxing, which causes the air passages to narrow or completely close upon inhalation. This reduces the amount of oxygen getting into the body. As a result, the brain may force the patient awake momentarily to unblock the airways. People with obstructive sleep apnea often snore, and may even sound as if they are choking.

Complex sleep apnea syndrome is diagnosed when a person experiences both central and obstructive sleep apnea.

Symptoms

Symptoms of apnea include snoring, shortness of breath upon waking, fatigue, and briefly waking at night. Another person may see the cessation of breathing and report it to the patient.

Treatments

Less severe forms of apnea may require less drastic forms of treatment, such as losing weight. In more severe forms, a person may be instructed to wear a CPAP(continuous positive airway pressure) machine during sleep, which increases air pressure in the airway, keeping the airways open enough for adequate oxygen intake to occur.

If other treatments are ineffective, surgery may be performed to remove tissue in and around the airway, which can increase the passageway for air to travel through.

Asthma

Asthma is a chronic respiratory disease that causes **constriction of the airways**, restricting oxygen intake. Asthma usually begins in childhood, but may disappear with age. Other times, it remains a chronic condition. Other factors such as smoking or obesity may lead to the development of asthma.

Causes

Asthma affects the **smooth muscle in the walls of the bronchial tubes**. Typically, when a person inhales an irritant(such as dust or smoke), the smooth muscle spasms and constricts in an effort to reduce the irritant moving further into the lungs. The bronchi will also produce an **excessive amount of mucous**, which further restricts the flow of oxygen into the lungs.

Symptoms

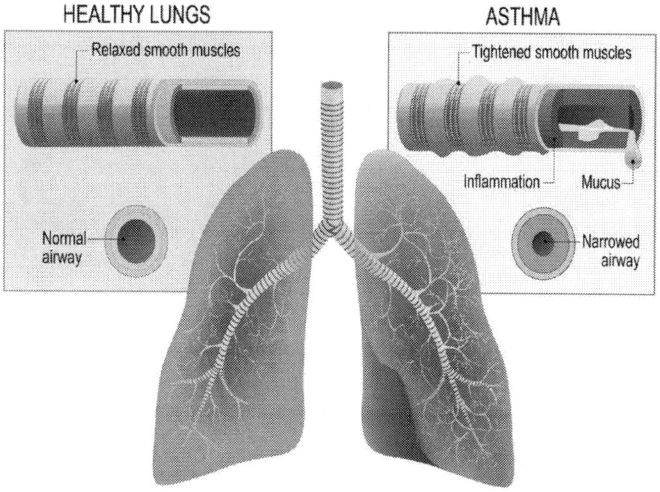

Symptoms include wheezing, chest tightness, and shortness of breath. Treatment varies depending on the severity in acute stages. If it is mild, medication may not be required. If symptoms are more severe, bronchodilators may be required to calm and open the airways. In extreme cases, where regular bronchodilators do not work, medical attention should be sought. A nebulizer, with inhalable steroids, should be used with asthma attacks.

Treatments

Treatment for asthma primarily consists of the use of steroids and bronchodilators administered directly to the lungs via inhalers. If a person suffers from an asthma attack or has more severe forms of asthma, a nebulizer(which turns medication into a mist) may be required. Corticosteroids may also be used to lessen the chances of having an asthma attack.

Bronchitis

(bronch-: bronchi; -itis: inflammation)

Bronchitis is an inflammatory disease of the Respiratory System, restricting oxygen intake.

Causes

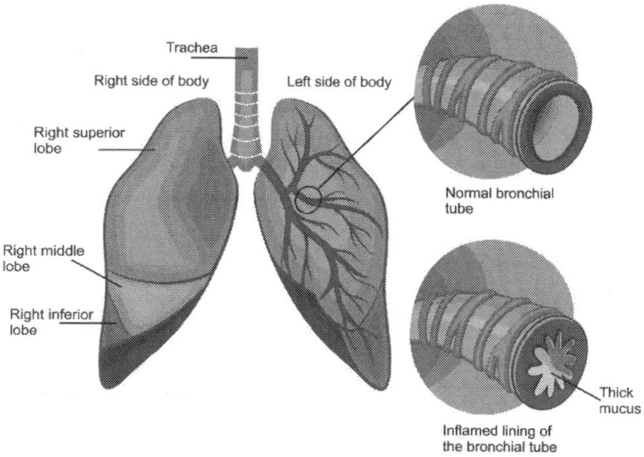

There are two different types of bronchitis: acute bronchitis and chronic bronchitis. **Acute bronchitis** is the result of a **primary infection** of the Respiratory System, such as influenza or pneumonia. These diseases affect the bronchial tubes, causing them to become irritated and inflamed. When these diseases resolve, the bronchitis will also resolve. **Chronic bronchitis** is the result of **constant irritation to the bronchial tubes**, caused by exposure to things such as **cigarette smoking or dust**. When exposure to the irritant ceases, the bronchitis will also cease.

Symptoms

With both forms of bronchitis, there is an increased amount of mucous produced in the lungs, which makes breathing difficult. Increased coughing may be a side effect of the increase in mucous.

Treatments

Treatments vary depending on which type of bronchitis is involved. Acute bronchitis may require nothing more than a bronchodilator or cough suppressant. Because acute bronchitis is usually caused by a viral infection, antivirals may be prescribed to stop the advancement of the virus. Chronic bronchitis often requires the use of a bronchodilator, but not much else.

Emphysema

(emphyso: inflate)

Emphysema is a chronic condition of the lungs, resulting in difficulty bringing oxygen into the body and eliminating carbon dioxide from the body.

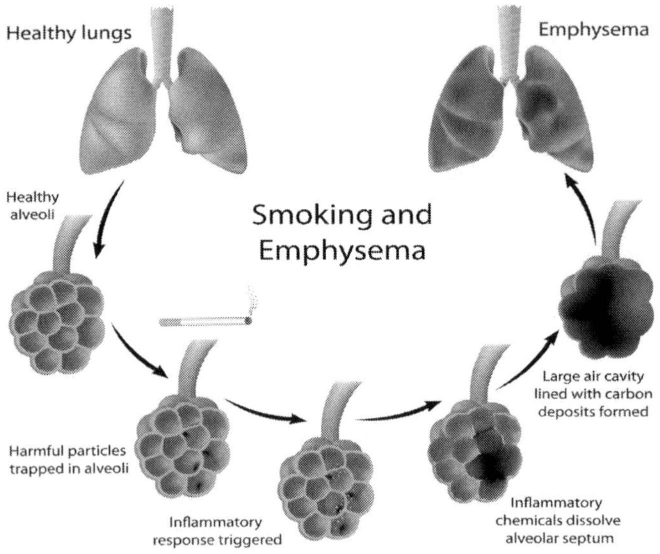

Causes

Emphysema is caused by over-exposure to substances such as **cigarette smoke**. Constant irritation of the lungs by smoke can lead to **degeneration of the alveoli**, air sacs at the end of bronchial tubes where gas exchange takes place. When the alveoli degenerate, they lose surface area, which is what capillaries move across to eliminate carbon dioxide from the body and bring oxygen into the body. Lack of sufficient alveoli surface area makes gas exchange extremely difficult.

Symptoms

Emphysema causes shortness of breath. A person with emphysema may be much more likely to develop a collapsed lung due to damage to the lungs.

Treatments

Breathing exercises and oxygen supplementation may help control emphysema. If needed, bronchodilators can help relax the airways. If infections such as pneumonia occur, antibiotics may help.

Influenza

(Italian "influenza": influence)

Influenza is a **highly contagious viral infection** that primarily affects the lungs.

Causes

There are many different strains of the flu virus. It is constantly mutating, so treatment can be difficult. **Vaccinations** are the primary form of prevention for influenza.

During acute stages, influenza results in fever, general malaise, body aches, runny nose, and cough. Symptoms generally last no more than a week. Depending on the person involved, it can be a moderate infection, or can be life-threatening. Children and the elderly are much more likely to have serious cases of influenza than the general population.

Symptoms

Influenza typically has a sudden onset of symptoms, including fever, body ache, fatigue, sore throat, nasal congestion, body chills, and sweating.

Treatments

Treatment for influenza is usually nothing more than rest and increased fluid intake. Antiviral medication may be prescribed, and may help reduce the length of the infection. Influenza usually clears up on its own.

Laryngitis

(laryng-: larynx; -itis: inflammation)

Laryngitis is **inflammation of the larynx**, also known as the voice box. Laryngitis may affect one's **ability to speak** due to the presence of the vocal cords inside the larynx.

Causes

There are many different causes of laryngitis. There are two main types of laryngitis: acute and chronic. **Acute laryngitis** is commonly the result of trauma to the larynx caused by yelling, or caused by an acute infection. Once the larynx has had time to heal, or the infection goes away, the inflammation should dissipate and the voice should return to normal. In **chronic laryngitis**, common causes include smoking and acid reflux.

Symptoms

Symptoms include difficulty speaking, pain in the throat, and dry coughing. In some cases, the voice may be completely lost, and in others, the voice is only hoarse.

Treatments

If laryngitis is not caused by an infection, resting the voice is extremely helpful. If bacterial infection is the cause, antibiotics may aid in destroying bacteria causing the inflammation. Most cases of infectious laryngitis are viral, however, and won't be helped by antibiotics.

Lozenges may aid in soothing the throat, as well as using humidifiers.

Pneumonia

(pneumo: lung)

Pneumonia is a **highly contagious infection of the lungs**, resulting in a **buildup of fluid in the alveoli**.

Causes

The primary cause of pneumonia is **bacterial infection** (staphylococci), but may also be caused by a virus or fungi. The bacterium enters the body through breathing, which then infects the lungs.

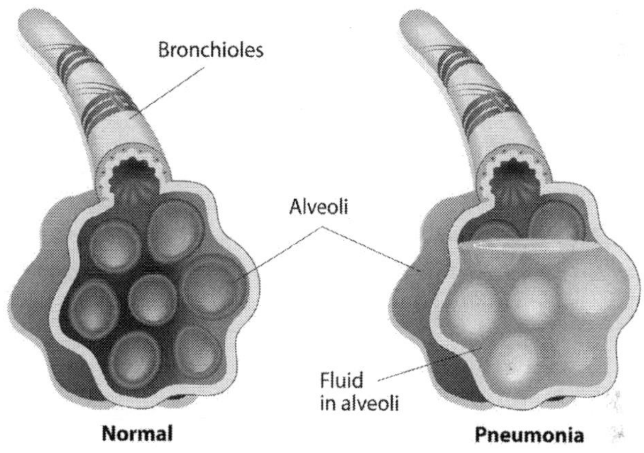

Symptoms

Mild cases of pneumonia usually present with symptoms similar to those of influenza. Other symptoms may include pain in the chest upon breathing, coughing which may produce phlegm, fever, nausea, and shortness of breath. Symptoms can range from mild to severe, and even life threatening, based on the overall health and age of the person infected.

Treatments

Pneumonia is typically treated with antibiotics. Cough medicine and antipyretics may be prescribed to aid with coughing and to lower fever.

Sinusitis

(sinus: sinus; -itis: inflammation)

Sinusitis is an acute condition causing **inflammation and swelling in the nasal sinuses**, which can result in **excessive mucous production**. It can also prevent mucous from properly draining from the sinuses, causing a person to feel a lot of pressure in the face around the nose and eyes. Bacterial infection may result, which can increase the amount of fluid present in the sinuses.

Causes

The most common cause of sinusitis is an acute viral infection, such as the common cold, which may in turn cause bacterial infection to take place.

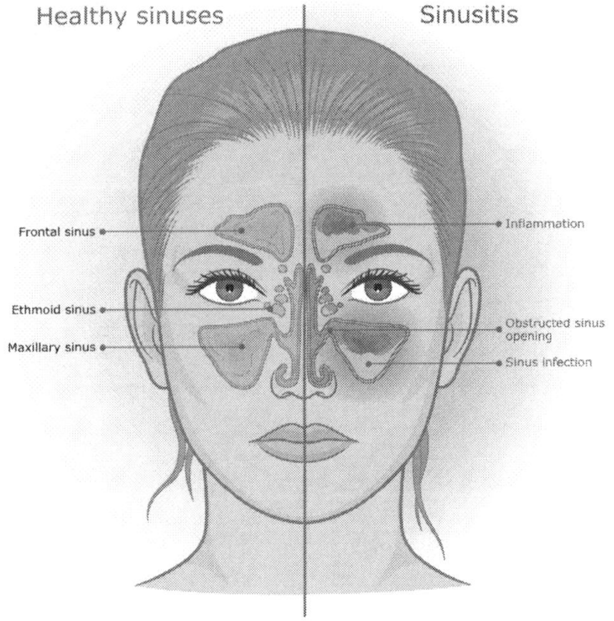

Symptoms

A person with sinusitis may experience pressure in the face around the nose, eyes, and ears, headache, a thick mucous produced by the nose usually presenting with a yellow or green color, and congestion in the nasal cavity.

Treatments

Decongestants are effective at helping to drain the nasal cavities, which can help ease pressure in the area. Nasal sprays can help alleviate inflammation and clean out the nasal cavity, further helping to reduce pressure. If bacterial infection is present, antibiotics may be prescribed.

Tuberculosis

(tubercul/o: tubercle; -osis: condition)

Tuberculosis is a **serious bacterial infection** of the Respiratory System, and is contagious. Exposure to tuberculosis may cause a person to acquire either **latent tuberculosis or active tuberculosis.** In latent tuberculosis, the bacteria enters the body but does not cause any problems or symptoms. This type is not contagious. However, if it becomes active tuberculosis, it becomes contagious. Active tuberculosis is when the bacteria is activated and symptoms of a tuberculosis infection are present.

Causes

Tuberculosis is contracted from another person through **microscopic droplets** spread through the air. This can be caused by actions such as **coughing and sneezing.**

Tuberculosis may have a better chance of becoming active in a person with HIV/AIDS, due to the compromised immune system.

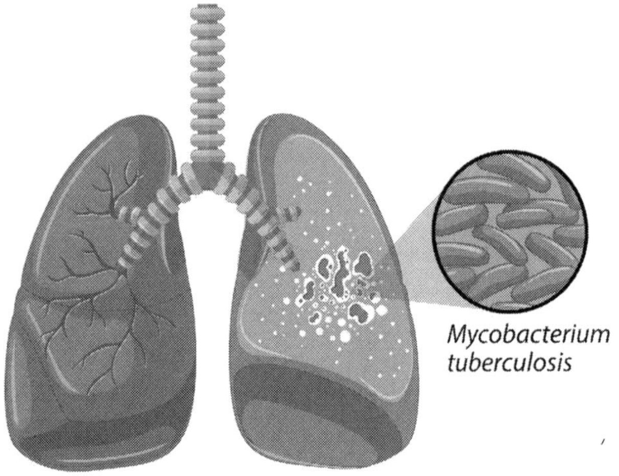

Symptoms

Symptoms include chronic coughing, pain in the chest when breathing, fatigue, fever, and producing blood upon coughing. Night chills, sweating, and unexplained loss in weight may also be signs of an active tuberculosis infection. Tuberculosis may, in some instances, also affect structures and organs in the body such as the kidneys.

Treatments

The bacteria responsible for tuberculosis is extremely hard to destroy, so a person afflicted with the condition will need to take antibiotics for an extended period of time. This ensures the bacteria is completely destroyed and there is no chance of the bacteria becoming immune to the antibiotics being used.

Skeletal Pathologies

Ankylosing Spondylitis

(ankyl/o: crooked; spondyl-: spine; -itis: inflammation)

Ankylosing Spondylitis is an **autoimmune disorder**, similar to rheumatoid arthritis, in which the body's immune system attacks and destroys the **annulus fibrosus of the intervertebral discs.** Over time, the curvature in the vertebrae is lost. Because the intervertebral discs are destroyed, the space between vertebral bodies lessens, eventually allowing the vertebral bones to sit directly atop one another. Movement between these bones is severely reduced, and eventually the bones can fuse together, which eliminates any movement between the bones at all.

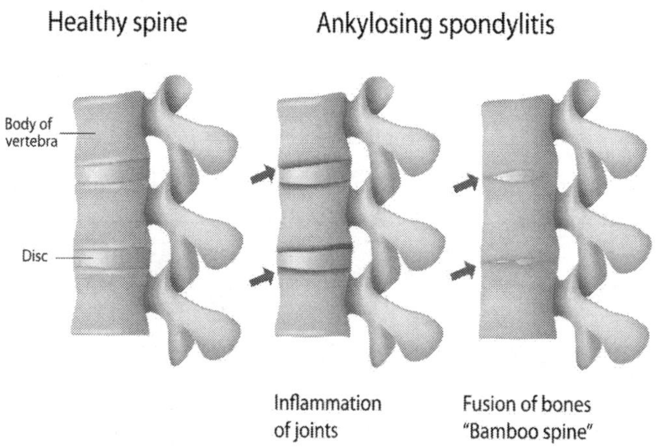

A person with ankylosing spondylitis may appear to be hunched forward, and may present with kyphosis as a result. Another name for ankylosing spondylitis is "**Bamboo Spine**" because after fusion, the **vertebrae resembles a bamboo stalk.**

Causes

Ankylosing spondylitis is caused by the body's immune system attacking the intervertebral discs for unknown reasons.

Symptoms

Pain is an extremely common symptom of ankylosing spondylitis, especially in the neck, base of the skull, and lumbar region. Lack of mobility is a secondary symptom, usually the result of pain.

Treatments

Non-steroidal anti-inflammatory medications may be prescribed to help reduce pain and inflammation in affected areas. Physical therapy, massage therapy, stretching, and range-of-motion exercises are all helpful in maintaining mobility in the vertebral joints and preventing bones from fusing together.

If the condition is severe, surgery may be performed to remove fused bone, or to insert metal rods to correct posture.

Bunion

A bunion is a **subluxation of the big toe**, the result of the toe pushing back against the first metatarsal. Excessive force against this bone causes the **big toe to turn laterally**, with the **first metatarsal turning medially**, creating a **large bump**.

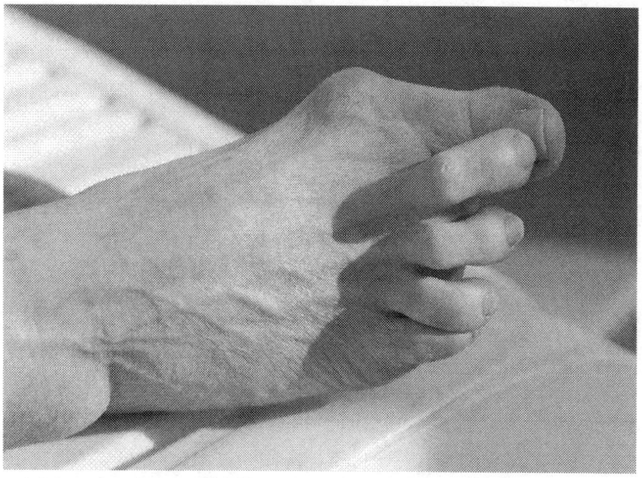

Subluxation forcing the big to laterally, creating a large bump

Causes

Tight fitting shoes may contribute to the development of bunions. Rheumatoid arthritis may also contribute. Foot injuries may also play a role.

Symptoms

Pain and swelling may present in the area of the bunion. With bunions, the big toe may cross under the second toe. This may cause calluses or corns to form on the area where these toes rub together. Movement in the big toe may reduce.

Treatments

How severe the bunion is determines the treatment. Less severe bunions may require only changing shoes or applying a splint to help reset the toe. More severe forms of a bunion may require surgery to correct the placement of the toe.

Bursitis

(burs-: bursa; -itis: inflammation)

Bursitis is a condition that results in **inflammation of a bursa**, a small sac filled with synovial fluid.

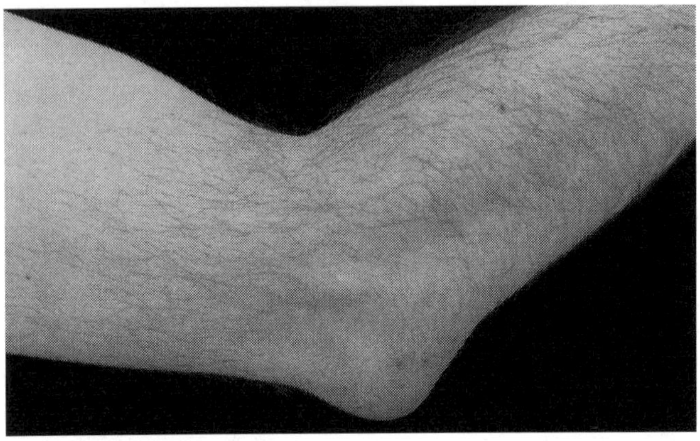

Causes

Bursae are located all over the body, typically between a tendon and bone to prevent friction and irritation. When there is **repeated stress** placed on the bursa, it can become inflamed. Bursitis may affect many different joints, including the knee, shoulder, elbow, hip, and ankle.

Bursitis is most often caused by repetitive motions in the affected joint, which may irritate the bursa. **Trauma** may also result in bursitis, such as fractures or tendonitis.

Symptoms

Typically, a joint affected with bursitis will be inflamed and painful to move. The inflammation may be moderate or severe.

Treatments

Bursitis is easily treatable, primarily with rest and ice. Depending on the severity, the bursa may also need to be surgically drained or removed, or injected with corticosteroids to reduce the inflammation.

Dislocation

A dislocation is when a **bone at an articulation becomes displaced** from its normal location. A dislocation, in the acute stage, results in immobilization of the joint and temporary deformation. It may also be painful and result in inflammation around the joint.

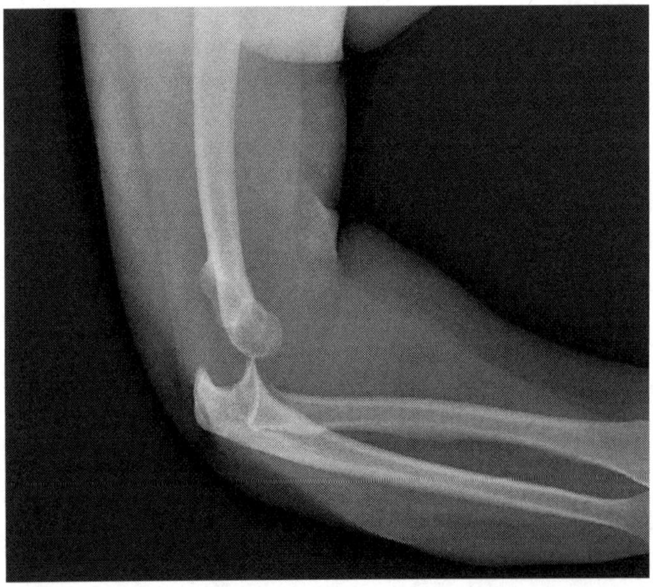

Dislocation at the elbow joint

Causes

Dislocations are most commonly the result of trauma to the joint, which pushes a bone out of place. The most common areas for dislocations are the fingers and shoulder, but dislocations may occur in many other joints as well, such as the knee or hip.

Dislocations may result in tearing of tendons, ligaments, muscles, or in the case of the shoulder or hip, the labrum(-circular cartilage surrounding the joint). The dislocated joint, while most commonly returns to normal strength and function after being relocated, may become prone to dislocations in the future. This may cause arthritis to develop.

Symptoms

Dislocations are extremely painful, and often present with deformity of the joint and an inability to move the joint. Inflammation may be present in some cases.

Treatments

Treatment of a dislocation in the acute stage primarily involves trying to get the bone back to its normal position, known as reduction. After the joint has returned to its normal position, it is typically immobilized for a number of weeks to reduce recurrence of dislocation and to help the tissues around the joint to heal. If the dislocation is severe and unable to be returned to position, surgery may be required.

Fracture

A fracture is a **break in a bone**. There are several different types of fractures, including transverse, greenstick, oblique, and spiral.

Causes

Fractures are the result of trauma to a bone. Despite many different types of fractures, every fracture is categorized as one of the following: Simple or Compound. A **simple fracture** is a fracture that **does not break through the skin**, and does not generally damage any surrounding tissue. A **compound fracture**, which is much more severe, **breaks through the skin and damages surrounding tissues**. Compound fractures are much more prone to infection due to exposure to the outside environment.

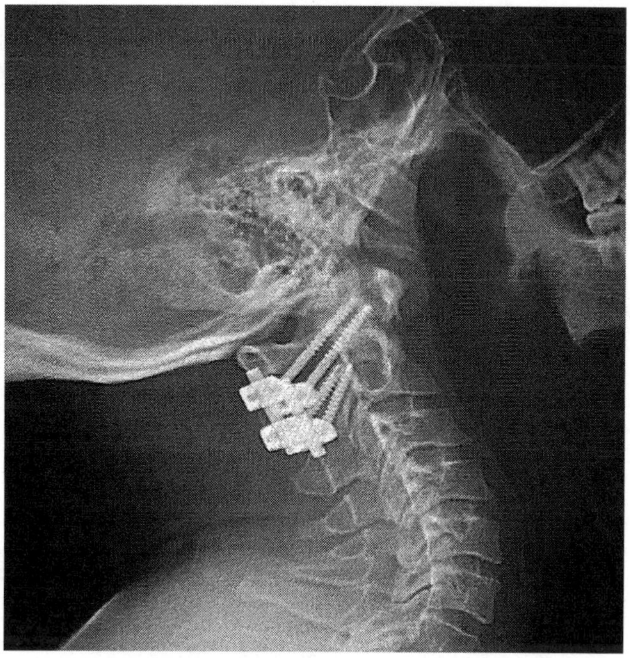

Spinal fusion surgery to repair fracture at C1-C2

Symptoms

Fractures result in deformity of the affected bone, pain, immobilization of the area, and inflammation. In the case of compound fractures, external bleeding may also occur.

Despite most fractures being the result of blunt trauma, certain diseases that weaken the bones may also cause fractures, such as osteoporosis.

Treatments

Fractures should be treated immediately. A cast or splint may be applied, depending on which bone is fractured. Other fractures, such as vertebrae fractures, may need more extensive treatment, including metal plates or bone grafts.

Gout

Gout is a form of arthritis, mostly seen around the **base of the big toe**, but may also affect other joints in the body, such as the hands and fingers.

Causes

Gout is the result of an **over-abundance of uric acid crystals** in the body. Gravity pulls the uric acid crystals down the body, where they collect in the most distal points in the limbs, the big toes, hands and fingers. Gout is typically the result of the kidneys not excreting enough uric acid, or the body producing too much uric acid.

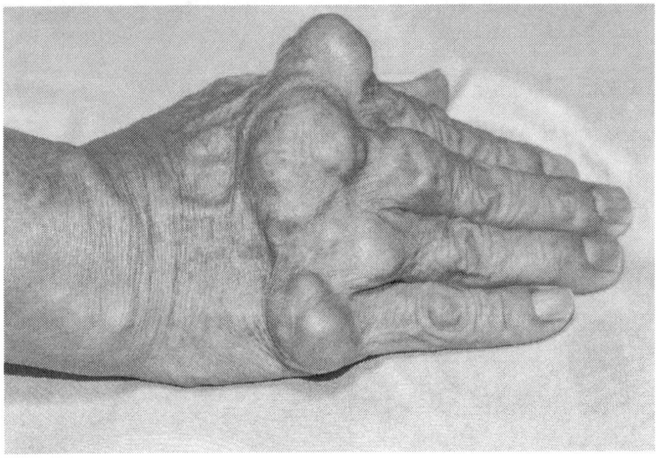

Symptoms

Gout may be extremely painful in the acute stage as the crystals collect in the joints. Inflammation may set in, which can increase the pressure and pain in the joint. Loss of range-of-motion may also occur. Untreated, gout may result in kidney stones.

Treatments

Treatments for gout include non-steroidal anti-inflammatory drugs and/or corticosteroids to reduce pain and inflammation. Gout may also require the use of certain medications that prevent the creation of uric acid in the body.

Herniated Disc

A herniated disc is a condition affecting the vertebral column, which may cause intense pain and numbness.

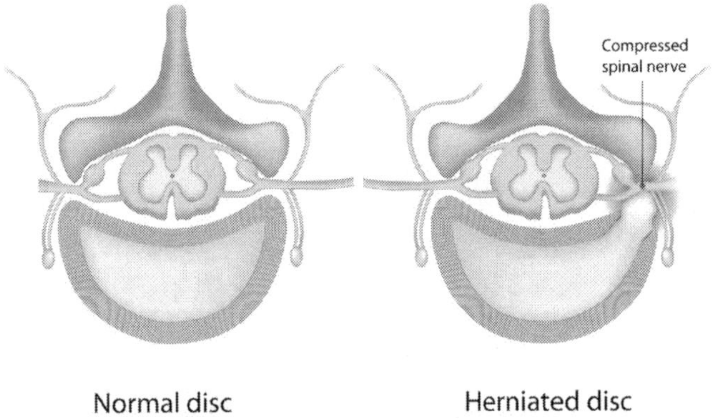

Causes

An intervertebral disc, located between two vertebrae, is made of two parts: the nucleus pulposus, and the annulus fibrosus. The nucleus pulposus is a gelatinous substance located in the center of the disc. The annulus fibrosus is the part of the disc made of thick cartilage. If a **tear occurs in the annulus fibrosus**, the **nucleus pulposus may protrude through the torn section**, which may place pressure on spinal nerves emerging from the spinal cord. This is a herniated disc.

A herniated disc is primarily caused by degeneration of a disc, which takes place gradually. This makes injury of the disc much easier in actions such as lifting and twisting. Other times, trauma may cause a herniated disc, such as in car accidents.

Symptoms

Herniated discs may result in pain and/or numbness due to the disc placing pressure on the spinal nerves. Because numbness may occur, weakness in the muscles innervated by the nerves may also set in due to impaired function.

Treatments

Treatment for a herniated disc varies depending on the severity. Pain medication may help control pain. Muscle relaxers may help take pressure off the area of the herniation. Physical therapy may also contribute to lessening the effects of the herniated disc. Very rarely, surgery may be required.

Kyphosis

(kyph-: hill; -osis: condition)

Kyphosis is a condition affecting the **thoracic vertebrae**, resulting in **hyper-curvature**. Another name for kyphosis is "**Dowager's Hump**".

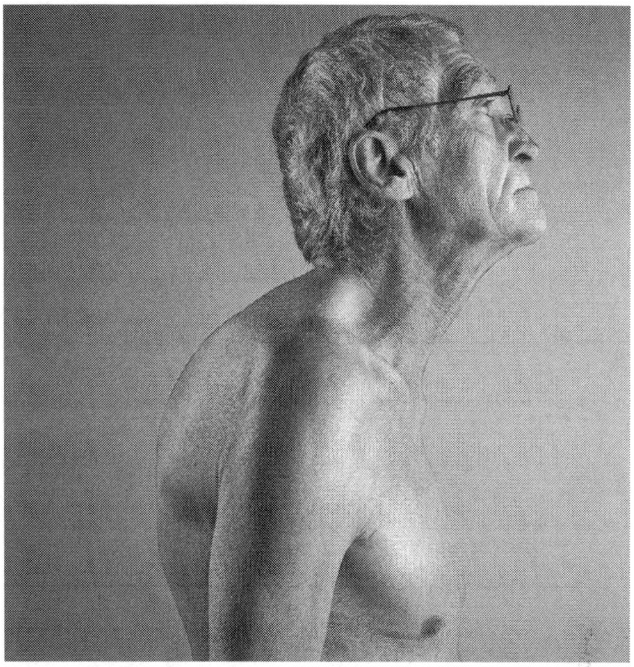

Causes

A kyphotic curvature in the vertebrae is a curvature that moves posteriorly. If the curvature is exaggerated, it is known as kyphosis. Kyphosis has many different causes. Kyphosis may be caused by extremely tight muscles(such as **pectoralis minor and serratus anterior**) pulling the scapulae anteriorly, which rounds the back. It may also be the result of bone degeneration(osteoporosis), disc degeneration(ankylosing spondylitis), or even birth defects.

Symptoms

Kyphosis may cause pain in the back, and difficulty in movement and breathing as a result. It may also result in the lumbar vertebrae losing its curvature, a condition known as **flat back**.

Treatments

Kyphosis may vary from mild to severe, depending on the cause. Treatments include exercises that strengthen the muscles of the back, stretching of tight muscles that may contribute to kyphosis, braces to keep the vertebrae properly aligned, and possibly even surgery if it's warranted.

Lordosis

(lord-: curve; -osis: condition)

Lordosis is a condition affecting the **lumbar vertebrae**, resulting in **hyper-curvature**. Another name for lordosis is "**Swayback**".

Causes

A lordotic curvature in the vertebrae is a curvature that moves anteriorly. If the curvature is exaggerated, it is known as lordosis. Lordosis has many different causes. Lordosis may be caused by tight muscles(such as **psoas major**, **iliacus**, **quadratus lumborum**, and rectus femoris), weak muscles(such as **rectus abdominis and the hamstrings**), obesity, or bone diseases (such as osteoporosis). Pregnancy is also a common cause of lordosis, but the condition typically subsides post-pregnancy.

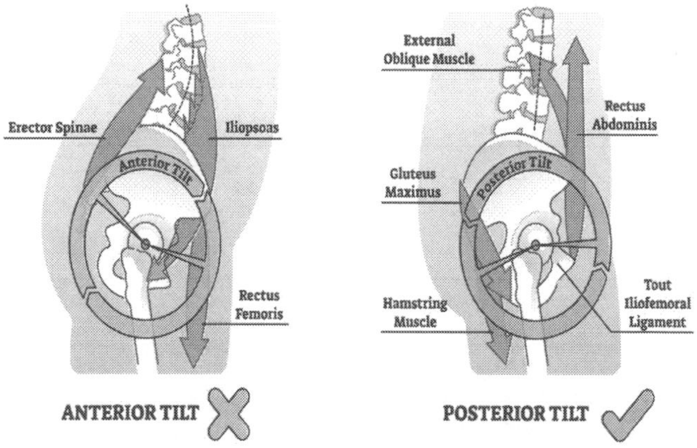

Symptoms

Lordosis may place excessive pressure on the vertebrae, and alter a person's stance and gait. Lordosis may result in pain in the back, and cause difficulty moving.

Treatments

Treatment primarily includes strengthening weak muscles, stretching tight muscles, and lifestyle changes such as adjusting posture, diet, and exercise.

Lyme Disease

Lyme Disease is a **bacterial infection spread by deer ticks**, and contracting the infection is much more common in grassy or wooded areas where deer ticks are found. The condition may affect a person for months, and lead to symptoms that may last for years afterwards.

Causes

The bacteria responsible for Lyme Disease is spread through a bite from deer ticks. The bacteria is usually only transmitted if the bite lasts longer than **36 hours.**

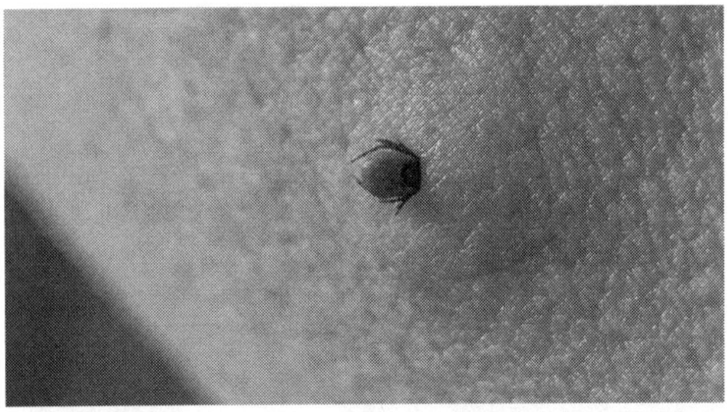

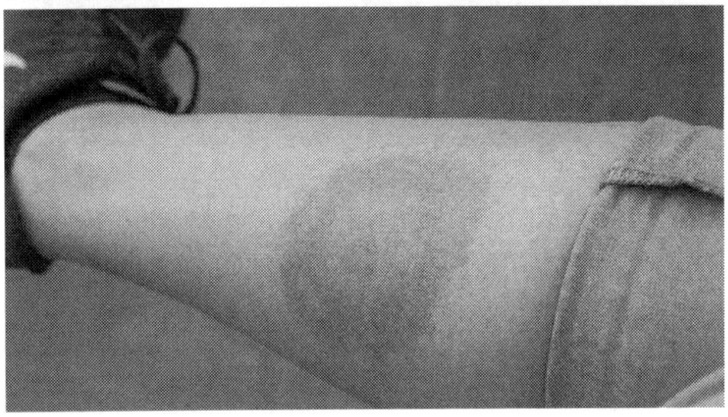

Symptoms

Symptoms of Lyme Disease vary depending on the stage of infection. In the early stages, a bump may appear where the person has been bitten. Sometime later, within 30 days, a rash may appear that forms a bullseye pattern. It may spread outward from that area over a few days. A person may experience flu-like symptoms when the rash appears. In advanced stages, conditions may begin occurring such as pain and inflammation in joints, meningitis, and paralysis in different parts of the body such as the face.

Treatments

Lyme Disease is a bacterial infection, and therefore is treated with antibiotics. Advanced stages of Lyme Disease, where there may be some sort of paralysis, require the use of intravenous antibiotics. Otherwise, oral antibiotics may be taken. The course of treatment usually lasts up to three weeks to completely destroy all bacteria.

Osgood-Schlatter Disease

Osgood-Schlatter Disease is a repetitive strain injury, caused by **over-use of the patellar tendon**.

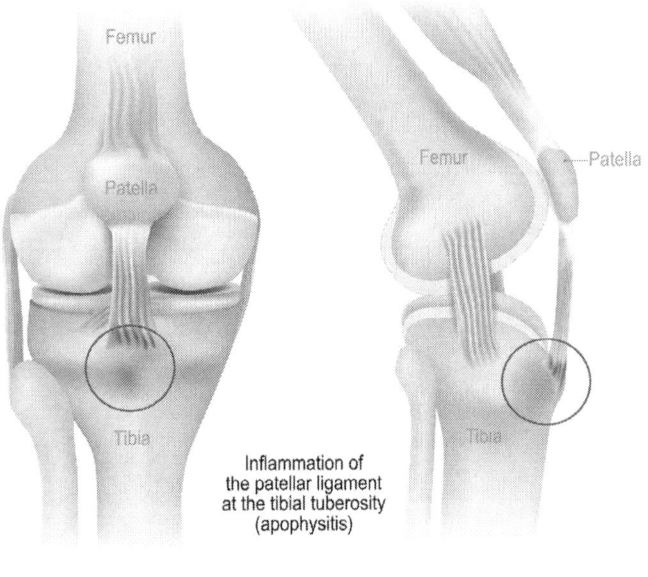

Causes

Osgood-Schlatter Disease primarily affects **adolescents**, particularly those involved in sports. **Over-use of the quadriceps** during activities such as running and jumping can cause tightness in the patellar tendon. When the patellar tendon tightens, it pulls proximally on the tibial tuberosity. Because the bone is still growing, the force of the patellar tendon on the tibial tuberosity can cause an **over-growth of bone**, resulting in a bony lump. Males are more likely to develop this condition than females, but instances in females are increasing as participation in sports by females increases.

Symptoms

Osgood-Schlatter Disease may cause pain, but it varies from person-to-person. The pain may be mild, or it may be more intense in some cases, making movement of the knee difficult.

Despite complications from Osgood-Schlatter Disease being rare, inflammation of the area may persist over time. The bony lump produced by increased bone production may also remain.

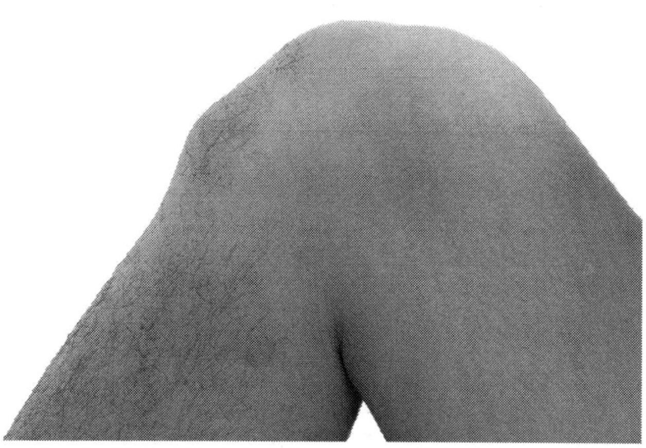

Treatments

Treatment is mild, usually nothing more than pain relievers, rest, and ice. Exercises that stretch the quadriceps are recommended.

Osteoarthritis

(osteo-: bone; arthr-: joint; -itis: inflammation)

Osteoarthritis is the most common form of arthritis, which is **inflammation of a joint**.

Causes

Osteoarthritis, also known as "**wear-and-tear arthritis**", is caused by damage to the **hyaline cartilage** separating one bone from another. The cartilage between bones reduces friction between the bones, and absorbs shock in the joint. Over time, the articular cartilage may begin to break down and wear away. This causes irritation in the joint and increases friction between the bones, which causes inflammation. As this persists, damage to the bone may take place. The most common location of osteoarthritis is the knee.

Symptoms

Osteoarthritis may cause pain, difficulty moving the affected joint, and bone spurs in the joint due to increased friction between the bones. When the condition advances to the point of the joint being mostly unusable, joint replacement surgery may be recommended.

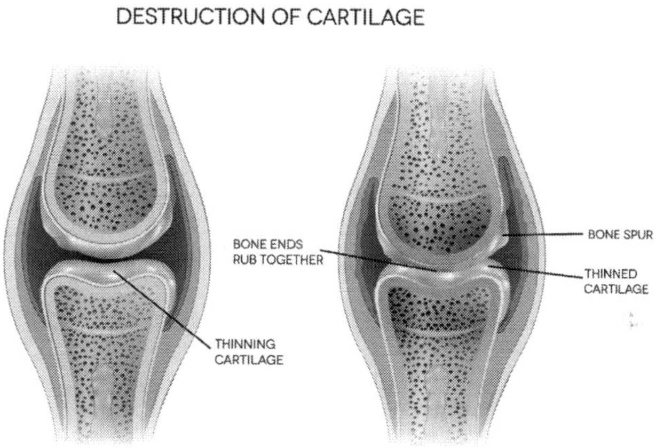

Treatments

Treatment includes non-steroidal anti-inflammatory drugs, lifestyle and dietary changes if caused by obesity, and alternative methods such as yoga.

Osteoporosis

(osteo-: bone; por-: porous; -osis: condition)

Osteoporosis is a condition that causes **weakness and degeneration in the bones**.

Causes

Osteoporosis mainly affects **post-menopausal women**. After menopause, a woman's body produces **less estrogen**. During growth stages of a person's life, estrogen helps the bones grow and mature. When estrogen levels drop post-menopause, osteoclast levels increase and more bone is destroyed than is created. When this occurs, the bones become brittle, weak, and prone to fracture.

In addition to making bones brittle, osteoporosis may also contribute to the development of kyphosis and back pain. One of the most common places for fracture to occur is in the neck of the femur. The femur, which is normally the strongest bone in the body, should be able to support roughly 2,000 pounds of pressure per square inch. When the femur becomes weakened,it makes it incredibly easy to break. If a fracture takes place around the hip joint, joint replacement surgery is often required.

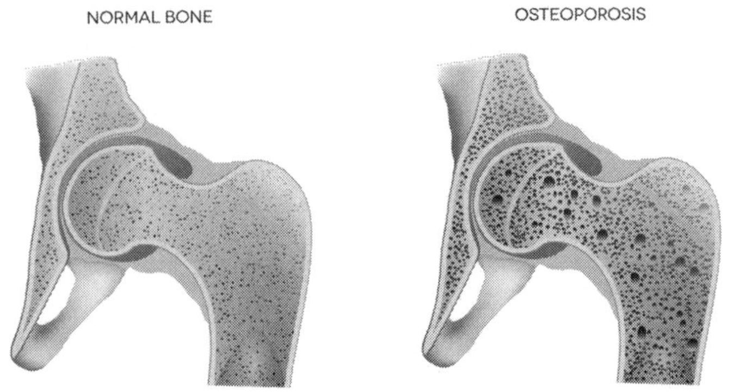

Symptoms

In the early stages of osteoporosis, there are usually no symptoms. As bone loss increases over time, a person may experience back pain, hunched posture(kyphosis), and bones that fracture easier than usual. These symptoms often become worse as the disease progresses and more bone tissue is lost.

Treatments

Treatments for osteoporosis include estrogen replacement therapy, and weight-bearing exercise earlier in life before any symptoms of osteoporosis surface. Weight-bearing exercise, such as squats and dead-lifts, helps to strengthen the bones, which substantially reduces the risk of developing osteoporosis in older age.

Rheumatoid Arthritis

Rheumatoid Arthritis is an **autoimmune disorder**, resulting in **inflammation**, **pain**, and **deformity of the joints around the hands and wrists**.

Causes

Around synovial joints, there is a membrane called the synovial membrane, which supplies joints with synovial fluid. In rheumatoid arthritis, the body's immune systems attacks the **synovial membranes**, destroying them. This is especially common in the metacarpophalangeal joints. After the synovial membranes have been destroyed, extremely thick, fibrous material replaces them, which not only makes movement painful and difficult, but can also cause deformity, turning the fingers into an adducted position.

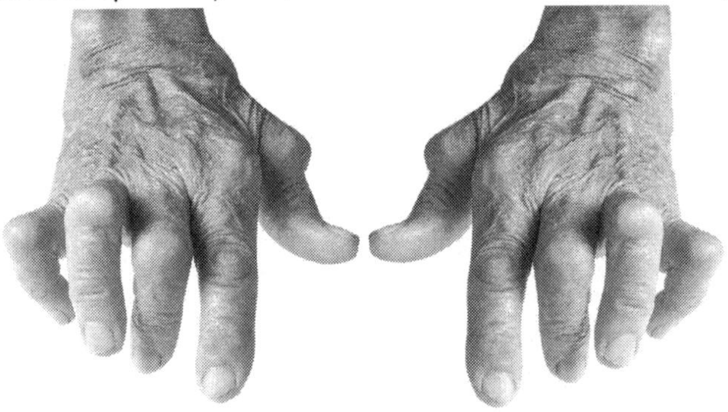

Symptoms

Rheumatoid arthritis can produce pain and discomfort in the affected joints, as well as cause pain and stiffness after long periods of inactivity in the joints. Fever and fatigue may also be symptoms of general rheumatoid arthritis. Less commonly, some people may experience symptoms in structures completely unrelated to the affected joints, such as the eyes, heart, lungs, and kidneys.

Treatments

There is no cure for rheumatoid arthritis, but treatments include non-steroidal anti-inflammatory drugs, corticosteroids, and physical therapy.

Scoliosis

(scoli-: crooked; -osis: condition)

Scoliosis is a condition causing the vertebral column, usually in the thoracic region, to be pulled into a **lateral position**.

Causes

The causes of scoliosis are unknown, but there may be a hereditary link. Scoliosis typically develops around the beginning stages of puberty. Scoliosis is mostly mild in severity, but can become much more prominent, which can put incredible strain on the ribs, vertebrae, and hips. With scoliosis, one hip may be higher than the other, which causes a discrepancy in gait. Tight muscles may also contribute to the development of scoliosis, as seen in cases such as a hypertonic rhomboid major and minor unilaterally, which pulls the vertebrae to one side.

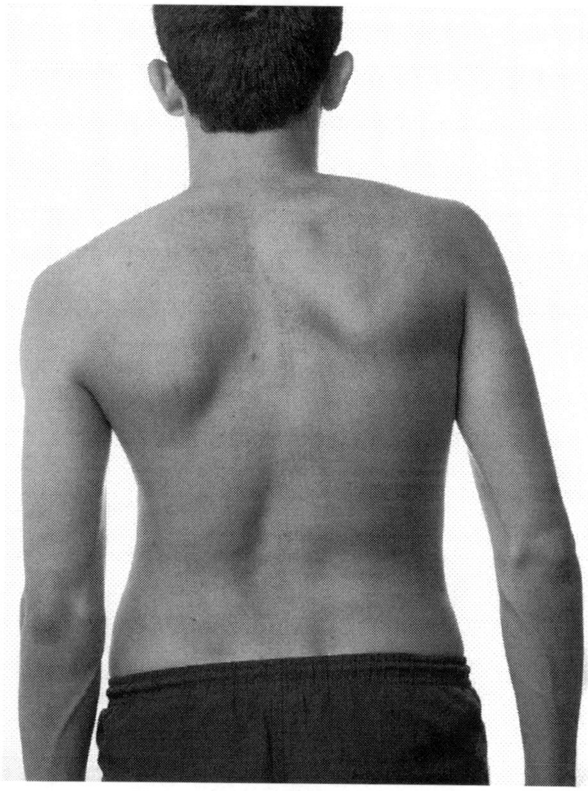

Symptoms

If scoliosis is severe, damage to the heart or lungs may occur, due to the deformity of the rib cage. Back pain may also persist.

Treatments

Treatment, while commonly unnecessary, may include the use of braces to correct posture, the use of chiropractic therapy, massage therapy, or in severe cases, surgery with metal rod implantation.

Sprain

A sprain is an **injury to a ligament.**

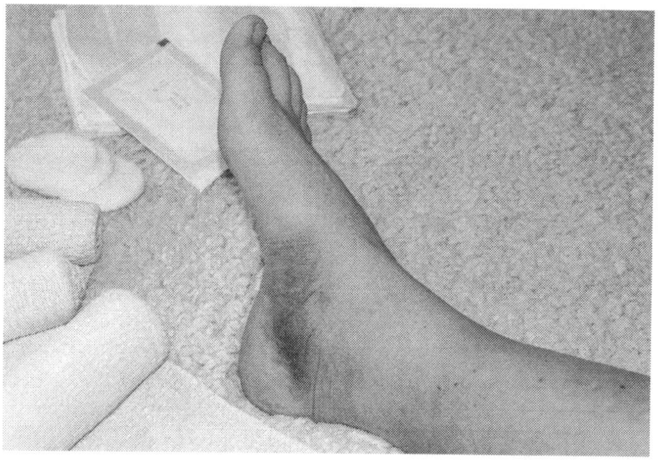

Causes

Sprains are much less likely to be caused by repetitive motions, unlike strains. Sprains typically occur quickly, causing tears in a ligament. Like strains, sprains may be broken down in severity by using grades: grade 1, grade 2, and grade 3.

A **grade 1 sprain** is caused by **stretching of a ligament**, but does not cause major tearing. Common grade 1 sprains may be caused by activities such as running. After 24-48 hours, the ligament should return to normal, and any pain and/or inflammation should subside.

A **grade 2 sprain**, such as a high ankle sprain, causes **tearing of a ligament** and presents with **bruising and inflammation.** Grade 2 sprains may require surgery to repair, or they may heal on their own, depending on the severity of the tear.

A **grade 3 sprain** is a **complete rupture of a ligament**, and much like a grade 3 strain, **does require surgery to repair.** The most common form of grade 3 sprain is a torn anterior cruciate ligament(ACL, the ligament holding the femur and tibia together), most commonly caused by sports or automobile accidents.

Symptoms

Symptoms of sprains are very similar to symptoms of strains, including inflammation, pain, and potential bruising depending on the grade of sprain. If the sprain is severe, a pop in the joint may be heard or felt at the time of injury.

Treatments

Sprains take much longer to heal than strains, due to ligaments being avascular, compared to muscles and tendons, which have a rich blood supply. Treatment for sprains vary depending on the severity of the sprain. The less severe, the more likely it is that rest, ice, and elevation will suffice. Surgery is only required when there is no chance of the ligament repairing itself.

Temporomandibular Joint Dysfunction

Temporomandibular Joint Dysfunction(TMJD) is a condition affecting the mandible, causing simple tasks such as **chewing to become painful and difficult**.

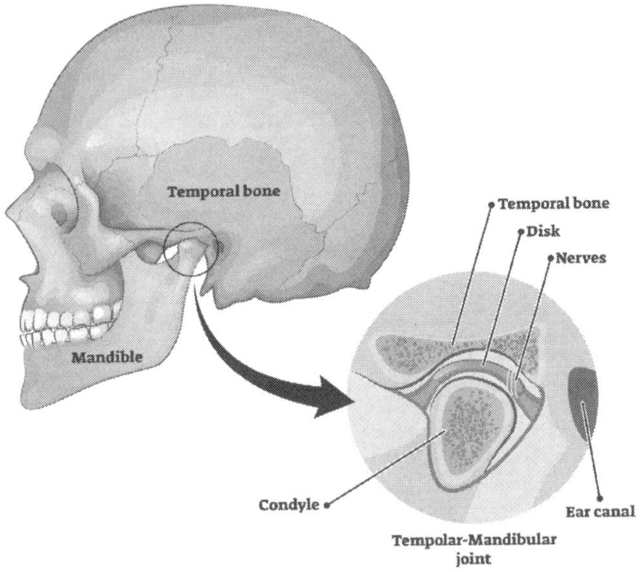

Causes

The temporomandibular joint is the joint that connects the mandible to the temporal bone. Between the bones, there is a small disc of cartilage, used to prevent friction between the bones and to make movement smooth. If there is arthritis in the joint, or the disc is damaged, it can result in temporomandibular joint dysfunction. This can cause pain, difficulty in moving the jaw, and produce a clicking sensation when the jaw opens. Often times, the muscles that connect to the mandible(temporalis, lateral pterygoid) may tighten and pull the mandible out of place.

Symptoms

Temporomandibular joint dysfunction can produce pain in the face, a clicking or popping sound when closing the mouth, and difficulty in opening the mouth. The jaw may become locked while open.

Treatments

Treatments vary depending on the primary cause, ranging from prescription muscle relaxants and pain relievers, to physical and massage therapy.

Whiplash

Whiplash is an **injury to the neck**, resulting from a **quick, forceful movement of the head forward and back**. This results in the **tendons and ligaments in the neck to become stretched further than normal**, damaging the tissue and reducing neck stability.

Causes

The most common cause of whiplash is a car accident. Injuries during sport or physical abuse may also cause whiplash. Shaking a baby may result in whiplash, and is one of the reasons shaking a baby should never happen.

Symptoms

The neck can become stiff and painful, especially upon movement. Headaches may occur. Pain may radiate to the shoulders, and range-of-motion may be restricted. Numbness may be experienced in the upper limbs due to possible injury to nerves emerging from the brachial plexus.

Treatments

Rest and ice are effective treatments for whiplash. The use of pain relievers can help eliminate pain associated with the condition. Inflammation in the area may be present, and contrast therapy on the neck may be performed to assist with reduction of inflammation. Physical therapy may also be performed to help strengthen the tendons and ligaments affected.

Urinary Pathologies

Cystitis

(cyst-: bladder; -itis: inflammation)

Cystitis is a **bacterial infection** resulting in **inflammation of the bladder**. It can often involve the entire Urinary System, and is then known as a Urinary Tract Infection(UTI). Cystitis is most common in women, as the female urethra is shorter than the male urethra, giving bacteria a shorter passage to the bladder.

Causes

Cystitis is caused most commonly by E. Coli entering the urethra, then reproducing. The increased amount of bacterium in the urethra causes the infection to spread upwards into the bladder. Cystitis can cause numerous symptoms, including blood in the urine, burning sensations while urinating, and a frequent urge to urinate. If untreated, the infection may spread to the kidneys. When this happens, it is known as pyelonephritis.

Symptoms

Symptoms of cystitis include a frequent urge to urinate, a painful burning sensation upon urination, urinating small amounts at a time, fever, and blood in the urine.

Treatments

Because cystitis is a bacterial infection, it is treated with antibiotics.

Kidney Stones

Kidney Stones, also known as Nephroliathiasis, are **deposits of salts and minerals** created inside the kidney, which are hard and rough. Stones vary in size, and may cause many differing health complications.

Kidney stones are more common in people who are obese or have a family history of kidney stone development. Diet may play a role as well.

Causes

Kidney stones may be caused by numerous factors. Most commonly, they are caused by increased amounts of calcium oxalate, which is found in many types of food. Excessive amounts of calcium oxalate can cause stones to develop. Uric acid may also produce stones if a person does not drink enough fluids. A high protein diet may contribute to the development of uric acid stones.

Less commonly, struvite stones may form, which are the result of bacterial infections of the urinary tract.

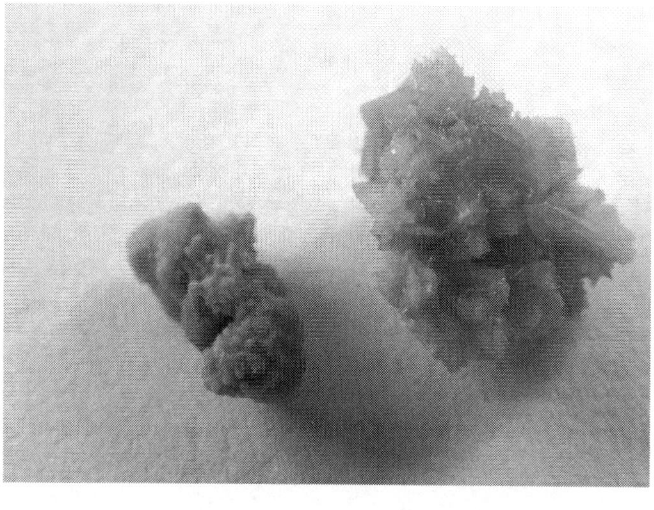

Symptoms

Kidney stones are largely asymptomatic until they leave the kidney and enter the ureter. When this occurs, pain may be felt around the abdomen, groin, back, and sides. Painful urination may take place as the stone blocks the ureter. The urine may have a pink or brown appearance due to blood in the urine. An inadequate amount of urine may be produced due to blockages.

Treatments

Many treatment options are available. In less severe cases, increasing water intake can help flush the kidneys of the increased calcium and help move the stones out of the body.

To aid in moving the stone out of the body, a doctor may prescribe medications that help to relax the smooth muscle in the ureter, known as alpha blockers.

In more severe cases, stones may be destroyed while still inside the body using a treatment known as **extracorporeal shock wave lithotripsy**. The stones are broken down using sound waves, and then are able to be passed out of the body easier. If the stones are too big to be destroyed using sound waves, they may be removed surgically.

Pyelonephritis

(pyel/o: renal pelvis; nephr/o: kidney; -itis: inflammation)

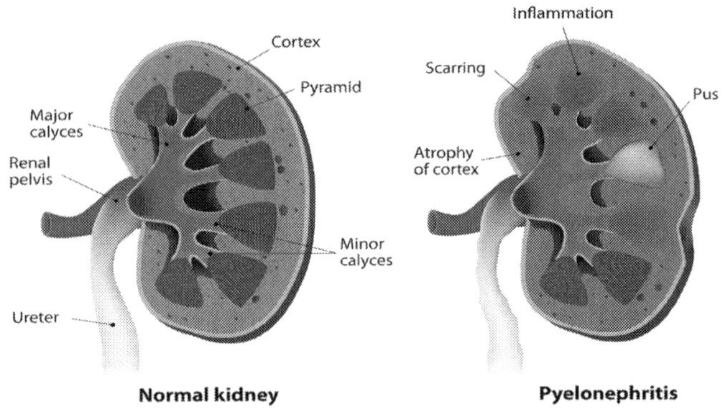

Pyelonephritis is a **bacterial infection of the kidney**, usually beginning in the urethra or bladder. The infection spreads upwards through the ureters and **into the kidneys**. Pyelonephritis is considered a serious condition, and if suspected, should be seen by a doctor immediately for treatment.

Causes

Bacteria enters the urethra. Usually, urinating cleans out the urethra. Rarely, it does not, and bacteria can reproduce in the urethra. The bacteria then can spread upwards into the bladder, then move further up into the ureters and kidneys. Women are more likely than men to develop urinary tract infections due to a shorter urethra.

Symptoms

Symptoms of an acute infection in the kidneys include pain in the back, groin, or abdomen, nausea, vomiting, fever, blood in the urine, burning during urination, and an urge to constantly urinate. Cloudy urine may also be a sign of an infection, especially if there is a foul odor.

Treatments

Antibiotics are used to combat pyelonephritis. They are typically administered orally, but in more severe cases that require hospitalization, they may be administered via IV. Pain relievers may be used to aid with associated pain.

Renal Failure

Renal failure is **kidney failure**, where the kidneys stop functioning properly. This can lead to the body being **unable to eliminate waste**, **electrolytes**, and **excessive fluid**. This can lead to dangerous, even fatal levels of these substances in the body.

Causes

Renal failure is commonly the result of another condition damaging the kidney enough to impair function. Examples are hypertension, glomerulonephritis, pyelonephritis, diabetes, and polycystic kidney disease.

Symptoms

Usually, renal failure occurs gradually, and symptoms become more known as the kidney begins to lose function. Fatigue, nausea, vomiting, hypertension, increased fluid accumulation in the lower limbs, and loss of appetite are common symptoms.

Treatments

As the kidneys begin failing, treatment usually revolves around treating the symptoms to try and slow the disease. Once thekidneys have experienced too much damage and the body is unable to eliminate waste and fluid effectively, dialysis may be performed to remove these substances, either through the blood or through the peritoneum.

Kidney transplants may be performed. Instead of removing the damaged kidneys, a doctor will leave the damaged kidneys in the body and attach another kidney. Despite not functioning optimally, the damaged kidneys can still assist the new kidney in filtering waste and fluid, even though it may only be a small amount.

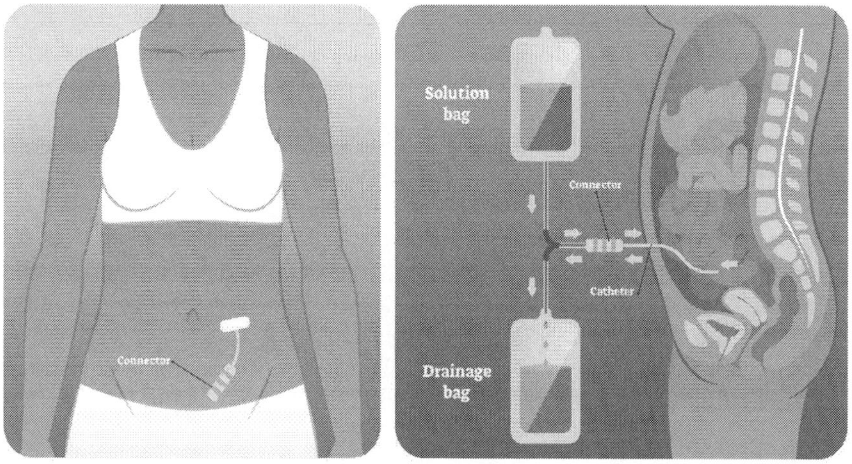

Peritoneal dialysis

Urethritis

(urethr/o: urethra; -itis: inflammation)

Urethritis is **inflammation of the urethra**, usually caused by a **bacterial infection**. It is extremely treatable.

Causes

Urethritis is caused by a bacterial infection. Bacteria enters the urethra and reproduces, resulting in an infection. The infection may spread up the urinary tract, and may lead to cystitis or pyelonephritis if left untreated.

Less commonly, urethritis may be caused by herpes simplex.

Symptoms

Pain upon urination is the primary symptom of urethritis. A less common symptom is inability to effectively urinate, known as dysuria. Discharge from the vagina may present, and the urine may contain blood.

Treatments

Because urethritis is most commonly caused by bacterial infection, antibiotics are prescribed to destroy the bacteria and prevent the infection from moving further into the Urinary System.

Cancer

When the body produces an **abnormal amount of a specific tissue**, it develops what is known as a **tumor**. Tumors are also known as neoplasms. Tumors may be either benign or malignant. **Benign tumors** are considered noncancerous, and do not spread to other areas of the body. **Malignant tumors** are considered **cancerous**, and will **spread to other areas of the body**. The most common type of cancer is skin cancer.

Benign tumors typically **grow slowly.** These tumors do not invade other tissues or structures in the body. Benign tumors may cause harm, however, by placing pressure on regions of the body that contain major blood vessels, lymph vessels, or nerves. Benign tumors are often removed before they get to this point if there is a risk of damaging other structures. Other benign tumors may be left alone if they do not cause problems.

Malignant tumors spread through the body and affect other tissues and structures through a process known as metastasis. Cancerous cells spread through the body by entering into the **blood stream and lymph vessels**, allowing the cells to easily transport to another region. Once these cells settle in another region or structure, they continue to reproduce at a rapid, uncontrolled rate. The **original site** of the tumor is known as the **primary tumor**, while the tumor that has **developed elsewhere** is known as a **secondary tumor**. Some cancers, such as leukemia, do not result in any tumor growing. Malignant cancers commonly spread through the Lymphatic System and can result in tumors in major lymph nodes. This is especially common in areas like the breasts and neck.

There are three main classifications for cancer: carcinoma, sarcoma, and cancers of the blood stream/Lymphatic System. **Carcinoma** is cancer that occurs in the **epithelial tissue**, which can be found in the skin, digestive tract, and respiratory tract. A common form of carcinoma is basal cell carcinoma. **Sarcoma** is cancer that occurs in the body's **connective tissues**, such as bone and cartilage. Examples include bone cancer and Kaposi's Sarcoma. Examples of cancers that involve the blood stream and Lymphatic System include leukemia and Non-Hodgkin's Lymphoma.

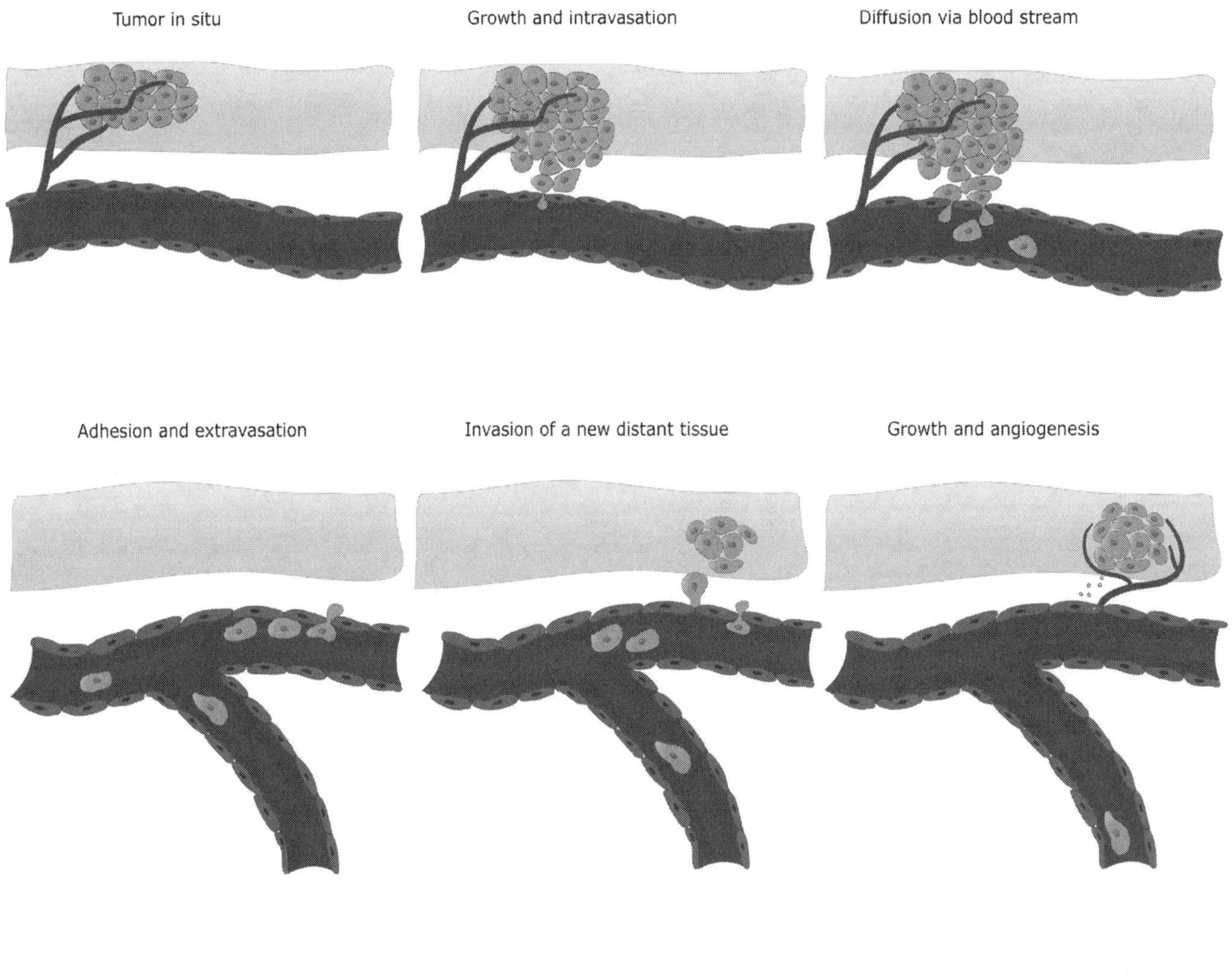

Basal Cell Carcinoma

(carcin-: cancer; -oma: tumor)

Basal Cell Carcinoma is a type of **skin cancer** typically seen around the **face**, **head**, **neck**, and **arms**.

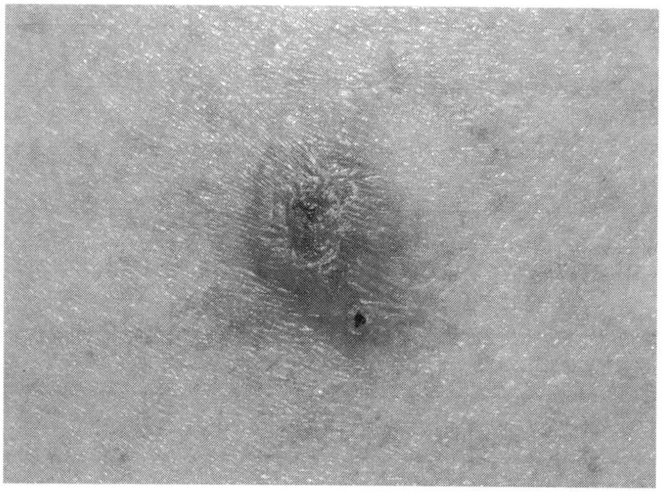

Causes

Basal cell carcinoma is the **most common form of skin cancer**, caused by exposure to **ultraviolet light**. The tumor grows **extremely slowly**, which makes basal cell carcinoma much more treatable than other types of skin cancer. Because it is much more treatable, it is considered the **least serious form of skin cancer**.

Basal cell carcinoma is considered a malignant form of cancer, due to its ability to spread to the tissues immediately surrounding it, but rarely spreads to other organs.

Symptoms

Basal cell carcinoma tumors may appear to have blood vessels in them, and vary in color from black to brown to pink. These growths may bleed easily.

Treatments

Treatment for basal cell carcinoma includes surgical excision of the tumor, freezing the tumor, or in more serious cases, medications that prevent the cancerous cells from spreading to other tissues.

Breast Cancer

Breast cancer is cancer of **breast tissue**, including **lymph nodes and vessels** in the **breast and axillary region**. Breast cancer is the second most common form of cancer diagnosed in women, behind skin cancer. Breast cancer is much more common in women, but it can also occur in men.

Breast cancer can spread throughout the breast and to other regions of the body, and is considered a malignant form of cancer.

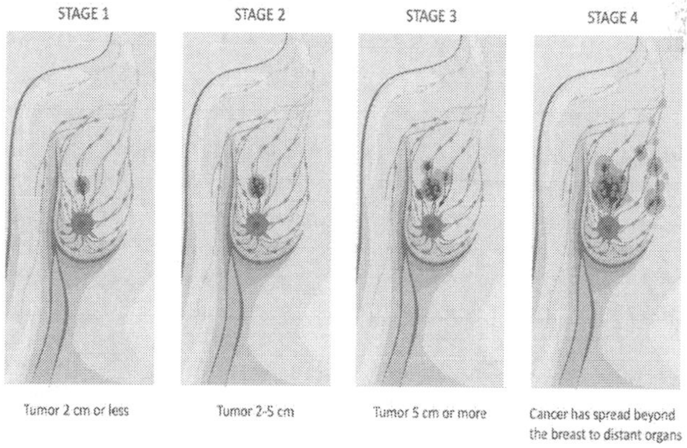

Causes

Breast cancer occurs when breast tissue begins growing abnormally, forming a tumor that feels like a lump under the skin. Breast cancer may be a genetic disorder, or may be the cause of unspecified environmental factors. Women who are older in age tend to develop breast cancer more often than younger women.

Symptoms

Symptoms include a lump in the breast that does not feel the same as tissue surrounding it, a nipple that has recently become inverted, change in size or appearance of the breast, dimpling of the skin of the breast, the skin of the breast and/or areola becoming scaly or flaky, and the skin of the breast becoming red. If any of these symptoms occur, a person should be seen by a medical professional.

Treatments

Treatment is based on the severity of the tumor growth. Surgery to remove the tumor will likely be performed after locating it via mammogram and ultrasound. If a large amount of breast tissue is involved, the breast may be completely removed, known as a mastectomy. Lymph nodes may also be removed to prevent any cancerous tissue from spreading to other parts of the body. Chemotherapy and radiation therapy are performed to kill the remaining cancerous cells.

Hodgkin's Lymphoma

(lymph-: lymph; -oma: tumor)

Hodgkin's Lymphoma is a **malignant cancer** affecting the Lymphatic System, specifically the **lymph nodes in the upper limb, chest, and neck.** Hodgkin's Lymphoma usually follows lymph channels in a predictable manner, moving from one lymph node to the next.

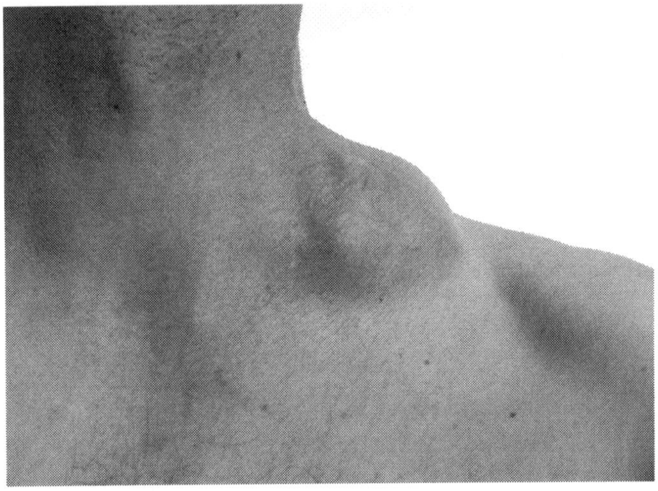

Causes

Hodgkin's Lymphoma is caused by an excessive amount of B-cells being produced. These cells, known as **Reed-Sternberg cells**, are larger than normal and contain multiple nuclei, as opposed to non-cancerous B-cells, which are smaller and only contain one nucleus.

Symptoms

Symptoms of Hodgkin's Lymphoma include swelling of lymph nodes in the neck, upper limb, and axilla that may be painless, weight loss, fever, and fatigue. A person may also experience sensitivity to alcohol.

Treatments

Surgery isn't usually performed for a patient with Hodgkin's Lymphoma. Instead, chemotherapy and radiation therapy are used to destroy the cancerous lymphocytes. Bone marrow transplants may also be performed to stimulate the production of non-cancerous cells.

Leukemia

(leuk/o: white; -emia: blood condition)

Leukemia is a cancer of the **bone and lymph** involving **excessive production of non-functioning leukocytes**. These leukocytes do not function the way normal leukocytes should, leaving the body with a compromised immune system. These cancerous cells may spread to other parts of the body such as the liver and brain.

Causes

There is no known cause for the development of leukemia.

Symptoms

Common symptoms of leukemia include pain in the bone, swollen lymph nodes, fatigue, fever, chills, increased likelihood of developing infections, the appearance of small red spots in the skin, and bruising or bleeding easily. A doctor should be seen if any of these symptoms persist.

Treatments

Treatment for leukemia largely depends on the advancement of the condition. If the cancer has metastasized to other parts of the body, treatment would be performed on those areas in conjunction with treating the leukemia. Chemotherapy and radiation therapy are used to target and destroy cancerous cells through out the body. After chemotherapy and/or radiation therapy, stem cell transplant may be performed to supply the bone with stem cells that grow healthy marrow, which produces functioning leukocytes. Bone marrow itself may also be transplanted into the patient to accomplish the same goal.

Lung Cancer

Lung cancer is the development of **tumors in the lung**. People who **smoke cigarettes** are at a much higher risk to develop lung cancer than anyone else. Lung cancer is the **leading cause of cancerous death** in the United States.

Causes

Lung cancer is primarily caused by exposure to carcinogens being inhaled. Carcinogens that cause lung cancer may be found in cigarette smoke. Other carcinogens may include radon and asbestos. These substances damage the tissue of the lungs, which in turn may begin reproducing unnaturally, causing cancer.

Lung cancer may spread to other areas and organs of the body, including the liver and brain.

Symptoms

Lung cancer is usually asymptomatic in early stages. As the condition progresses, however, symptoms may begin to appear and worsen over time. Symptoms include coughing that may produce blood, shortness of breath, and chest pain. Hoarseness may occur due to excessive coughing.

Treatments

Treatment largely depends on the stage of the cancer. The earlier stages of cancer may only require surgical removal of a small portion of the lung to take out the tumor. Advanced stages involving larger tumors may require an entire lobe of a lung to be removed, or in extreme cases, having the entire lung removed.

After the tumor is removed, radiation and chemotherapy may be performed to destroy any remaining cancerous cells.

Malignant Melanoma

(melan-: black; -oma: tumor)

Malignant Melanoma is a type of **skin cancer** that may affect any part of the skin, and can also affect other tissues such as the eyes and internal organs.

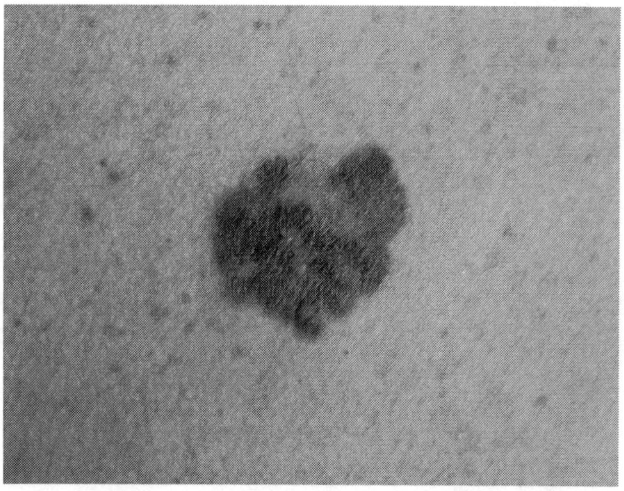

Causes

Malignant melanoma is the **least common** form of skin cancer, but it is the **most serious**. It is caused by exposure to **ultraviolet light**. The cells in the body that produce skin pigment, **melanocytes**, become stimulated by exposure to ultraviolet light and reproduce, causing darker skin. In malignant melanoma, the melanocytes reproduce uncontrolled. This uncontrolled reproduction results in a tumor, and these cancerous cells can easily spread throughout the body and damage other organs and tissues.

Dermatologists use the ABCDE method to diagnose malignant melanoma:

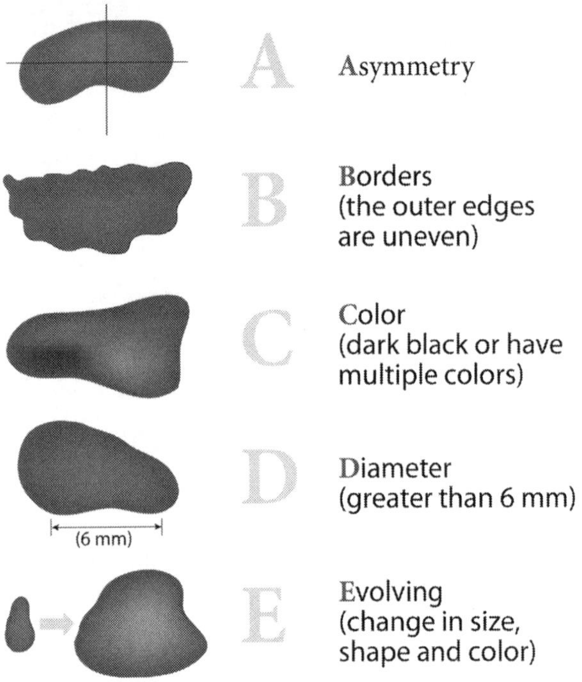

A: Asymmetrical; moles are typically symmetrical, but melanoma tumors have an unusual shape, and the sides don't match.

B: Borders; the borders of the growth change over time and are uneven. This is a sign of significantly increased melanin production.

C: Color; moles are typically some shade of brown. If there are multiple shades or colors, or if the tumor is black, this may be a sign of increased melanin production.

D: Diameter; if a growth is 6mm or greater in diameter(the distance through it), this may be a sign of melanoma.

E: Evolving; moles typically look the same over time. If a mole or growth begins to evolve or change in any way, this may be a sign of melanoma.

Malignant melanoma most commonly begins to appear on a part of the body that doesn't have any prior lesions, like moles. If a new growth appears where there was nothing prior, this may be a sign of melanoma. Less commonly, moles may become cancerous.

Symptoms

Symptoms of melanoma are all included in the ABCDE's.

Treatments

Malignant melanoma, if caught early enough, is easily treatable. Later stages, where it has grown beyond the skin, need more advanced treatments, including surgery to remove any tumors or cancerous lymph nodes, chemotherapy, and radiation therapy.

Non-Hodgkin's Lymphoma

(lymph-: lymph; -oma: tumor)

Non-Hodgkin's Lymphoma is a type of cancer of the Lymphatic System, caused by the development of **tumors by lymphocytes**.

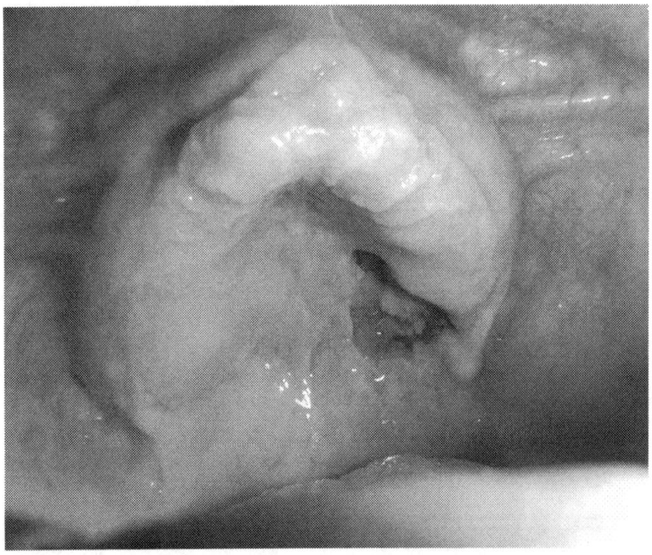
Tumor appearing in the hard and soft palate of the maxilla

Causes

In the body, lymphocytes, like every cell, go through their normal life cycle, and die when they are supposed to. In Non-Hodgkin's Lymphoma, the **lymphocytes don't die**, but **continue reproducing**. This causes an **excessive amount of lymphocytes** to build up in the lymph nodes.

Symptoms

People with Non-Hodgkin's Lymphoma may experience swollen lymph nodes around the neck, groin, and axilla, fatigue, weight loss, and fever.

Treatments

Often times, Non-Hodgkin's Lymphoma isn't serious, and treatment is only required when it becomes advanced. Advanced Non-Hodgkin's Lymphoma is treated with chemotherapy and radiation therapy to destroy the cancerous cells.

Pancreatic Cancer

Pancreatic cancer is cancer that grows in the **pancreas**, which can metastasize rapidly into other tissues and organs, such as the liver.

Causes

The exact cause of pancreatic cancer is unknown. People who are more likely to develop pancreatic cancer include those who **smoke**, are **obese**, have **diabetes**, and have **chronic pancreatitis.**

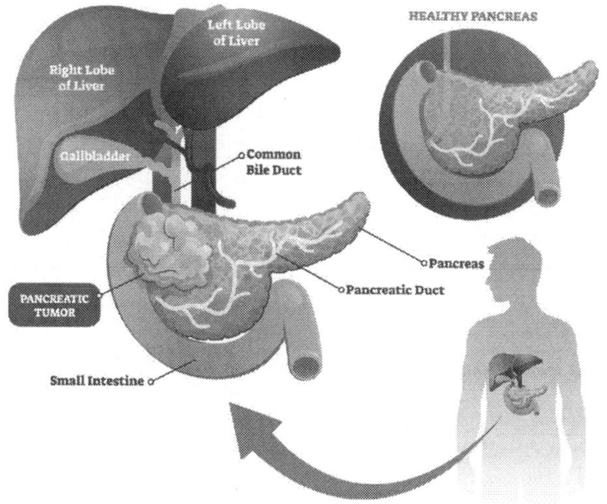

Symptoms

Early stages of pancreatic cancer may be asymptomatic. As the cancer progresses, a person may experience pain in the abdomen, loss of appetite, loss of weight, fatigue, jaundice, and diabetes.

Treatments

Treatment largely depends on the stage of the cancer. Typical treatment focuses on removing the tumor from the pancreas. If the tumor is too large, or has affected too much of the pancreas, the entire pancreas may be removed. The spleen may also be removed, as it may contain cancerous cells. After the tumor has been removed, chemotherapy and radiation therapy may be performed to destroy any remaining cancerous cells.

Squamous Cell Carcinoma

(carcin-: cancer; -oma: tumor)

Squamous Cell Carcinoma is a form of **skin cancer** that in many cases is not serious, but has the ability to spread to other parts of the body. Squamous cell carcinoma is **more serious and less common than basal cell carcinoma**, but **not as serious and more common than malignant melanoma.**

Causes

Squamous cell carcinoma, much like basal cell carcinoma and malignant melanoma, is most often caused by exposure to ultraviolet light. Tumors most commonly develop on areas of the body commonly exposed to sunlight, such as the head, neck, arms, and hands. Tumors may be flat, scaly, and firm, and appear around the mouth, in the mouth, and on the lips.

Symptoms

Squamous cell carcinoma tumors are typically shaped like a dome, and tend to bleed easily. They appear red and scaly, with a rough texture. If the tumor is large, pain may be present around the area.

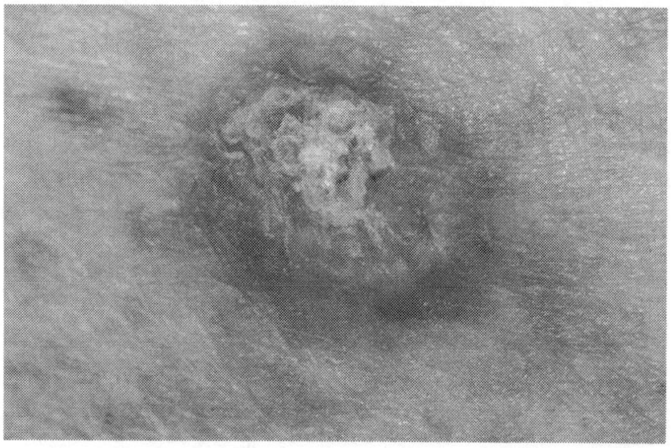

Treatments

Much like basal cell carcinoma, treatment for squamous cell carcinoma is relatively easy, with several different methods, from surgical excision and freezing of the tumor, to radiation therapy for more advanced tumors.

Psychological Pathologies

Addiction

Addiction is the repeated use of a substance or behavior that makes the person feel as if they need to constantly repeat this behavior by providing a rewarding sensation. Examples include alcohol addiction, nicotine addiction, opioid addiction, and gambling addiction. A behavior becomes an addiction when a person is unable to stop themselves from doing the action.

A person with substance or behavioral addiction may carry an increased risk of developing depression or anxiety.

Causes

Family history may contribute to the development of addiction. Anxiety and depression may lead a person into addictive behaviors.

Symptoms

Addiction may lead to many health issues, including poor hygiene, and damage to the body and its organs by substance abuse. If a person stops taking the addictive substance or performing the addictive behavior, they may experience withdrawal symptoms such as seizures, sweating, change in personality and anger, depression, and increased likelihood of violence.

A person who is addicted may distance themselves from others and give up certain things in their life that may cost money in order to keep themselves supplied with their substance of choice. Commonly, an addict will deny that they are addicted, and may experience problems with personal relationships because of the addiction.

Treatments

Addiction is a mental health disorder, and is highly treatable with psychotherapy. Going to self-help and recovery groups may help a person cope with overcoming the addiction.

Anorexia Nervosa

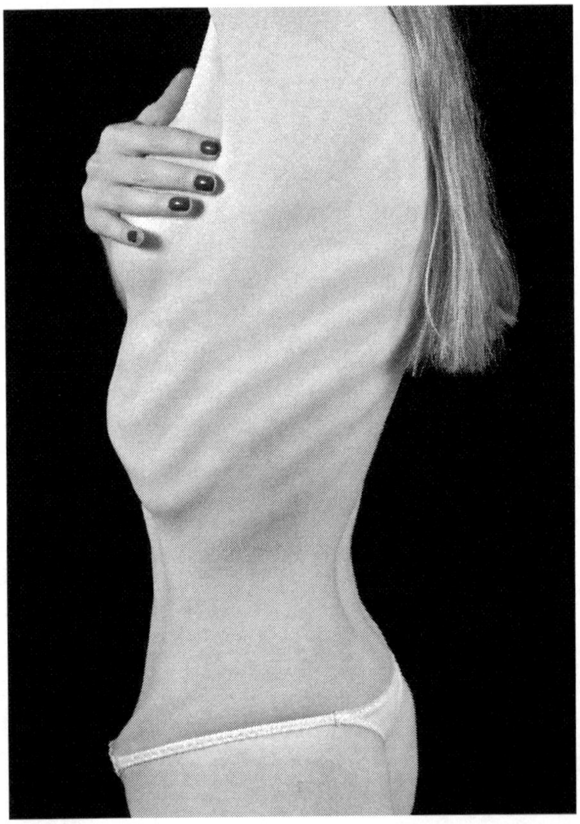

Anorexia nervosa is a condition marked by **severe weight loss** resulting from an **unhealthy restricting of caloric intake**. In conjunction with eating an inadequate amount of food, a person with anorexia may also try losing weight by taking diuretics, laxatives, and vomiting after eating. This can cause a severe lack of nutrition, resulting in the body thinning far beyond a healthy level.

Causes

Anorexia is a psychological disorder in which a person's perception of their weight is distorted. Contributing factors towards the development of anorexia include environmental influences that put an over-emphasis on being thin, and psychological issues such as obsessive compulsive disorder that make it easier to not eat by sticking to set goals.

Symptoms

Symptoms are wide-ranging, from severe thinness and weight loss, to problems with tooth decay from excessive vomiting.

A lack of proper nutrition can lead to fatigue, weakness, thinning hair, and dehydration. A person with anorexia may develop anemia, osteoporosis, abnormalities in hormone production and regulation, issues with kidney function, and muscle atrophy.

Psychologically, a person may withdraw socially, and try to hide their anorexia by wearing clothing to hide their weight loss. A person may become irritable and skip meals. When confronted, a person may deny skipping meals or lie about how much food they have eaten.

Treatments

Treatment for anorexia may include hospitalization in severe cases, where the body is not receiving adequate nutrition over a long period of time. While in the hospital, a person will be given fluids to balance dehydration and electrolyte levels, and be treated for issues possibly relating to the heart, liver, and kidneys. A feeding tube may be inserted to ensure a person is receiving enough nutrients.

Aside from a stay in the hospital, a person may be seen by a mental health professional to deal with underlying causes of anorexia. A person may work closely with a dietician to maintain a healthy diet.

Anxiety Disorders

Anxiety disorders are a group of disorders in where a person experiences an **increased amount of anxiety**, often at a level where the person feels they are in a **life-or-death situation**. These anxious moments can adversely affect a person's daily life and relationships. Different types of anxiety disorders include panic disorder, social anxiety disorder, and general anxiety disorder. A person with an anxiety disorder may also suffer from addiction, depression, chronic pain, or even attempt suicide.

Causes

Often times, underlying medical issues may be the cause of anxiety disorders. Some examples include cardiovascular diseases, substance withdrawal, asthma, and hyperthyroidism. Medications may also induce anxiety.

Symptoms

Symptoms vary depending on the type of anxiety a person suffers from. General symptoms include nervousness, increased breathing and heart rate, shaking, trembling, digestive issues, and the inability to stop thinking about whatever it is that is putting a person into a state of anxiety.

Panic anxiety may leave a person with a feeling of fear or terror, and lead to chest pain, shortness of breath, and a rapid heart beat. Social anxiety may lead a person to avoid contact with others as a means to protect themselves from situations they might find themselves being embarrassed or self-conscious in.

Treatments

Psychotherapy is the primary treatment for anxiety disorders. Cognitive Behavioral Therapy is used to help treat social anxiety by exposing a person to situations they may experience in real life, giving them exposure and helping them learn how to cope with the situation when it arises. Medications may be prescribed, such as antidepressants, that can help a person from feeling anxious.

Bulimia

(Greek "boulimia": ravenous hunger)

Bulimia is a psychological disorder in which a person ingests **abnormally large portions of food**, followed by **purging of the food ingested**. Purging of food can be caused by **self-induced vomiting, consuming laxatives or diuretics**, and/or **excessive exercise**. This is all done in an effort to avoid weight gain.

The use of self-induced vomiting and laxatives/diuretics is known as Purging Bulimia. These involve ridding the body of the ingested food in some way that doesn't allow it to be properly digested. The use of excessive exercise is known as Non-Purging Bulimia.

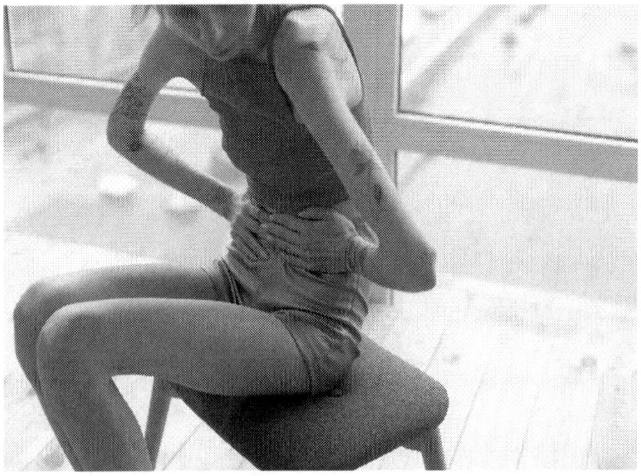

Causes

The exact cause of bulimia is unknown, although there are several contributing factors that may lead to the development of the condition. Stress, history of abuse, trauma, low self-esteem, and having a negative image of one's body can all be contributing factors.

Symptoms

Common symptoms may include dehydration, imbalances in electrolyte levels, fluctuating weight, lesions in the mouth due to excessive vomiting, chronic heart burn, and infertility.

People with bulimia may exhibit some of the following traits and behaviors: frequent bathroom usage after eating, eating privately, smelling of vomit, and lacking control when eating.

Treatments

Bulimia is most commonly caused by low self-esteem and negative body image. Therefore, the primary treatment is therapy to help the patient overcome these psychological issues.

Depression

Depression is a disorder affecting **mood**, causing a person to feel **sad**, usually over a **prolonged period of time**. A person may become disinterested in normal daily activities, and become more distant. Depression usually develops during teenage years, but may occur at any time. If a person is experiencing depression, they should seek help from a mental health professional.

Causes

There are many different causes for depression, and no one person is the same as another. Causes include a change in the body's hormone levels, such as during and after pregnancy, changes in the function of neurotransmitters in the brain, and even may be genetically passed down.

Symptoms

Symptoms are wide-ranging, and people experience depression differently. Symptoms may include a feeling of sadness, fatigue, disinterest in eating, anxiety, insomnia, irritability, and consistently thinking about death and suicide. A person with depression may attempt suicide.

Treatments

If a person is diagnosed with depression, antidepressants known as selective serotonin reuptake inhibitors, or SSRIs, are usually prescribed to help manage hormone levels and increase serotonin levels in the blood. Talking with a mental health professional may help a person feel better. Exercise and a healthy diet may help with hormone imbalances and increase a person's self esteem, which can aid in lowering depression. Other relaxation techniques, such as massage therapy and yoga, may be sought.

Insomnia

(in-: not; somnus: sleep)

Insomnia is a disorder causing a **lack of sufficient sleep**. This may be the result of a person having **difficulty falling asleep**, **staying asleep**, or **waking too early**. This can lead to many health complications.

Causes

There are many reasons a person's sleep may be affected. Stress is the most common cause of insomnia, making it difficult to "turn off" thoughts when it's time to sleep. Having an irregular sleep schedule may make it difficult for the body to adjust when it's time to sleep. Jet lag may also cause insomnia. Certain medications may interfere with normal sleep. Pain associated with medical conditions may also keep a person from sleeping.

Symptoms

Common symptoms include trouble falling asleep, trouble staying asleep, waking too early, general fatigue, irritability, increased stress and anxiety, and depression. A person with insomnia may develop other health conditions as a result of not getting enough sleep, such as hypertension.

Treatments

Determining and treating the root cause of the insomnia is the primary treatment for insomnia. Reducing stress, getting a person on a set sleep schedule, increasing exercise, meditation, yoga, and massage therapy can all aid in eliminating insomnia. If these methods do not accomplish the goal, medications to help a person sleep may be prescribed. Over-the-counter sleep aids may help a person sleep, but should not be used long-term as a person may develop a dependency on them.

Sensory Pathologies

Conjunctivitis

(conjunctiv/o: conjunctiva; -itis: inflammation)

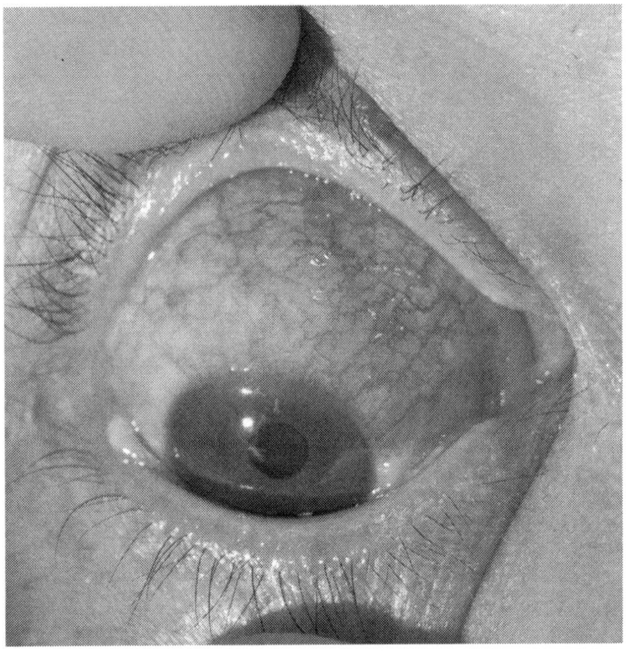

Conjunctivitis is **inflammation and/or infection of the conjunctiva**, the clear membrane that lines the inner eyelid and covers the sclera of the eye. Conjunctivitis is also known as **pinkeye**, due to the appearance of the conjunctiva when the blood vessels inside become irritated and inflamed.

Causes

The most common cause of conjunctivitis is a **bacterial or viral infection**. In infants, conjunctivitis may occur if tear ducts become blocked. Allergens may also cause conjunctivitis.

Symptoms

The affected eye may appear red, producing a **discharge**. This discharge may crust over and make it difficult to open the eye in the morning after sleep. The eye may feel itchy. Vision is not affected by conjunctivitis, but an increased amount of tears may be produced.

Treatments

Treating conjunctivitis is dependent on the cause. If it is caused by bacteria, antibiotic eye drops are prescribed. Antiviral medications may be prescribed in certain cases, such as a herpes simplex outbreak. If conjunctivitis is caused by an irritant such as contact lenses, a person will stop using contacts until the conjunctivitis clears up.

Glaucoma

(Greek glaukos: bluish-green; -oma: tumor)

Glaucoma is a **degenerative eye disorder** in which the **optic nerve is progressively damaged by increased pressure** in the eye, eventually resulting in blindness. It is more common in people over the age of 60.

Causes

Inside the eye, there is fluid known as aqueous humor that is normally produced and drained from the eye. In people with glaucoma, this fluid does not properly drain, but keeps being produced, which adds pressure inside the eye. This pressure damages the optic nerve. When the optic nerve is damaged extensively, vision is lost.

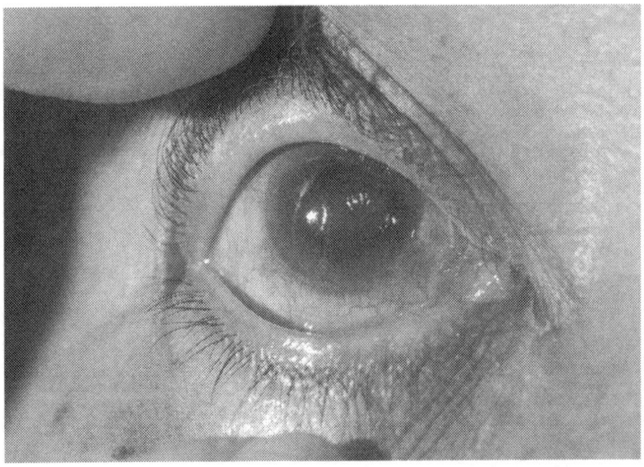

Symptoms

Symptoms vary depending on the advancement of the condition. Earlier stages may be relatively asymptomatic. Advanced stages can see a person develop tunnel vision, lose vision in the peripheral edges, experience headaches, nausea, vomiting, pain in the eye, and blurred vision.

Treatments

Treatment for glaucoma mainly focuses on reducing pressure inside the eye. Eyedrops can be prescribed that increase the amount of fluid being drained from the eye. Other eye drops may reduce the production of fluid in the eye. If these aren't useful, surgery may be performed. Laser surgery helps to open any blocked fluid draining channels. Small tubes may be put into the eye itself to help drain excess fluid.

Tinnitus

(Latin "tinnire": to ring like a bell)

Tinnitus is the presence of a **sound in the ear**, typically **ringing, without an external auditory source**. Tinnitus is usually related to another cause, such as an injury to the ear or hearing loss. It is usually not serious, but may be somewhat irritating. Tinnitus may always be present, or may come and go. The volume and pitch of the sound may be low or high, and may be loud enough to interfere with a person's ability to hear properly.

Causes

Common causes of tinnitus include exposure to loud noises, such as music, machinery, and firearms, hearing loss related to aging, and Meniere's disease. Less commonly, conditions that affect the Cardiovascular System may contribute to tinnitus, such as atherosclerosis and hypertension. With these conditions, more pressure is being placed on the blood vessels, which can harm the blood vessels in the ears, making them more susceptible to developing tinnitus.

Symptoms

The main symptom is a sound in the ear that only the person can hear. This sound can be a ringing, clicking, humming, roaring, or buzzing sound. Depending on the cause, it may be heard in one or both ears.

Treatments

Treatment for tinnitus is often treating the underlying cause, which should alleviate the ringing in the ear. If a cardiovascular issue is suspected, medications may be prescribed to help treat these, which can eliminate the tinnitus. Less commonly, excessive ear wax may produce tinnitus. If this is the case, impacted ear wax may be removed. Avoiding loud noises will also alleviate tinnitus.

Vertigo

Vertigo is the sensation that a person's **surroundings are moving or spinning**, which may cause **dizziness**. This can be especially prevalent if a person is looking down from a tall height.

Causes

Commonly, vertigo is the result of a problem with the **inner ear. Meniere's disease**, which causes **fluid buildup that changes pressure inside the ear**, is a common cause. A buildup of calcium deposits in the inner ear can alter balance. Viral infections, such as vestibular neuritis, may also cause vertigo. Less commonly, tumors in the ear may cause vertigo.

Symptoms

Vertigo presents with a feeling of the environment around a person spinning, moving, swaying, or tilting. A person may become unbalanced, become nauseated, vomit, or develop headaches.

Treatments

Treatment for vertigo is usually dependent on the cause. If calcium is present in the inner ear, certain head and neck movements may be performed to aid the calcium in leaving the inner ear, allowing it to be broken down by the body. Medications may be prescribed to aid with nausea and fluid build up associated with Meniere's disease. Surgery may be performed if there is a tumor present. Often times, no treatment is necessary, as the brain becomes acclimated to vertigo and the symptoms lessen or disappear.

Pathology Matching

______: Hyper-curvature of the thoracic vertebrae caused by tight pectoralis minor and serratus anterior

______: Protrusion of the nucleus pulposus through the annulus fibrosus

______: Inflammation of the liver

______: Swelling of veins due to malfunctioning valves

______: Injury to a ligament caused by over-stretching

______: Lack of cortisol production caused by damage to the adrenal cortex

______: Epidermal growth caused by the human papilloma virus

______: Fungal infection of the skin causing a circular rash

______: Autoimmune disorder causing dry, scaly patches to form on the skin

______: Bacterial infection of the kidneys presenting with back pain and fever

______: Swelling of a limb due to excessive interstitial fluid in an area

______: Subluxation of the distal phalange of the big toe forcing the first metatarsal to turn medially and the big toe to turn laterally

______: Bacterial infection causing inflammation of the bladder

______: Paralysis of one side of the face due to damage to the facial nerve

______: Necrosis of heart tissue

______: Compression of the brachial plexus and blood vessels caused by tight scalenes and pectoralis minor

______: Bacterial infection of a hair follicle, also known as a furuncle

______: Form of tendonitis causing inflammation at the lateral epicondyle of the humerus

______: Highly contagious viral infection of the respiratory tract

______: Degeneration of alveoli, reducing gas exchange

A: Varicose Veins
B: Emphysema
C: Thoracic Outlet Syndrome
D: Kyphosis
E: Psoriasis
F: Boil
G: Hepatitis
H: Myocardial Infarction
I: Bunion
J: Wart
K: Tennis Elbow
L: Bell's Palsy
M: Cystitis
N: Sprain
O: Pyelonephritis
P: Herniated Disc
Q: Influenza
R: Lymphedema
S: Ringworm
T: Addison's Disease

Answer Key on Page 292

Pathology Crossword

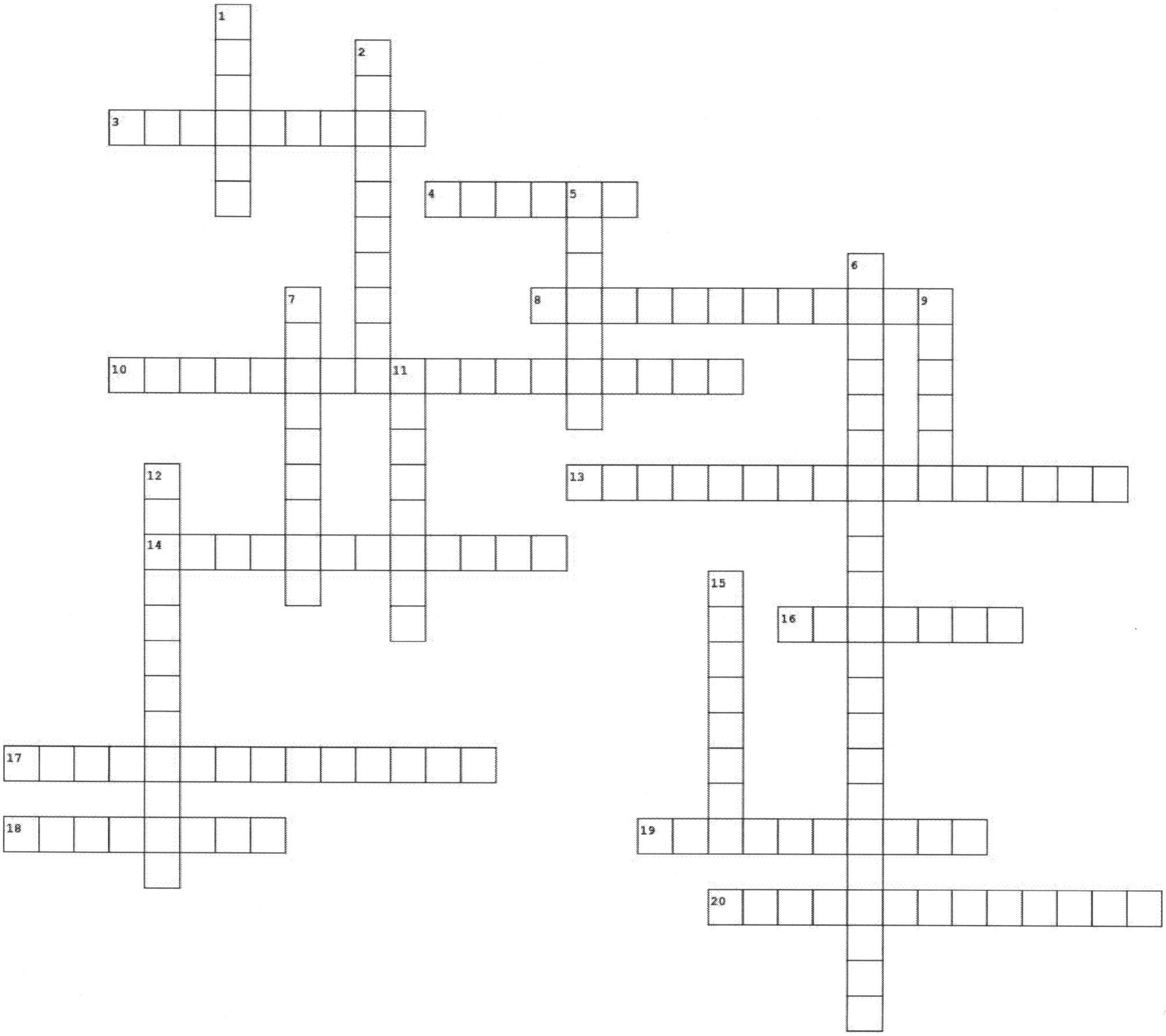

Across

3. A cancer that spreads to other tissues/regions in the body
4. Scar raised off the skin due to excessive scar tissue production
8. Bacterial infection in the lungs causing coughing with blood, fever, and chills
10. The most common, slowest growing, least serious form of skin cancer
13. Constriction of blood vessels in the fingers, reducing circulation
14. Fungal infection affecting the feet
16. Medications used to lower cholesterol and assist in lowering hypertension
17. Bacterial infection in kidneys, beginning in the urethra
18. Disease a person obtains at some point after birth
19. Substances released by damaged tissue to dilate blood vessels in an area and produce inflammation
20. Inflammation of the gallbladder typically caused by the development of gallstones that block the bile duct

Down

1. Subluxation causing the big toe to turn laterally and the first metatarsal to turn medially, producing a large bump
2. Disease a person is born with
5. In a person with diabetes, this hormone is either not produced in enough quantity, or the body becomes desensitized to it
6. Overgrowth of bone at the tibial tuberosity
7. Medical device used to regulate heart rhythm in a person with arrhythmia
9. An injury to a muscle or tendon
11. Hypercurvature of the lumbar vertebrae
12. The process of a cell eating another structure
15. Hypercurvature of the thoracic vertebrae

Answer Key on Page 293

Pathology Practice Test

1. A patient is experiencing nausea, pain in the low back, and bloody urine. After performing imaging, the doctor diagnoses the patient with kidney stones. The kidney stones appear large, and are unable to pass without treatment. Which treatment is utilized to break the kidney stones into smaller pieces to allow the stones to pass easier
A. Dialysis
B. Arthroscopy
C. Lithotripsy
D. Chemotherapy

2. Rapid production of epithelial cells resulting in thick silvery patches, caused by an autoimmune response
A. Psoriasis
B. Rosacea
C. Melanoma
D. Papilloma

3. Sean is baking a delicious cake, and the timer goes off, letting him know the cake is done baking. Sean reaches in to the oven and accidentally touches the side of the oven with his forearm. He immediately pulls his arm out, and sees skin has already begun peeling away in the area. After a trip to the emergency room, Sean's wound is bandaged, and he is sent home to recover. Several months pass, and the wound has healed, but scar tissue has formed to fill in the area where tissue has suffered necrosis. What is this type of scarring known as
A. Keloid
B. Contracture
C. Striae
D. Hypertrophic

4. Which of the following describes meningitis
A. Paralysis of one side of the body due to infection of the Herpes Simplex virus
B. Inflammation of the brain, causing increased pressure placed on the cranium
C. Degeneration of brain tissue, resulting in loss of memory
D. Inflammation of the meninges, resulting in pressure being placed on the brain

5. A patient states they have been diagnosed with Meniere's disease, with vertigo as an associated symptom. Which of the following describes vertigo
A. Ringing in the ears
B. Bacterial infection of the mucous membranes
C. Dizziness
D. Abnormal lateral curvature of the cervical vertebrae

6. All of the following are forms of parasites except
A. Pinworm
B. Tapeworm
C. Hookworm
D. Ringworm

7. Substances released by T cells and B cells after binding to an antigen that communicate with the immune system to bring other T cells and B cells to the area of infection
A. Paratopes
B. Immunoglobulins
C. Antibodies
D. Cytokines

8. Anemia, scurvy, and osteoporosis may all be considered
A. Hereditary diseases
B. Idiopathic diseases
C. Deficiency diseases
D. Autoimmune diseases

9. In a patient with renal failure, blood may need to be filtered through the following machine to eliminate harmful substances
A. Pacemaker
B. Centrifuge
C. Dialyzer
D. Defibrillator

10. A patient was recently on a walk in the desert when they were attacked by a coyote. The coyote managed to bite the patient twice in the forearm, but the patient was able to fight off the coyote and scare it away. The patient went to the hospital for treatment, suffering only a couple puncture wounds but nothing too severe. What type of healing would be required for this type of wound
A. Primary intention healing
B. Secondary intention healing
C. Quadrilateral intention healing
D. Tertiary intention healing

Answer Key on Page 295

Pharmacology

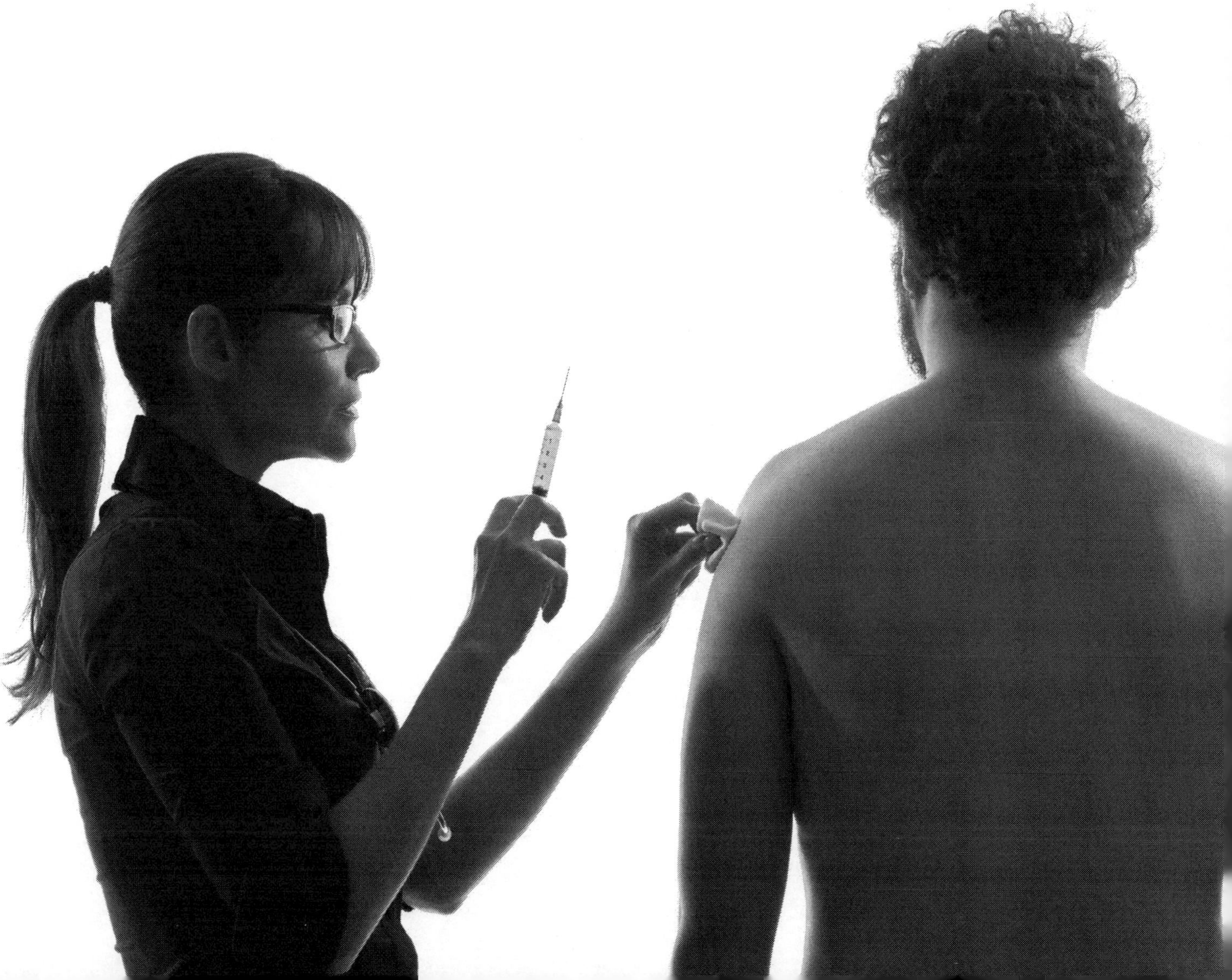

Medications

There are many different types of medications used to treat many types of illnesses, diseases, and infections. Among the most common are:

Analgesics, which help to **relieve pain**. Examples include acetaminophen and non-steroidal anti-inflammatory drugs. These help treat symptoms of conditions that cause pain, such as cancer.

Antacids, which **reduce the activity of acids** in the stomach. These help treat conditions such as Gastroesophageal Reflux Disease.

Antibiotics, which are used to **combat bacterial growth**. Examples include penicillin, amoxicillin, and erythromycin. These are used to treat infections in the body, such as cellulitis, impetigo, and strep throat.

Anticoagulants, which are used to **reduce the formation of blood clots**. Examples include aspirin, heparin, and warfarin. These are used to treat conditions such as deep vein thrombosis and phlebitis.

Antidepressants, which are used to **combat depression**. Common forms include selective serotonin reuptake inhibitors(SSRIs), serotonin and norepinephrine reuptake inhibitors(SNRIs), and tricyclic antidepressants.

Antidotes, which are used to **counteract the effects of poison** on the body. These are used when too much of a substance has entered the body that can result in harmful, or even fatal effects.

Antifungals, which aid in **destroying fungus**. Examples include terbinafine and fluconazole. These are used to treat any type of fungal infection, such as Tinea Pedis(Athlete's Foot) or Tinea Capitis.

Antihistamines, which **reduce the effects of histamines** on the body, including runny nose and itching. These are used to treat allergic reactions.

Anti-inflammatory agents, which help to **reduce inflammation**. Examples include non-steroidal anti-inflammatory drugs such as ibuprofen. These are used to help treat inflammation in conditions such as bronchitis, and potentially Alzheimer's Disease.

Antipyretics, which help to **reduce fever**. Examples include ibuprofen and aspirin. These are used to treat symptoms of fever and other systemic infections.

Antivirals, which aid in **preventing virus reproduction**. Examples include amantadine and rimantadine. These are used to combat virus reproduction in conditions such as encephalitis.

Beta blockers, which help to **reduce blood pressure**. Examples include acebutolol, nadolol, and nebivolol. These are used to treat conditions such as hypertension, arrhythmia, and myocardial infarction.

Bronchodilators, which aid in **dilation of the bronchial tubes**. Examples include albuterol and salmeterol. These are used to treat conditions such as asthma and bronchitis.

Decongestants, which **reduce inflammation in the nasal cavity**. Examples include pseudoephedrine and phenylephrine. These are used to treat congestion caused by allergies.

Expectorants, which are used to help a person **expectorate**, or cough/spit mucous from the lungs. Common forms include over-the-counter brand names such as Mucinex and Robitussin. These are commonly used to treat chest congestion.

General anesthetics, which are used to **numb the entire body**. Examples include propofol, ketamine, and etomidate. General anesthetics are primarily used when a person is having surgery performed that requires them to be in an unconscious state. These can be administered via needle injection or may be inhaled.

Insulin, which **lowers the amount of sugar in the blood stream**. Insulin is primarily used to treat diabetes.

Laxatives, also known as stool softeners, which are used to help **loosen and eliminate feces from the digestive tract**. Common forms include mineral oil and milk of magnesia. These are used to treat constipation.

Local anesthetics, which are used to **numb an area**. They are most commonly administered via needle injection. Examples include lidocaine and nitracaine. These are typically used before performing a surgical procedure around the area of incision.

Sedatives, which are used to **calm and relax the body**. Examples include diazepam and clonazepam. These are typically used to calm a person before a painful or uncomfortable procedure is performed, such as a colonoscopy.

Statins, which aid in **lowering cholesterol levels in the blood stream**. Examples include atorvastatin, rosuvastatin, and lovastatin. These are used to treat and/or prevent heart disease and its various symptoms, including hypertension and stroke.

Steroids, which are primarily used to **combat inflammation in specific areas**. Common forms include corticosteroids and anabolic steroids. Corticosteroids are useful in treating conditions such as asthma, arthritis, and lupus.

Thrombolytics are used to **dissolve a blood clot** that is already present in the body, which can prevent major complications in conditions such as stroke, myocardial infarction, and pulmonary embolism. Common forms include anistreplase, reteplase, and streptokinase.

Vaccines, which are used to **prevent a contagious disease from developing** in a person. Common vaccines include MMR(Measles-Mumps-Rubella), DTaP(Diphtheria, Tetanus, and Pertussis), influenza, and human papilloma virus. Vaccines are commonly administered via intramuscular needle injection.

Drug Actions and Adverse Reactions

Drug actions occur when an administered medication interacts with its **intended target** on a molecular level. When the drugs interact with their target, it causes **desired effects**. For example, if a patient is administered a drug, it interacts with its intended receptors. This interaction then produces an effect in the body, such as reduced pain. If a medication is used for a certain disease or condition, it is considered indicated for use. A drug that is indicated for use of a specific condition will be known to help treat, cure, or prevent the condition.

Adverse reactions may occur with medications. Adverse reactions are **unintended or unexpected effects** of the administration of medication that may be harmful to the patient. The severity of each adverse reaction is dependent on the patient and their overall health, the dosage of the medication, and the type of medication administered. Adverse reactions can range from mild to lethal. Any adverse reactions should be treated and documented to prevent further instances from occurring. Adverse reactions differ from **side effects** in that side effects are often **temporary reactions** that are commonly known to occur, and usually not life threatening.

Allergic reactions to drugs may occur, and these reactions are caused by an **immune response** to the administered medication. Rash, fever, and hives are the most common signs and symptoms of a drug allergy. Drug allergies should be treated immediately, as they have the potential to be result in extreme reactions such as anaphylaxis. This can be fatal.

Contraindications

Medications often are **inadvisable** for certain people to use. These circumstances result in **contraindications** for medications.

An **absolute contraindication** occurs when it is **completely inadvisable** for a patient to utilize a certain type of medication, because it may harm the patient. For example, for a patient with hemophilia, blood thinners such as aspirin would be an absolute contraindication, because the patient already has problems with blood clotting, and it could endanger the patient to receive blood thinning medication.

A **relative contraindication** occurs when there is **potential** for a medication to be inadvisable for use by the patient, but may still be administered if it is necessary. For example, if a pregnant patient develops some sort of bacterial infection, it may be inadvisable for the patient to use antibiotics due to the risk it poses to the fetus. However, if the infection results in septicemia, then antibiotics would be administered, because the benefits of taking the medication outweigh the risks.

Storage of Drugs/Inventory Control

The **Food and Drug Administration**, also known as the **FDA**, is a government agency responsible for ensuring public safety and health in regards to **food, medications, vaccines, medical devices**, and more. The FDA regulates the production and overall safety of products such as medications by performing inspections of production facilities. The requirements to pass inspection are typically published by the FDA and distributed.

New drugs that are developed are tested by the FDA, in a process known as a **new drug application**. The new drug is tested, and either approved or denied for use by the FDA. This process only concerns prescription medications.

The Food and Drug Administration has specific requirements for the storage of prescription drugs. Drugs should be stored in areas with adequate lighting, temperature, ventilation, humidity, sanitation, space, and equipment. Any drug that is outdated, damaged, misbranded, or deteriorated should be kept in a quarantined area to prevent these drugs from being distributed to patients. Drugs should be kept in a clean area, and should be secured from access by outside personnel.

Drug inventory should be recorded, including where the drugs were shipped from, quantity of drugs distributed, quantity of drugs disposed of, and dates of all events. These records are made available at request of federal, state, or local law enforcement agencies, and may be photocopied and inspected by all these parties up to three years after the recorded date.

Preparing and Administering Oral and Parenteral Medications

Six Rights of Medical Administration

When administering medication to a patient, it is important to remember the **six rights of medication administration**: right patient, right drug, right route, right time, right dose, right documentation. **Right patient** refers to making sure you are giving medication to the correct patient, and not a patient who was not prescribed the medication. **Right drug** refers to making sure you are giving the patient the right drug that they have been prescribed. **Right route** refers to making sure you are using the correct means of medical application, such as injection, transdermal, or oral. **Right time** refers to making sure you are providing the patient with the medication at the correct time, as some medications require a prescribed dose at specific time intervals. **Right dose** refers to making sure the patient is receiving the correct dosage of the medication. **Right documentation** refers to making sure the administration of medication is properly documented, and documented only after the medication has been administered. Documenting before medication is administered is considered falsification of documentation.

Dosage

A **prescribed dosage** is the **size or frequency** of a dose of medication. The **regimen** is **how frequently** a dose is meant to be taken, such as once a day. Factors that determine the dosage of a medication include the disease or condition being treated, the age of the person, the weight of the person, any other conditions the person may have, and any other medications the person may be taking that can influence the medication's desired effects.

Metric Conversions

Weight
1 gram(g) = 1000 milligrams(mg)
1 kilogram(kg) = 1000 grams(g)

Metric Volume
1 cubic centimeter(cu cm) = 1000 cubic millimeters(cu mm)
1 cubic decimeter(cu dm) = 1000 cubic centimeters(cu cm)
1 cubic meter(cu m) = 1 million cubic centimeters(cu cm)
1 cubic meter(cu m) = 1000 cubic decimeters(cu dm)

Liquid Volume
1 milliliter(ml) = 1 cubic centimeter(cc)
1 milliliter(ml) = 1000 microliters(mcl)
1 cubic centimeter(cc) = 1000 microliters(mcl)
1 liter(L) = 1000 milliliters(ml)
1 liter(L) = 1000 cubic centimeters(cc)
500 milliliters(ml) = 1 pint(pt)
1000 milliliters(ml) = 1 quart(qt)

Calculations

Solid dosage forms: tabs, troches, suppositories, caps, lozenges, etc.

An ordered dose is the dose given by physician, and it is often the job of the allied health professional to determine the correct amount to give. For example, the ordered dose is 50mg, and the amount in stock is 25mg tab.

The order is written as such:

$$\frac{50mg}{x\ unit} = \frac{25mg}{1\ tab}$$

To determine the amount of medication to give, solve for x by cross multiplying, and dividing. 50 x 1 ÷ 25 = 2 tabs
Capsules and extended release drugs cannot be split, because it will alter the effectiveness of the medication.

Liquid dosage forms: sol, enemas, suspensions, injections, emulsions, magmas.

Liquid dosages are often are expressed as an amount of drug contained within an amount of liquid, as mg/ml, %, or a ratio. For example, the ordered dose is 500mg, and the amount in stock is 125mg/15ml. The order is written as such:

$$\frac{125mg}{5\ ml} = \frac{500mg}{xml}$$

To determine the amount of medication to give, solve for x by cross multiplying, and dividing. 500 x 5 ÷ 125 = 20ml

Percentages are used when discussing the amount of grams or ml of active pharmaceutical ingredient in 100g/ml of base. For example, if 5% lidocaine is given, that means that there are 5 grams of lidocaine in 100 grams of the base. To convert a percentage to a decimal amount, divide the percentage by 100.

Examples:
100% ÷ 10 = 1.0
75% ÷ 10 = 0.75
50% ÷ 10 = 0.5
25% ÷ 10 = 0.25

Ratios are used when talking about parts of an active pharmaceutical ingredient in a base. For example, if a ratio is given of 1:100, the 1 references the amount of active pharmaceutical ingredient, and 100 references the amount of base. 1:100 ratio of lidocaine means there is one gram of lidocaine and 100 grams of base.

Injections

Injections are used to administer **liquid medications**. These medications may be **drugs, vaccines,** or even **contraceptives**. Injections are delivered using a **needle and syringe**, which should always be sterile. The **gauge** of a needle is its **diameter**. The **higher** the gauge number, the **smaller** the needle's diameter is. The **lower** the gauge number, the **larger** the needle's diameter.

The location of an injection is dependent on many factors, such as the age of the patient, the medication being administered, and the frequency of the medication being administered. If a patient is a child, injections such as immunizations are often administered in the thigh. Certain medications require different types of injection routes, and these routes change the location of injections. For example, in adults, immunizations are often administered via intramuscular injection located at the deltoid. The frequency of medication administration can also change the location, because repeated injections in the same location can cause complications. For example, a patient who injects insulin will often rotate the location of the injection site to allow each injection site to heal and prevent infection.

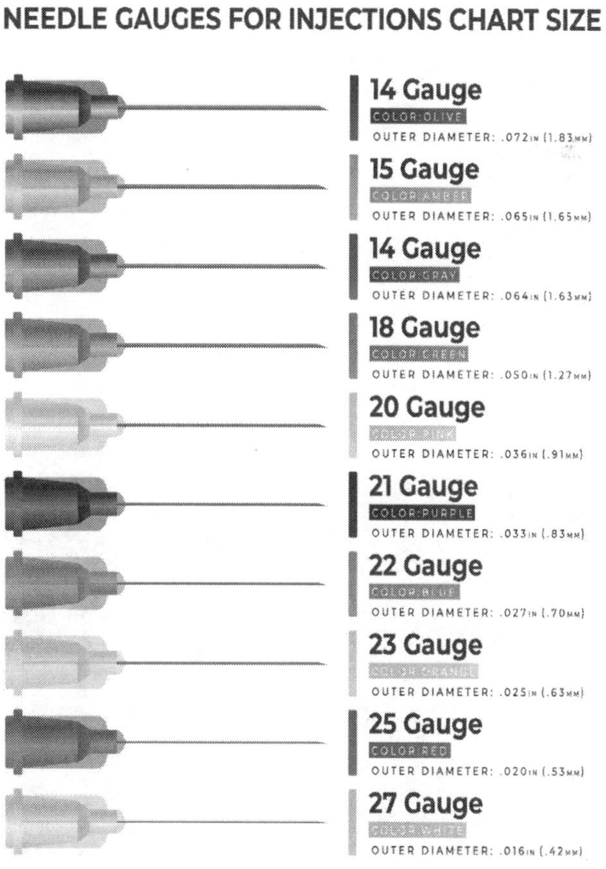

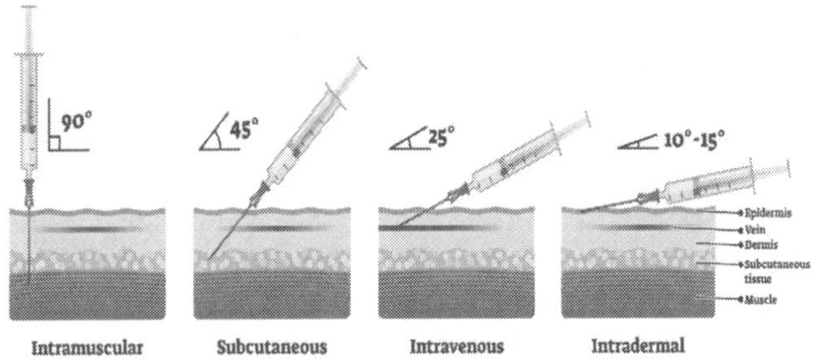

There are four types of injections: intradermal, intramuscular, subcutaneous, and intravenous.

An **intradermal injection** enters **into the skin**, but moves no further. This is performed with the needle at a **10-15 degree angle**. Common locations for intradermal injections are the **anterior forearm, posterior arm, thorax, and scapular region.** An intradermal injection is most commonly used when performing tuberculin skin test, but may also be used when performing local anesthesia, or for allergy testing.

An **intramuscular injection** enters the body **into the muscle**. Intramuscular injections are performed with the needle at a **90 degree angle**, and are most commonly performed into the **deltoid, vastus lateralis, the ventrogluteal region, and dorsogluteal region**.

Intramuscular injections may require the use of the **Z-track method**, which is helpful in preventing medication from **leaking** into the subcutaneous layer of the skin. During the injection, the skin will be pulled away from the injection site, and the injection will take place. The skin is then released, leaving the track the injection took in a Z shape. Z-track is not commonly used, but can be useful when injecting medication that needs to be absorbed into the muscle.

Subcutaneous injections enters into the **subcutaneous layer**, just deep to the dermis, but above the muscle. Subcutaneous injections are performed with the needle at a **45 degree angle**, most commonly at the **posterior and lateral arms, the abdomen around the umbilicus, and the anterior thigh**.

An **intravenous injection** enters into a vein, most commonly at an angle of **25 degrees**. Intravenous injections are usually performed in several locations such as the **cubital fossa, doral hand, and volar aspect of the wrist**.

Oral/Sublingual/Buccal Medication

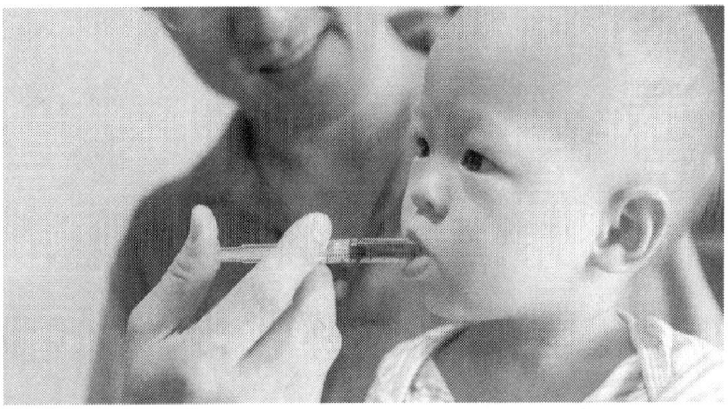

Oral medication is medication administered **into the mouth**, designed to be **swallowed.** These types of medications come in different forms, including liquid, chewable tablets, and pills. **Sublingual administration** requires the medication to be held **under the tongue**, where it will dissolve and be absorbed into the blood stream. **Buccal administration** requires the medication to be held **between the gums and the cheek**, where it is also dissolved and absorbed into the blood. Sublingual and buccal administration is useful in people who may have difficulty swallowing medication, or if the medication needs to enter the blood stream quickly.

Topical/Transdermal Medication

Topical medication is administered by placing medication on a **surface of the body**, such as the **skin or mucous membranes**. These medications are usually found in gel, lotion, or cream form. Types of topical medications include corticosteroid creams that treat conditions such as eczema, anti-itch creams, and iodine.

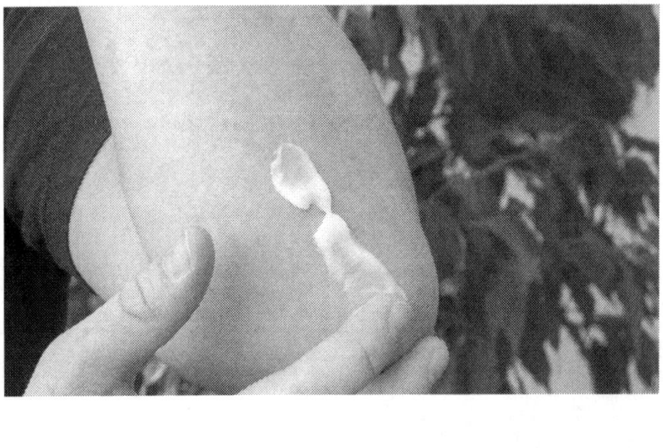

Transdermal administration is using a medication **directly on the skin** to achieve a systemic result. Transdermal administration typically takes place using a **transdermal patch**, in which medication is placed on one side of an **adhesive patch** that is then absorbed into the body through the skin, often over an **extended period of time**. An example of a medication used this way is birth control or pain relievers. Gels may also be used. Transdermal administration allows the medication to enter the blood stream without being filtered through the liver first.

Inhalation Medication

Inhalation is medication that is administered by **inhaling** it into the body. These medications are commonly found in **vapor or powder form**, and are useful for treating conditions such as asthma or chronic bronchitis. Bronchodilators are types of medication that are used via inhalation.

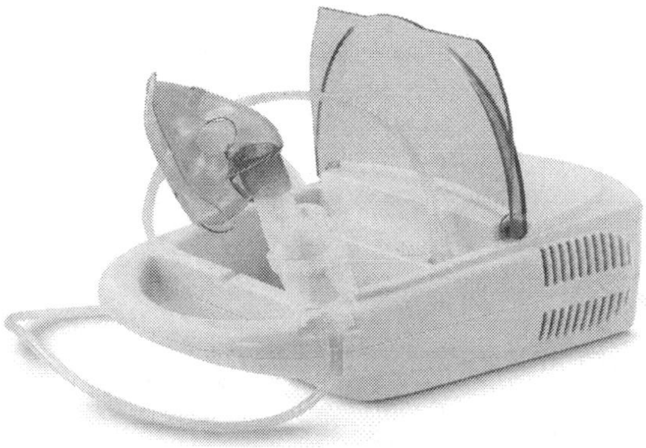

Instillation

Instillation refers to administering a medication onto a specific surface with the use of a **dropper**. These medications are used with **eye drops, ear drops, and nose drops**. Ear infections, sinus infections, or eye infections are treated with antibiotics directly into the area, and may also require oral antibiotics.

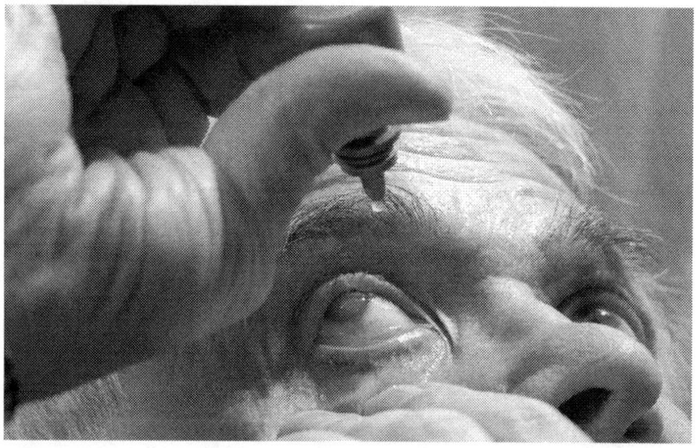

Vaginal and Rectal Medication

Administering medication into the vagina is used to treat conditions specific to the vagina that do not have systemic implications. These medications are administered directly into the vagina, most commonly with the use of **suppositories**. These medications can help treat hormonal problems relating to estrogen or progesterone, or bacterial or fungal infections that may be present.

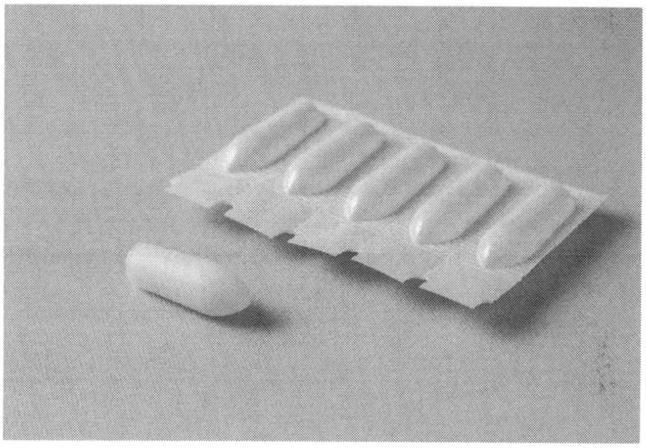

Administering medication into the rectum is used to treat conditions of the intestinal tract or rectum, to allow medication to react and enter the blood stream quicker than oral medication, and to prevent nausea associated with certain oral medications. These medications are administered via **suppositories**, with the use of an **enema**, or with use of a **catheter**.

Multidose Vial

A **vial** is a small glass or plastic container, sealed by a **rubber stopper** at the top, that may be punctured by the needle through the rubber stopper to access medication. Multi-dose vials contain medication for multiple doses. The vial usually contains some sort of antimicrobial agent that prevents bacterial growth inside the vial. The vial is labeled by the manufacturer with the type of medication inside. These vials are primarily only used for one patient.

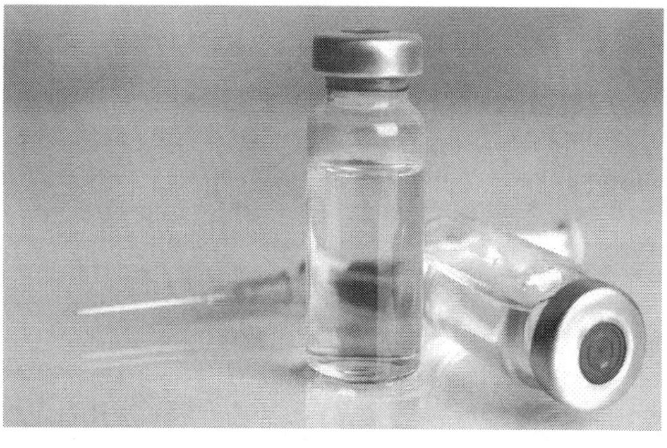

Ampule

An **ampule** is a **small glass container** that must be **broken at the top** to access the medication. The top is sealed shut by using a flame, enclosing the medication inside. To open an ampule, the neck of the ampule should be scored, then broken off. Ampules typically contain enough medication for a single injection.

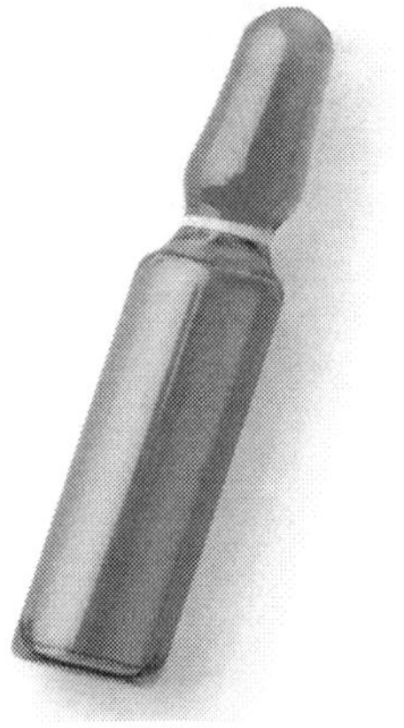

Pre-filled Cartridge Needle Unit

A **prefilled cartridge-needle unit** is a **single dose** of medicine delivered in a **syringe**, most commonly **insulin** for injection for a person with diabetes. Cartridges that contain the medication can be replaced, and the needle may be re-used in these instances. If the needle is unable to be re-used, it should be properly disposed of in a sharps container.

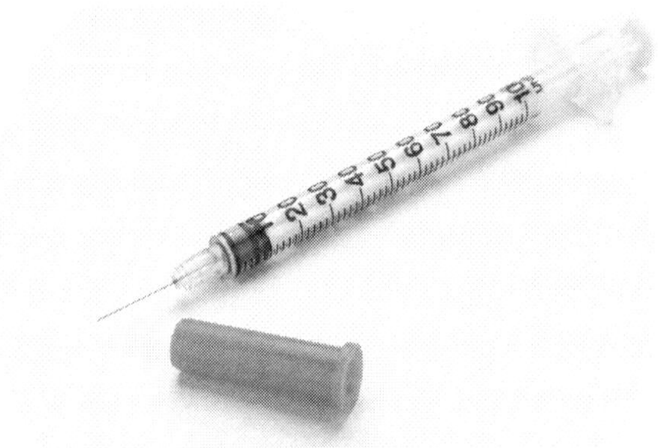

Unit Dose

A **unit dose** is a single dose of a medication that has been **prepared and packaged** by the pharmaceutical company. These can be found in **blister cards, strips, and pre-filled syringes**. These are used in a hospital setting to ensure a patient receives only the amount of medication prescribed, and nothing more. These can also be seen in over-the-counter medications, such as cold medicine.

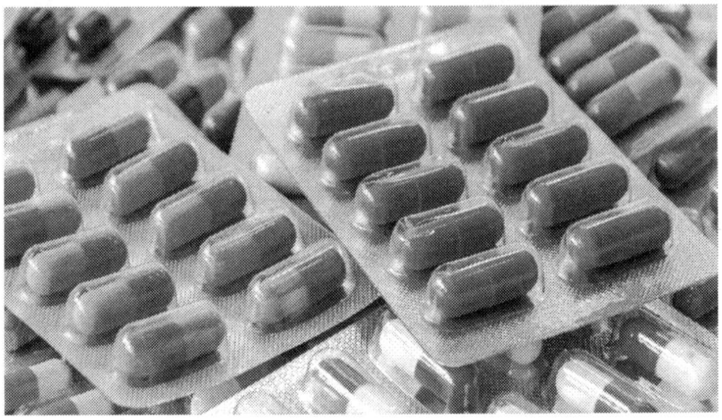

Powder for Reconstitution

Some medications are unable to be stored once they are added to a liquid. If this is the case, the medication will be kept in a powder form. When the medication is required, it is then mixed with a liquid known as a **diluent** in specific quantities, which then becomes usable medication. The diluent is most commonly water or saline. The powder and diluent are mixed in a vial.

Physician's Desk Reference

A **Physician's Desk Reference(PDR)** is a book released annually that details **all available medications** that may be prescribed. Information provided about each medication includes actions of the medication, adverse reactions, contraindications and indications, side effects, and warnings.

Medication Record Keeping

When an error occurs in providing a patient with medication, the error must be **reported and documented**. Reporting and documenting errors helps to improve safe practices through ownership, accountability, and ensuring errors do not happen again in the future. Documentation is also extremely important in lawsuits, as it shows exactly what error was made.

If an error in medication administration occurs, the error should be reported. These errors can be reported internally in most instanced, but may also be reported to agencies such as the Food and Drug Administration or the Institute for Safe Medication Practices. The error should be reported on an incident report. Examples of items that may be listed in an incident report include incorrect medication administered, incorrect dosage, incorrect route of administration, medication being administered to the wrong patient, and medication being administered at the incorrect time.

Immunization Resources

Immunizations should be administered at specific times in a person's life, or in certain situations where a person may be exposed to things such as blood-borne pathogens on a consistent basis. Immunizations help a person develop an immunity to certain diseases that may otherwise be life-threatening.

Centers for Disease Control and Prevention

The **Centers for Disease Control and Prevention**, also known as the **CDC**, is a government agency that promotes **health**, and **disease prevention**. The CDC is used to monitor disease outbreaks, and provide the public with information on how to combat the spread of certain diseases. The CDC promotes the use of vaccines, safe working conditions and environments, and injury prevention.

Immunizations

Vaccines are administered several times throughout **childhood**. Vaccines commonly administered throughout childhood include Tetanus, diphtheria, & acellular pertussis(Tdap), hepatitis B, inactivated poliovirus, influenza, measles, mumps, rubella, and pneumococcal conjugate. These are administered at different times in a child's development, and some of these are often administered numerous times over several years to ensure proper immunity has formed.

During **adulthood**, common vaccines administered include influenza, human papilloma virus, tetanus, diphtheria, & acellular pertussis(Tdap), and in cases where a person may have exposure to certain viruses, hepatitis A, hepatitis B, and pneumococcal conjugate. These too are administered at differing portions of an adult's life, and may correspond to the birth of a child.

When a person receives any type of immunization, it should be documented. Documenting immunizations gives health care professionals information about patients in regards to overall health, and when a person should receive another immunization in the future. Failure to properly document immunizations may lead to a patient receiving an un-needed immunization, or influence their ability to do things such as travel to other countries that may require certain immunizations to be completed.

Any time a vaccine is given, the patient or their legal guardian should receive a **vaccine information statement**. This statement is given before the vaccination, and provides the patient or guardian information on the vaccine, what it is used for, and any potential side effects that may be caused by receiving the vaccine. Distribution of the vaccine information statement should be documented, including the edition of the VIS and the date the VIS was distributed.

The **Vaccine Adverse Event Reporting System(VAERS)** is used to report any **adverse events** that occur to a patient resulting from administration of a vaccine. Adverse events may include **allergic reaction** to the vaccine, and **injuries** the patient sustains from receiving the vaccine. Information provided in a report includes the names of vaccines administered, dosage form, concentration strength, route of administration, etc. Essentially any information about the event that can be provided should be provided.

Like any medication, vaccines should be properly stored to prevent degradation of the vaccine, which may make it unusable. Vaccines should be stored in a **freezer or refrigerator**, with enough room around it to prevent the motor unit from breaking or overheating. The vaccines should be kept at a proper temperature, which should be handled using a temperature monitoring device. These devices give an accurate reading of temperature inside the refrigerator or freezer, and are especially useful when trying to keep the vaccine within a specified temperature range.

Pharmacology Matching

______: Medications used to combat bacterial infections

______: A medication that is completely inadvisable for a patient to use

______: Agency responsible for promoting health, and disease prevention

______: Used to report any adverse events resulting from administration of a vaccine

______: Ensuring a patient is receiving the correct drug that has been prescribed

______: The size or frequency of a dose of medication

______: The diameter of a needle

______: Medication designed to be placed on the surface of the body

______: Book released annually detailing all available medications that may be prescribed

______: Unintended or unexpected effects of administration of medication that may be harmful to the patient

______: Potential for a medication to be inadvisable for use, but may be administered if necessary

______: A drug interacting with its intended target

______: Medication used to numb the entire body

______: Temporary reactions commonly known to occur with medications that are typically not serious

______: Agency responsible for ensuring public safety and health regarding food, medications, vaccines, and medical devices

______: How frequently a dose of medication is meant to be taken

______: Injection administered at a 90 degree angle

______: Small glass container that must be broken at the top to access medication inside

______: Single dose of medication prepared and packaged by the pharmaceutical company

______: Injection administered at a 45 degree angle

A: VAERS
B: Prescribed dosage
C: Desired effects
D: Antibiotics
E: Intramuscular
F: Physician's Desk Reference
G: Absolute contraindication
H: FDA
I: Regimen
J: Gauge
K: Right drug
L: Subcutaneous
M: Ampule
N: CDC
O: Relative contraindication
P: Adverse reactions
Q: General anesthetic
R: Unit dose
S: Topical medication
T: Side effects

Answer Key on Page 292

Pharmacology Crossword

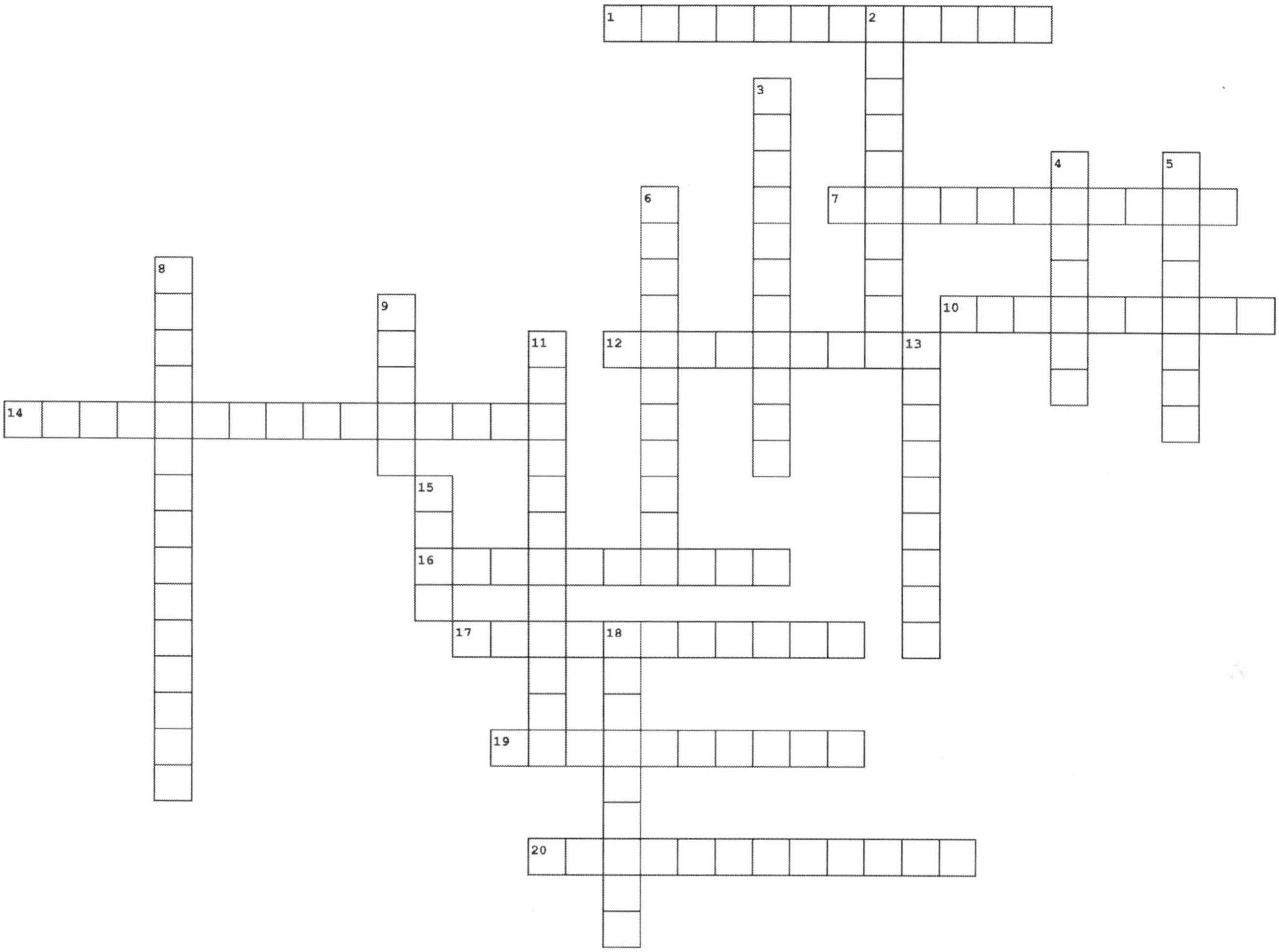

Across

1. Medications used to loosen phlegm in lungs
7. Medication administered by being placed directly on the skin, usually using a patch
10. Medications used to increase the production of urine
12. Medications used to help loosen and eliminate feces from the digestive tract
14. Medications used to aid in dilation of the bronchial tubes
16. Medications used to relieve pain
17. Injection administered at an angle of 10-15 degrees
19. Medications used to prevent a virus from reproducing
20. Medications used to combat fever by lowering body temperature

Down

2. Making sure the correct means of medical application is being utilized
3. Medications used to combat bacterial infection
4. Type of anesthetic used to numb the entire body
5. Medications used to prevent a contagious disease from developing in a person
6. Injection administered at an angle of 25 degrees
8. A medication known to help treat, cure, or prevent a condition
9. Type of anesthetic used to numb an area of the body
11. Administering a medication onto a surface using a dropper
13. Medications used to calm and relax the body
15. Medication administered into the mouth, designed to be swallowed
18. Medications used to counteract the effects of poison on the body

Answer Key on Page 294

Pharmacology Practice Test

1. The size or frequency of a dose of medication
A. Prescribed dosage
B. Method of administration
C. Metric conversion
D. Recommended dosage

2. Ibuprofen is commonly used to treat which condition
A. Anemia
B. Fever
C. Bacterial infection
D. Constriction of bronchial tubes

3. 1 ml is equal to
A. 1 liter
B. 1 cubic centimeter
C. 1 quart
D. 1 gram

4. Which type of injection utilizes an angle of 90 degrees
A. Intradermal
B. Epidermal
C. Subcutaneous
D. Intramuscular

5. Reporting system used to document adverse events resulting from administration of a vaccine
A. VAERS
B. PDR
C. DARF
D. CDCRS

6. All of the following medications are used to treat blood conditions except
A. Anticoagulants
B. Statins
C. Analgesics
D. Thrombolytics

7. Single dose of medication delivered in a syringe
A. Unit dose
B. Ampule
C. Suppository
D. Pre-filled cartridge needle unit

8. Of the following, which is not one of the six rights of medical administration
A. Right route
B. Right arm
C. Right dose
D. Right documentation

9. Gels, lotions, and creams are commonly used with which form of medication administration route
A. Instillation
B. Buccal
C. Topical
D. Inhalation

10. Sol, enemas, and injections are all forms of
A. Reconstitution dosage
B. Transdermal dosage
C. Liquid dosage
D. Unit dosage

Answer Key on Page 295

Legal and Ethical Issues

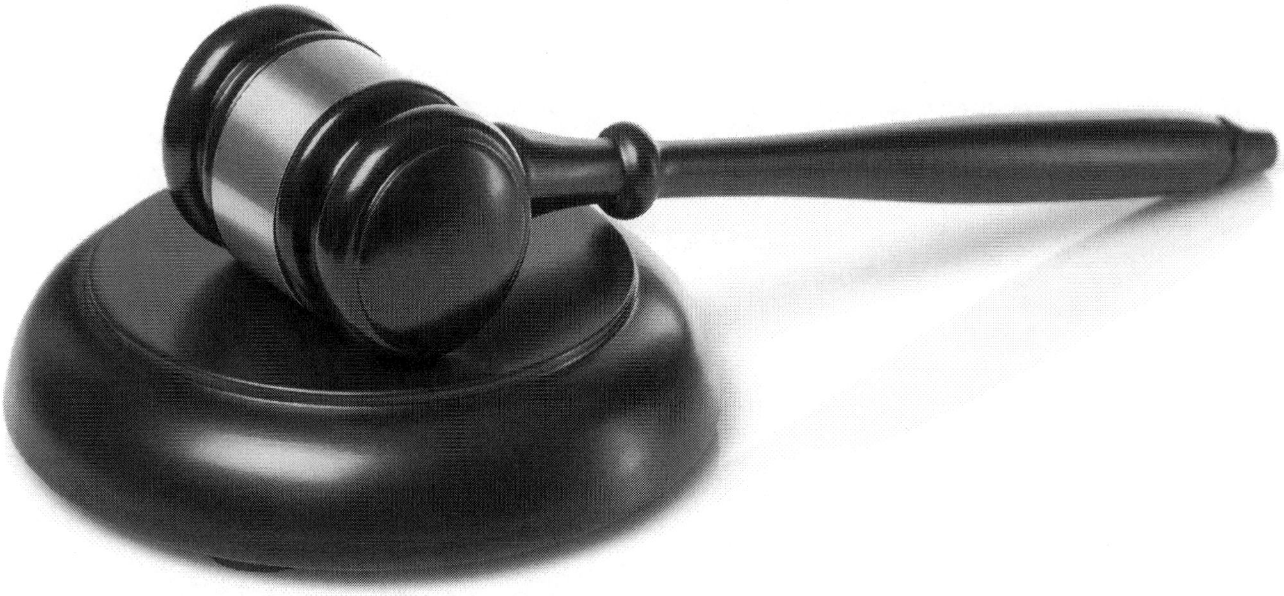

Health Insurance Portability and Accountability Act

The **Health Insurance Portability and Accountability Act**, also known as **HIPAA**, was enacted August 21st, 1996. It was created by the US Department of Health and Human Services. Inside HIPAA lies the **Privacy Rule**, which is used to **protect all individually identifiable health information**. The Privacy Rule ensures client/patient information is kept private. However, it does allow this information to be transferred between healthcare providers when necessary, which allows high-quality health care. Assessments and diagnoses do not need to be re-done, as the information is already present.

Title I of HIPAA provides protections for insured persons to transfer health insurance coverage from one place of employment to the next. It also prevents a person transferring health insurance from being denied coverage due to pre-existing conditions.

Title II of HIPAA helps to prevent health care abuse and fraud by establishing national standards for health care transactions transmitted electronically.

Title III of HIPAA provides certain deductions to be implemented into medical insurance, and provides guidelines for medical spending accounts.

Title IV of HIPAA provides guidelines for group health plans, specifically in regards to coverage of pre-existing conditions.

Title V of HIPAA regulates company-owned life insurance policies. It also governs treatment of people who lose US citizenship due to issues with income tax, and repeals the financial institution rule to interest allocation rule.

The **Security Rule** specifies **protection** of patient information via **computers and internet**.

Confidentiality

Confidentiality is an extremely important part of the medical field, and is one of the defining factors of HIPAA. In order to ensure a business is abiding by HIPAA and confidentiality laws, whether it be small such as an independent practice, or large such as a hospital, activity logs may be utilized. Electronic access logs are able to log every person that has had access to a patient's medical files, and the time and date the person logged in to the network. Other events may also be recorded, such as log-in attempts, software updates, and changed passwords.

Health Information Technology for Economics and Clinical Health Act

The **Health Information Technology for Economics and Clinical Health Act**, also known as **HITECH**, was enacted in 2009 to **incentivize** the use of **electronic health record systems** amongst healthcare providers. The act also helps to strengthen privacy of information covered by HIPAA, furthering the liability a person or company has regarding being non-compliant of HIPAA regulations. It also gives the patient the ability to inspect, amend, or restrict access to their medical records for whatever reason they see fit.

Patients' Right to Inspect, Amend, and Restrict Access to Records

A patient has a right to inspect their medical records, amend their medical records, and restrict access to their medical records if they feel it is in their best interest. For example, a patient may be willing to grant access to their medical records to one physician, but not another. In this case, the patient may state that they wish to restrict access to medical records for a specific physician. A patient is always in control of their own medical records.

Patient's Bill of Rights/Patient Care Partnership

A patient's bill of rights are rights that a patient is assured of having. It is similar to the US Constitution's Bill of Rights. A patient's bill of rights includes being provided with **information** on health services, being able to **choose their own plan** or providers, having access to **emergency services** such as ambulances, having **informed consent**, information being kept **confidential**, and **prevents discrimination**.

The **Patient Care Partnership**, developed by the American Hospital Association, was developed to help a patient **understand their benefits and rights** during a hospital visit or stay. While similar to a patient's bill of rights, it differs in some areas that are more hospital specific, such as ensuring the patient has help with billing for services, and the patient is provided with a clean and safe environment.

Security of Electronic Transmission of Information

Security is vital in protecting patient information and maintaining confidentiality. One of the most important steps a medical office can take to protect confidential information on a computer is by using **passwords**. Any application or program that contains confidential information should be password protected. The program should keep track of login information to determine who is using the application and what information they are accessing.

Every computer should have a **screen saver** active when it is not being actively used. Screen savers block the information on the computer monitor from being viewed, instead showing some sort of image or text that may be animated or static. Screen savers become activated after a set number of minutes of inactivity on a computer. The time allotted before the screen saver becomes active can be changed manually in a computer's settings.

Encryption is the process of **encoding information** during transmission to make it impossible to be stolen. While it does not prevent the information from being accessed, the information is changed into a **cipher** that cannot be understood or read.

Firewalls are used to create a **barrier** between **secure and unsecured networks**. It is a form of gatekeeper that prevents unwanted or unsafe data transmission from entering the computer or network.

Protected Health Information

Protected health information, or **PHI**, is information about the patient that is protected by HIPAA. This information includes medical history, demographic information, laboratory results, and insurance information. While this information may not be used with identifiable information attached unless approved by the patient, it may be used with the identifiable information removed. This may help manage an entire population's health by looking at certain demographic factors in correlation with others to identify patterns in diseases and treatment outcomes, such as age, race, and gender.

Under the Privacy Rule, a patient may give consent, or authorization, to a health care provider to release protected health information. This information is only given to that specific provider, and no one else. If for whatever reason the information may need to be distributed to other parties, an authorization is required. Authorizations to release information are acquired by the patient signing a form or document that will detail the exact information being released, which is far more detailed and specific than a consent. Authorization forms may also include the reason for the information to be shared.

Drug and alcohol treatment records are kept confidential at all times, due to the passing of the **Comprehensive Alcohol Abuse and Alcoholism Prevention, Treatment, and Rehabilitation Act of 1970** and the **Drug Abuse Prevention, Treatment, and Rehabilitation Act of 1972**. These laws were designed to help ensure a patient's identifiable information is kept confidential, which increases the likelihood that a person seeking treatment will be successful in their efforts to be treated.

HIV-related information is required to be kept confidential, unless authorization is granted by the patient to release information, or there is some form of risk to the patient or another person.

Mental health history should be kept confidential, unless the patient is deemed unable to make choices that determine treatments or medications. In this case, certain medical records may be released to specific friends or family members with whom the patient has intimate contact with to help with treatment. Information may also be given to law enforcement if deemed necessary, such as the patient posing a risk to themselves or others.

Genetic Information Nondiscrimination Act

The **Genetic Information Nondiscrimination Act of 2008**, also known as **GINA**, was enacted to **prevent discrimination** in employment or health insurance based on **genetic information**. Under this act, a person may not be discriminated against based on information genetics may provide, such as the likelihood of developing a disease in the future.

Authorization to Rescind Release

A patient is also assured the right to rescind any release they may have previously granted. The patient may rescind a release verbally or in writing, and the medical practice or physician who the release is being rescinded from must comply with the order.

Use and Disposal of Personal Health Information

When receiving treatment, information may be released for the means of treatment, payment, and operations, or TPO, without authorization from the patient. Services and care provided to the patient is known as treatment. Insurance company services, including billing, claims, and collections, are detailed under payment. Operations are any activity that is used to improve the functioning of the health care operation in some way. Examples include legal operations, financial operations, and administrative operations.

Disposing of PHI can be accomplished in many different means, depending on the type of record being disposed of. Paper records can be disposed of using a document shredder, or burning the documents to make the PHI unreadable. Digital PHI can be disposed of by destroying the equipment the PHI is stored on, or simply deleting all PHI from the device, ensuring no copies or backups exist elsewhere.

Consent

Consent to Treat

A **liability** is anything that makes a person **legally responsible** for every aspect of a medical practice. To help limit liabilities, consent and informed consent should be utilized, both verbally and written.

Consent is a patient giving **permission** for an examination, treatment, or diagnosis to be performed.

When a patient is receiving some sort of treatment, if they are able, they should be given **informed consent**. Informed consent provides the patient with all of the information about the treatment they will be receiving, including risks and side effects. This allows the patient to be informed about the procedure, and to give consent or decline the treatment based on the information provided.

In a medical situation, if a patient is unable to provide consent because they may be unconscious or in a compromised state, a medical professional may assume that consent would normally be given to help the patient if they were able to communicate. This is known as **implied consent**.

Expressed consent is a form of informed consent in which the patient gives their consent verbally or in writing to have procedures or treatments performed. This is in contrast to implied consent, in which the patient is unable to state whether consent is given. Expressed consent is usually given by the patient signing documents detailing the procedure or treatment being performed.

Exceptions

In certain cases, a minor may be considered mature enough to make medical decisions for themselves. These patients are called **mature minors**, and are granted the same legal rights as an adult in regards to making medical decisions and informed consent. These minors are not emancipated, and each is looked at on a case-by-case basis.

If a person under the age of 18 lives independently apart from their parents, they may request a court determine that they are an **emancipated minor**. If the court grants the request, the emancipated minor will have the same legal rights as an adult, and are able to make medical decisions and informed consent on their own behalf.

A person who is not a senior citizen, but still requires care, can be categorized as a **dependent adult**. These adults are unable to perform daily functions adequately, and require another person to help them function daily. Examples of dependent adults include people with developmental disorders or disabilities, and mental disorders or disabilities. Caretakers are used for dependent adults in cases where the dependent adult would be in some form of danger without care or support.

Emergency situations comply with the concept of implied consent, assuming a person would consent to treatment or care if they were not too incapacitated to do so.

In some cases, the patient may be considered incompetent either by the doctor or by a court. In these cases, the patient may be treated with consent of a **power of attorney**, a person who acts in good faith on behalf of the patient.

Federal and State Regulations

Torts

A **tort** is a **wrongful act** by one person that is responsible for an **injury or harm** to another person, and is considered a civil wrong that bears liability. An **injury** in this case refers to **invasion of a legal right**. A **harm** in this case refers to a person suffering some sort of **loss**. Torts are often used to provide **monetary compensation** to a person who has been injured or harmed in some way by the offending party or parties. A tort caused by **accidental means**, or is unintentional, is known as **negligence**. The offending party did not intend for injury or harm to be done.

Intentional torts are the result of one party **intentionally causing injury or harm** to another in some way, be it physical, emotional, or damaging a person's standing or reputation. Examples of intentional torts that do not physically harm a person are slander and libel. **Slander** is a person intentionally using **false statements verbally** in order to discredit or harm the reputation of a person. **Libel** is similar, but instead of the false statement being spoken, it is **written**. These are only considered intentional torts when the person saying the false claim knows the statement is false and will harm a person's reputation.

Abandonment

Abandonment is a form of **negligence** that refers to a medical professional **not providing suitable or adequate treatment** to a patient in their care. This can result in many complications to the patient, including death. The most common form of abandonment occurs when a physician terminates the relationship with the patient without providing the patient with adequate time to find a new physician or care.

Current Standard of Care

In order to prevent bodily harm, medical professionals should follow the **current standard of care** for each patient. The current standard of care is a general guideline for treatment of specific diseases or conditions. Standard of care ensures each patient coming into a hospital for care receives the same **quality of care**, regardless of professional standing or personal wealth.

Legal Terms and Doctrines

Subpoena

When a court requires a person to attend a hearing or trial and testify in some way, the person is issued a writ by the court known as a **subpoena**. Subpoena literally translates to "**under penalty**", and if the person does not appear, they will be in violation of law. There are two separate types of subpoenae. A **subpoena duces tecum** is a court summons in which the person being summoned is required to appear in court with documentation or other evidence used in a trial or hearing. A **subpoena ad testificandum** is a court summons in which the person being summoned is required to appear in court and testify.

Deposition

A **deposition** is a **statement given under oath** and **outside of court**. Depositions are used to determine what the person specifically knows about the case, and to document testimony for trial. Depositions are commonly used when there is a chance the witness will not appear in court. These cases are typically approved by a judge beforehand.

Respondeat Superior

Respondeat superior refers to an **employer** being held **legally responsible** for the actions of an **employee**. Plaintiffs who bring lawsuits will commonly try to hold both the employer and employee responsible for any damages the plaintiff has suffered. Independent contractors and federal employees are not included.

Good Samaritan Acts

Good Samaritan Laws were developed in order to protect anyone who is helping a person they believe are in immediate danger or peril, are ill, or are in some way incapacitated. These laws **prevent** the good samaritan from being **sued for alleged wrongdoing**.

Contracts

Physician-patient relationships are formed around **contracts**. These contracts can be expressly written, or can be implied, and state that a physician will treat a patient to the best of their abilities. A physician has a legal obligation to utilize their professional skills in a professional and legal manner to best treat the patient. Physicians are also legally obligated to provide all necessary information to the patient and gain consent from the patient to perform selected services or treatments.

If, during the course of treatment, a patient refuses to follow a certain prescription, take medication as instructed, or generally not follow a doctor's direction, the patient is considered **non-compliant**. Often times, patients are non-compliant because they may be confused about the instructions given by a doctor. Other times, they may feel as if they don't need to take a prescribed dose of medication, or follow through with treatment.

When there are circumstances in which the patient is not following through with treatment, or even purposefully making sure their condition does not improve, medical care may be **terminated**. Other reasons for terminating treatment may include failure to follow office policies, failure to attend follow-up appointments, and failure to pay medical bills. When terminating care, the patient should be notified via a written letter instructing them that treatment is terminated and they will need to seek another physician for care. The notice should contain the date of termination, and the reason for termination. Termination, the reason for termination, and the date of termination should all be documented.

Pharmaceutical Laws

Prescriptions/E-Prescribing

E-prescribing, also known as electronic prescribing, is using **electronic systems** to **write and send prescriptions** to pharmacies without having to write or fax the prescriptions. This allows the pharmacy to quickly receive the prescription, and have it prepared for the patient much quicker than if the patient physically brings in the prescription.

Drug Schedules

Certain drugs are considered controlled substances, and are rated under five schedules, based on accepted health benefits, potential for abuse or dependence, and danger the patient may face by using the drug.

Schedule I drugs are drugs that have no accepted medical benefits, and have a high potential for abuse. Examples include marijuana, heroin, and LSD.

Schedule II drugs are drugs that have an increased potential for abuse, with the development of dependence. Examples include vicodin, methamphetamines, oxycodone, and cocaine.

Schedule III drugs are drugs that are considered to have a moderate to low chance to develop dependence. Examples include ketamine, anabolic steroids, and Tylenol with codeine.

Schedule IV drugs are drugs that are considered to have a low risk of developing dependence and abuse. Examples include Xanax, Valium, and Tramadol.

Schedule V drugs are drugs that are considered to have the lowest risk of abuse and dependence. These drugs are commonly found in analgesics, antitussives, and antidiarrheals.

Controlled Substances

Controlled substances are regulated for use via the **Controlled Substances Act**. This act is part of the Comprehensive Drug Abuse Prevention and Control Act of 1970, and regulates the manufacture, import, possession, distribution, and use of narcotics. These narcotics include depressants, stimulants, anabolic steroids, opioids, and hallucinogens.

The Controlled Substances Act categorizes these drugs under one of five schedules, which helps to determine the frequency of prescriptions based on the likelihood a person develops a dependency on the drug and its likelihood of being abused.

Drug Enforcement Administration

The **Drug Enforcement Administration**, also known as the **DEA**, is a law enforcement agency responsible for combating **drug distribution** within the United States. Regulation of import, manufacture, or possession of illegal substances is covered in the Controlled Substances Act of 1970, of which the DEA is a part of. This act categorizes a drug in one of five schedules. A schedule I drug is considered highly addictive, and completely unsafe to use. A schedule V drug is not considered addictive and is safe to use.

Mandatory Reporting/Public Health Statutes

Communicable Diseases

A **communicable disease** is a disease that **spreads from one person to another** through means such as exposure to bodily fluids, blood, and through inhalation, which poses a threat to the population in some way. Examples of these diseases include hepatitis A, chlamydia, staphylococcus, and influenza. These diseases are required to be reported to help reduce transmission in a community.

Vital Statistics

Vital statistics are reported to keep accurate **stats** regarding the **population of an area**. Examples of vital statistics include birth records, death records, marriages, and divorces. Details expanding on each situation may also be provided, specifically in regards to death reporting.

Abuse/Neglect/Exploitation

Abuse, neglect, and/or exploitation of a child is required to be reported by the person who discovers the alleged wrongdoing. This is performed to help protect the victim, and does not require the person reporting to gain permission.

Elder abuse and domestic abuse are both able to be reported to authorities to help protect these people who are often in a vulnerable state.

Wounds of Violence

Wounds of violence are wounds that are caused by **intentional means.** Wounds of violence reporting varies from state-to-state, with some exceptions. Suspected child abuse is always reported in every state. Other forms of abuse, such as domestic abuse and elderly abuse, may be required to be reported based on circumstances surrounding the wounds. Gunshot wounds, stab wounds, and other wounds are commonly reported as well to local authorities.

Public Health and Welfare Disclosure

The **Privacy Rule** is designed to protect certain information from being distributed. However, in certain cases, information may be distributed to appropriate people or agencies in cases that involve health and welfare. If a person is diagnosed with a communicable disease, it may be reported to agencies such as the CDC. Birth and death are considered vital statistics, and are reported. If child abuse or elder abuse is suspected, child protective services or adult protective services may be notified. If domestic abuse is suspected, police may be notified. If a person has sustained wounds such as a gunshot or stabbing wound resulting from violence, the police may also be notified.

Ethical Standards

Ethics are **guiding moral principles** that are used to help a medical professional determine the best course of action when confronted with ethical dilemmas. There are four primary principles of medical ethics: autonomy, beneficence, justice, and non-maleficence.

Autonomy refers to the ability of the patient to think and make medical decisions for themselves. The patient is given all information available about medical treatments, and is able to make **informed consent** regarding these treatments.

Beneficence refers to the medical professional always working with the **best interest of the patient** in mind, and provides the best service and treatment possible. This includes consistently learning and training utilizing continued education.

Justice refers to new or experimental treatments being distributed and utilized on people from **all backgrounds**. These treatments must obey all existing laws in regards to patient distribution.

Non-maleficence refers to the treatment provided to the patient **not causing harm** to the patient or to others. Again, the physician must always work in the best interest of the patient, not only physically, but mentally as well.

An **ethical dilemma** is any situation a person finds themselves in which offers **differing choices that conflict with a person's ethics**. Ethics are guiding moral principles, and a person may find themselves in conflict with ethical choices in certain circumstances. Ethical dilemmas arise when there are conflicts regarding duties or rights. **Duties** are often categorized as **nonmaleficence**, or doing no harm, and **beneficence**, or acting in good faith. **Rights** refer to the patient having the ability to make **informed consent**, and having autonomy in making decisions that are in their best interest.

Resolving Ethical Dilemmas

The ability to resolve ethical dilemmas can be tricky, and is often confusing. When approached with an ethical dilemma, questions a person can ask themselves are "Is this situation a potential problem?", "What do the Code of Ethics say regarding this situation?", and "What do other people think of this situation and how would they handle it?"

Here is an example of an ethical dilemma: A patient states they are looking to buy a car for their child who has just graduated from high school. The physician has a car for sale. Let's break down this dilemma using one of the questions listed above:

Is this situation a potential problem?

- Can you think of any reasons this situation could be considered a problem?
- Are there any ways the physician's behavior, or the patient's behavior, might change as a result of this situation if the physician were to tell the patient they were selling their car?
- Could the patient potentially seek favors from the physician to try to influence the physician to sell the car to the patient?
- Could the physician treat the patient more favorably than other patients because the patient may want to purchase the car from the physician?

These are all questions that a medical professional must ask themselves when confronted with an ethical dilemma. My personal approach is, if I even have to question whether a certain situation is ethical or not, it's not a situation I want to be a part of. The question I always ask myself is, "What would I do if I wanted to keep my job or license? Would my employer or the state board approve or not?"

Factors Affecting Ethical Standards

Medical law often plays an important role in medical ethics. Ethical and legal situations are closely associated, and laws are often created that ensure the medical professional adheres to strict ethical standards. In cases where there is no law that governs a certain situation and how to respond, **moral** decisions are made that influence a medical professional's behavior. Morals are a person's belief system, and can be based on factors such as religion, politics, or other personal views.

Professional Behavior

While in the workplace, professional behavior should be adhered to at all times. There are many factors that contribute to an employee exhibiting professional behavior. When interacting with customers, clients, patients, and co-workers, an employee should display tact, diplomacy, courtesy, respect, and dignity. **Tact** is understanding how to deal with people or situations with sensitivity and respect. **Diplomacy** is the ability to manage relationships between people for the betterment of all parties. **Courtesy** is showing politeness and having a positive attitude when communicating with others. **Respect** is regarding another person's feelings and rights with some sort of appreciation or admiration. **Dignity** is a feeling of pride or self-respect.

Employees in the workplace should always demonstrate responsibility in acting in the best interest of the business, the employee, and the customer, patient, or co-workers. Employees should always display integrity and honesty in every situation, and not try to pass blame on to others when mistakes are made.

Standards of Conduct

Standards of conduct are a set of general guidelines that ensure a physician acts with **honesty and integrity**, and works with the **best interest of the patient** in mind. These behaviors can be considered ethical behaviors, and may even cross into legal behaviors, such as releasing medical records without prior authorization from the patient.

Compliance Reporting

Compliance is **adhering to laws, regulations, and guidelines** that apply to a person or medical practice's operation. Compliance maintains safety, prevents potential violations in areas such as HIPAA, and provides the patient with the best care possible.

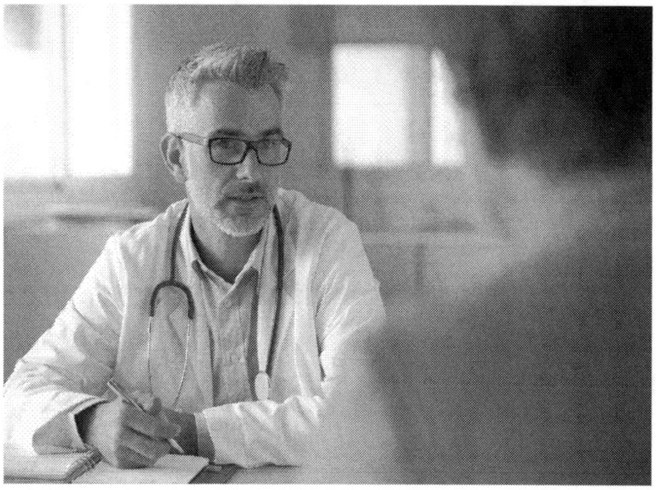

When an error occurs in care of a patient, the error must be reported. Disclosing errors is performed to the patient in person. The person who is responsible needs to disclose the error, explain how the error occurred, express remorse and apologize, and review corrective measures to fix the error. The error should also be reported to appropriate agencies. When a medical error occurs, a medical facility may offer some sort of compensation to the patient to reimburse them for the error, which is a form of settlement.

Medical Directives

Advance Directives

If a person is unable to properly communicate their wishes in medical cases that involve end-of-life care, an **advance directive**, or **living will**, may be developed. The advanced directive allows a person to preemptively determine what kind of care they agree to receive, such as palliative, or to assign a medical durable power of attorney.

Living Will(DNR and DNI)

End-of-life care preferences on behalf of the patient can involve not only an advance directive, but also Do-Not-Resuscitate and Do-Not-Intubate orders. A **DNR order** instructs physicians and other medical personnel that if the patient loses consciousness, is unable to breathe, or otherwise face a disease or disorder that presents with complications that could lead to quality of life impairment, the patient **will not be resuscitated**. **DNI orders** are given to instruct physicians and other medical personnel to **not intubate** a patient in cases where a patient **cannot breathe** on their own. Patients may be able to use other forms of breathing support that do not involve intubation.

Medical Durable Power of Attorney

A **durable power of attorney** document allows a patient to identify **another person** to **make decisions** regarding the patient's healthcare if the patient is unable to do so for whatever reason. The person assigned to make decisions may be referred to as an agent, health care surrogate, or health care proxy. A medical durable power of attorney differs from a living will, or advance directive, in that a living will is established by the patient and most commonly determines care provided at the dying and death stages, while a medical durable power of attorney's goal may be to improve the patient's health and facilitate recovery.

Patient Self Determination Act of 1990

The **Patient Self Determination Act of 1990** was enacted to inform patients of their rights in regards to their own medical care. The act ensures that any hospital a patient is admitted to is up-front about the rights the patient has. This gives the patient the knowledge that they are capable of refusing any medical treatment or surgery, make their own health care decisions, or prepare a living will.

Legal and Ethical Issues Matching

______: Encoding information during transmission to make it impossible to be stolen

______: Rights a patient is assured of having, such as information on services, being able to choose a plan or providers, and having access to emergency services

______: Anything that makes a person legally responsible for every aspect of a medical practice

______: Form of consent in which the patient gives consent verbally or in writing to have treatments or procedures performed

______: A minor being considered mature enough to make medical decisions for themselves

______: A person who acts in good faith on behalf of a patient, determined by a doctor or court

______: Doing no harm

______: Understanding how to deal with people or situations with sensitivity and respect

______: Set of general guidelines ensuring a physician acts with the honesty and integrity, working with the best interest of the patient in mind

______: Order instructing physicians that the patient will not be resuscitated if they lose consciousness, or are unable to breathe

______: Act designed to inform patients of their rights in regards to their own medical care

______: Using electronic systems to write and send prescriptions to pharmacies

______: Drugs that are considered to have the lowest risk of abuse and dependence

______: Agency responsible for combating drug distribution within the United States

______: Intentional tort in which a knowingly false statement is written

______: Writ issued by a court requiring a person to attend a hearing or trial and testify in some way

______: Statement given under oath and outside of court

______: Information about the patient such as medical history, demographic information, laboratory results, and insurance information

______: Drugs that have no accepted medical benefits, and have a high potential for abuse

______: Document allowing a person to preemptively determine what kind of care to receive, or to assign a medical durable power of attorney

A: Mature minor
B: Power of attorney
C: Standards of conduct
D: E-prescribing
E: Patient Self Determination Act
F: Subpoena
G: Patients' Bill of Rights
H: Schedule I drugs
I: Advanced directive
J: Tact
K: Schedule V drugs
L: Nonmaleficence
M: Encryption
N: Protected health information
O: DEA
P: Liability
Q: Libel
R: DNR order
S: Deposition
T: Express consent

Answer Key on Page 292

Legal and Ethical Issues Crossword

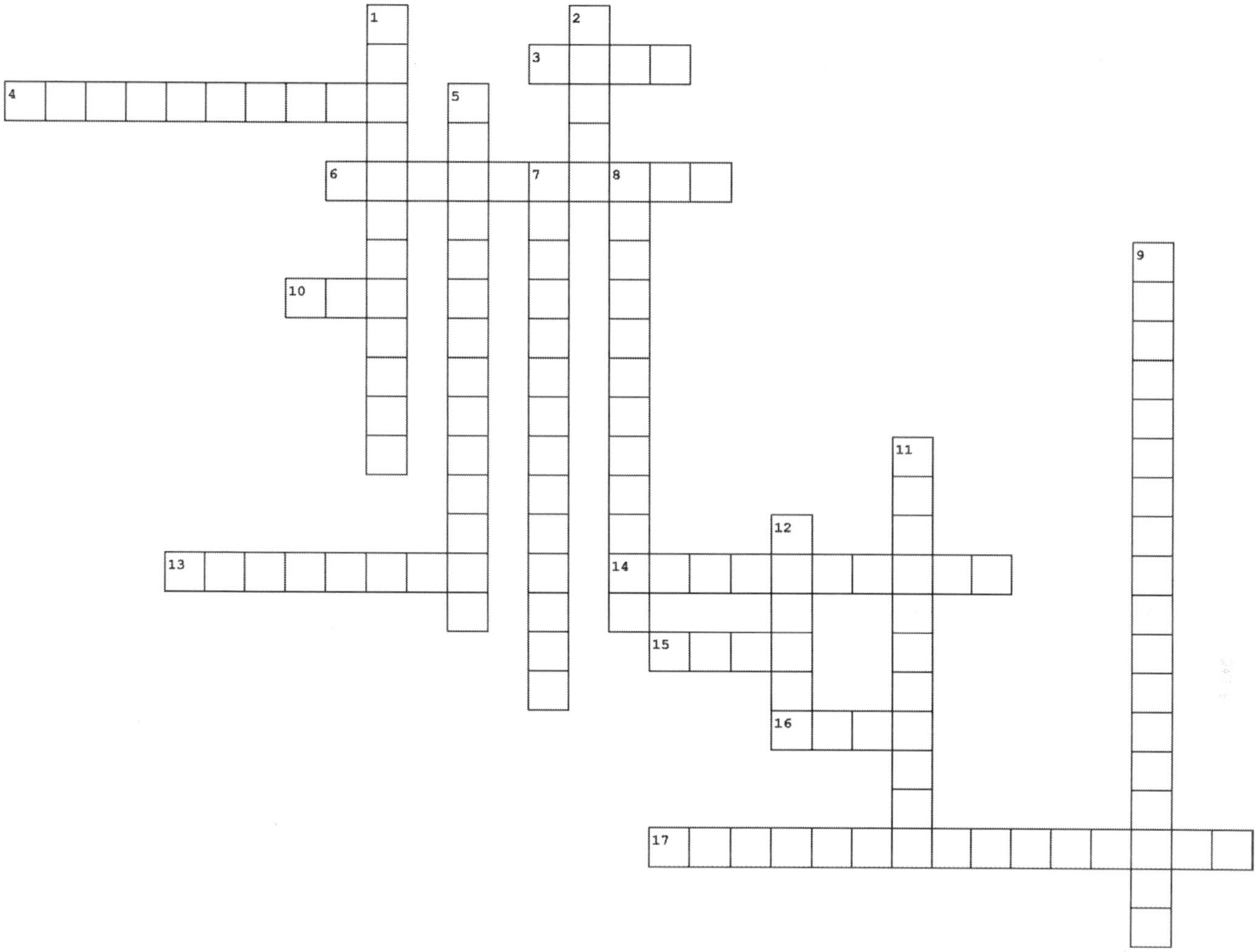

Across

3. Act designed to prevent discrimination in employment or health insurance based on genetic information
4. Alternate name for an advanced directive
6. Adhering to laws, regulations, and guidelines
10. Information protected by HIPAA, abbv.
13. Create barrier between secure and unsecured networks
14. A tort caused by accidental means
15. Number of schedules used to classify controlled substances
16. A person suffering some sort of loss
17. Information regarding the population of an area such as births, deaths, and marriages

Down

1. Rights a patient is assured of having, such as being provided information on services, choose their own plan or providers, and accessing emergency services
2. Act designed to protect all individually identifiable health information
5. A person who is not a senior citizen, but still requires care
7. Assuming a patient who is unable to provide consent would give consent in emergency situations
8. What a patient is considered if they do not follow a prescription, take medication as instructed, or not follow a doctor's direction
9. An employer being held legally responsible for the actions of an employee
11. A form of negligence referring to a medical professional not providing suitable or adequate treatment to a patient in their care
12. Act designed to incentivize the use of electronic health record systems amongst providers

Answer Key on Page 294

Legal and Ethical Issues Practice Test

1. Beneficence refers to
A. The treatment provided to the patient not causing harm to the patient or others
B. The ability of the patient to think and make decisions for themselves
C. New or experimental drugs being distributed and utilized on people from all backgrounds
D. A medical professional always working with the best interest of the patient in mind

2. A set of general guidelines that ensure a physician acts with honesty and integrity
A. Advance directive
B. Compliance
C. Standards of conduct
D. Current standard of care

3. The Patient Care Partnership was developed by the American Hospital Association in order to
A. Help a patient understand their benefits and rights during a hospital visit or stay
B. Providing a patient with information on health services, choose their own health insurance plan or providers, and having access to emergency services such as ambulances
C. Establish general guidelines for physicians to ensure they are acting with honesty and integrity
D. Ensure a patient's medical records are kept private and confidential at all times

4. A dependent adult is a person who
A. Is not a senior citizen but still requires care
B. A person who is under the age of 18 but considered mature enough to make medical decisions for themselves
C. A person who acts in good faith on behalf of another adult
D. A person who is under the age of 18 but lives separately from their parents

5. Which of the following is considered a schedule I drug
A. Tylenol
B. Heroin
C. Xanax
D. Ketamine

6. Which of the following is not considered an intentional tort
A. Negligence
B. Slander
C. Assault
D. Battery

7. Form of consent in which a patient gives their consent verbally or in writing to have procedures or treatments performed
A. Implied
B. Standards of conduct
C. Express
D. Advance directive

8. A patient refusing to follow a certain prescription, take medication as instructed, or generally not follow a doctor's direction results in the patient being considered
A. Libelous
B. Autonomous
C. Negligent
D. Non-compliant

9. HITECH is an act designed for the following
A. Allows a patient to move health insurance from one company to another without interruption of service
B. Incentivize the use of electronic health record systems amongst healthcare providers
C. Prevents discrimination against patients based on age, race, religion, or disabilities
D. Ensures a patient has access to healthcare and will be charged fairly based on standards of care

10. Which of the following must be obtained in order for personal health information to be released to a person who is not the patient
A. Doctor's note
B. Verbal approval by the party who is not the patient
C. Release form signed by the patient
D. Request from the patient's employer

Answer Key on Page 295

Communication

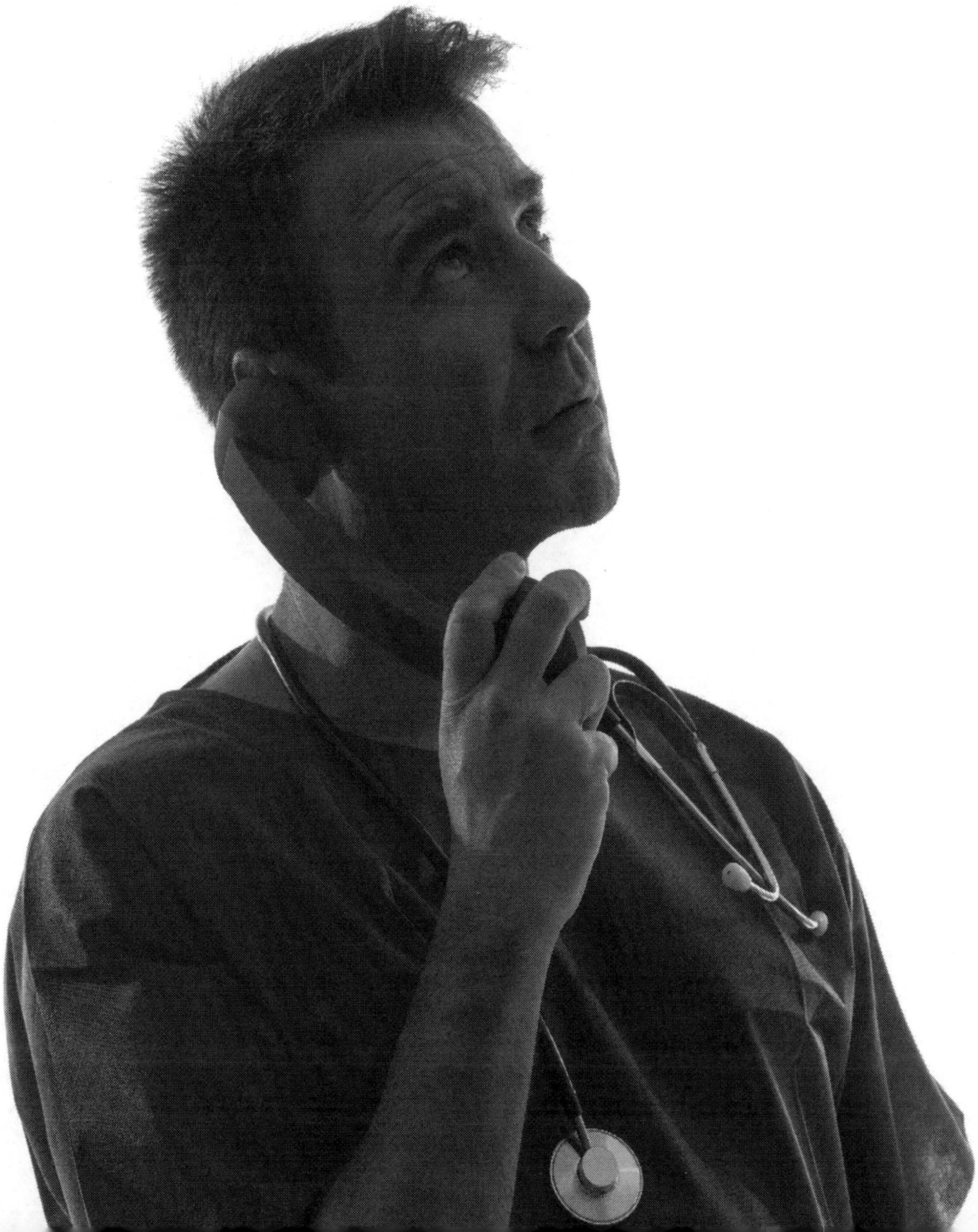

Interpersonal Relationship Skills/Customer Service

Behavioral Theories

Abraham Maslow was an American psychologist who developed the theory known as **Maslow's Hierarchy of Needs**. This theory states that a person has needs that must be fulfilled, starting with the most basic of needs such as food, water, and sleep, to self-actualization.

Physiological Needs: These needs include food, water, sleep, shelter, and sex. These needs are required by the body for survival. If these needs are not met, the other needs in the hierarchy will become more of a secondary thought. Once the needs are met, the other needs are tended to. According to Maslow, physiological needs are considered the most important needs.

Safety Needs: Safety needs primarily pertain to a person feeling a sense of security, order, and stability in their lives.

Love and Belongingness Needs: These needs pertain to social issues, such as friendship, affection, love, and trust. Examples of these needs include friends and family connections.

Esteem Needs: These needs are mostly driven by ego, in which a person seeks respect, status, or recognition in some way. This can involve the person themselves, or they can seek these things from others. Esteem sought from others is considered "lower" esteem, while self-esteem is considered "higher" esteem.

Self-Actualization Needs: Self-actualization is a person realizing their full potential, having a desire for betterment, personal growth, and a desire to learn. These give a person the desire to be the most they can hope to be.

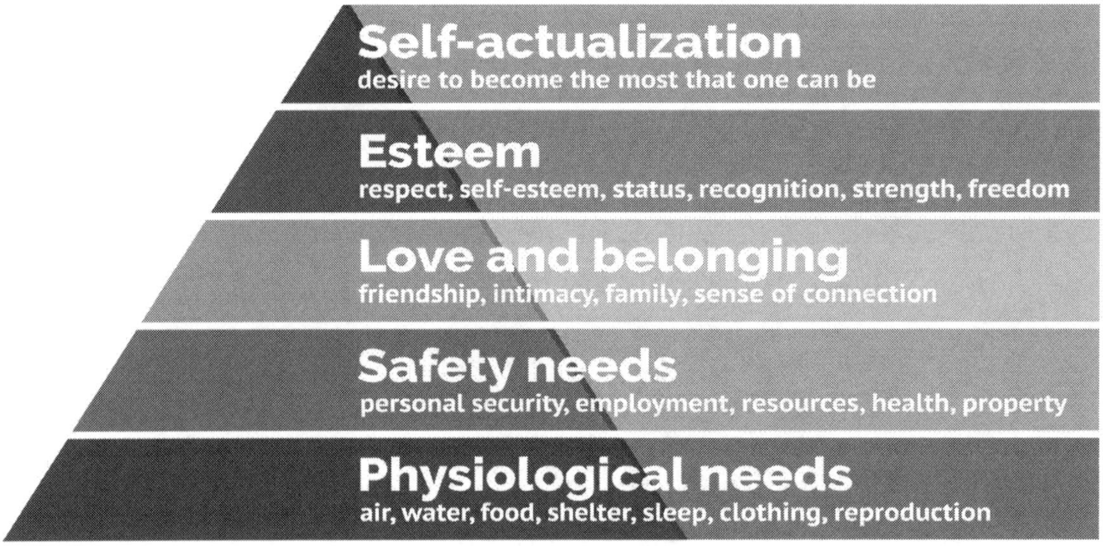

Erik Erikson was a German-American psychologist who developed a theory which states there are **eight stages of psychological development**, developing in a pre-determined order as a person ages. The theory states that completing a stage of psychological development successfully leaves a person with a healthy personality, and the person will have acquired basic virtues. If a person is unable to successfully complete a stage, it may hinder their ability to successfully complete other stages, and the person may develop an unhealthy personality.

Stage 1. Trust vs Mistrust: This stage occurs during the ages of **birth to 18 months**. During this stage, trust is developed by the infant, in which the caregiver provides a stable, consistent environment for the infant to grow in. If this stage is successfully completed, the infant will gain the virtue of **hope**.

Stage 2. Autonomy vs Shame and Doubt: This stage occurs during the ages of **18 months to three years**. During this stage, children are focused on establishing independence and personal control over themselves. Examples may include a child trying to dress themselves or walk on their own. The parent should provide a supportive environment for the child to establish some independence while still seeking help if they need it. If this stage is successfully completed, the child will gain the virtue of **will**.

Stage 3. Initiative vs Guilt: This stage occurs during the ages of **three years to five years.** During this stage, children develop interpersonal skills by interacting with other children during activities such as play. This gives children the confidence to make their own decisions. If a child is discouraged from interacting in this way, a sense of guilt may develop, in which the child may feel bothersome to others. If this stage is successfully completed, the child will gain the virtue of **purpose.**

Stage 4. Industry vs Inferiority: This stage occurs during the ages of **five years to 12 years.** During this stage, the child is inclined to demonstrate their knowledge and ability to complete certain tasks and skills. These skills are seen as valuable to the child, and being able to perform them gives the child a sense of pride and accomplishment. If performing these tasks is not encouraged, the child may begin feeling inferior and doubt may enter the child's mind about their abilities. If this stage is successfully completed, the child will gain the virtue of **competence.**

Stage 5. Identity vs Role Confusion: This stage occurs during the ages of **12 years to 18 years.** During this stage, children search for a sense of identity, exploring personal views and beliefs. This helps the child develop morals and ethics, and learn the role they will play in adulthood. If this stage is successfully completed, the child will gain the virtue of **fidelity.**

Stage 6. Intimacy vs Isolation: This stage occurs during the ages of **18 years to 40 years.** During this stage, internal conflict primarily centers around creating intimate relationships. If intimacy is avoided, a person may become isolated and depressed. If this stage is successfully completed, the person will gain the virtue of **love.**

Stage 7. Generativity vs Stagnation: This stage occurs during the ages of **40 years to 65 years.** During this stage, a person is focused on leaving a lasting mark on the world through things like helping others, raising children, and being successful. Failure to accomplish these goals may lead to a person feeling stagnant, disconnected, or unproductive. If this stage is successfully completed, the person will gain the virtue of **care.**

Stage 8. Ego Integrity vs Despair: This stage occurs during the ages of **65 years to death.** During this stage, a person looks back at their life and accomplishments. While looking back, a person may feel as if their life cycle was as it was, and is accepting of this fact. If a person experiences doubt about their life experiences, or guilt relating to things that happened during life, they may have a sense of dissatisfaction and enter a stage of despair. If this stage is successfully completed, the person will gain the virtue of **wisdom.**

Defense Mechanisms

Denial, a common defense mechanism, is a refusal to acknowledge a given situation, or acting as if something didn't happen.

Displacement is often negative. Displacement is satisfying an impulse by **substitution.** An example could be, you have a very bad day at work or school, you go home, and instead of being upset at school or work, you lash out at a significant other. Releasing your pent-up emotions at something other than what is causing the emotions.

Projection is placing one's own internal feelings onto **someone else.** An example could be my wife: when she gets hungry, she becomes easily agitated. She'll then accuse me of being in a bad mood, even though I'm feeling great. This is projection. For the record, this happens a lot.

Regression is taking a **step back** psychologically when faced with stress. An example could be quitting smoking. A person doesn't smoke for a few days, and then they are presented with a stressful situation, which causes them to regress and smoke again.

Repression is subconsciously **blocking out** unwanted emotions. Not even knowing you have something to be upset about. Your mind can erase certain memories to help protect you from stress.

Adapting Communication for Terminally Ill Patients

During the death and dying stage, it is important to understand that people come from many different backgrounds and cultures, and have many different views and beliefs in regards to death and grieving. There is no right or wrong way for a person to grieve, and it is appropriate for the medical professional to allow a person to process the death of a loved one in the way that they choose. Religion may play a role in the death/dying stages of a person's life, with religious figures providing comfort or aid to the grieving party or ill person. These practices should be respected.

Medical professionals who work in settings with terminally ill patients should understand their own views on death and dying, to form a better working relationship with those they treat. Self-reflection of one's own personal views on death and dying can also bring forth views the medical professional may personally disagree with, allow the medical professional to understand personal biases they may hold, and develop the ability to adapt one's own views when placed in a situation with others who are not like-minded.

When working specifically with a terminally ill patient, it is important that medical professionals carefully navigate their communication. Honestly is an important aspect of communication with terminally ill patients. Optimism may be appreciated, but false hopes and promises should never be given to the patient, and realistic expectations should be identified. Terminally ill patients should be treated with compassion and sympathy. In addition, these communication techniques should also extend to the patient's family, and helping the family understand the situation is important to help them find comfort and prepare for the passing of the patient.

Adapting Communication for Visually Impaired Patients

A person who is visually impaired may require special attention when receiving care. Verbal communication is key. Speaking the patient's name informs the patient that they are being spoken to. The patient may need to be physically touched or moved by a medical professional to perform specific actions that are easier understood visually. The patient should also be verbally notified when the medical professional is entering or leaving the room.

Adapting Communication for Hearing Impaired Patients

Patients who are hearing impaired also require special attention. Some patients may utilize hearing aids, while others may not. Some patients may have partial hearing impairment, or impairment in one ear, while others may have total hearing impairment. For hearing impaired patients, visual cues are the most effective forms of communication. Some patients with hearing impairment may be able to read lips. Others may utilize sign language. Others may simply write their thoughts on paper or electronic devices to communicate. Body language may be an effective form of communication. Proper lighting should be utilized when communicating with a hearing impaired patient so they can properly read lips, expression, and body language. An interpreter may be utilized if the patient uses sign language, but the medical professional does not.

Adapting Communication for Non-English Speaking Patients

Patients may utilize an interpreter if the medical professional they are communicating with cannot understand the language the patient is using. When communicating, the medical professional should be looking at the patient instead of the interpreter. Questions being relayed through an interpreter should be easy to understand, and be short to allow the interpreter to properly translate the question for the patient. A family member may act as the interpreter for the patient. A good strategy for communicating effectively with patients who speak another language is to research and learn relevant words in the patient's native language, easing the burden placed upon interpreters and forming a stronger relationship with the patient.

Illiteracy

There are different forms of illiteracy a medical professional may encounter. **Reading illiteracy** occurs when a patient is unable to **read and/or write**, or has a certain level of difficulty with these tasks. Communicating with these patients may present certain challenges. Medical professionals using simple terms when speaking, and asking open-ended questions may assist the patient in understanding and properly communicating. Pictures may be utilized in certain circumstances to obtain information, such as with pain scales.

Medical illiteracy occurs when a patient is **unable to understand and utilize medical information** given to them. This can be detrimental to the patient's health and outcomes. A patient who is unable to understand their own healthcare may lead the patient to misinterpreting directions given, or simply ignore prescriptions and suggestions from their physicians. When communicating with a person who may be medically illiterate, simple terms should be utilized, and examples should be given that help the patient understand their healthcare more appropriately.

Adapting Communication for Intellectually Challenged Patients

Communication with a patient who is intellectually challenged requires patience on behalf of the medical professional. Any instructions or questions presented to the patient should be worded simply. Communicating effective treatment planning with the patient's caregiver can assist in the patient understanding what is being said. Patients should be treated the same as any other. Communication should be slower, but not louder.

Adapting Communication for Geriatric Patients

Communication with geriatric patients offers different challenges. Geriatric patients should be communicated with by using active listening, and allowing the patient to expand upon aspects of their health. Geriatric patients enjoy respectful conversation, without feeling overwhelmed with the use of expansive medical language. Some geriatric patients may have difficulty understanding technology, and medical equipment, devices, or patient portals the patient is charged with using should be carefully explained to the patient with instructions on proper usage. Written directions may be beneficial to the patient.

Adapting Communication for Pediatric/Adolescent Patients

Pediatric/adolescent patients may be communicated with by developing a rapport with the patient. With pediatric patients, having a positive, up-beat attitude can help put the patient's mind at ease. When talking with a pediatric patient, the medical professional may squat down to eye level with the patient, helping the patient feel as if they are on equal ground as the medical professional. Smiling, laughing, joking, and using the patient's name can help a pediatric/adolescent patient feel more comfortable and instill trust and familiarity with the medical professional. Laying out each step of the appointment may be beneficial due to some patients feeling more comfortable with the knowledge of each step involved.

Americans with Disabilities Act Amendments Act

The **Americans with Disabilities Act Amendments Act**, also known as **ADAAA**, was originally enacted in 1990, but has since been amended as of 2009. ADAAA was enacted to **prevent discrimination** against people with **disabilities** in the workplace or school settings. It states a person with a disability is to be given reasonable accommodations to help the person function or learn optimally in a specific environment. It prevents a person who is disabled from being discriminated against in the hiring or firing process, or potential advancement in a company.

Non-Verbal Communication

Body language is a form of **unspoken communication**, in which a person is able to communicate through conscious or subconscious gestures. **Facial expression** can convey a person's current emotion, such as happiness. **Posture** can express whether a person is open and willing to engage or closed and hostile or anxious. **Eye contact**, avoiding eye contact, the space a person leaves between others while communicating, and **crossing the arms** across the chest are all other examples of body language, and can be interpreted in many different ways.

Personal Boundaries

Personal boundaries are **limitations** a person sets in their own life regarding numerous aspects. Examples of these examples are topics of conversation, physical touch, time boundaries, and more. These boundaries should be implied, as assumptions can be made that the majority of people have similar personal boundaries. Violation of a person's personal boundaries may lead to loss of business, loss of respect, loss of employment in cases such as sexual harassment and bullying, and up to incarceration in cases such as sexual assault.

De-escalation Techniques

De-escalating occurs when there is an person or professional issue that is becoming more aggressive, and a person helps to **calm the situation**. These techniques can be vital in numerous aspects, from retaining customers to preventing litigation efforts. When communicating with a patient and attempting to de-escalate a situation, consideration should be made to moving the conversation to a private area. Remaining calm can help the patient calm themselves and think rationally and logically about the situation. Empathy should be utilized to help build trust with the patient. Any body language utilized should remain as neutral as possible, and not appear aggressive. Active listening should be utilized. Solutions may be sought, or a patient may just want to have their voice heard. Eye contact should be utilized when possible to let the patient know they have full and undivided attention.

If criticism is made of the employee in regards to their work, the employee should not take it personally or become deeply offended. The employee should consider things from an unbiased point of view, see how the criticism may be valid, and try to change the behavior being criticized if necessary.

Listening Skills

Active listening is listening to what the patient is saying, and **actively interpreting** the information being given. The patient's statements are being paid attention to, and the patient has the full focus of the medical assistant while they are speaking. This allows the medical assistant to respond to and remember what is being said.

Passive listening is listening to a patient **without responding.** Passive listening does not require the listener to engage the talker in conversation or ask questions in response. This can result in the mind wandering, and details being provided by the patient to be forgotten.

Service Recovery/Patient Satisfaction

Many aspects form the basis of patient satisfaction. The primary way of ensuring patient satisfaction is properly caring for the patient. This involves proper diagnosis, treatment, after-care, listening, and communicating with the patient.

Customer service is an important priority for a medical office to retain patients. Treating patients with kindness, respect, sympathy, understanding, and compassion can lead to the patient feeling that their time, money, and health are all important to the medical office. Patients who feel desired by the medical office often return, and refer others to the practice. This increases profit and sustainability for the office.

Empathy and Sympathy

During conversation, a person may exhibit empathy or sympathy in response to another person and their situation. **Empathy** is when a person puts themselves in the shoes of another, viewing a situation from the other person's point of view. **Sympathy** is when a person feels compassion or pity for the other person and the situation they are in.

Therapeutic/Adaptive Responses

Cultural Diversity and Beliefs

Patients vary in many aspects, including in culture and belief systems. With any patient, beliefs and cultural diversity should be respected. Asking questions is an appropriate method of obtaining information if the proper course of action in dealing with different cultures is not apparent. Every patient should be treated equally, and each patient should be respected regardless of their background or beliefs.

Recognize Stereotypes and Biases

Stereotypes and biases exist within every person in some way. It is important to understand that these stereotypes and biases can influence behavior, and to ensure that care of a patient is not affected. Self-reflection can determine what biases exist, and how a person can better respond to ensure that these biases to not influence the care provided to a patient who may be different than the medical professional in some way. Every patient should be treated the same, and respect should be given to every patient.

Learning Styles

Assessing and Adapting to Level of Understanding

Communication is a key factor in properly treating a patient. Understanding in communication begins with an initial statement or idea made by a sender. The sender presents the statement or idea to a receiver. The receiver is then responsible for providing feedback. This process may loop many times until an understanding has been reached between the sender and receiver.

Overcoming Barriers to Communication

At times, a person may have difficulty properly communicating due to varying barriers. Some barriers may include the patient dealing with pain or hunger, the surrounding environment being too loud or distracting, the patient thinking about something and not paying attention, or the current situation making the patient upset. Assessing the situation and what is preventing the conversation from flowing optimally is vital, and should be managed to allow proper dialogue to occur. An example, if the patient is not communicating because they are hungry, offering them some sort of snack may lead to the patient being more open and willing to converse.

Health Care Team Roles

Understanding/Communicating Plan of Care

An example of an appointment protocol would be a **doctor referral**. Many insurances will require a referral for most any provider or service other than the PCP. Sometimes it is the individual provider, usually a specialist, that will require a referral regardless of the insurance. The provider will not see the patient without first **authorizing the referral**, or without first having the insurance authorize the referral. It is important to follow the protocol and not schedule an appointment without an authorized referral. This will ensure that the provider will see the patient and/or that the insurance will cover the appointment costs.

Patient Navigator/Advocate

A **patient navigator** is a person who works within a medical system and **helps patients** with their needs within that system. Patient navigators help patients gain access to numerous healthcare related tests and screenings. Navigators can help explain financial information, legal information, finding healthcare providers and physicians, and explaining treatments and options the patient has. Many navigators are nurses, and many navigators have no medical background and are trained by different medical associations to be an effective navigator.

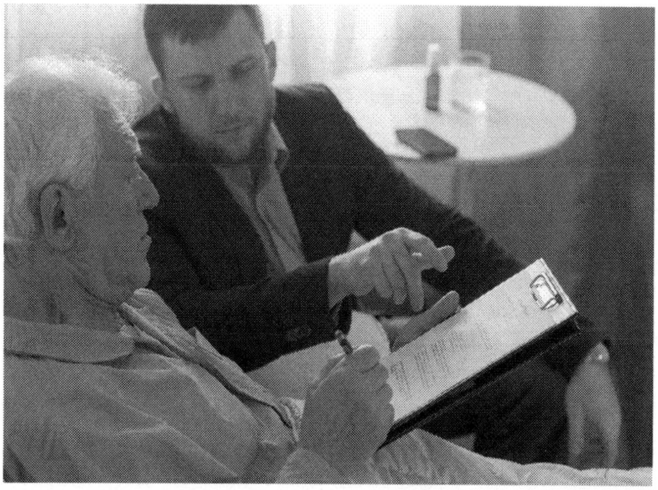

Utilizing Team Approach to Patient Care

Operating and functioning effectively as a team, in which each person has their specific roles in the running of the medical office, are a vital step in patient care management. Communication between team members is vital. A hierarchy in which one person leads the team can be beneficial.

Teams do not just extend to the immediate office, but can also involve other offices and specialists. A patient who has surgery to repair a torn ACL would also likely require the help of a physical therapist. The surgeon, primary care physician, and physical therapist working together as a team and sharing patient information agreed upon by the patient can help the patient have a positive outcome with their treatment.

Medical Specialties

Anesthesiology is the use of medications that cause a patient to **lose sensation** while performing surgery. These types of medications can be used **locally** or **generally**. Examples of medications administered by anesthesiologists include ketamine, propofol, and diazepam. The type of medication administered is dependent on the type or surgery, the length of surgery, and the overall health of the patient.

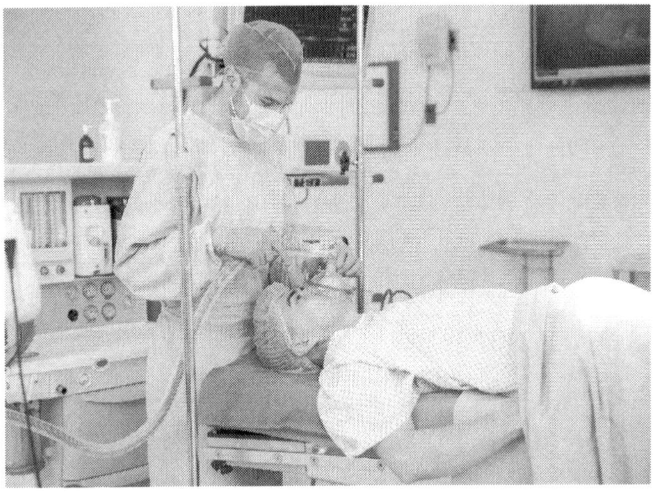

Dermatology is the study of the **skin**. Treatment of skin diseases is the primary function of a dermatologist. Examples of skin diseases include skin cancers such as basal cell carcinoma, acne, warts, and other forms of growths and lesions that may damage the skin or harm the body in some way. Abnormal growths may be surgically removed by a dermatologist.

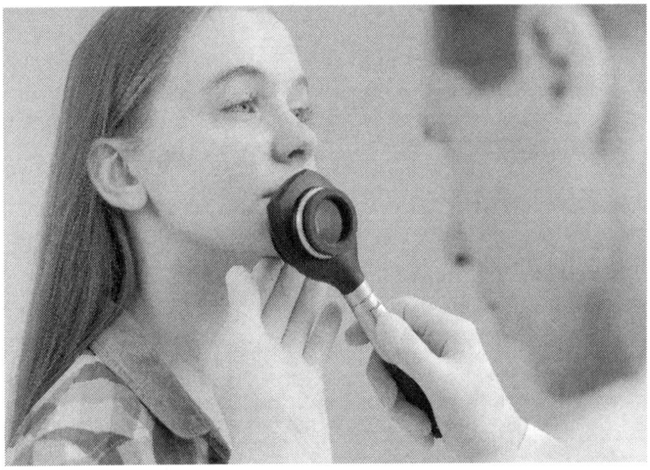

Cardiology is the study of the **heart** and diseases associated with the **heart** or **blood vessels**. A primary function of a cardiologist is to administer and interpret ECG/EKGs, which give the cardiologist an overall view of the function of the heart. Patient education is an important factor of cardiology, with a focus on proper health and nutrition to reduce the likelihood of the development of heart disease.

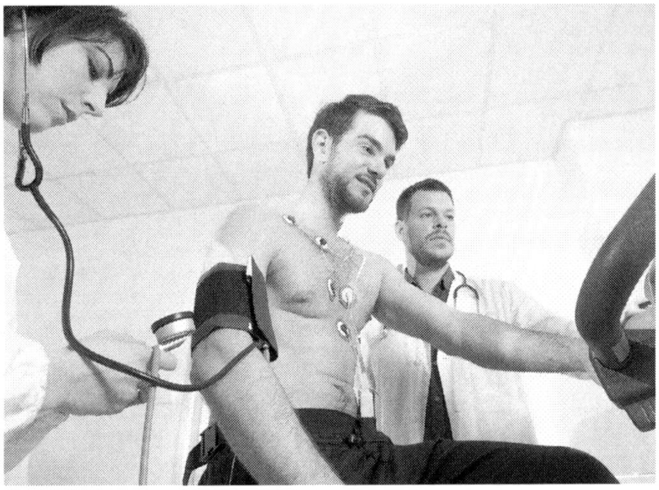

Emergency Medicine is practiced by a physician who specializes in **emergency situations**. These doctors work in a hospital's emergency room, dealing with conditions such as physical trauma and injuries that may be life-threatening if not treated quickly.

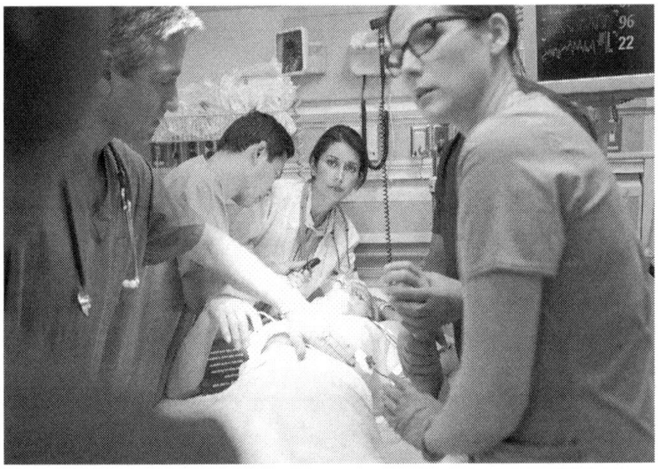

Endocrinology is the study of the **endocrine glands** and diseases that may be involved with the glands. Examples may include hyperthyroidism, which may produce a goiter, Addison's disease, and Graves' disease. Endocrinologists may work with other specialists to determine if there may be tumors present on any glands that are affecting hormone production.

Gastroenterology is the study of the **digestive tract**. Gastroenterologists specifically deal with digestive disorders and problems, ranging from GERD to Crohn's disease. Gastroenterologists utilize endoscopy to view the inner walls of organs such as the esophagus, stomach, and large intestine. This allows a view of potential issues such as ulcers or tumors that may be causing digestive problems.

Gerontology is the study of the **aging process**. A branch of gerontology is geriatrics, which is the diagnosis and treatment of aging related medical conditions.

Gynecology is the study of the **female reproductive system**. Gynecologists check the health of the female reproductive system by performing general examinations, performing testing such as Pap smears, and providing medication when needed. Gynecologists are often also obstetricians, who deal with pregnancy, labor, delivery, and post-labor.

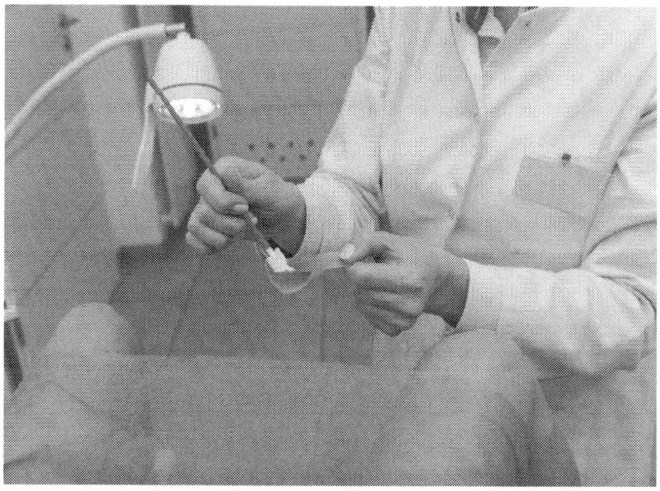

Obstetrics is the study of **pregnancy**, **labor**, **child delivery**, and **postpartum**. Obstetrics is commonly practiced by gynecologists. A person who practices both gynecology and obstetrics is known as as obstetrician/gynecologist(OB/GYN).

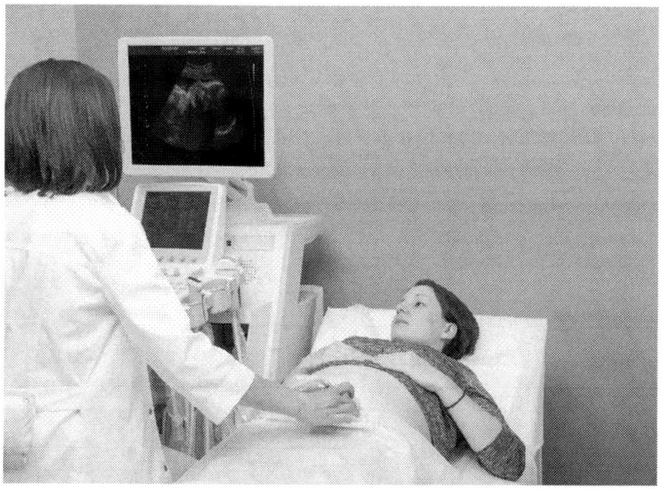

Ophthalmology is the study of the **eye**. An ophthalmologist is a person who diagnoses medical conditions associated with the eye. There are numerous tests an ophthalmologist may perform to test a person's vision, ranging from the use of Snellen and E charts to physical examination of the eyeball itself.

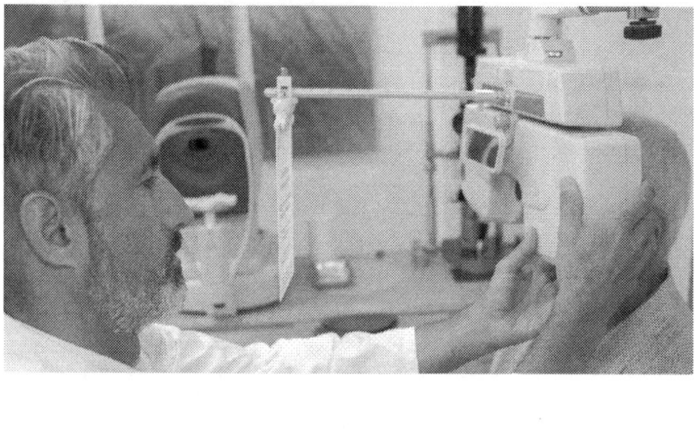

Internal Medicine is specializing in the **internal organs** of the body. Examples of internists include cardiologists, endocrinologists, nephrologists, and gastroenterologists.

Nephrology is the study of the **kidneys**. Nephrologists diagnose any medical conditions that occur with the kidneys, from kidney failure to infections such as pyelonephritis. Nephrologists administer **dialysis** in cases of kidney disease, both peritoneal dialysis and hemodialysis. If the patient is located further away from the medical office where dialysis is to take place, the nephrologist may assist the patient with education on operating a mobile dialysis machine.

Neurology is the study of the **nerves** and **nervous system**. Neurologists diagnose any medical condition that occurs with the nerves or brain, such as strokes, neuropathy, and paralysis. Neurologists may implement tools such as reflex hammers to test the reflexes in joints, and electroencephalograms to monitor brain wave activity.

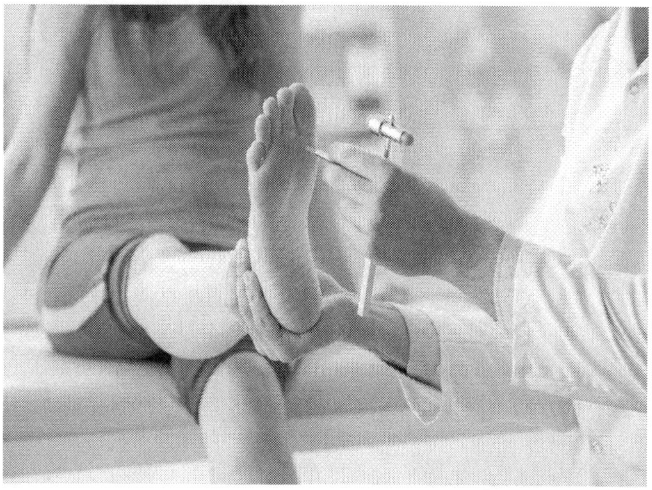

Oncology is the study of **tumors**. An oncologist studies tumors to determine the type of tumor, whether benign or malignant. Oncologists also treat patients who have cancer. Treatments an oncologist administers includes chemotherapy or radiation therapy.

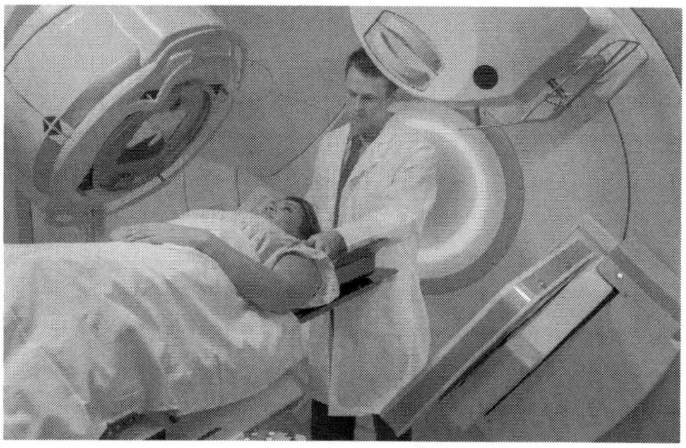

Orthopedics is a branch of surgical medicine that deals specifically with the **muscles** and **bones**. Orthopedic surgeons may specialize in a certain type of patient, such as sports medicine specialists. Orthopedic surgeons commonly perform joint replacements, repair of soft tissues, and spinal fusion surgeries.

Otorhinolaryngology is the study of the **ear**, **nose**, and **throat**. Otorhinolaryngologists may also be called **ENT**(Ear, Nose, and Throat) specialists. ENT specialists diagnose and treat medical conditions associated with the ear, nose, and throat such as tinnitus, sinusitis, and laryngitis.

Pediatrics is the study of the development of **children**. A pediatrician will primarily focus on a child's development, measuring whether or not the child is meeting certain developmental milestones in weight, height, and mentally. Pediatricians will also diagnose and treat medical conditions a child may experience, and educate parents on how to keep their child healthy.

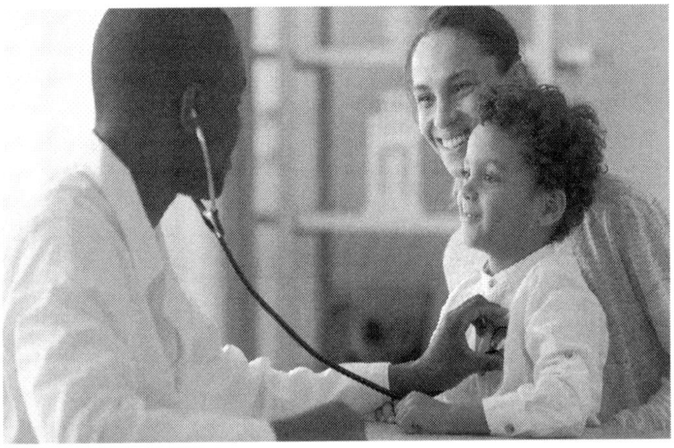

Plastic Surgery is a branch of surgery performed by plastic surgeons that involves **correction** or **reconstruction** of body parts that have not formed properly or have been damaged in some way. Plastic surgery may also be cosmetically beneficial to the patient, which may help with mental health. Common plastic surgeries include breast augmentation, rhinoplasty, abdominoplasty, and hair transplantation.

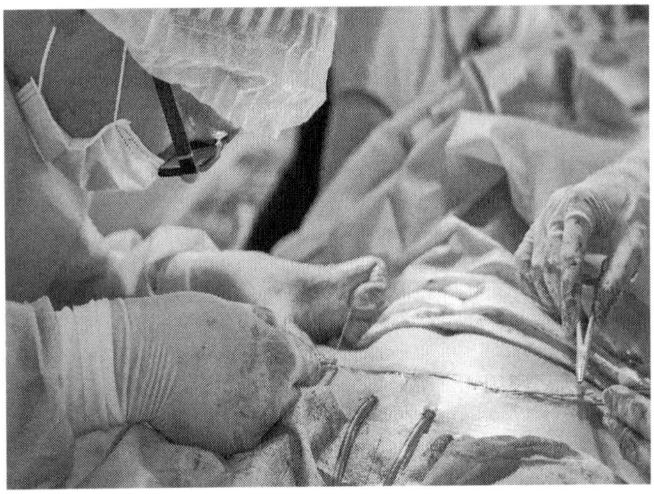

Radiology is the use of **X-rays** and radioactive substances to view internal structures. Viewing internal structures may help to diagnose certain diseases and develop treatment plans. A radiologist is a person who administers the X-ray, and they then read the X-ray.

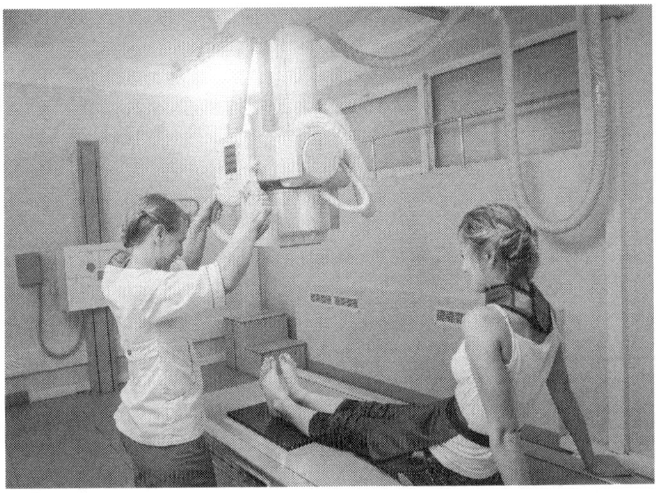

Urology is the study of the **kidney**, **bladder**, and entire **urinary tract**. A urologist will diagnose medical conditions associated with the urinary tract, commonly by collecting urine samples and performing urinalysis on the sample.

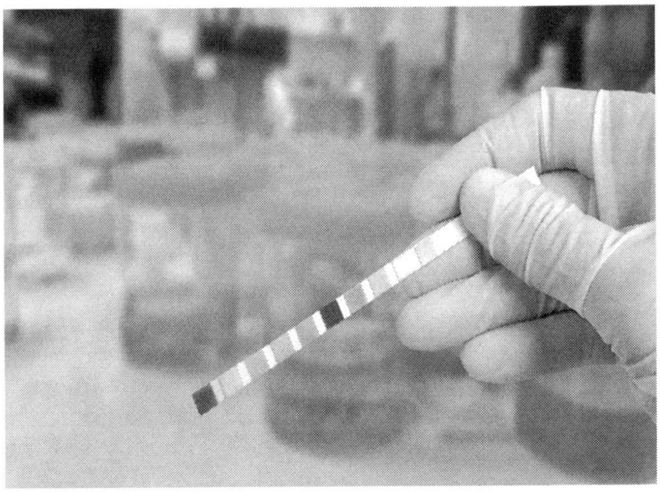

Professional Telephone Etiquette/Techniques

Message Protocols

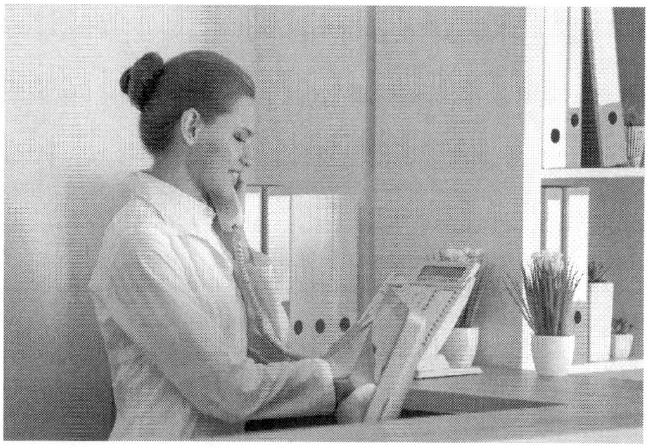

Taking correct messages is extremely important. Each medical office has their own system in place for taking messages. PHI should always be met with caution. It is vital that the message is sent to the correct person in the medical office. Messages should be taken using precise and condensed language, which allows the message to be understood quickly and easily. If the message is urgent, it should be noted as such. The caller's name and phone number should be double checked to ensure the information is correct.

Leaving messages properly is just as important as taking messages. The person leaving the message should clearly identify themselves and the office they are calling from, leave the correct number to return the call, and the hours of operation for the office. The message may contain a generalized statement, such as requesting an appointment be rescheduled, or to confirm the time of an appointment. Messages should be brief, polite, and spoken clearly and slowly so the person receiving the message can understand and take notes if needed.

Screening/Gathering Data

Occasionally a patient will call to make an appointment or ask for advice on dealing with symptoms that require emergency care. The person scheduling appointments should be familiar with signs and symptoms of stroke, heart attack, substance abuse withdrawal, and traumatic events. If the patient or the person they are calling for is exhibiting any of these signs or symptoms, they should be transferred to emergency medical services or 911. The caller's permission must be obtained beforehand, and the permission or refusal needs to be documented. Upon transfer, the person should stay connected with the 911 operator until they approve the transfer of the phone connection. If the caller disconnects before the connection can be transferred, the 911 operator should be made aware of the situation.

Communication Matching

______: A person who works within a medical system and helps patients with their needs within the system

______: Refusal to acknowledge a given situation

______: Limitations a person sets in their own life regarding numerous aspects, such as topics of conversation, physical touch, and time

______: Needs detailed by Maslow involving friendship, affection, love, and trust

______: A patient being unable to understand and utilize medical information given to them

______: A person putting themselves in the shoes of another, viewing a situation from the other person's point of view

______: Study of the endrocrine glands and diseases involved with the glands

______: Stage of psychological development detailed by Erikson occurring from birth to 18 months

______: Unspoken communication performed using conscious and subconscious gestures

______: Study of pregnancy, labor, child delivery, and postpartum

______: Study of the development of children

______: Needs detailed by Maslow mostly driven by ego, such as respect, status, and recognition

______: Act designed to prevent discrimination against people with disabilities in the workplace or school setting

______: Satisfying an impulse by substitution

______: A person being unable to read and/or write, or has a certain level of difficulty with these tasks

______: The use of medications that cause a patient to lose sensation while performing surgery

______: Stage of psychological development detailed by Erikson occurring from the ages 65 years to death

______: Subconsciously blocking out unwanted emotions

______: A person feeling compassion or pity for another person and the situation they are in

______: Listening to what a patient is saying and interpreting the information being given

A: Empathy
B: Repression
C: Displacement
D: Trust vs Mistrust
E: Sympathy
F: Esteem Needs
G: Reading illiteracy
H: Denial
I: ADAAA
J: Pediatrics
K: Personal boundaries
L: Endocrinology
M: Obstetrics
N: Love and Belongingness Needs
O: Ego Integrity vs Despair
P: Anesthesiology
Q: Body language
R: Patient navigator
S: Active listening
T: Medical illiteracy

Answer Key on Page 292

Communication Crossword

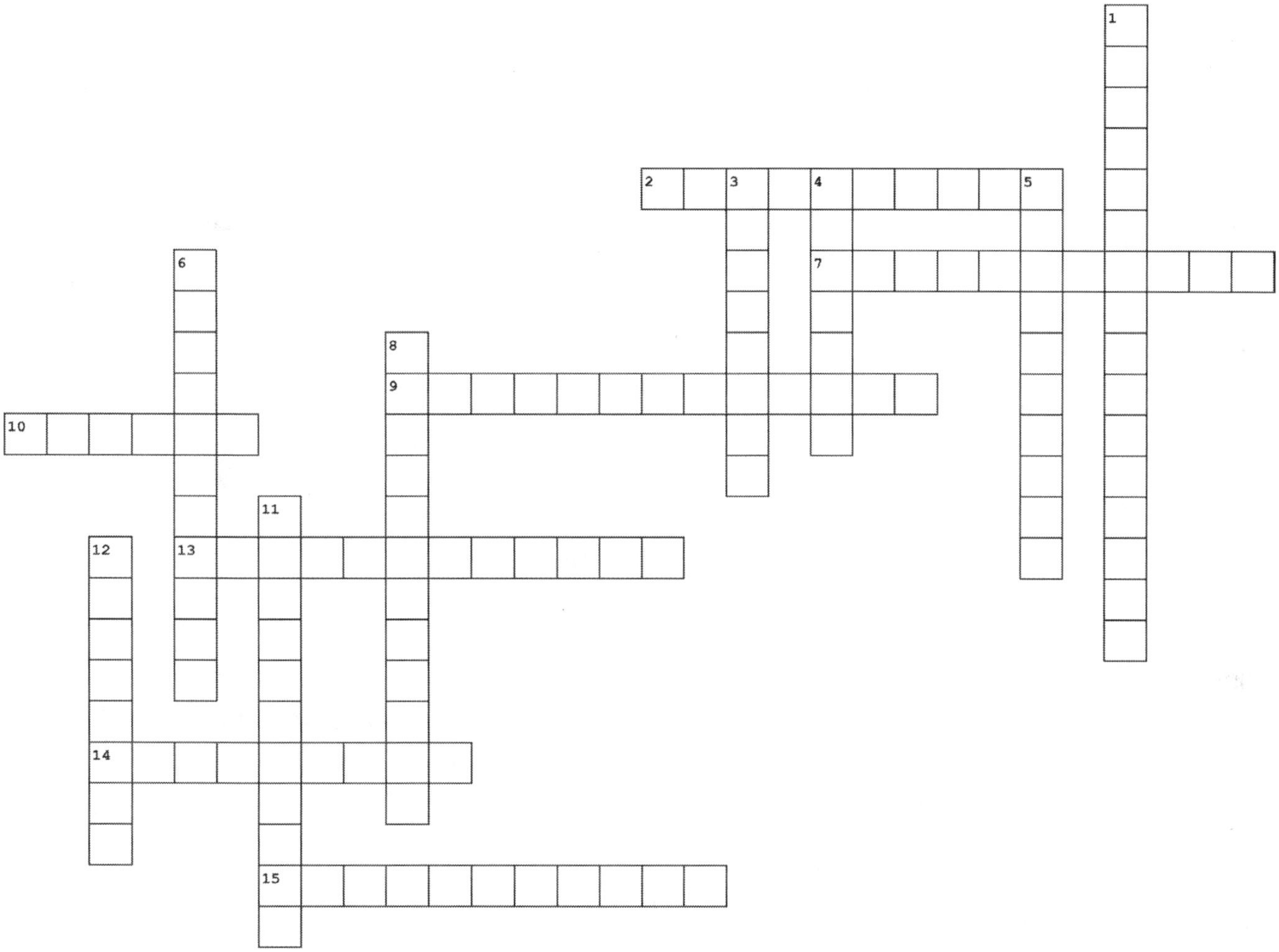

Across

2. Placing one's own internal feelings onto someone else
7. A person who translates one language to another as an intermediate party
9. The study of the eye
10. American psychologist who developed the Hierarchy of Needs
13. Calming a situation that is becoming increasingly more aggressive
14. The use of X-rays and radioactive substances to view internal structures
15. The study of the aging process

Down

1. Listening to a patient without responding
3. The study of tumors
4. German psychologist who developed the eight stages of psychological development
5. The study of the kidneys
6. Branch of surgical medicine that deals specifically with the muscles and bones
8. Facial expression, posture, and eye contact are all forms of this
11. The study of the skin
12. Document received from a doctor to have a specific test or treatment performed by another specialist

Answer Key on Page 294

Communication Practice Test

1. Of the following, which is not one of the eight stages of psychological development proposed by Erik Erikson
A. Identity vs Role Confusion
B. Ego Integrity vs Despair
C. Love vs Loneliness
D. Trust vs Mistrust

2. All of the following are effective means of communication with intellectually challenged patients except
A. Giving simple instructions
B. Slower communication
C. Relaying information to the patient's caregiver
D. Using extensive explanations

3. Gerontology is the study of
A. The female reproductive system
B. The aging process
C. The kidneys
D. Tumors

4. A medically illiterate patient is a patient who
A. Is unable to understand and/or utilize medical information
B. Is unable to administer prescription doses effectively
C. Is unable to or has difficulty in reading or writing
D. Is unable to describe symptoms they are experiencing

5. Which of the following best describes the defense mechanism of projection
A. Taking a step back psychologically when faced with stress
B. Satisfying an impulse by substitution
C. Placing one's own internal feelings onto someone else
D. Subconsciously blocking out unwanted emotions

6. Act designed to prevent discrimination against people with disabilities in the workplace or school settings
A. HIPAA
B. CLIA
C. ADAAA
D. GINA

7. Which psychological stage proposed by Erik Erikson details a child exploring personal views and beliefs, helping the child develop morals and ethics, and learn the role they will play in adulthood
A. Generativity vs Stagnation
B. Initiative vs Guilt
C. Industry vs Inferiority
D. Identity vs Role Confusion

8. A person who helps another person who does not speak a specific language communicate with others who do
A. Navigator
B. Interpreter
C. Advocate
D. Custodian

9. Specialists who work specifically with the eye
A. Ophthalmologists
B. Urologists
C. Obstetricians
D. Nephrologists

10. Needs detailed by Maslow that are primarily driven by ego, such as respect, status, or recognition
A. Safety
B. Esteem
C. Self-actualization
D. Physiological

Answer Key on Page 295

Billing, Coding, Insurance, and Scheduling

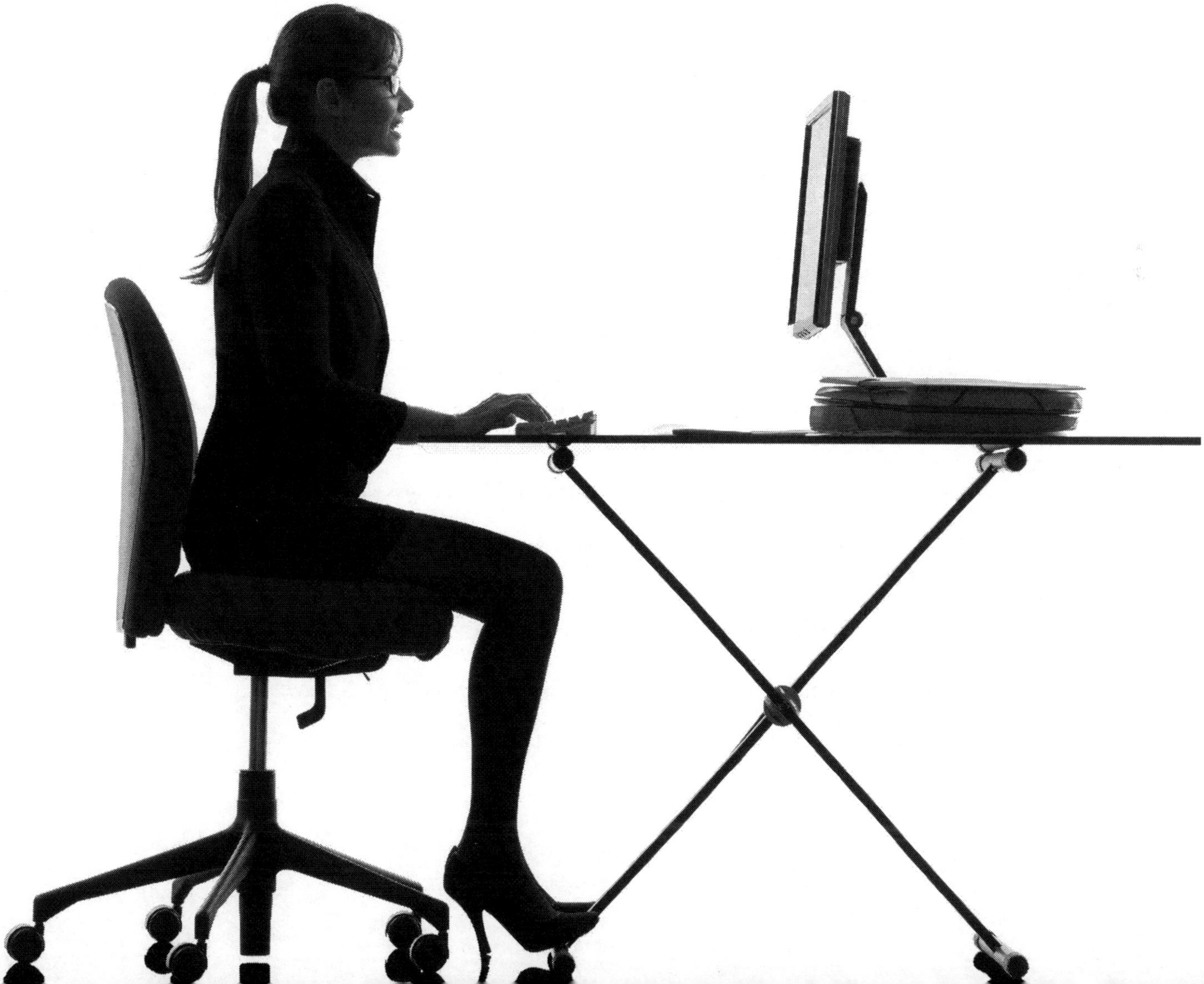

Coding Applications

Procedural Coding

Medical coding is translating medical diagnoses, equipment, and procedures into an **alphanumerical code**. This is done to provide correct claims to insurance companies. Medical codes are able to be utilized across medical fields. There are several different types of codes, which are utilized for different types of diagnoses.

CPT, which stands for **Current Procedural Terminology**, is a coding set used for reporting medical procedures such as **surgeries**. Modifiers are used to further describe these procedures, adding an additional two digits to the code.

CPT modifiers are used to add information to an original code. Modifiers typically involve additional information about surgical procedures, and provide details that cannot be described just using the original code. CPT modifiers are two digits. Some of the most common CPT modifiers are 25(physician provides another completely separate service to a patient on the same day as another service), 59(distinct procedural service when no other modifier can apply), and 91(repeat laboratory tests on the same day for the same patient). Modifiers are updated annually.

Upcoding is a **fraudulent and illegal act**, in which a bill for a health service **costs more** than is necessary based on the service or treatment provided. This is usually performed by the code being sent for a **different service** than the service the patient received. For example, if a patient's order calls for a routine physical examination, but it is billed for the examination with tests performed that were not called for nor performed, it is considered upcoding.

Downcoding is the alternate of upcoding, in which a provider bills for services at rates **lower** than what should be charged. Downcoding may involve certain parts of service **not being reported** in an effort to get the claim approved. This may be done in instances where certain aspects of a service or treatment would most likely have the claim denied. This can be harmful to the patient because incorrect coding is being used, and the full details of services, treatments, and/or diagnostic testing are not being submitted.

Bundling of charges is performed to make it easier to manage payments for the treatment received. An example, if a patient is receiving an injection, that is one code. What is being injected is another code. The reason for the injection may be another code. Bundling these all together creates one payment instead of three separate payments.

Unbundling occurs when multiple codes are used for a service or treatment that has been provided, which increases the cost of the service or treatment, and provides a larger reimbursement for the facility. This is a form of fraud, and is similar to upcoding.

Diagnostic Coding

ICD-11(International Classification of Diseases, created by the World Health Organization) is utilized to code for **morbidity**, or **cause of death**.

E-codes, which stands for **external cause of injury**, is used to detail the cause of an injury, poisoning, or adverse reactions to drugs or medications.

M-codes, which stands for **morphology**, are used by tumor registries to identify **tumors and abnormal growths**.

Z-codes, formerly V-codes under ICD-9-CM, are used to describe circumstances other than disease or injury. Examples include **preventative care**, **chemotherapy**, or **radiation therapy**.

CMS-1500 is a claim form used to **bill Medicare providers**.

Healthcare Common Procedure Coding System(HCPCS Level II)

Products, **services**, and **supplies** that are not generally included in CPT coding are detailed in HCPCS Level II coding. Examples of items coded are ambulance services, medical supplies and equipment for use outside of a healthcare facility by the patient, prosthetics, and more. These codes are used by healthcare providers and suppliers of medical equipment.

Linkage of Procedure and Diagnostic Coding

When submitting claims to insurance or Medicare, coding must be utilized. ICD coding must be utilized with CPT codes to determine the medical condition a patient has been diagnosed with, validating the claim for the service the patient has received.

Insurance Fraud and/or Abuse

Insurance fraud is when a person or company intentionally attempts to deceive an entity by **miscategorizing or falsifying an insurance report**. Examples include billing for services that were never rendered, and charging more for services than necessary.

Insurance waste is the **over-utilization of services** that are **unnecessary**, and drive up the cost of medical plans such as Medicare. Insurance waste is not the result of negligence, but by misuse of available resources. Examples include prescribing too much of a medication such as an antibiotic, or performing numerous tests that all accomplish the same goal when only one test should suffice.

Insurance abuse is the result of **billing practices** that cause an **inappropriate increase in costs**. Examples can include billing for unnecessary services, improper coding, and charging an excessive amount for services, treatments, or supplies.

Coverage for Patient Services and Waivers

Insurance Eligibility Verification

Before a patient receives treatment, the **insurance eligibility** for the treatment should be verified. Verification is obtained by submitting information provided by the patient to the insurance company. The insurance company will **provide costs** of co-pays, deductible information, services and costs not covered by insurance, and eligibility based on the date of the service being provided. This gives both the medical facility and the patient the expected cost of the service.

Insurance Claims

Insurance claims are submitted by the policy holder to the insurance company for **compensation of a covered event or procedure**. Submission of an insurance claim typically involves receiving an itemized bill from the health care provider, filling out a claim form, and emailing/mailing the documents to the insurance company. After the insurance company has received all the documentation, it is reviewed, and a determination is made in regards to whether the insurance company will accept or deny the claim.

Claims submitted should be checked for accuracy in all areas, including the patient's personal information, diagnoses, coding, deductibles, payments, etc. Any information submitted incorrectly may cause delays in processing claims, or result in claim rejection.

Explanation of benefits(EOB) is a form that is mailed to an insured person after a medical procedure has taken place, showing a break down of all the **medical costs** for the specific procedure, and how much has been **paid off by the insurance company**. EOBs often resemble medical bills, but will state that they are explanations of benefits only, and that they are **not a bill**.

Remittance advice is some sort of **proof**, usually documentation, that a **customer** has **paid their bill** to a provider. The payment may come directly from the patient, or may also come from insurance providers covering the cost of care. Information provided on remittance advice documents include the patient's name, any claim number associated, type of service provided, the amount billed, the amount allowed to be billed, the amount that has been paid, and the amount of the deductible the patient has.

Certain circumstances may arise that result in a claim being rejected. Rejection of a claim requires the claim be followed-up on. These claims may need extra information, documentation, or other material to be provided for the claim to be approved. Reasons for claim rejection are included in remittance advice, which helps speed the process of resubmitting the claim with extra documentation, increasing acceptance of the claim in the future.

Unpaid claims should be tracked to help ensure payment is received. Claims should be filed to insurance in a timely manner. When a payment is unpaid, the party responsible for payment should be contacted to inquire about the unpaid claim, and to encourage payment to be sent, reducing the chances of revenue being lost.

Advance Beneficiary Notices(ABN) are forms provided to those with Medicare before a procedure is performed, letting the person know that the procedure may not be covered by Medicare. This allows the person to make a determination on whether or not to receive the treatment, as they may be required to pay for the full amount of the procedure.

Diagnostic Related Groups are used by medicare and health insurance groups to **determine the amount of money** to pay for a person's **hospital stay**, and to categorize costs associated with hospitals. Factors that contribute to categorization include the patient's age, diagnosis, and any procedures performed. DRGs were designed to minimize the ability of a hospital to keep a patient longer than necessary, driving up the amount a hospital would charge Medicare for board and supplies such as bandages.

Relative value units(RVUs) are used to provide **pricing** for a **physician's services** based on the **level of skill** and **amount of time** the service requires. For example, a surgical procedure that may take the same amount of time as a basic check-up will cost more because of the skill and training involved in performing the surgical procedure.

Insurance Types/Third-Party Payers

Health insurance is used to cover the cost of a person's medical expenses. These expenses may include hospital visits, medication, check ups, and surgical procedures, amongst others. Insurance may be included in employee benefits, or may be individually purchased. The purchaser of the insurance may have the cost of expenses completely covered, or pay a portion of the expense, depending on the type of insurance obtained.

Commercial Plans

A **Health Maintenance Organization**, or **HMO**, is a form of health insurance plan that limits an insured person's coverage to **doctors who contract with the HMO**. This typically will not allow care out of network.

A **Preferred Provider Organization**, or **PPO**, is a form of health insurance plan in which doctors and other medical professionals provide **discounted services to plan subscribers.** A person subscribed to a PPO may see doctors outside of their network, but will be charged an increased amount.

Medicare

Medicare is a type of insurance designed for **elderly citizens** over the age of 65, **young people** with certain **disabilities**, and people with **end-stage renal failure**. Medicare is sponsored by the **government**, and is split into three parts. **Part A** covers **hospital expenses**, such as hospice, inpatient hospital stays, and nursing facility stays. **Part B** covers **physician fees**, **immunizations**, **screening tests**, and **diagnostic tests. Part D** provides **prescription drug coverage** to Part A and Part B plans. **Part C** is an **all-encompassing plan**, which includes Part A, Part B, and Part D, and can include additional benefits such as having a lower out-of-pocket cost than the usual Medicare.

Medicaid/State Children's Health Insurance Program(SCHIP)

Medicaid, which is regulated by both state and federal governments, provides health insurance to **low-income persons**, **children**, the **elderly**, people with **disabilities**, and **pregnant women**.

If families earn more than the limit to qualify for Medicaid, they may be able to gain insurance for children utilizing **SCHIP**, or **State Children's Health Insurance Program**. This program typically allows coverage for doctor's visits, hospitalization, emergency room visits, and immunizations. Each state has different requirements for SCHIP eligibility.

TRICARE/CHAMPVA

TRICARE is health insurance only offered to **military personnel**, both active and retired, and their dependents.

CHAMPVA, the **Civilian Health and Medical Program of the Department of Veterans Affairs**, is a health care program established by the Department of Veterans Affairs(VA) to share the cost of health care services with veterans who are eligible for the program. Any persons eligible for CHAMPVA cannot be eligible for TRICARE.

Managed Care Organizations

Managed care organizations, also known as **MCOs**, are organizations that offer managed care health plans in order to help reduce costs accrued by the insured person. MCOs are often made up of physicians, hospitals, and specialists. HMOs and PPOs are examples of MCOs.

Workers' Compensation

Workers' compensation is a form of insurance that is used to **replace lost wages** and **provide insurance** to any worker who is **injured on the job.** Workers' compensation is often utilized to prevent negligence lawsuits. If workers' compensation is agreed upon, the injured employee will receive lost wages and repayment of any medical costs accrued.

Authorizations and Resources

Precertification/Prior Authorization

Precertifications may be required to receive certain treatments, screenings, medications, and tests. **Precertifications**, also known as **prior authorizations**, are provided by the patient's physician, and are determined based on **necessity**. For example, a child would not likely need to be seen by a dermatologist for a skin cancer screening, while a middle aged adult who has a family history of skin cancer would be more likely to need a screening performed. Prior authorizations can help open appointments for those who require them, and reduce unnecessary insurance claims.

Prior authorization is needed when performing diagnostic testing. These tests include MRIs, CT scans, nuclear scans, and prenatal testing, among others. Surgical procedures also necessitate prior authorization, depending on the medical necessity of the surgical procedure.

Prior authorization also covers medications. **Medications covered** by an insurance plan is known as the plan's **formulary**. Insurance companies may only cover specific medications to help lower the cost of prescriptions for the patient, providing coverage for generic medication instead of expensive brand name medication, which is often the exact same medication as generic.

Denials/Appeals

If an insurance company **does not accept** an insurance claim, it is known as a **denial**. If this is the case, the insured may request an appeal of the decision. The claim may then be reviewed by a separate third party, who will make the final determination.

Financial Terminology

Accounts Payable

Accounts payable is the amount of money the **office owes** to a person or company for services rendered. If an office places an order for a specific type of equipment, they have accrued an amount of money in accounts payable. Once the balance has been paid to the merchant for the equipment, the amount of money in accounts payable for that specific transaction returns to a zero balance.

Accounts Receivable

Accounts receivable are credits granted to a customer for goods already delivered, but not yet paid back. In short, it is **money owed to the office.** If a patient is billed later for services already rendered, this money is placed in accounts receivable. Once payment has been received, the balance of this specific transaction returns to a zero balance.

Debits

Debit is the **amount of money** a business is **reporting as an expense**, usually in relation to a bank account. The amount debited should be the exact same amount being credited to another account, which ensures proper accounting is taking place.

Credits/Credit Card Balance

Credit is **debt** allowed to be **borrowed** by a person to be **paid back at a later date**. There are four main types of credit: revolving credit, installment credit, service credit, and charge cards. **Revolving credit** involves a maximum line of credit, not allowing charges to be made past that limit. Payments are usually made monthly, with some sort of interest applied. **Installment credit**, such as a mortgage, is a set amount of debt that is paid back over a period of time. These also involve interest added on, and are often paid back over a lengthy period of time. **Service credit** is debt billed for services such as power and water. These are credited and expected to be paid monthly. **Charge cards** are similar to credit cards, but require the balance to be paid off each month.

Deductible

Deductibles are the amount **required to be paid** by the policy holder **before insurance payments begin**. Typically, the amount a person pays for insurance is based on the deductible and covered expenses. The lower the deductible, the higher the payment.

Assets

Assets are **property owned** by the business that has some sort of **tangible value**, and are available to use as collateral for **debts**. Common assets include accounts receivable, cash, office equipment, intellectual property such as trademarks, and physical property.

Patient Account Financial Procedures

Post Charges

Anything that is charged to the patient should be posted to the patient's account, and should be checked for accuracy to ensure the patient is paying the proper amount for each service, treatment, item, or medication received. Insurance, coverage, and proper coding should all be checked.

Post Payments

Any payments received from the patient should be documented, including determining what service, treatment, item, or medication the payment is paying for at that specific time. After the payment has been received, the patient should receive a statement containing the remaining balance owed with a receipt.

Post Adjustments/Write-offs

Post adjustments, also known as **write-offs**, are the amount of money the hospital or physician has agreed to **not charge** for a service or treatment. The insurance company then pays the amount they are **contractually obligated to pay**, leaving the insured with the remaining balance for the service/treatment. If the amount owed is in excess of the amount contractually agreed to, then the excess amount is written-off and not charged.

End-of-Day Reconciliation

End-of-day reconciliation is the process of **calculating all monetary transactions** that occurred during a day. Payments received for services and treatments should be calculated and compared against all bills issued to patients and claims submitted to insurance companies. The totals of each should match.

Billing/Collections

Itemized Statements

An **itemized statement** is a document detailing the **cost of all treatments and procedures** performed. These costs can include the cost of items, tools, and medicines utilized during a treatment. This provides the patient with an exact cost breakdown for every aspect of the treatment or procedure, providing transparency.

Aging of Accounts

Accounts receivable is used to document all money owed to a medical office. This is done by keeping a record of each patient who owes money, including the date payment is due. When payment has **not been received** by the due date, the payment is considered **past due**, and efforts should be made to obtain payment. If payment is not received, and the amount of money attempting to obtain is substantial enough, it may be sent to a collection agency, who will work to obtain payment for the office for a fee.

Collecting Payments

There are several different means of obtaining payment from a patient, including co-pay, pre-pay, co-insurance, and self-pay.

Co-pay is the amount a patient will pay for a procedure that has been **predetermined** by the patient's insurance coverage. For example, if a patient's co-pay for a mental health treatment is $40, then the patient will pay $40 up front for the treatment, and the rest of the treatment is billed to the insurance company.

Pre-pay is used when collecting funds from a patient **before** a treatment has been performed. Pre-pay is an option utilized to ensure funds are received for the treatment. The cost of the treatment may be less than what the patient pays beforehand, however, and the patient would then receive a refund for the difference.

Co-insurance is the amount a patient pays for treatment **after meeting the deductible**. If a patient has a $2000 deductible on health insurance, they will pay the first $2000 of all health care related expenses in a year. Any procedures or treatments required after the $2000 deductible has been paid will require the patient to pay only a fixed percentage of the cost of care, as opposed to the entire cost of the procedure. The insurance company covers the remaining cost of the treatment or procedure.

Self-pay is utilized when a patient is **not using insurance** to help pay for a treatment or procedure. A patient may choose not to utilize insurance for many reasons, leaving them solely responsible for paying for each treatment or procedure. A payment policy should be utilized with all self-pay patients to help ensure payment is received.

Preplanned Payment Options/Credit Arrangements

When receiving a treatment or procedure that incurs a large financial obligation on behalf of the patient, the medical facility understands that the patient will likely be unable to pay the entire balance due either beforehand or immediately after. Establishing a preplanned payment schedule is a viable option for these patients, allowing patients to pay their bills due over a longer period of time, usually in monthly intervals. Interest may apply if using credit, or the payment may only need to be a simple division of the overall funds due and number of months to pay.

Preplanned payment options may be utilized for an account that is behind on payments to establish payment of the account. These payment options may include paying cash, check, or having the funds debited from a bank account directly. Credit arrangements may be made to further assist in making payment on the account.

Use of Collection Agencies

Collection is **acquiring funds or payments owed to the office**. If payment is unable to be collected and is past due, a **collection agency** is utilized. After the collection agency has obtained the past due payments, they are awarded with a percentage of the money in exchange for services rendered.

If a business has accounts receivable it does not expect to be paid back, it looks at the aging of the accounts to determine the appropriate steps to take. The longer the account has aged, the more likely it is the account will be sent to a collection agency to recoup some sort of payment.

Account Collection Rules

Consumer Protection Acts are designed to **protect consumers** from **unfair**, **misleading**, or **fraudulent business practices**. Complaints may be filed, investigations may take place, and lawsuits may arise from activities that harm consumers.

The **Fair Debt Collection Practices Act** was enacted to **prevent abusive** and **unfair collection practices** by collection agencies. It limits the time and place a debt collector may attempt to contact a debtor, and prevent any form of harassment of the debtor and/or family members. A debt collector must cease contact if a written request is submitted.

Scheduling Appointments

Appointment Matrix is the way to determine **what type** of appointment is needed and **what information** is required to make the correct appointment. Each provider will have set lengths of time for each type of appointment. There are new patient appointments and established patient appointments.

New Patient Appointments

A **new patient** is someone who has **never been seen** by the provider or within their network, such as a large medical group with a central patient database. Required information for creating the chart of a new patient would include the patient's full legal name, a notation of the patient's preferred name, the date of birth, social security number if applicable, the legal gender, a notation of the patient's preferred gender, a current mailing address, phone number, and current email if available. All of these things are used to confirm the patient's identity, ensuring there can be no mistake as to which chart belongs to which patient. The insurance information is needed for billing, and the insurance card and a photo ID will need to be added to the chart. The patient will need to complete any and all required paperwork for the initial appointment. This usually includes a health history survey, forms for patient demographics and insurance information, a privacy protection form, and possibly a release of information form at the patient's discretion. This form is needed to discuss any PHI with someone who is not the patient or another healthcare provider involved in the patient's care.

Established Patient Appointments

Established Patient Appointments fall into two categories: routine care and urgent appointments. **Routine care** can include things like annual physicals and wellness exams, and well child visits. Routine care can also include regular follow-up visits, such as six month follow-up for chronic issues such as diabetes. Regular medication refill appointments may also be considered routine care, as many controlled substances require a handwritten prescription, and therefore require an appointment for each refill. Annual preventative care appointments are set by insurance, and that is usually 366 days from the last annual preventative. Follow-up appointments at regular intervals for various reasons are at the discretion of the provider.

Routine versus Urgent

Urgent appointments include things like sick visits, emergency room or hospital follow-up appointments that need to be completed within a set amount of time. For example, some emergency room providers require a patient to follow up within two days or within two weeks for things like removal of stitches.

Coordinate Facility/Equipment/Personnel Requirements

When making appointments, it is important to ask **in-depth questions** to get all the information necessary to schedule correctly within both the providers preferences and the patient's preferences, and to keep a good patient flow. A **patient flow** is keeping the schedule balanced between routine care, new patients, and room for urgent appointments. If a provider has nothing but new patients and annual preventative appointments, that provider cannot accommodate patients who are sick or injured or in need of an immediate medication refill for that day.

This is where the **provider/physician preferences** come into play. Many providers have session limits, meaning they will only see a set number of new patients and/or annual preventative appointments per day/week. This allows for the majority of the provider's schedule to be open for urgent appointments and various other routine care appointments such as test result follow-ups.

The other key to a good patient flow is also the **patient's preferences**. Many patients call ahead of time for things like routine care, so it is important to ask questions like "When will you be out of medication?" to determine an adequate appointment date. If the patient says they will run out in three days, then a same day/next day appointment is required. However, if the patient states that they will not be out of medication until the middle of next month, then they do not need to be seen immediately, and the appointment can be scheduled the week they will need the refill. This will prevent the provider from being fully booked the first two days of the work week, where sick patients cannot be seen until later in the week. The first appointment available of the date needed should always be offered, as this will prevent the provider from having large gaps in their schedule and create a better flow.

Some appointments will need to be scheduled only on specific dates and certain times due to equipment availability for testing or speciality consultants available in office. These will be set by the office.

Ancillary Services

Ancillary services are **diagnostic treatments or tests** that can help a physician in treating a patient. Examples of ancillary services are X-rays, blood tests, physical therapy, and dialysis, among others. These are treatments an average physician is unable to provide in-office. Ancillary services often require appointments. When scheduling these services, the patient's identifying information should be verified. Many ancillary services require prior authorization, which also needs to be verified. Insurance coverage should also be verified, and if the service is not covered by insurance, the patient should be notified so they are able to make an informed decision about their options. Certain ancillary services require patient preparation beforehand, such as fasting, and these details should be discussed with the patient upon scheduling the appointment. The date, time, and location should also be reviewed with the patient to ensure the patient understands all the particulars about the appointment, minimizing confusion and possible no-shows.

Cancellations/No-Shows/Physician Delay

Another important appointment protocol are those regarding appointment no-shows and the office cancellation policies. Many offices will hold to a 24-hour cancellation policy, in which a fee will be imposed for any no-shows or late cancellations, such as canceling an appointment 24 hours or less prior to. Some offices will not charge for these, but instead inform the patient that a set number of no-shows or a set number of late cancellations will result in dismissal from the office. It is important to mark the no-show or late cancellation correctly in order to track these instances per the office protocols.

When the provider is unavailable, out of the office, sick, or on vacation, it will be the responsibility of the medical assistant to follow the protocols and call each patient scheduled on the day the provider will be out and let the patient know they will need to be rescheduled or leave an appropriate message to call back to be rescheduled. If the provider is delayed, late to start due to weather, late to an individual appointment due to the previous appointment running over, or other unforeseen circumstances, each circumstance will have its own set of protocols to follow. The medical assistant may be asked to notify the patient that they will need to reschedule or advise them of the projected time they will be seen and offer them to reschedule if needed.

Appointment cards and **reminder calls** are protocols that help to minimize the instances of no-shows and late cancellations. An appointment card is generally a handwritten card with the provider's name and the office phone number on one side, and the appointment date and time on the other. A reminder call is generally made 1-2 days before the appointment date and generally includes a reminder of the cancellation/no show policy.

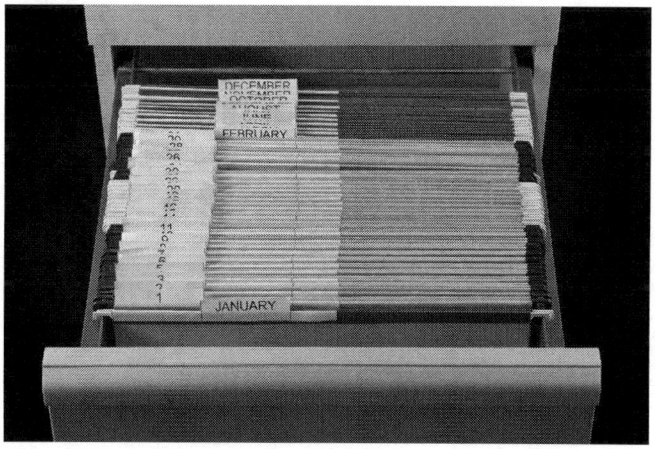

Tickler file systems, also known as **43 folders systems**, are used as a reminder system. These reminders are sorted chronologically as a way to remind a person of upcoming events. The tickler file is a folder system, which contains **12 folders for each month**, and **31 folders for each day**. This allows specific events, like the re-scheduling of appointments, to be performed without forgetting. Supply orders and follow-up appointments are other examples of things a tickler file may help with.

Practice Information Packet

A **practice information packet** is a packet that gives a patient **relevant information** about the medical practice they are visiting. This packet may contain **office policies**, such as cancellation or no-show policies, and will most likely detail the **financial responsibilities** of the patient. This can include insurance and billing policies. Other information that may be found in a practice information packet includes biographies about each physician, confidentiality statements, and office hours.

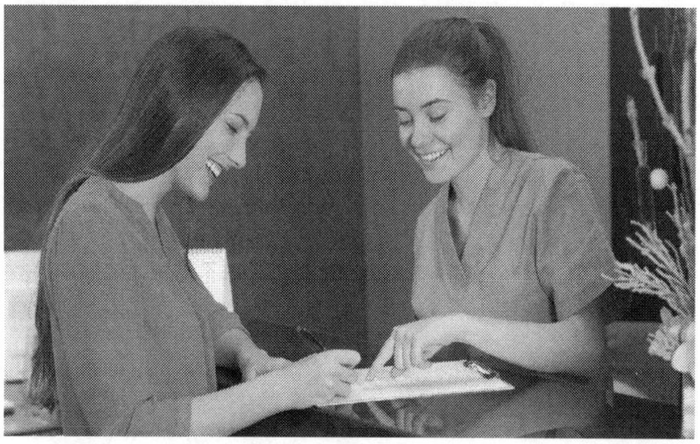

Medical Reception/Patient Registration

Appointment protocols are an important and unique aspect to each provider and/or office that are important and necessary to the office and patient flow. Always adhere to any federal HIPAA laws and all protocols set by the office. This is important for various legal aspects. By following all federal HIPAA regulations in regards to all PHI, the provider and all who interact with the PHI will remain in compliance and free from breach of confidentiality legal concerns. By following all office regulation and protocols, the medical assistant can ensure that the PHI is protected and in HIPAA compliance. This is the main reason for appointment protocols. If all appointments follow the same protocol, then the risk of being non-compliant is greatly reduced.

Identity Theft Protection

Demographic data is reviewed for many reasons, an example of which is **identity theft prevention**. Medical identity theft is one person stealing another person's identity by obtaining personal health information to illegally obtain or bill for medical services. Demographic data should always be reviewed, such as the patient's driver's license, to ensure they are the correct patient and not stealing someone's identity.

All federal HIPAA and place of business policies and procedures should be followed when discussing protected health information over the phone. Per HIPAA, the caller must verify two forms of identifying information before PHI can be released. Forms of identifying information can be full name, date of birth, phone number, the last four digits of the social security number, an email address, street address, and member ID number from the patient's insurance card.

Protected health information callers may request can include appointment times and dates, appointment locations, the provider of the appointment, and what the appointment is for. Medical assistants may also be asked about any labs or testing the patient has had performed, test results, and prescription information.

If the caller is not the patient, a release form needs to be checked to ensure the patient has given permission for information to be released to the caller.

Obtain Accurate Billing Information

Accurate billing information is vital in preventing issues with billing, treatments, and efficient functioning of the medical facility. Information obtained from the patient should be carefully checked and documented, including name, contact information, coding, charges for treatments and procedures, and any payments the patient has already made.

Electronic Health Records

Patient Portals

Patient portals are websites a patient has access to that give the patient all of their **personal health information** and history, medical records, upcoming and past appointments, and more. Patients are able to send messages to their healthcare providers, request refills of prescriptions, and view lab results. Patient portals and the information are secured with the use of passwords.

History and Physical Reports

History and physical medical records are basic documents used when admitting a new patient. After the patient's initial visit, they are considered an **established patient**, and the history and physical records are referenced in each subsequent visit. Information documented includes the chief complaint, history of the present illness, any past medical or psychological history, family history, a list of medications, a review of systems, and a physical examination. An overall assessment and plan is also detailed.

Discharge Summary

Discharge summary forms are given when a patient is **discharged** from a medical facility, and discuss numerous aspects of the patient's visit. Information typically seen on a discharge form includes the date the patient was admitted, the date of discharge, a history of the patient's visit, the diagnosis upon admittance, any procedures or surgeries that were performed, any complications that arose, and instructions on follow-up care post-discharge. The discharge form should be signed by the physician discharging the patient.

Operative Note

Operative notes are produced by **surgeons** during operations and detail exactly what was done during the procedure, what devices were used, and any post-operative orders. Operative notes are extremely useful in transferring care from the operating room to the recovery room. Operative notes also allow for proper billing and coding to take place.

Diagnostic Test/Laboratory Report

Diagnostic tests are performed by **collecting samples of bodily fluids** such as blood, urine, feces, saliva, and semen, then performing specific tests on the fluid to help diagnose medical conditions, check the content of the fluid, and more. The results of the findings are presented to the patient by way of a test/lab report. These reports detail what was tested, what was being examined in the test, and the ultimate results of the test. For example, if a person has blood drawn to test cholesterol levels, the amount of HDL and LDL in the blood will be listed on the report per the testing or laboratory findings.

Clinic Progress Note

Clinic progress notes are used to **document a patient's care and progress** during a **hospital stay** or **outpatient care**. Documenting this information can help determine if treatment is successful, if it needs to be altered, what the patient's physical condition is during a course of treatment, and more. Examples of progress notes are SOAP and DART.

Consultation Report

Consultation reports are reports that detail **professional advice or opinions** given by a person who is not the primary care physician to a patient. The consultation can involve developing a treatment plan. An example is an ER physician consulting with a patient, then referring the patient to a specialist based on the consultation findings. Consultation reports contain several pieces of information, such as the reason for the consultation, symptoms the patient is experiencing, physical findings, laboratory or testing findings, and any treatments recommended.

Growth Charts, Graphs, and Tables

Charts, graphs, and tables are used to give the patient and physician a visualization of information. Giving a visual representation of information may help the person reading the information have a better grasp on what is being presented. An example of a chart is a pie chart. An example of a graph is a bar graph.

Medical Record Preparation

Medical records should be drawn **before the patient arrives** at the office to help the flow of appointments. If the patient has an electronic medical record, the record may be printed. If it is a paper system, the medical record should be located, and the patient's information should always be cross-referenced to ensure the correct patient is being seen, as some patients may have the same name. Information that is used to check for the correct patient can be **date-of-birth, social security number, telephone number, and address on file**. Any new records, such as lab work, should be obtained and attached to the medical record. Finally, the medical records should be placed in order of appointment, which allows the physician to quickly view the next patient's file without having to search through each file to find the correct records.

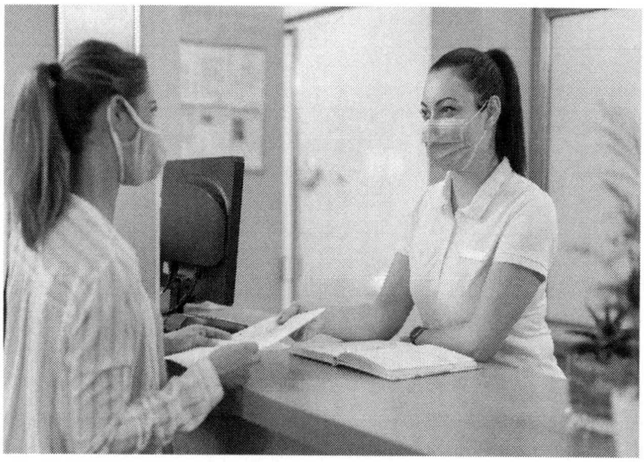

Billing, Coding, Insurance, and Scheduling Matching

______: Codes used to describe circumstances other than disease or injury, such as preventative care, chemotherapy, or radiation therapy

______: Coding system used to detail products, services, and supplies

______: Diagnostic treatments or tests designed to help a physician in treating a patient

______: The amount required to be paid by the policy holder before insurance payments begin

______: Medications covered by an insurance plan

______: Notes produced by surgeons during operations detailing what was done during the procedure, devices used, and post-operative orders

______: A bill for a health service costing more than is necessary based on the service or treatment provided

______: Codes used to detail the cause of an injury, poisoning, or adverse reactions to drugs or medications

______: The amount of money a business is reporting as an expense, usually in relation to a bank account

______: A person or company intentionally attempting to deceive an entity by miscategorizing or falsifying an insurance report

______: Type of health insurance designed for elderly citizens over the age of 65, young people with certain disabilities, and people with end-stage renal failure

______: Form of insurance that is used to replace lost wages and provide insurance to any worker who is injured on the job

______: Form mailed to an insured person after a medical procedure showing a breakdown of all the medical costs for the specific procedure and amount paid off by the insurance company

______: Form provided to those with Medicare before a treatment is performed, to inform the patient the procedure may not be covered by medicare

______: Money owed to the office

______: Insurance company not accepting an insurance claim

______: Property owned by the business that has some sort of tangible value

______: Billing practice causing an inappropriate increase in costs

______: The amount of money the hospital or physician has agreed to not charge for a service or treatment

______: The amount of money the office owes to a person or company for services rendered

A: Drug formulary
B: Z-codes
C: Post adjustment
D: Deductible
E: Accounts payable
F: Insurance fraud
G: Debit
H: Insurance abuse
I: HCPCS Level II coding
J: Medicare
K: E-code
L: Accounts receivable
M: Asset
N: Upcoding
O: Worker's compensation
P: Denial
Q: Operative notes
R: Explanation of benefits
S: Advance Beneficiary Notice
T: Ancillary services

Answer Key on Page 292

Billing, Coding, Insurance, and Scheduling Crossword

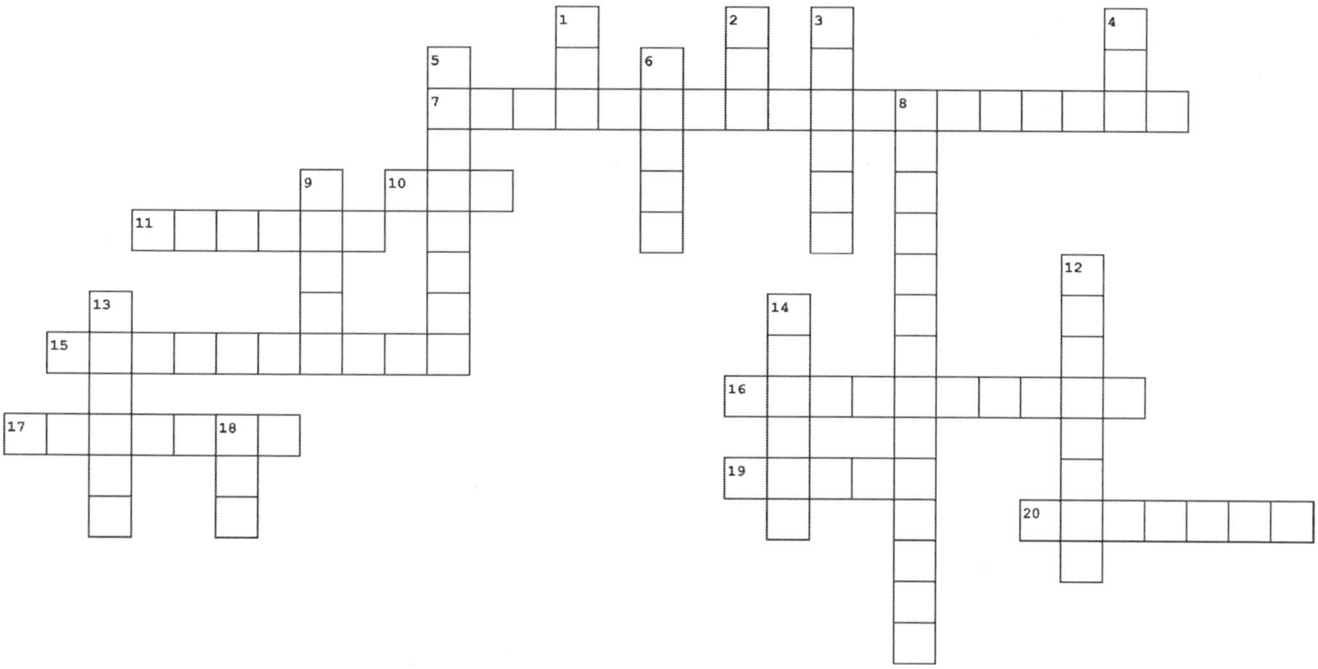

Across

7. A determination by the insurance company provided to the physician stating a treatment or test is necessary
10. Form mailed to an insured person after a procedure breaking down all medical costs and amount paid off, abbv.
11. An insurance company not accepting an insurance claim
15. Billing for a health service at a lower rate than what should be charged
16. The amount required to be paid by the policy holder before insurance payments begin
17. Health insurance plan only offered to military personnel and their dependents
19. Part of Medicare that covers hospital expenses
20. A patient paying for a treatment or procedure without using insurance

Down

1. Form of health insurance that limits an insured person's coverage to doctors who contract with the group, abbv.
2. Coding set used for reporting medical procedures such as surgeries, abbv.
3. Codes used by tumor registries to identify tumors and abnormal growths
4. Form of health insurance in which doctors provide discounted services to plan subscribers, abbv.
5. Billing for a health service at a higher rate than necessary
6. Part of Medicare that covers physician fees, immunizations, and tests
8. Billing practices that cause an inappropriate increase in costs
9. Part of Medicare that covers prescription drug coverage to other parts
12. Type of people who may be covered by Medicaid
13. Translating medical diagnoses, equipment, and procedures into an alphanumeric code
14. Collecting funds from a patient before a treatment has been performed
18. Provide pricing for a physician's services based on level of skill and amount of time the service requires, abbv.

Answer Key on Page 294

Billing, Coding, Insurance, and Scheduling Practice Test

1. Of the following, which form of code is used to detail external cause of injury, poisoning, or adverse reactions to drugs or medications
A. E codes
B. CMS-1500
C. Z codes
D. M codes

2. Which form of credit is a set amount of debt that is paid back over a lengthy period of time, usually adding interest
A. Service credit
B. Installment credit
C. Charge cards
D. Revolving credit

3. Form of health insurance plan in which doctors and other medical professionals provide discounted services to plan subscribers
A. PPO
B. TRICARE
C. HMO
D. Medicare

4. What is a patient considered after their initial visit has been completed
A. Established patient
B. Recurrent patient
C. Discharged patient
D. Compliant patient

5. Medicaid is regulated by both state and federal government and provides health insurance to all of the following demographics except
A. Low-income persons
B. Military personnel
C. People with disabilities
D. Pregnant women

6. Which of the following forms of debt requires the balance to be completely paid off each month
A. Installment credit
B. Revolving credit
C. Charge cards
D. Service credit

7. Which code is utilized to detail circumstances other than disease or injury such as preventative care
A. E codes
B. M codes
C. CMS-1500
D. Z codes

8. Which of the following describes a drug formulary
A. Medications considered absolute contraindications for specific conditions
B. Medications produced by introducing a liquid to a powder
C. Medications covered by an insurance plan
D. Medications classified under schedules

9. Proof via documentation that a customer has paid their bill to a provider
A. Relative value unit
B. Advanced beneficiary notice
C. Explanation of benefits
D. Remittance advice

10. All of the following are means of identifying a patient for a scheduled appointment except
A. Patient's name
B. Patient's hair color
C. Patient's phone number
D. Patient's social security number

Answer Key on Page 295

Answer Keys

Matching Answer Keys

Clinical Workflow		Word Roots		Prefixes		Suffixes	
L	T	R	H	S	D	I	R
Q	C	M	A	C	K	L	C
M	B	G	D	F	I	K	Q
F	G	J	E	B	O	S	J
O	D	K	S	A	E	O	D
K	R	L	I	J	H	A	F
S	E	P	F	R	N	P	T
A	N	Q	O	T	Q	H	E
P	J	B	N	G	L	B	N
I	H	C	T	M	P	G	M

Safety and Infection Control		Procedures/ Examinations		Anatomy and Physiology		Pathology	
B	S	O	T	C	O	D	R
J	I	S	R	K	A	P	I
L	K	L	J	E	H	G	M
H	D	Q	C	T	S	A	L
T	P	N	A	M	J	N	H
R	A	I	M	L	F	T	C
Q	N	P	E	B	G	J	F
E	G	D	H	Q	I	S	K
O	C	G	K	P	R	E	Q
F	M	F	B	N	D	O	B

Pharmacology		Legal/Ethical Issues		Communication		Billing, Coding, Insurance, Scheduling	
D	O	M	E	R	J	B	J
G	C	G	D	H	F	I	O
N	Q	P	K	K	I	T	R
A	T	T	O	N	C	D	S
K	H	A	Q	T	G	A	L
B	I	B	F	A	P	Q	P
J	E	L	S	L	O	N	M
S	M	J	N	D	B	K	H
F	R	C	H	Q	E	G	C
P	L	R	I	M	S	F	E

Crossword Answer Keys

Clinical Workflow

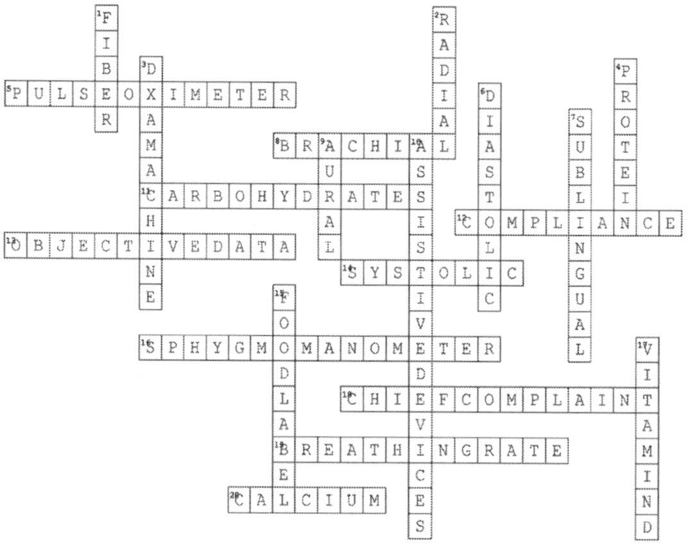

Medical Terminology

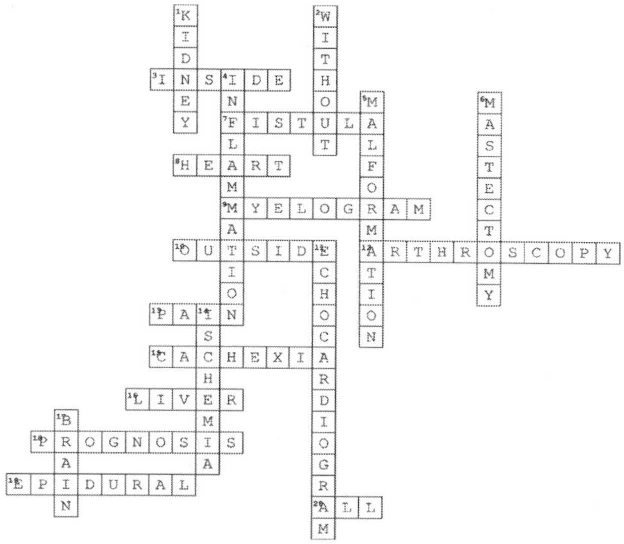

Safety and Infection Control

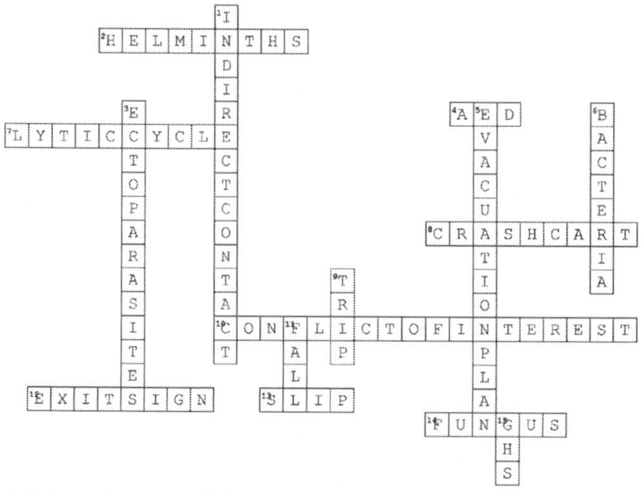

Procedures/Examinations

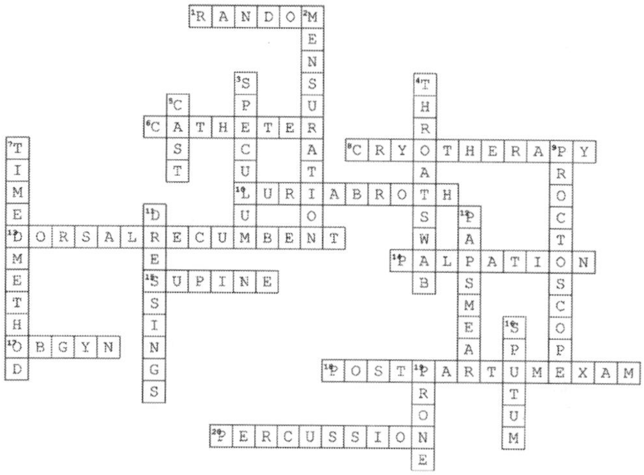

Anatomy and Physiology

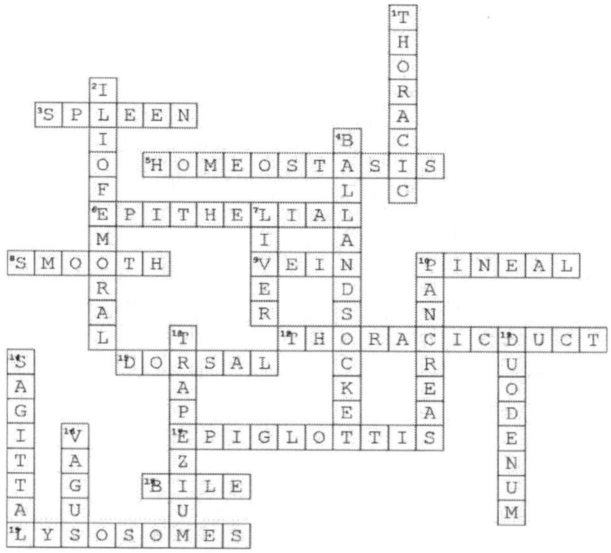

Pathology

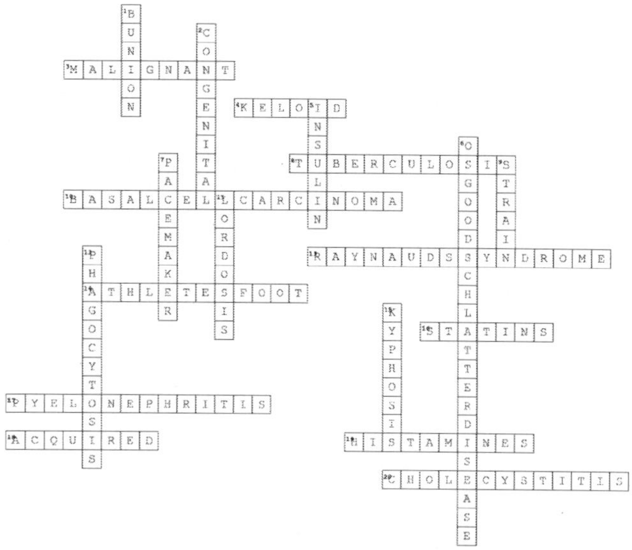

Pharmacology

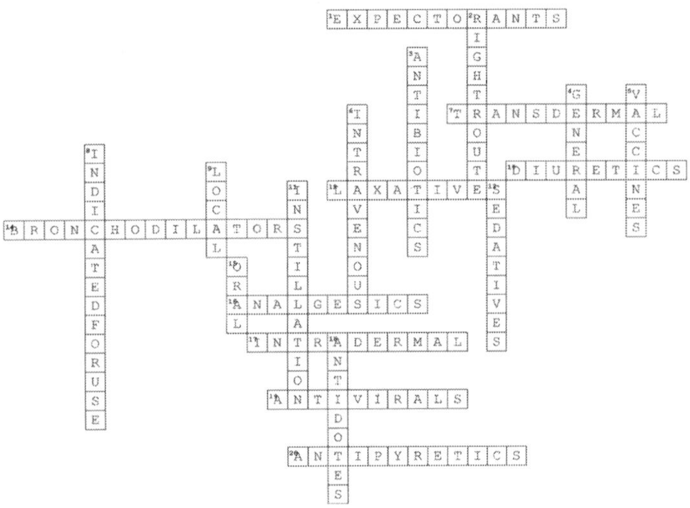

Legal and Ethical Issues

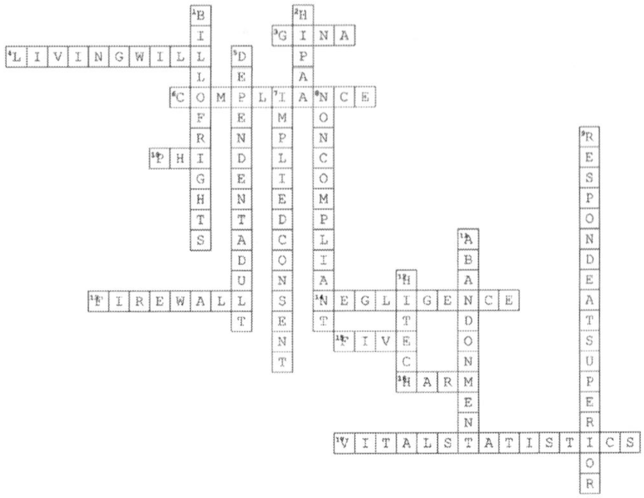

Communication

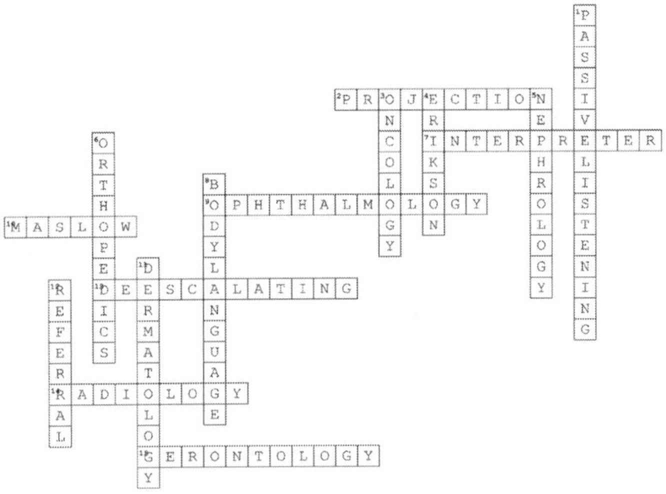

Billing, Coding, Insurance, and Scheduling

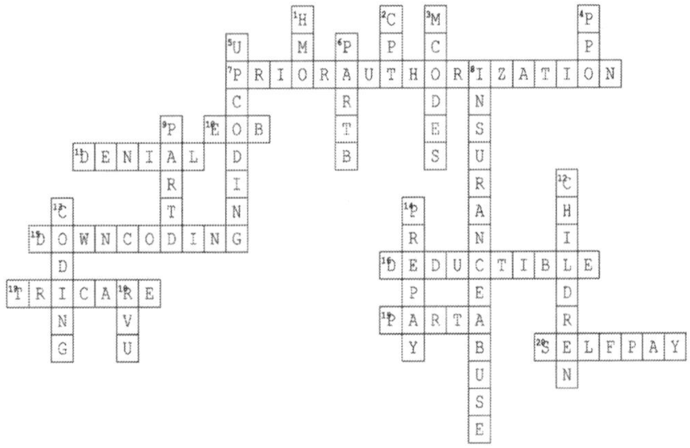

Medical Terminology Breaking Down/Building

Breaking Down:

1. Artery/hard/condition
2. Renal pelvis/kidney/inflammation
3. Brain/inflammation
4. Lymph/swelling
5. Excessive/thyroid/condition
6. Bile/bladder/inflammation
7. Liver/inflammation
8. Vein/inflammation
9. Twisted/neck
10. Skin/plant/condition
11. Extremity/irregular enlargement
12. Muscle/heart/blood flow obstruction
13. Not/sleep
14. Nerve/pain
15. Tendon/synovial/inflammation

Building:

1. An/emia
2. Athero/scler/osis
3. Gastr/itis
4. Melan/oma
5. Fibro/my/algia
6. Osteo/arthr/itis
7. Cyst/itis
8. A/pnea
9. Onycho/myc/osis
10. Dermat/itis
11. Hyper/tension
12. Ar/rhythmia
13. Leuk/emia
14. Kyph/osis
15. Cellul/itis

Anatomy and Physiology Muscle Identification

1. Temporalis
2. Masseter
3. Sternocleidomastoid
4. Splenius capitis
5. Levator scapulae
6. Pectoralis major
7. Deltoid
8. Biceps brachii
9. Infraspinatus
10. Rhomboids
11. Trapezius
12. Triceps brachii
13. Latissimus dorsi
14. Psoas major
15. Iliacus
16. Tensor fascia lata
17. Sartorius
18. Gracilis
19. Rectus femoris
20. Gluteus maximus
21. Biceps femoris
22. Semitendinosus
23. Semimembranosus
24. Tibialis anterior
25. Gastrocnemius
26. Soleus
27. Peroneus longus
28. Pectoralis minor
29. Serratus anterior
30. Rectus abdominis

Anatomy and Physiology Bone Identification

1. Temporal
2. Sphenoid
3. Frontal
4. Ethmoid
5. Lacrimal
6. Nasal
7. Vomer
8. Maxilla
9. Mandible
10. Zygomatic
11. Parietal
12. Occipital
13. Clavicle
14. Sternum
15. Ribs
16. Sacrum
17. Coccyx
18. Scapula
19. Cervical vertebrae
20. Thoracic vertebrae
21. Lumbar vertebrae
22. Humerus
23. Radius
24. Ulna
25. Ilium
26. Ischium
27. Pubis
28. Metacarpals
29. Proximal phalanges
30. Intermediate phalanges
31. Distal phalanges
32. Femur
33. Fibula
34. Tibia
35. Metatarsals
36. Proximal phalanges
37. Intermediate phalanges
38. Distal phalanges
39. Scaphoid
40. Lunate
41. Triquetrum
42. Pisiform
43. Trapezium
44. Trapezoid
45. Capitate
46. Hamate
47. Calcaneus
48. Talus
49. Cuboid
50. Navicular
51. Cuneiform I
52. Cunieform II
53. Cuneiform III

Individual Subject Practice Test Answer Keys

Clinical Workflow	Medical Terminology	Safety and Infection Control	Procedures/ Examinations
01. C	01. B	01. C	01. B
02. B	02. A	02. A	02. A
03. D	03. D	03. D	03. D
04. C	04. B	04. B	04. B
05. B	05. D	05. C	05. D
06. A	06. C	06. D	06. C
07. B	07. D	07. A	07. D
08. A	08. B	08. B	08. C
09. D	09. C	09. D	09. A
10. C	10. A	10. B	10. C

Anatomy and Physiology	Pathology	Pharmacology	Legal/Ethical Issues
01. D	01. C	01. A	01. D
02. A	02. A	02. B	02. C
03. C	03. B	03. B	03. A
04. B	04. D	04. D	04. A
05. A	05. C	05. A	05. B
06. B	06. D	06. C	06. A
07. A	07. D	07. D	07. C
08. D	08. C	08. B	08. D
09. D	09. C	09. C	09. B
10. C	10. D	10. C	10. C

Communication	Billing, Coding, Insurance, Scheduling
01. C	01. A
02. D	02. B
03. B	03. A
04. A	04. A
05. C	05. B
06. C	06. C
07. D	07. D
08. B	08. C
09. A	09. D
10. B	10. B

Greatness is setting ambitious goals that your former self would have thought impossible, and trying to get a little better every day.

- Tim Ferriss

Full Length Practice Tests

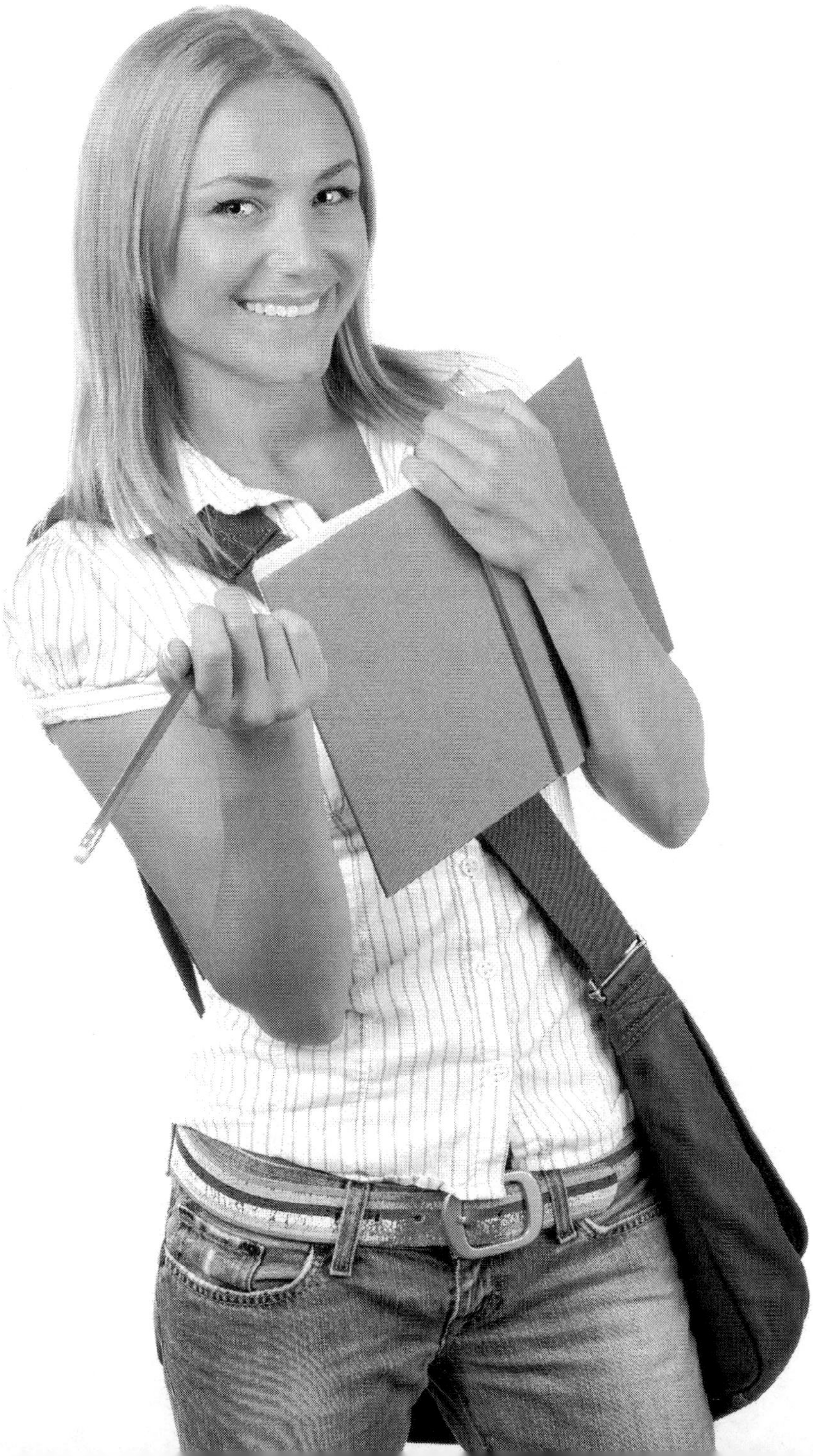

Welcome to the full length practice test section of the book! This is one of the most important parts of the study guide. This is where you get to finally put your knowledge to use and see what you know, what you don't know, what you need to study more of, and most importantly, using your test-taking techniques!

Just be aware: THESE ARE NOT THE EXACT SAME QUESTIONS YOU WILL SEE ON THE CMA EXAM. I DO NOT WORK FOR, NOR HAVE ANY ASSOCIATION WITH THE AAMA OR HAVE ANY INSIGHT INTO THE QUESTIONS ASKED ON THE EXAM. These questions were created by me, and only me!

These questions test you on the material you MAY see on the exam! There are even questions in these practice tests covering information not seen in this study guide. Just like the CMA exam, you will have questions on things you've never seen or learned before. This is where your test-taking techniques come in! Practice answering questions on things you've never learned before and it can help you do the exact same thing on the CMA exam! If you're tested on information you've never seen before, look it up! Learn about that information, and if that information comes up on the CMA exam, you'll be even more prepared!

What I always recommend my students do while taking their exams is, if they have access to a piece of paper, write down as many test-taking techniques as they can remember before trying to answer any questions. This way, while they're taking the CMA exam, they can look at their test-taking techniques and remind themselves to do them. Write things down like: Take your time, don't change answers, identify key words, eliminate answers, stay relaxed, and read the entire question. On the page to your right, you will see an example page that I have created for you to use. Make photocopies of this page and utilize it while taking the full-length practice tests. See if you can take notes on things you may need help remembering later on in the test. See if you can successfully draw structures in the body for reference. Write down any acronyms or mnemonic devices such as "Some Lovers Try Positions That They Can't Handle"(scaphoid, lunate, triquetrum, pisiform, trapezium, trapezoid, capitate, hamate). Spend a small amount of time preparing this document, and it will give you a chance to calm down, relax, and be even more prepared for the exam than before. Use all the tools at your disposal! You don't want to leave the test thinking "would I have passed if I had used that piece of paper?"

A common theme I see with students is a fear of taking the test. The test cannot hurt you. I do understand a fear of not succeeding, however, there are much better ways to view the test. This is the test you attended school to pass. This is the test that will help grant you licensure. This is a test you should be excited for! Here's how I've always approached important tests: when it comes time to test, I know what I know, I have become exceptionally adept at taking tests due to my use of test-taking techniques, and if I pass, awesome! If I don't pass, of course I'm not satisfied, but I know I can take the test again, and I immediately look at the test I just took as the best practice test I can ever take. I now have experience with the test, I know how the questions are worded, I know the kind of information the test is looking for, I still have my notes and I can go back and highlight every piece of information from the test that I recognize to ensure I study it more thoroughly just in case I get those questions on my test again, and I will be even more prepared the next time I take the test. Just because you don't pass the test doesn't mean you have failed. If you don't pass, do not get discouraged, get motivated to conquer it the next time! Preparing for the test isn't just going over information, it's also about your mindset, and your willingness to overcome the obstacle in front of you. Vince Lombardi, former professional football head coach, once said "I firmly believe that any man's finest hour, the greatest fulfillment of all that he holds dear, is that moment when he has worked his heart out in a good cause and lies exhausted on the field of battle, victorious." It's worth the time, it's worth the effort, it's worth the struggle to come out of the test victorious. I believe in you. Believe in yourself, and you can accomplish your goals.

For a reminder of your test-taking techniques, refer to page 4.

Make a photocopy of this page for use with every practice test you take! When you take the CMA exam, replicate this page on your own scratch paper provided by the testing center and put it to use!

Test-Taking Tips:
Read the entire question
Read all the answers
Identify key words
Eliminate answers
Take your time
Don't change answers
Breathe and stay relaxed

Important Information Found For Reference

Additional Notes

Illustrations

Practice Test 1

1. CMS-1500 is used to
A. Document procedures
B. Identify tumors
C. Classify cause of injury
D. Bill Medicare providers

2. Primary function of a gland
A. Secretion
B. Protection
C. Absorption
D. Contraction

3. Branching muscle tissue is also called
A. Smooth
B. Skeletal
C. Cardiac
D. Striated

4. The leading cause of lung, oral, and esophageal cancer
A. Industrial dust
B. Cigarette smoking
C. Asbestos
D. Cystic fibrosis

5. Which of the following is not utilized in a medical dress
A. Shoe covers
B. Face masks
C. Ear plugs
D. Surgical glasses

6. Operative notes are
A. Notes prepared by a surgeon after a procedure that document every action and device used during a surgery
B. Notes prepared by a physician detailing the surgery to be ordered, including date, time, and procedure
C. Notes prepared by a physician the details post-operative care, treatment, and medications the patient is required to take
D. Notes prepared by a surgeon before a procedure that instructs a patient on fasting, waste elimination, and cleanliness

7. Blood pressure is measured using which of the following instruments
A. Spirometer
B. Hemocytometer
C. Sphygmomanometer
D. Electrocardiograph

8. Depolarization of the right atrium and left atrium in an EKG is represented by
A. PR Interval
B. QRS Complex
C. P Wave
D. ST Segment

9. Universal precautions are
A. Considering every fluid and person as contaminated or infectious
B. Noting all emergencies involving patients
C. Classifying an injury based on urgency, location, and severity
D. Protecting a person performing first aid from potential lawsuits

10. The pulmonary arteries carry blood from the right ventricle to
A. Left atrium
B. Rest of the body
C. Aorta
D. Lungs

11. Nausea, vomiting, fatigue, and yellowing of the skin may be the result of
A. Hepatitis
B. Food poisoning
C. Diarrhea
D. Meningitis

12. T lymphocytes are produced by which gland
A. Thymus
B. Thalamus
C. Pituitary
D. Pineal

13. PPE is known as
A. Professional priorities in emergencies
B. Personal protective equipment
C. People profiting from the environment
D. Pulse performed in the ear

14. Dual energy X-ray absorptiometry machines are utilized to test for which specific medical condition a patient may be experiencing
A. Breast cancer
B. Osteomyelitis
C. Osteoporosis
D. Rheumatoid arthritis

15. Classifying an injury by severity, urgency, and location is known as
A. Universal precautions
B. Emergency triage
C. Documentation
D. Sterilization

16. Breaking the skin resulting in exposure of underlying tissue
A. Incision
B. Laceration
C. Abrasion
D. Open wound

17. A sedative has what effect on the body
A. Increases urine production
B. Relaxes and calms
C. Reduces body temperature
D. Reduces inflammation

18. Blood, saliva, vomit, urine, and feces are all categorized as
A. Body membranes
B. Body excretions
C. Body fluids
D. Body secretions

19. LSD, heroin, and peyote are all classified under which drug schedule
A. Schedule IV
B. Schedule V
C. Schedule I
D. Schedule III

20. A blood pressure reading of 140/90 results in a person being diagnosed with
A. Hypertension
B. Hypotension
C. Hyperemia
D. Myocardial infarction

21. Acknowledging a patient's behaviors, utilized in the OARS interviewing technique
A. Affirming
B. Reflecting
C. Summarizing
D. Open-ended questioning

22. Another name for a leukocyte is
A. Thrombocyte
B. Red blood cell
C. Platelet
D. White blood cell

23. Diagnosis Related Groups
A. Provide pricing for a physician's services based on the level of skill and amount of time the service requires
B. Type of insurance designed for elderly citizens over the age of 65, young people with certain disabilities, and people with end-stage renal failure
C. Organizations that offer managed care health plans in order to help reduce costs accrued by the insured person
D. Determine the amount of money to pay for a person's hospital stay, and to categorize costs associated with hospitals

24. Device used to sterilize medial instruments
A. Retractor
B. Nebulizer
C. Autoclave
D. Centrifuge

25. Temperature reading taken in the ear
A. Sublingual
B. Aural
C. Axillary
D. Oral

26. Which of the following best describes a communicable disease
A. A disease that spreads from one person to another
B. A disease a person develops due to genetic factors
C. A disease that emerges in response to changes the body experiences in DNA
D. A disease that has an unknown cause or origin

27. Meningitis is best defined as
A. Inflammation of the meninges, resulting in pressure being placed on the brain
B. Inflammation of the brain, causing increased pressure placed on the cranium
C. Degeneration of brain tissue, resulting in loss of memory
D. Paralysis of one side of the body due to infection of Herpes Simplex virus

28. Breathing is also known as
A. Respiration
B. Systolic pressure
C. Heart rhythm
D. Blood pressure

29. Vital signs are read using all of the following except
A. Pupil constriction
B. Blood pressure
C. Temperature
D. Respiration

30. Which of the following is not one stage of human growth and development
A. Senescence
B. Midlife
C. Death and Dying
D. Adolescence

31. TRICARE provides health care to
A. Dependents of active military personnel
B. Elderly
C. Low-income persons
D. High-income persons

32. Coding system used to code morbidity
A. CPT
B. ICD-9-CM
C. E Codes
D. V Codes

33. Repolarization of the right ventricle and left ventricle
A. ST Segment
B. QRS Complex
C. T Wave
D. PR Interval

34. Medication used to numb a localized area
A. Antacid
B. Local anesthetic
C. Antihistamine
D. Insulin

35. An ampule is
A. A small glass container
B. A type of tumor
C. A type of needle
D. A diabetic medication

36. An intradermal injection should enter the dermis at what angle
A. 15 degree
B. 20 degree
C. 45 degree
D. 90 degree

37. A patient being unable to understand or utilize medical information that has been given to them
A. Medical illiteracy
B. Medical non-compliance
C. Termination of care
D. Medical de-escalation

38. All of the following carry blood away from the heart except
A. Capillaries
B. Arteries
C. Arterioles
D. Veins

39. Dopamine is an example of a
A. Neurotransmitter
B. Synapse
C. Neuron
D. Dendrite

40. Money owed to the office is known as
A. Credit
B. Collection
C. Accounts receivable
D. Chapter 7 Bankruptcy

41. The metric conversion of one gram is
A. 1 kg
B. 1000 mg
C. 100 kg
D. 100 mg

42. Identification of tumors and growths is coded using
A. V Codes
B. E Codes
C. CMS-1500
D. M Codes

43. An ST Segment is
A. Depolarization of the right ventricle and left ventricle
B. Repolarization of the right ventricle and left ventricle
C. Time it takes for a nerve impulse to travel from the SA node through the atria into the ventricles
D. Depolarization of the right atrium and left atrium

44. Gravity of urine is measured using a
A. Refractometer
B. Sphygmomanometer
C. Spirometer
D. Urinometer

45. Which of the following is not a structure in the digestive system
A. Gallbladder
B. Spleen
C. Liver
D. Pancreas

46. The trachea lies directly inferior to the
A. Lungs
B. Pharynx
C. Bronchus
D. Larynx

47. Pepsin is located in the
A. Stomach
B. Small intestine
C. Pancreas
D. Gallbladder

48. Volume of intake and output of air is measured by
A. A spirometer
B. A centrifuge
C. A refractometer
D. An otoscope

49. A P Wave represents
A. Depolarization of the right atrium and left atrium
B. Time taken for an impulse to travel from the SA node through the atria into ventricles
C. Depolarization of the right ventricle and left ventricle
D. Conduction of electrical impulse from bundle of His through ventricles

50. Analgesics help relieve
A. Inflammation
B. Congestion
C. Pain
D. Virus reproduction

51. Of the following, which best describes empathy
A. A person feeling compassion or pity for another person and the situation they are in
B. A person offering to assist another in resolving a conflict
C. A person viewing a situation from another person's point of view
D. A person actively listening to another and reflecting on the information being provided in a constructive manner

52. Crutches, walkers, wheelchairs, and canes are all forms of
A. Surgical tools
B. Patient-administered treatments
C. Assistive devices
D. Home monitoring devices

53. Bone found in the region of the forearm
A. Radius
B. Humerus
C. Fibula
D. Hamate

54. The gauge of a needle is its
A. Length
B. Width
C. Diameter
D. Sharpness

55. A microscope allows a person to
A. View objects visible to the naked eye
B. View objects not visible to the naked eye
C. View objects that are inside the body
D. View objects that are being electrically stimulated

56. A hemocytometer is used to count
A. Blood cells and thrombocytes
B. Levels of urine in the blood
C. Amount of acidity or alkalinity in a substance
D. Heart beats per minute

57. A thrombus is also known as
A. Aneurysm
B. Embolus
C. Blood clot
D. Platelet

58. An abnormality in an EKG reading that is caused by non-cardiac origins
A. Articulation
B. Arrhythmia
C. Artifact
D. Atrial Fibrillation

59. The most common form of local anesthetic is
A. Lidocaine
B. Aspirin
C. Insulin
D. Glucose

60. Conduction of electrical impulse from bundle of His through ventricles
A. P Wave
B. PR Interval
C. T Wave
D. QRS Complex

61. If an ordered dose is 50mg, and the amount in stock is 25mg tab, how many tabs will be prescribed
A. One
B. Two
C. Four
D. Eight

62. A patient giving permission for examination, treatment, or diagnoses is known as
A. Conformity
B. Liability
C. Consent
D. Confidentiality

63. Active listening is
A. Listening to the patient and replying to statements being made
B. Listening to the patient without offering a reply
C. Questions used when asking for feedback
D. Questions that require only a yes or no response

64. CPT is used to
A. Document procedures
B. Identify tumors and growths
C. Document up to four different conditions
D. Describe circumstances other than disease

65. Cramping and abdominal pain, associated with rectal bleeding, may be a sign of
A. Hiatal hernia
B. Crohn's disease
C. Diverticulosis
D. Ulcerative colitis

66. One part lidocaine and 100 grams of base gives which ratio
A. 100:1
B. 1:99
C. 1:100
D. 99:100

67. The use of multiple codes for a service or treatment that increases the cost, providing a larger reimbursement for the facility
A. Unbundling
B. Downcoding
C. Upcoding
D. Bundling

68. Vitamin K contributes to
A. Blood clotting
B. Absorption of calcium
C. Production of hemoglobin
D. Production of erythrocytes

69. The time it takes for nerve impulses to travel from the SA node through the atria into ventricles
A. PR Interval
B. QRS Complex
C. T Wave
D. ST Segment

70. Inspection of the inner portions of the eyes is performed using which instrument
A. Proctoscope
B. Otoscope
C. Stethoscope
D. Ophthalmoscope

71. Temperature reading taken in the armpit
A. Aural
B. Oral
C. Axillary
D. Rectal

72. A laceration is a cut that produces
A. Jagged edges
B. Scraping of skin
C. Clean cut
D. A hole

73. Developmental stage beginning after infancy, ending when puberty no longer takes effect
A. Adulthood
B. Senescence
C. Adolescence
D. Childhood

74. Non-verbal communication is known as
A. Listening
B. Body Language
C. Active Talking
D. Inactive Talking

75. A patient presents with a non-healing wound in the skin located on the foot. Which of the following is the most common cause of a non-healing wound
A. Increased circulation in the area of the wound
B. Bacterial growth in the area of the wound
C. Neuropathy in the area of the wound
D. Lack of elastic fibers in the area of the wound

76. The manner in which an infectious agent leaves its host
A. Portal of entry
B. Reservoir
C. Immune response
D. Portal of exit

77. Classification of causes of injury, poisoning, or adverse reaction to drugs is coded using
A. E Codes
B. M Codes
C. V Codes
D. CPT

78. Injection that enters into the muscle
A. Intradermal
B. Subcutaneous
C. Submuscular
D. Intramuscular

79. The most abundant mineral in the body is
A. Sodium
B. Magnesium
C. Potassium
D. Calcium

80. A single dose of a medication that has been prepared and packaged by the pharmaceutical company, found in blister cards, strips, and pre-filled syringes
A. Prescribed dose
B. Unit dose
C. Dose ratio
D. Ordered dose

81. Which of the following is not one of the six rights of medication administration
A. Right patient
B. Right route
C. Right location
D. Right documentation

82. Intentional artifacts may be caused by
A. Beta-Blockers
B. Pacemakers
C. Nebulizers
D. Blood thinners

83. Antipyretics are used to
A. Dilate bronchial tubes
B. Reduce inflammation
C. Reduce body temperature
D. Relieve pain

84. Blood passes from the right atrium through the tricuspid valve into the
A. Left ventricle
B. Left atrium
C. Right ventricle
D. Pulmonary artery

85. The study of tumors
A. Pathology
B. Etiology
C. Cardiology
D. Oncology

86. Degeneration of myelin sheaths in the central nervous system
A. Multiple sclerosis
B. Myasthenia gravis
C. Parkinson's disease
D. Alzheimer's disease

87. Breathing rate is described as
A. The amount of air a person is able to take in during inspiration and expel during expiration
B. The amount of carbon dioxide being exhaled in a single breath
C. The amount of breaths a person takes during a one minute span
D. The amount of oxygen being inhaled in a single breath

88. Vitamin D allows the body to absorb
A. Sodium
B. Beta-carotene
C. Potassium
D. Calcium

89. Unintended or unexpected effects of the administration of medication that may be harmful to the patient
A. Adverse reactions
B. Expected side effects
C. Dissociated effects
D. Inverse reactions

90. Advanced directives allow a patient to
A. Receive all information related to a medical procedure and provide implied consent
B. Determine the right course of treatment and medication options in a post-operative setting
C. Preemptively determine what kind of care they agree to receive, such as palliative, or to assign a medical durable power of attorney
D. Seek autonomy and be self-governed in relation to taking prescribed medication and performing physical therapy

91. The auricle, external acoustic meatus, and tympanic membrane are all parts of the
A. Ear
B. Eye
C. Esophagus
D. Small intestine

92. Valve found between the left atrium and left ventricle
A. Pulmonary
B. Tricuspid
C. Aortic
D. Bicuspid

93. The deltoid is a common injection site for which type of injection
A. Subcutaneous
B. Intradermal
C. Intramuscular
D. Submuscular

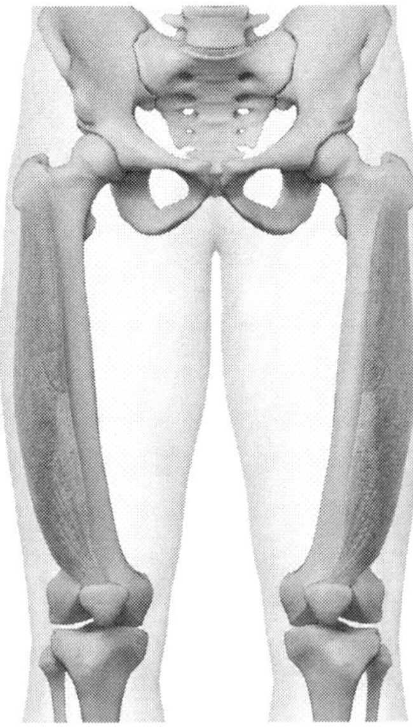

94. Identify the pictured muscle
A. Tensor fascia lata
B. Sartorius
C. Gracilis
D. Vastus lateralis

95. Acquiring funds owed to the office
A. Credit
B. Collection
C. Accounts receivable
D. Bankruptcy

96. An example of a close ended question is
A. "When was your last check-up?"
B. "How often do you take your medication?"
C. "Have you been prescribed antifungal medication?"
D. "Where was your last injection site?"

97. A spouse or child may be considered a
A. Dependent
B. Liability
C. Organization
D. Deductible

98. Depolarization of the right atrium and left atrium in an EKG is represented by
A. PR Interval
B. QRS Complex
C. P Wave
D. ST Segment

99. Catheters are most commonly responsible for
A. Draining bile from the gallbladder
B. Bringing food into the stomach
C. Draining urine from the urinary bladder
D. Draining pus from an abscess

100. The largest artery in the body
A. Aorta
B. Brachial
C. External iliac
D. Femoral

101. Bradycardia is a form of
A. Aneurysm
B. Heart murmur
C. Infarction
D. Arrhythmia

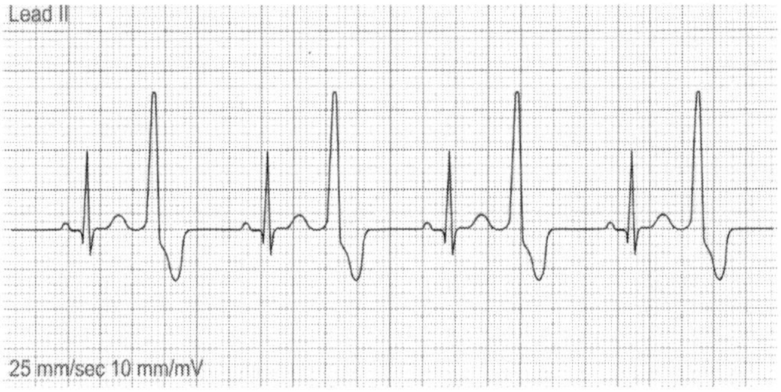

102. Identify the pictured form of arrhythmia
A. Couplet PVC
B. Complete heart block
C. Sinus bradycardia
D. Second-degree AV block

103. Injection administered into the dermis
A. Subcutaneous
B. Intradermal
C. Intramuscular
D. Subdermal

104. A statement given under oath and outside of court, used to determine what the person specifically knows about the case, and to document testimony for trial
A. Subpoena
B. Deposition
C. Arbitration
D. Mediation

105. Being legally responsible for every aspect of a medical practice is known as
A. Consent
B. Confidentiality
C. Liability
D. Malpractice

106. Instrument used to pull, grasp, or handle tissues or equipment
A. Scissors
B. Retractor
C. Scalpel
D. Forceps

107. A centrifuge is responsible for
A. Draining the urinary bladder
B. Separating solids from liquids
C. Delivering medication in vapor form
D. Measuring blood pressure

108. A puncture produces
A. Scraping of skin
B. Jagged edges
C. A hole
D. A clean cut

109. Temperature reading taken under the tongue
A. Sublingual
B. Axillary
C. Rectal
D. Aural

110. The carotid pulse, popliteal pulse, and dorsalis pedis pulse all help to measure the following vital sign
A. Blood pressure
B. Heart rate
C. Respiration
D. Temperature

111. An employer being held legally responsible for the actions of an employee
A. Respondeat superior
B. Subpoena ad testificandum
C. Res ipsa loquitor
D. Locum tenens

112. An error in diagnosis or treatment
A. Liability
B. Malpractice
C. Code of Ethics
D. Scope of Practice

113. All of the following are functions of the Digestive System except
A. Elimination of feces
B. Absorption of nutrients
C. Break-down of food
D. Elimination of urine

114. A nephrologist would be the type of specialist referred to in all of the following conditions except
A. Lupus
B. Pitting edema
C. Pyelonephritis
D. Uremia

115. M Codes are used to
A. Identify tumors and growths
B. Describe diseases other than disease or injury
C. Classify causes of injury
D. Document up to four different conditions

116. Of the following, which describes the numbered stroke method
A. Each area being scrubbed has a set amount of strokes used to ensure the area is cleaned
B. Each area being scrubbed is scrubbed for a set amount of time, usually three to five minutes
C. Each area being scrubbed is scrubbed three times utilizing providone-iodine to sanitize the area
D. Each area being scrubbed has five separate types of strokes utilized to ensure the area is fully cleaned

117. Ishihara tests are used to determine if a patient suffers from the following
A. Arrhythmia
B. Colorblindness
C. Glaucoma
D. Hearing loss

118. A subcutaneous injection should enter the subcutaneous layer at what angle
A. 45 degree
B. 90 degree
C. 10 degree
D. 35 degree

119. A spirometer measures
A. Volume of urine
B. Refraction of light through a liquid
C. Volume of air intake and output
D. Amount of acidity in a substance

120. Retractors are instruments used to
A. Perform incisions
B. Grasp, pull, or handle tissue or equipment
C. Cut bandages or sutures
D. Hold tissues open

121. Information on safely handling hazardous materials, health risks associated with handling materials, safely transporting, and safely storing materials is found in which of the following
A. Safety data sheets
B. Compliance reports
C. Emergency response plans
D. Public health disclosures

122. A nebulizer is used to
A. Prevent introduction of microorganisms
B. Deliver medication in vapor form
C. Drain urine from the bladder
D. Separate solids from liquids

123. Medication used to prevent the formation of blood clots
A. Anticoagulant
B. Antihistamine
C. Antipyretic
D. Analgesic

124. Which of the following is not a common injection site for an intramuscular injection
A. Deltoid
B. Abdomen
C. Ventrogluteal
D. Vastus lateralis

125. Which of the following is not one of the seven nutrients
A. Amino acids
B. Protein
C. Carbohydrates
D. Fiber

126. Act used to regulate the manufacture, import, possession, distribution, and use of narcotics
A. Genetic Information Nondiscrimination Act
B. Truth in Lending Act
C. Controlled Substances Act
D. Health Insurance Portability and Accountability Act

127. 500ml converts to
A. 1 quart
B. 100 liters
C. 1 pint
D. 5 liters

128. Group Health Benefits are offered by all of the following except
A. Employers
B. Unions
C. Associations
D. Government

129. In a blood pressure reading, the higher number represents
A. Heart rate
B. Diastolic pressure
C. Arterial contraction
D. Systolic pressure

130. Which of the following best describes a patient portal
A. A website a patient has access to that gives the patient all of their personal health information and history
B. The means in which a patient submits an insurance claim and appeal in case of claim denial
C. A form presented to the patient upon discharge discussing aspects of the patient's visit and follow-up care
D. Notes produced by surgeons detailing all aspects of a surgical procedure after the procedure has been completed

131. Alpha cells in the pancreas produce
A. Glycogen
B. Insulin
C. Glucagon
D. Bile

132. Arteries carry blood in which direction
A. Between the heart chambers
B. Towards the heart
C. Away from the heart
D. Between the heart valves

133. Signs of inflammation include
A. Heat, pain, redness, coldness
B. Pain, edema, swelling, redness
C. Swelling, heat, redness, pain
D. Redness, pain, heat, dehydration

134. The most common form of hemocytometer is
A. Nebulizer
B. Newcastle
C. Neopathic
D. Neubauer

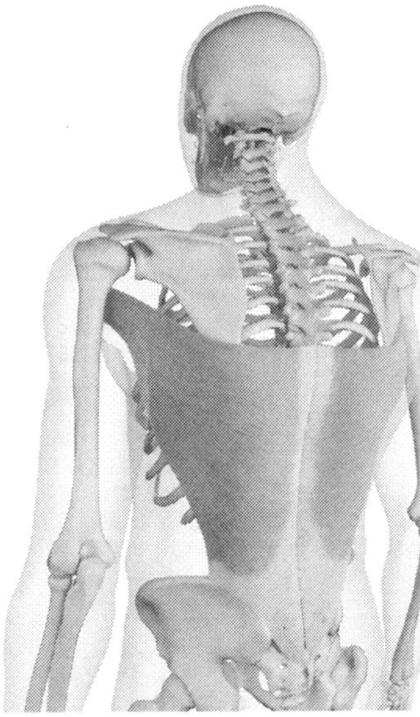

135. Identify the pictured muscle
A. Latissimus dorsi
B. Quadratus lumborum
C. External obliques
D. Rectus abdominis

136. Main type of cell that creates nervous tissue
A. Axon
B. Neuron
C. Dendrite
D. Astrocyte

137. Which of the following is not one of the four types of tissue
A. Nervous
B. Connective
C. Epithelial
D. Skeletal

138. Ringworm is a form of .
A. Fungus
B. Bacteria
C. Virus
D. Parasite

139. A myelogram is performed to test for
A. Improper functioning of the heart chambers
B. Problems in the spinal canal such as herniated discs, or meningitis
C. Possible presence of breast cancer
D. Proper functioning of muscles and nerves that innervate the muscles

140. The anterior thigh is a common injection site for which type of injection
A. Intramuscular
B. Subcutaneous
C. Intradermal
D. Submuscular

141. Which of the following needles has the largest diameter
A. 18 gauge
B. 14 gauge
C. 21 gauge
D. 27 gauge

142. A tort is
A. A wrongful act by one person that is responsible for an injury or harm to another person, and is considered a civil wrong that bears liability
B. An illegal act that carries less severe punishment than a felony, which carries a jail sentence of no longer than one year, but usually does not result in jail time
C. A form of alternative dispute resolution, in which both sides agree to come together and negotiate a form of settlement
D. A statement given under oath and outside of court, used to determine what the person specifically knows about the case, and to document testimony for trial

143. A scalpel is used to
A. Perform incisions
B. Close wounds
C. Pull, grasp, or handle equipment
D. Hold layers of tissue open

144. The fight or flight response is also known as
A. Sympathetic
B. Parasympathetic
C. Autonomic
D. Peripheral

145. All of the following are contagious conditions except
A. Mononucleosis
B. Herpes Simplex
C. Psoriasis
D. Impetigo

146. Blockage of a pore may result in the development of
A. Melanoma
B. Wart
C. Lupus
D. Acne

147. Deoxygenated blood enters the heart into which chamber
A. Right ventricle
B. Right atrium
C. Left atrium
D. Left ventricle

148. The diaphragm separates which body cavities from each other
A. Abdominal and pelvic
B. Thoracic and abdominal
C. Pelvic and thoracic
D. Dorsal and ventral

151. Debt borrowed to be paid at a later date
A. Collection
B. Credit
C. Bankruptcy
D. Accounts Receivable

152. Sutures are used to
A. Hold tissues open
B. Prevent introduction of microorganisms
C. Cut bandages
D. Close wounds

153. An autoclave sterilizes instruments by utilizing
A. Steam
B. Bleach
C. Gravity
D. Rubbing alcohol

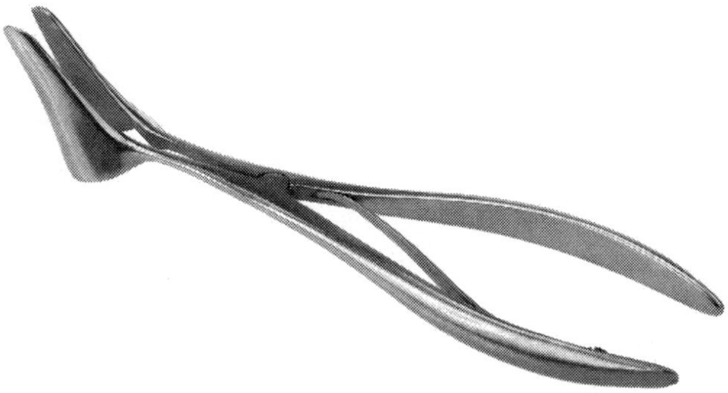

154. Identify the pictured instrument
A. Speculum
B. Retractor
C. Forceps
D. Laryngoscope

155. The bones of the wrist are also called
A. Carpals
B. Tarsals
C. Metacarpals
D. Phalanges

156. Insulin is produced by which organ
A. Pancreas
B. Liver
C. Gallbladder
D. Stomach

157. Dilation of blood vessels during the inflammatory stage is controlled by
A. Histamines
B. Leukocytes
C. Neutrophils
D. Fibrosis

158. Of the following which describes a relative risk
A. Comparing two demographics in relation to probability that a disease will develop
B. Examining a person's genetic profile to determine the likelihood a person will develop a disease
C. Determining a person's likelihood of contracting a viral infection based on their location
D. Comparing two different people and the diseases they have developed over a set period of time

159. Blood in the right ventricle is
A. Oxygenated
B. Deoxygenated
C. Clotted
D. Going backwards

160. The right and left sides of the heart are separated by the
A. Pulmonary veins
B. Tricuspid valve
C. Bicuspid valve
D. Septum

161. Instrument designed to open the nasal passages for further examination
A. Ophthalmoscope
B. Nasal speculum
C. Laryngoscope
D. Autoclave

162. Instrument used to listen to sounds throughout the body
A. Electrocardiogram
B. Laryngoscope
C. Stethoscope
D. Otoscope

163. Blood in the urine, usually a result of renal failure
A. Hyperemia
B. Pyelonephritis
C. Cystitis
D. Uremia

164. Amoxycillin and methicillin are forms of
A. Macrolides
B. Penicillin
C. Cephalosporins
D. Tetracyclines

165. Acute viral infection affecting the respiratory tract
A. Influenza
B. Pneumonia
C. Pneumothorax
D. Bronchitis

166. Instrument used to test the loss of hearing
A. Stethoscope
B. Audioscope
C. Laryngoscope
D. Otoscope

167. Collection is
A. Acquiring funds owed to the office
B. Liquidation of assets
C. Debt borrowed to be paid at a later date
D. Money owed to the office

168. HIPAA was enacted in
A. 1992
B. 1986
C. 1964
D. 1996

169. The large intestine converts chyme into
A. Bolus
B. Feces
C. Water
D. Bile

170. Heat creation is produced by which type of muscle tissue
A. Smooth
B. Cardiac
C. Skeletal
D. Adipose

171. An OB/GYN is a doctor who practices
A. Ophthalmology and gerontology
B. Otorhinolaryngology and gastroenterology
C. Oncology and genetics
D. Obstetrics and gynecology

172. A person who is not a senior citizen, but still requires care
A. Mature minor
B. Emancipated minor
C. Patient navigator
D. Dependent adult

173. A 90 degree angle is used when administering which injection
A. Intradermal
B. Intramuscular
C. Subcutaneous
D. Submuscular

174. Pacemakers are commonly implanted in patients who suffer from
A. Arrhythmia
B. Emphysema
C. Angina pectoris
D. Heart murmur

175. Mammary glands produce what substance
A. Oil
B. Sweat
C. Milk
D. Testosterone

176. An injury to a ligament
A. Sprain
B. Strain
C. Fracture
D. Dislocation

177. Vein found in the region of the armpit
A. Inguinal vein
B. Brachial vein
C. Femoral vein
D. Axillary vein

178. The pulmonary veins carry blood from the lungs to
A. The aorta
B. The body
C. The vena cava
D. The heart

179. The body of a letter is placed how many lines below the subject
A. Two lines
B. Three lines
C. Five lines
D. One line

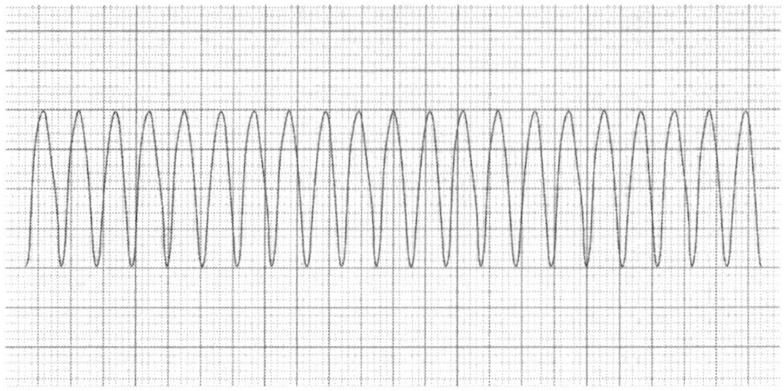

180. Identify the pictured form of arrhythmia
A. Ventricular tachycardia
B. Sinus arrest
C. Bigeminy PVC
D. Atrial flutter

181. Guiding moral principles
A. Code of ethics
B. Scope of practice
C. Liability
D. Negligence

182. An average range of blood sugar content over a three month span is tested using
A. Lipid profile test
B. Thyroid function test
C. Hemoglobin A1c test
D. Liver function test

183. Certain leukocytes perform phagocytosis, which is when cells perform what action
A. Eat substances
B. Absorb nutrients
C. Move from an area of high concentration to an area of low concentration
D. Transportation of oxygen and carbon dioxide

184. Cancer of connective tissue is known as
A. Sarcoma
B. Melanoma
C. Carcinoma
D. Lymphoma

185. The formation of scar tissue
A. Hypoplasia
B. Hyperplasia
C. Fibrosis
D. Inflammatory response

186. Inflammation of a joint
A. Osteoporosis
B. Arthritis
C. Dislocation
D. Subluxation

187. Scissors are used to
A. Perform incisions
B. Hold layers of tissue open
C. Close wounds
D. Cut tissue or bandages

188. The extent of a burn by total body area involved is determined by
A. First degree
B. The Rule of 9's
C. Quadrants
D. Contacting EMS

189. Expiration is also known as
A. Tidal volume
B. Blood pressure
C. Exhaling
D. Inhaling

190. The skin produces the following type of vitamin
A. Vitamin K
B. Vitamin A
C. Vitamin D
D. Vitamin B12

191. Insurance waste is defined as
A. Billing practices that cause an inappropriate increase in costs
B. Not reporting services or treatments on an insurance report in order to lower costs
C. Over-utilization of services that are unnecessary and drive up the cost of medical plans
D. Miscategorizing or falsifying an insurance report

192. An electroencephalogram measures
A. Muscle contractions
B. Heart rhythm
C. Blood pressure
D. Brain wave activity

193. A lack of hemoglobin in erythrocytes may result in
A. Decreased immune response
B. Raynaud's syndrome
C. Myocardial infarction
D. Anemia

194. Of the following, which condition is contagious
A. Ankylosing spondylitis
B. Osteoporosis
C. Trigeminal neuralgia
D. Mononucleosis

195. A wart is caused by
A. Parasite
B. Bacteria
C. Fungus
D. Virus

196. The inferior chambers of the heart are known as
A. Atria
B. Ventricles
C. Vena Cava
D. Aorta

197. Instrument used to test reflexes
A. Otoscope
B. Stethoscope
C. Percussion hammer
D. Forceps

198. An open-ended question is
A. Used when asking for feedback from a patient
B. Used to ask a patient if they have a heart condition
C. Used when only looking for a yes or no response
D. Used when a patient has allergies

199. The most abundant form of connective tissue found in the body
A. Fascia
B. Bone
C. Cartilage
D. Blood

200. The amount of money a business is reporting as an expense, usually in relation to a bank account
A. Debit
B. Credit
C. Asset
D. Debt

Answer Key on Page 321

Practice Test 2

1. The second phase of inflammation is called phagocytosis, which is the responsibility of
A. Leukocytes
B. Erythrocytes
C. Thrombocytes
D. Histamines

2. In a patient with herpes simplex, exposure to sunlight, stress, or hormonal changes may result in the development of
A. Impetigo
B. Decubitus ulcers
C. Cold sores
D. Acne

3. Inhalation and expiration contribute to which vital sign
A. Respiration
B. Blood pressure
C. Pulse
D. Temperature

4. The apical pulse helps to read heart rhythm and rate at what point in the body
A. Medial wrist
B. Apex of the heart
C. Proximal anterior thigh
D. Back of the knee

5. Natural pacemaker of the body, responsible for contracting the right and left ventricles
A. Phrenic nerve
B. Papillary muscles
C. SA node
D. Coronary arteries

6. The Rule of 9's is used to
A. Determine the nine regions of the body used to divide the abdomen
B. Determine the nine sections of the tongue that taste
C. Determine the extent of burns by total body area involved
D. Determine the gauge of a needle used for injections

7. E Codes are used to
A. Identify tumors and growths
B. Document procedures
C. Circumstances other than disease or injury
D. Classify cause of injury, poisoning, or adverse reaction to drugs

8. An incision produces
A. A hole
B. Jagged edges
C. Scraped skin
D. A clean cut

9. Which type of gland has no ducts
A. Endocrine
B. Exocrine
C. Eccrine
D. Mammary

10. Follicle-stimulating hormone, produced by the pituitary gland, affects what other structure in the body
A. Ovaries
B. Testes
C. Pancreas
D. Thyroid

11. A percussion hammer is used to test
A. Reflexes
B. Blood pressure
C. Electrical activity in the heart
D. Hearing loss

12. Which device assists in performing auscultation
A. Syringe
B. Sphygmomanometer
C. Stethoscope
D. Speculum

13. Melanoma is what type of tumor
A. Benign
B. Malignant
C. Idiopathic
D. Lymphatic

14. Swelling of the following gland results in a goiter
A. Pituitary
B. Thyroid
C. Thymus
D. Adrenal

15. The function of the mouth
A. Absorption
B. Mastication
C. Excretion
D. Secretion

16. Treating every person and fluid as infectious is known as
A. Emergency triage
B. Documentation
C. Contamination
D. Universal precautions

17. Thin connective tissue surrounding the brain and spinal cord, primarily responsible for providing protection
A. Pericardium
B. Serous membrane
C. Meninges
D. Peritoneal membrane

18. Visual acuity is defined as
A. The ability a person has to detect colors
B. The sharpness of a person's vision
C. The presence of cloudy lenses
D. A person's field of view, such as peripheral vision

19. Form of consent in which the patient gives consent verbally or in writing to have procedures or treatments performed
A. Implied consent
B. Returned consent
C. Denied consent
D. Expressed consent

20. A bacterial infection that enters the blood stream results in
A. Septicemia
B. Anemia
C. Gout
D. Leukemia

21. Vomiting is also known as
A. Defecation
B. Reflux
C. Emesis
D. GERD

22. Melatonin levels in the body fluctuate in response to the
A. Circadian rhythm
B. Heart rhythm
C. Circulatory system
D. Lymphatic system

23. Alveoli are located at the ends of
A. Pulmonary veins
B. Bronchial tubes
C. Bronchioles
D. Trachea

24. Adding information to an original code is achieved by utilizing
A. CPT bundlers
B. CPT upcoders
C. CPT addendums
D. CPT modifiers

25. The most common form of Vitamin A is
A. Calcium
B. Beta-carotene
C. Iron
D. Sodium

26. Which of the following part of blood is responsible for clotting of the blood in response to physical trauma
A. White blood cells
B. Red blood cells
C. Platelets
D. Plasma

27. An intradermal injection is administered into the
A. Subcutaneous layer
B. Epidermis
C. Dermis
D. Muscle

28. Which of the following is a visualization of the firing of an SA node
A. PR Interval
B. T Wave
C. P Wave
D. QRS Complex

29. A sphygmomanometer measures
A. Blood pressure
B. Heart rate
C. Volume of intake and output of air
D. Gravity of urine

30. The small intestine
A. Breaks down food into usable parts for absorption
B. Absorbs water from feces and eliminates waste
C. Absorbs nutrients from chyme into the blood
D. Transports food from the mouth to the stomach

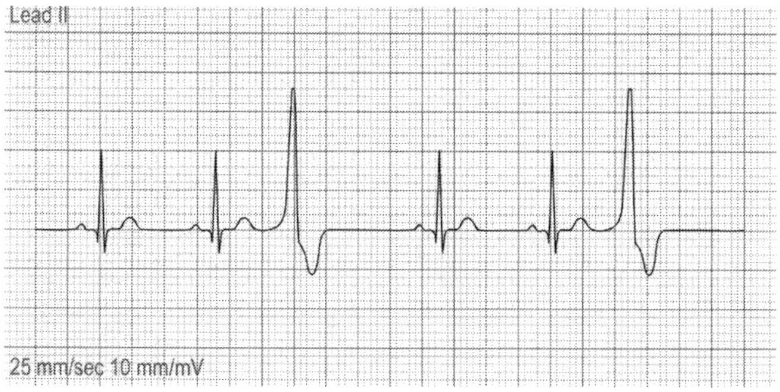

31. Identify the pictured form of arrhythmia
A. ST depression
B. Trigeminy PVC
C. ST elevation myocardial infarction
D. Bigeminy PVC

32. SCHIP is a form of health insurance specifically designed for which demographic
A. Dependent adults
B. Senior citizens
C. Military personnel
D. Children

33. Medication given to people who suffer from asthma to relax smooth muscle in the respiratory system
A. Bronchodilators
B. Expectorants
C. Decongestants
D. Statins

34. Part of the ear separating the outer ear and inner ear
A. Antihelix
B. Helix
C. Malleus
D. Tympanic membrane

35. Which of the following is not a common injection site for a subcutaneous injection
A. Scapula
B. Abdomen
C. Posterior and lateral arm
D. Anterior thigh

36. Vitamin D allows the body to absorb
A. Sodium
B. Beta-carotene
C. Potassium
D. Calcium

37. Secretions expelled by the lungs
A. Ammonia
B. Sputum
C. Saliva
D. Pus

38. A contusion is also known as
A. Bruise
B. Wart
C. Fracture
D. Hives

39. The kidneys
A. Reabsorbs urea into the blood stream and removes water
B. Eliminates waste from the bladder
C. Filter waste from the blood and reabsorb substances into the body
D. Produces norepinephrine to assist with the sympathetic nervous response

40. Sympathy is best described as
A. A person feeling compassion or pity for the other person and the situation they are in
B. A person puts themselves in the shoes of another, viewing a situation from the other person's point of view
C. A person actively listening to another person, asking questions and giving feedback when warranted
D. A person passively listening to another person, not responding but taking in information and possibly documenting the information

41. Which of the following is considered one of the four types of tissue in the body
A. Nervous
B. Smooth
C. Skeletal
D. Hair

42. Removing dead or damaged tissue from a wound to promote proper healing and scar tissue formation
A. Dilation and curettage
B. Hysterectomy
C. Debridement
D. Biopsy

43. Pseudo-epinephrine is a substance found in the following medications
A. Antihistamines
B. Expectorants
C. Bronchodilators
D. Decongestants

44. Necrosis of myocardium due to blockages in the coronary arteries leads to
A. Aneurysm
B. Heart murmur
C. Myocardial infarction
D. Arrhythmia

45. Urine flows from the kidneys through the ureters on its way to the
A. Urethra
B. Bladder
C. Bloodstream
D. Liver

46. The smallest type of blood vessel
A. Capillary
B. Artery
C. Vein
D. Arteriole

47. Malpractice is
A. An error in diagnosis or treatment
B. Being legally responsible for every aspect of a medical practice
C. Keeping information private and protected
D. Guiding moral principles

48. Medicare provides health insurance to
A. Low-income persons
B. Elderly
C. Dependents of active military personnel
D. Retired military personnel

49. Which of the following is not a main group of food
A. Lipids
B. Protein
C. Carbohydrates
D. Insulin

50. Vitamin A is produced and stored by the
A. Gallbladder
B. Liver
C. Spleen
D. Small intestine

51. Which of the following is used to bill Medicare
A. M Codes
B. ICD-9-CM
C. E Codes
D. CMS-1500

52. A collection of pus, usually localized
A. Psoriasis
B. Lesion
C. Wart
D. Abscess

53. Agency responsible for combating drug distribution within the United States
A. Occupational Safety and Health Administration
B. Drug Enforcement Administration
C. Food and Drug Administration
D. Substance Abuse and Mental Health Administration

54. Failure to perform essential actions that results in harm to a patient
A. Malpractice
B. Negligence
C. Liability
D. Consent

55. Inflammation of the kidneys
A. Hepatitis
B. Nephritis
C. Cystitis
D. Gastritis

56. Bronchodilators, expectorants, and decongestants all affect the
A. Respiratory system
B. Endocrine system
C. Nervous system
D. Cardiovascular system

57. Diarrhea may result in
A. Diverticulosis
B. Constipation
C. Ulcerative colitis
D. Dehydration

58. Type of drug that combats bacterial infection
A. Morphine
B. Antibiotics
C. Non-steroidal anti-inflammatory drugs
D. Immunizations

59. Of the following, which properly describes mensuration
A. Measuring structures or areas of the body
B. Tapping on areas of the body
C. Using the hands to physically move, adjust, or alter the location of a structure in the body
D. Listening to internal body sounds

60. Patient position simply requiring the patient to be seated, with the seat back set at an angle of 45 to 60 degrees
A. Fowler's
B. Lithotomy
C. Dorsal recumbent
D. Knee-chest

61. Allergic reactions in the body may be controlled with use of
A. Vasodilators
B. Statins
C. Antihistamines
D. Beta-blockers

62. Proper sputum collection technique
A. Patient coughs hard enough to dislodge phlegm, and phlegm spit into collection tube, which can be repeated over several days
B. Patient opens the mouth, the back of the throat is swabbed, then the swab is placed into a collection tube for testing
C. The patient sits upright, leans the head back, a swab is inserted into the nasal cavity, and the swab is then placed in a collection tube for testing
D. A person uses a tongue depressor to collect a saliva sample, and wipes the saliva on a card with spaces for collection of saliva on different days

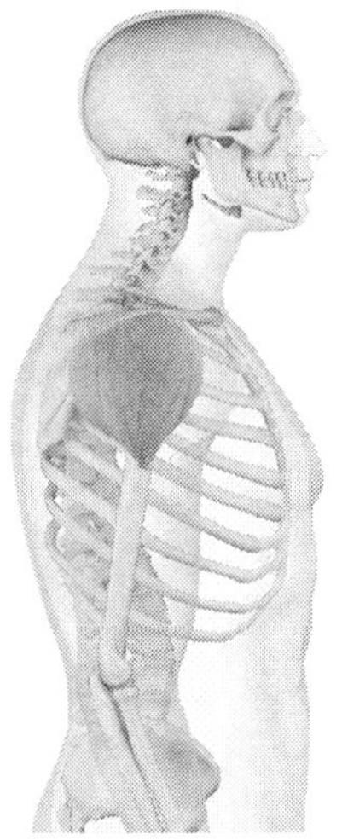

63. Identify the pictured muscle
A. Deltoid
B. Biceps brachii
C. Trapezius
D. Infraspinatus

64. The four types of tissue found in the body are
A. Muscular, smooth, skeletal, cardiac
B. Epithelial, connective, nervous, muscular
C. Epithelial, skeletal, connective, nervous
D. Connective, epithelial, nervous, smooth

65. Ureters transport what substance
A. Blood
B. Urine
C. Lymph
D. Feces

66. The aorta carries blood to the liver via the
A. Carotid artery
B. Renal artery
C. Hepatic artery
D. Pulmonary artery

67. The diameter of a needle is known as
A. Gauge
B. Stopper
C. Plunger
D. Point

68. Papillae are responsible for
A. Giving the tongue a rough texture
B. Detecting chemicals used for olfaction
C. Vibrating bones inside the ear to produce auditory sensation
D. Covering the eye to prevent penetration of light in areas other than the pupil

69. Portal of entry refers to
A. The route taken to administer intravenous injections
B. The manner in which an infectious agent enters its new host
C. The means to administer a suppository
D. The manner in which an endoscope is performed

70. Pressure felt as blood passes through an artery
A. Diastolic
B. Systolic
C. Venous
D. Cardiac

71. During the fight or flight response, what body function shuts down
A. Movement
B. Circulation
C. Respiration
D. Digestion

72. Keeping patient information private and protected
A. Liability
B. Confidentiality
C. Malpractice
D. Informed consent

73. Medicaid provides health care to
A. Elderly
B. Dependents of active military personnel
C. Low-income persons
D. Active military personnel

74. A T Wave is
A. Depolarization of the right ventricle and left ventricle
B. Repolarization of the right ventricle and left ventricle
C. Depolarization of the right atrium and left atrium
D. Time taken for a nerve impulse to travel from an SA node through atria into ventricles

75. Pain relievers are also known as
A. Antibiotics
B. Broncho-dilators
C. Diuretics
D. Analgesics

76. Utilizing active listening techniques and engaging with the patient to determine if the statements given are accurate is an important part of which OARS step
A. Open-ended questioning
B. Summarizing
C. Reflecting
D. Affirming

77. An artifact in an EKG reading is
A. An abnormality of non-cardiac origin
B. An abnormality caused by a pacemaker
C. A medical instrument that sends electrical impulses through the heart
D. A flatline

78. A refractometer measures
A. Volume of air intake and output
B. Gravity of urine
C. Refraction of light through a liquid
D. Blood pressure

79. A patient has been diagnosed with iron-deficient anemia. Which of the following medications would be considered an absolute contraindication for this patient
A. Analgesics
B. Expectorants
C. Diuretics
D. Anticoagulants

80. The tough, white portion of the eye, preventing light from penetrating the eye in locations other than the pupil
A. Retina
B. Sclera
C. Iris
D. Ciliary body

81. The most common form of cancer is found in the
A. Breast
B. Lungs
C. Pancreas
D. Skin

82. The presence of a fever
A. Cachexia
B. In Situ
C. Febrile
D. Pallor

83. Collecting a stool sample, a urea breath test, or in more serious cases, performing endoscopy and biopsy of the stomach are tests performed if a patient is suspected of the following infection
A. H. pylori
B. Herpes simplex
C. Strep throat
D. Influenza

84. Sublingual, axillary, rectal, and aural are all regions used to measure
A. Temperature
B. Blood pressure
C. Pulse
D. Respiration

85. Form of tort referring to invasion of a legal right
A. Injury
B. Negligence
C. Harm
D. Abuse

86. The left atrium receives blood from the
A. Pulmonary arteries
B. Pulmonary veins
C. Superior vena cava
D. Inferior vena cava

87. Atrial fibrillation is a form of
A. Heart murmur
B. Arrhythmia
C. Infarction
D. Aneurysm

88. Ibuprofen and acetaminophen are examples of
A. Antihistamines
B. Anti-inflammatory
C. Diuretics
D. Antipyretics

89. Lack of calcium entering into the bone can lead to
A. Scoliosis
B. Osteomyelitis
C. Dowager's hump
D. Osteoporosis

90. Contraction of the ventricles causes
A. Systole
B. Diastole
C. Dilation
D. Embolism

91. Inspiration is also known as
A. Inhaling
B. Exhaling
C. Tidal volume
D. Blood pressure

92. Hormone responsible for increasing heart rate and moving blood from digestive organs into the muscles
A. Aldosterone
B. Oxytocin
C. Growth hormone
D. Norepinephrine

93. Normal cells growing uncontrollably results in
A. Inflammation
B. Cyst
C. Cancer
D. Edema

94. Osteomyelitis and the most serious form of meningitis are the result of
A. Fungus
B. Bacteria
C. Virus
D. Parasite

95. Personal protective equipment helps to
A. Protect against lawsuits
B. Protect against infectious agents
C. Protect against weather
D. Protect against confidentiality

96. A QRS Complex is
A. Repolarization of right ventricle and left ventricle
B. Depolarization of the right atrium and left atrium
C. Conduction of an electrical impulse from the bundle of His through the ventricles
D. Depolarization of right ventricle and left ventricle

97. The amount required to be paid by a policy-holder before insurance payment begin
A. Dependent
B. Malpractice
C. Deductible
D. Bankruptcy

98. The inferior chambers of the heart are known as
A. Atria
B. Ventricles
C. Vena Cava
D. Aorta

99. Endocrine glands secrete their substances where
A. Into the respiratory passages
B. Onto a surface
C. Into the blood
D. Into the digestive organs

100. Accounts receivable
A. Money owed to the office
B. Acquiring funds or payment owed to the office
C. Debt borrowed to be paid at a later date
D. Assets sold off and funds distributed to creditors

101. Passive listening is
A. Listening to the patient and replying to statements being made
B. Questions used when asking for feedback
C. Questions that require only a yes or no response
D. Listening to the patient without offering a reply

102. Urea, ammonia, and creatinine are filtered from the body and form
A. Urine
B. Sweat
C. Oil
D. Feces

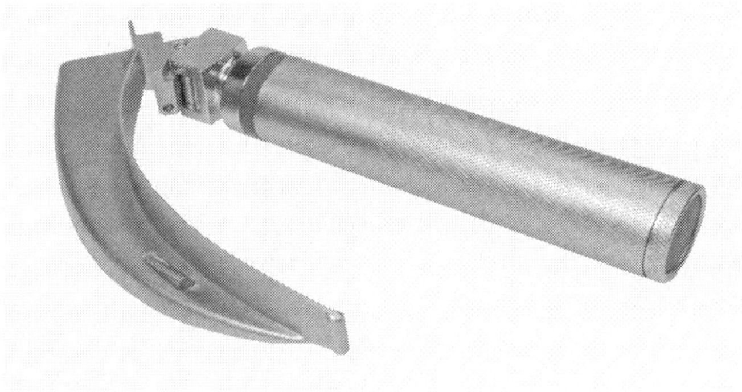

103. Identify the pictured instrument
A. Proctoscope
B. Anoscope
C. Endoscope
D. Laryngoscope

104. Shortness of breath
A. Dyspnea
B. Apnea
C. Asthma
D. Bronchitis

105. Health insurance provided to the elderly which is sponsored by the government
A. Medicaid
B. TRICARE
C. Medicare
D. PPO

106. Which of the following describes a biopsy
A. Attaching a portion of an artery to the base of the aorta and to the coronary artery that is suffering from a blockage to return blood to the heart muscle
B. Removing dead tissue to clean a wound
C. Removal of a small amount of bone tissue and placing it on another bone that may be lacking in sufficient tissue
D. Removal of tissue for microscopic examination

107. Antibodies play what role in the body's defense against pathogens
A. Destroy foreign substances
B. Engulf particles
C. Carrier cells for immunity
D. Create leukocytes

108. Function of cardiac muscle
A. Movement
B. Heat creation
C. Peristalsis
D. Transportation

109. Cholelithiasis is also known as
A. Gallstones
B. Kidney stones
C. Blood clot
D. Aneurysm

110. An antipyretic is a type of medication responsible for
A. Eliminating increased glucose
B. Decreasing inflammation
C. Destroying bacteria
D. Lowering fever

111. Infection of the skin by staphylococcus or streptococcus bacteria, forming yellowish scabs and sores around the mouth and nose
A. Psoriasis
B. Cold sore
C. Impetigo
D. Cellulitis

112. An increase of non-functioning leukocytes entering into medullary cavities may result in
A. Leukemia
B. Anemia
C. Melanoma
D. Non-Hodgkins Lymphoma

113. DNI stands for
A. Do not intubate
B. Do not inject
C. Do not intervene
D. Do not irradiate

114. The thorax is a common injection site for which type of injection
A. Intradermal
B. Intramuscular
C. Subcutaneous
D. Submuscular

115. Evacuated collection tubes may contain different colored rubber stoppers for which reason
A. To signify how much blood to collect
B. To signify which additive is in each tube
C. To signify which patient the blood sample belongs to
D. To signify the time of day the collection was taken

116. Temporary reactions to medications that are commonly known to occur, which are typically not life threatening
A. Side effects
B. Adverse reactions
C. Allergic reactions
D. Absolute contraindications

117. Of the following, which is not a primary way to reduce plaque accumulation in arteries
A. Increasing protein intake
B. Decreasing carbohydrate intake
C. Increasing sodium intake
D. Increasing vegetable intake

118. Sebum is produced by which type of gland
A. Mammary
B. Sudoriferous
C. Adrenal
D. Sebaceous

119. A catheter is
A. A tube inserted into the bladder
B. A tube inserted into the large intestine
C. A tube inserted into the esophagus
D. A tube inserted into the trachea

120. Forms provided to those with Medicare before a procedure is performed, instructing the patient a procedure may not be covered by Medicare
A. Remittance advice
B. Relative value unit
C. Advanced beneficiary notice
D. Explanation of benefits

121. A patient with Crohn's disease would be referred to which doctor
A. Gastroenterologist
B. Nephrologist
C. Neurologist
D. Dermatologist

122. Chronic bronchitis and emphysema are examples of
A. Chronic obstructive pulmonary disease
B. Asthma
C. Pleurisy
D. Congestive heart failure

123. Part of the brain split into two hemispheres
A. Cerebellum
B. Cerebrum
C. Brain stem
D. Diencephalon

124. Which of the following is considered a Schedule V drug
A. LSD
B. Analgesics
C. Oxycodone
D. Tramadol

125. A PR Interval represents
A. Conduction of electrical impulse from bundle of His through ventricles
B. Depolarization of the right atrium and right ventricle
C. Depolarization of the right ventricle and left ventricle
D. Time taken for an impulse to travel from the SA node through the atria into ventricles

126. A 45 degree angle is used in which type of injection
A. Submuscular
B. Intradermal
C. Subcutaneous
D. Intramuscular

127. An ophthalmoscope is used to inspect
A. The ears
B. The eyes
C. The large intestine
D. The mouth

128. Cytokines are created by B-cells and T-cells to allow the following
A. Communication between cells
B. Phagocytosis
C. Binding of an epitope with a paratope
D. Production of antibodies

129. Proteins are broken down into the following via digestive enzymes
A. Glucose
B. Amino acids
C. Lipids
D. Fructose

130. Peripheral vascular disease is usually the result of what other condition
A. Atherosclerosis
B. Myocardial infarction
C. Aneurysm
D. Muscular dystrophy

131. Thinning of mucous in the respiratory passages can be aided by which type of medication
A. Bronchodilator
B. Decongestant
C. Expectorant
D. Anticoagulant

132. Needles are used to
A. Administer injections
B. Contain pathogens
C. Relieve pain
D. Store medications

133. Part A of Medicare covers
A. Physician fees
B. Hospital expenses and inpatient stays
C. Prescription drug coverage
D. Diagnostic tests and screening tests

134. Bone located in the thigh
A. Tibia
B. Femur
C. Fibula
D. Talus

135. Thrombosis is defined as
A. Creation of a blood clot within a blood vessel
B. Blood clot blocking a valve in the heart
C. Weakening of an arterial wall, resulting in necrosis
D. Blockage of coronary arteries in the heart, producing an infarct

136. Instrument used to perform auscultation
A. Stethoscope
B. Anoscope
C. Vaginal speculum
D. Sphygmomanometer

137. Instrument used to hold layers of tissue open, allowing access to underlying tissue
A. Forceps
B. Scalpel
C. Retractor
D. Scissors

138. The emergency triage is
A. Classifying injuries by treatment urgency, treatment location, and severity
B. Noting all patient emergencies
C. Treating any fluid as contaminated
D. Wearing gloves and protective equipment

139. Obstetrics is a medical branch specifying in
A. Nerves and the nervous system
B. Muscles and bones
C. Pregnancy, labor, child delivery, and post-partum
D. Kidney, bladder, and urinary tract

140. Bacterial infection affecting the kidneys as a result of a urinary tract infection
A. Necrotising fasciitis
B. Cystitis
C. Pancreatitis
D. Pyelonephritis

141. Rupture of a cerebral aneurysm results in
A. Thrombosis
B. Stroke
C. Embolism
D. Myocardial infarction

142. A container sealed by a rubber stopper at the top is known as
A. Ampule
B. Insulin
C. Needle
D. Vial

143. Instrument used to deliver medication in vapor form
A. Bronchodilator
B. Beta-Blocker
C. Nebulizer
D. Electrocardiograph

144. Blood pressure is one of the primary means used to measure
A. Respiration
B. Temperature
C. Heart rhythm
D. Vital signs

145. Epithelial tissue is found in all of the following parts of the body except
A. Skin
B. Lungs
C. Heart
D. Intestines

146. The organization of a structure in the body
A. Organ → Tissue → Cell
B. Cell → Tissue → Organ
C. Cell → Organ → Tissue
D. Tissue → Cell → Organ

147. Pain in the chest and left arm resulting from myocardial ischemia
A. Angina pectoris
B. Atherosclerosis
C. Arteriosclerosis
D. Phlebitis

148. Which of the following is not a normal site to measure heart rate
A. Radial pulse
B. Brachial pulse
C. Axillary pulse
D. Femoral pulse

149. A stethoscope is used to
A. Inspect inner portions of the eye
B. Inspect the tympanic membrane
C. Open the nasal passages
D. Listen to sounds throughout the body

150. Nasopharyngeal swabs are primarily performed to test for the presence of
A. Fungal growths
B. Parasites
C. Throat cancer
D. Respiratory infections

151. Epinephrine and norepinephrine are produced by the
A. Thalamus
B. Pineal gland
C. Pituitary gland
D. Adrenal glands

152. Of the following, which condition is contagious
A. Influenza
B. Osteoarthritis
C. Raynaud's disease
D. Sebaceous cyst

153. An otoscope allows visual inspection of
A. Ears
B. Eyes
C. Nose
D. Mouth

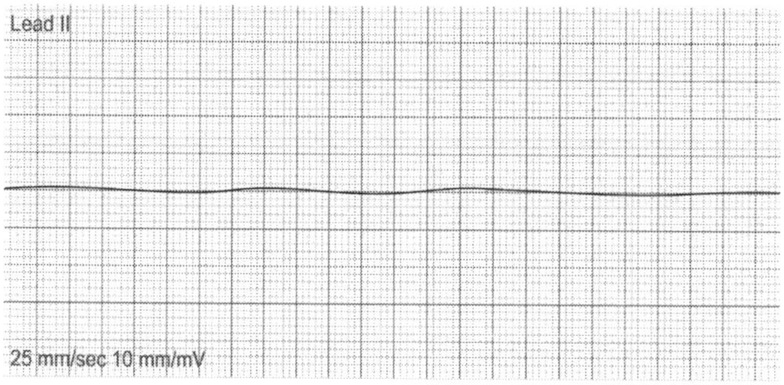

154. Identify the pictured arrhythmia
A. Cardiac asystole
B. Premature artial contraction
C. Complete heart block
D. Ventricular fibrillation

155. The regularity of a heart beat is known as
A. Heart rate
B. Systolic pressure
C. Heart rhythm
D. Diastolic pressure

156. Temperature, blood pressure, pulse, and respiration contribute to the reading of
A. Heart rhythm
B. Vital signs
C. Systolic pressure
D. Diastolic pressure

157. The pulmonary arteries carry
A. Deoxygenated blood
B. Oxygenated blood
C. Clotted blood
D. No blood

158. Upon stimulation of the sympathetic nervous response, the following reaction takes place in the heart
A. No change
B. Decreased heart rate
C. Increased heart rate
D. Cardiac arrest

159. Forceps are used to
A. Handle, pull, or grasp tissues or equipment
B. Hold layers of tissue open
C. Close tissues
D. Sterilization of equipment

160. Small knife used to perform incisions
A. Forceps
B. Scalpel
C. Retractor
D. Scissors

161. Ruffini corpuscles detect which of the following
A. Pain
B. Light sustained touch
C. Tension and stretching of skin
D. Warmth and cold

162. The sublingual salivary glands are located beneath the
A. Ears
B. Tongue
C. Nose
D. Mandible

163. Medical device used to view objects not visible to the naked eye
A. Centrifuge
B. Nebulizer
C. Microscope
D. Otoscope

164. Trauma to a vein may result in
A. Varicose veins
B. Phlebitis
C. Arteriosclerosis
D. Anemia

165. Ketamine, etomidate, and propofol are all forms of which medication
A. Steroids
B. Sedatives
C. Antidepressants
D. General anesthetic

166. Shaking of a part of the body that is involuntary
A. Tourette's syndrome
B. Paralysis
C. Tremor
D. Trigeminal neuralgia

167. Surgical procedure in which a baby is delivered after an incision is made in the mother's abdomen and uterus
A. Appendectomy
B. Abdominoplasty
C. Caesarian section
D. Bariatric surgery

168. Primary intention healing involves which of the following
A. A puncture being left open to prevent infection before being closed
B. Wound requiring granulated tissue to form to fill a wound in which the sides cannot be approximated
C. A wound that requires removal of tissue, in which tissue is replaced via grafts
D. A damaged area closed together via blood clots that allow new tissue to form underneath

169. The tricuspid valve is located between which two structures
A. Left ventricle and aorta
B. Left atrium and left ventricle
C. Stomach and esophagus
D. Right atrium and right ventricle

170. Bile is produced by the
A. Gallbladder
B. Liver
C. Stomach
D. Pancreas

171. Instrument used to cut tissue, bandages, or sutures
A. Scalpel
B. Forceps
C. Staples
D. Scissors

172. Low-density lipoprotein levels in the body can be reduced with the use of
A. Antihistamines
B. Beta-blockers
C. Statins
D. Expectorants

173. A heart murmur is described as
A. Necrosis of myocardium due to blockages in coronary arteries
B. Irregular heart rhythm due to random electrical impulses stimulating myocardium of ventricles
C. Hole in the ventricular septum, resulting in blood passing freely between ventricles
D. Blood flow moving backwards in the heart due to valve incompetence

174. Location of the sinoatrial node
A. Left ventricle
B. Right ventricle
C. Left atrium
D. Right atrium

175. Type of microscope used to count blood cells and thrombocytes
A. Hemocytometer
B. Centrifuge
C. Sphygmomanometer
D. Nebulizer

176. Which of the following contributes to the measurement of vital signs
A. Temperature
B. Injections
C. Skin rigidity
D. Pupil dilation

177. The ulnar pulse helps to read heart rhythm and rate at what point in the body
A. Lateral wrist
B. Back of the knee
C. Dorsal surface of the foot
D. Medial wrist

178. A doctor that specializes in the feet is known as a
A. Podiatrist
B. Oncologist
C. Radiologist
D. Rheumatologist

179. Mineral vital in the body's ability to transport oxygen and carbon dioxide
A. Iron
B. Potassium
C. Magnesium
D. Calcium

180. Mesentery is part of which serous membrane
A. Pleural
B. Pericardium
C. Peritoneal
D. Meninges

181. Ureters connect which two structures together
A. Liver and gallbladder
B. Bladder and urethra
C. Small intestine and pancreas
D. Kidneys and bladder

182. A vital sign reading of 120/80 mmHg measures
A. Pulse
B. Respiration
C. Temperature
D. Blood pressure

183. HMOs and PPOs are forms of
A. Worker's compensation
B. Government sponsored plans
C. Medicaid
D. Managed care organizations

184. Substance found in erythrocytes which attaches to oxygen and carbon dioxide, allowing transport of these molecules to parts of the body
A. Platelets
B. Leukocyte
C. Anemia
D. Hemoglobin

185. Heart activity is detected via an
A. Ophthalmoscope
B. Electroencephalogram
C. Audiometer
D. Electrocardiogram

186. Inflammation of the pleural membrane, resulting in chest pain
A. Bronchitis
B. Pneumonia
C. Pleurisy
D. Asthma

187. A patient is suspected of being affected by iron-deficient anemia. Which of the following tests is used to obtain an accurate reading of complete blood count
A. Erythrocyte sedimentation rate test
B. Prothrombin time test
C. Hematocrit test
D. Glucose test

188. Verifying a patient is covered by an insurance plan before a treatment or service is performed
A. Explanation of benefits
B. Insurance eligibility verification
C. Claim denial
D. Remittance advice

189. The primary reason a patient is seeking treatment
A. Family history
B. Chief complaint
C. Objective data
D. Subjective data

190. The urinary bladder is found in which body cavity
A. Cranial
B. Abdominal
C. Thoracic
D. Pelvic

191. Heart beats per minute is known as
A. Heart rate
B. Diastolic pressure
C. Systolic pressure
D. Heart rhythm

192. Osteoarthritis is also known as
A. De Quervain's disease
B. Rheumatoid arthritis
C. Wear-and-tear arthritis
D. Carpal tunnel syndrome

193. Neurotransmitter involved in the trembling movements involved with Parkinson's disease
A. Dopamine
B. Epinephrine
C. Norepinephrine
D. Melatonin

194. Blockage of the ureters by a kidney stone results in
A. Pyelonephritis
B. Cystitis
C. Uremia
D. Hydronephritis

195. Administering medication via a dropper into an area such as the eye or ear
A. Injection
B. Transdermal
C. Instillation
D. Intradermal

196. The cerebellum is formed by which type of tissue
A. Connective
B. Nervous
C. Epithelial
D. Muscular

197. Substance applied to a patient's skin before surgical procedures are performed to sterilize the skin and prevent post-operative infections
A. 10-1 bleach solution
B. Local anesthetic
C. Providone-iodine
D. 1-1 hydrogen peroxide solution

198. The final stage of an HIV infection is known as
A. AIDS
B. PPALM
C. ARC
D. HBV

199. The heart contains how many chambers
A. Four
B. Two
C. Three
D. Five

200. Glucagon is a digestive enzyme produced in the pancreas by
A. Alpha cells
B. Beta cells
C. Lymphatic tissue
D. Erythrocytes

Answer Key on Page 321

Congratulations! You've made it to the end of the study guide! How do you feel? How prepared are you? What do you still need to work on?

A common mistake a lot of people make is thinking they need to know EVERYTHING to pass the CMA exam. That's not the case at all. This line of thinking can make studying extremely stressful for some people.

Think about the amount of content you're actually studying when you crack open a book. It's a ton of information! It's extremely unlikely you're going to learn every bit of information. The key is to learn enough information where you can utilize test techniques like eliminating answers! You won't know everything on the test, but you can know enough where you'll likely recognize at least some piece of information in almost every test question. Even if you only see a term, identify that you've seen it, and that the term doesn't match with the information in the test question, that's still extremely helpful! Keep your head up, learn as much as you can, but don't get discouraged because you feel like you're not learning everything in this study guide. You'll be shocked at the amount of information you've learned, even when you feel like you haven't learned anything!

While grading the test, try to identify what strategies you incorporated that were successful, which strategies didn't work, information you may have been confused by or mixed up with other information, and do research on the questions you did not answer correctly. The way we learn is by challenging ourselves, breaking out of our comfort zones, and approaching each chance to engage with information as an opportunity to take one step closer towards passing the CMA exam.

Go forth with the determination necessary to conquer the CMA exam. You have the capability to do great things for yourself. Keep pushing, keep driving, keep enduring, and you will break through the wall ahead of you and vanquish the CMA exam.

I believe in you. Believe in yourself.

You can do this.

Full Length Practice Test Answer Keys

Practice Test 1				Practice Test 2			
1. D	51. C	101. D	151. B	1. A	51. D	101. D	151. D
2. A	52. C	102. A	152. D	2. C	52. D	102. A	152. A
3. C	53. A	103. B	153. A	3. A	53. B	103. D	153. A
4. B	54. C	104. B	154. A	4. B	54. B	104. A	154. A
5. C	55. B	105. C	155. A	5. C	55. B	105. C	155. C
6. A	56. A	106. D	156. A	6. D	56. A	106. D	156. B
7. C	57. C	107. B	157. A	7. D	57. D	107. A	157. A
8. C	58. C	108. C	158. A	8. A	58. B	108. D	158. C
9. A	59. A	109. A	159. B	9. A	59. A	109. A	159. A
10. D	60. D	110. B	160. D	10. A	60. A	110. D	160. B
11. A	61. B	111. A	161. B	11. A	61. C	111. C	161. C
12. A	62. C	112. B	162. C	12. C	62. A	112. A	162. B
13. B	63. A	113. D	163. D	13. B	63. A	113. A	163. C
14. C	64. A	114. A	164. B	14. B	64. B	114. A	164. B
15. B	65. D	115. A	165. A	15. B	65. B	115. B	165. B
16. D	66. C	116. A	166. B	16. D	66. C	116. A	166. C
17. B	67. A	117. B	167. A	17. C	67. A	117. C	167. C
18. C	68. A	118. A	168. D	18. B	68. A	118. D	168. D
19. C	69. A	119. C	169. B	19. D	69. B	119. A	169. D
20. A	70. D	120. D	170. C	20. A	70. B	120. C	170. B
21. A	71. C	121. A	171. D	21. C	71. D	121. A	171. D
22. D	72. A	122. B	172. D	22. A	72. B	122. A	172. C
23. D	73. D	123. A	173. B	23. C	73. C	123. B	173. D
24. C	74. B	124. B	174. A	24. D	74. B	124. B	174. D
25. B	75. C	125. A	175. C	25. B	75. D	125. D	175. A
26. A	76. D	126. C	176. A	26. C	76. C	126. C	176. A
27. A	77. A	127. C	177. D	27. C	77. A	127. B	177. D
28. A	78. D	128. D	178. D	28. C	78. C	128. A	178. A
29. A	79. D	129. D	179. A	29. A	79. D	129. B	179. A
30. B	80. B	130. A	180. A	30. C	80. B	130. A	180. C
31. A	81. C	131. C	181. A	31. B	81. D	131. C	181. D
32. B	82. B	132. C	182. C	32. D	82. C	132. A	182. D
33. C	83. C	133. C	183. A	33. A	83. A	133. B	183. D
34. B	84. C	134. D	184. A	34. D	84. A	134. B	184. D
35. A	85. D	135. A	185. C	35. A	85. A	135. A	185. D
36. A	86. A	136. B	186. B	36. D	86. B	136. A	186. C
37. A	87. C	137. D	187. D	37. B	87. B	137. C	187. C
38. D	88. D	138. A	188. B	38. A	88. D	138. A	188. B
39. A	89. A	139. B	189. C	39. C	89. D	139. C	189. B
40. C	90. C	140. B	190. C	40. A	90. A	140. D	190. D
41. B	91. A	141. B	191. C	41. A	91. A	141. B	191. A
42. D	92. D	142. A	192. D	42. C	92. D	142. D	192. C
43. A	93. C	143. A	193. D	43. D	93. C	143. C	193. A
44. D	94. D	144. A	194. D	44. C	94. B	144. D	194. D
45. B	95. B	145. C	195. D	45. B	95. B	145. C	195. C
46. D	96. C	146. D	196. B	46. A	96. C	146. B	196. B
47. A	97. A	147. B	197. C	47. A	97. C	147. A	197. C
48. A	98. C	148. B	198. A	48. B	98. B	148. C	198. A
49. A	99. C	149. B	199. D	49. D	99. C	149. D	199. A
50. C	100. A	150. B	200. A	50. B	100. A	150. D	200. A

R

S

References

This study guide was created with assistance from the following resources:

30 Second Anatomy: The 50 Most Important Structures and Systems in the Human Body, Each Explained in Half a Minute, 2013 – Gabrielle M. Finn, Judith Barbaro-Brown
ISBN: 978-1-4351-4065-3
Anatomica: The Complete Home Medical Reference, 2022 – Ken Ashwell
ISBN: 978-1-80242-058-6
The Four Hour Chef: The Simple Path to Cooking Like a Pro, Learn Anything, and Living the Good Life, 2013 – Timothy Ferriss
ISBN: 0-547-88459-1
Gray's Anatomy – Henry Gray
ISBN: 9781435145467
Essentials of Anatomy and Physiology(4th Edition), 2002 – Rod Seeley, Trent Stephens, Philip Tate
ISBN: 0-07-027260-3
Introducing Medical Terminology Specialties: A Medical Specialties Approach with Patient Records, 2003 – Regina Masters, Barbara Gylys
ISBN: 0-8036-0907-8
Exploring Medical Language: A Student-Directed Approach(5th Edition), 2002 – Myrna LaFleur Brooks
ISBN: 0-323-01218-3

Recommended Reading

The Obstacle is the Way: The Timeless Art of Turning Trials into Triumph, 2014 – Ryan Holiday
ISBN: 1591846358
Ego is the Enemy, 2016 – Ryan Holiday
ISBN: 1591847818
Outliers: The Story of Success, 2008 – Malcolm Gladwell
ISBN: 0316017930
Tools of Titans, 2016 – Timothy Ferriss
ISBN: 1328683788

The CMA Test Prep App

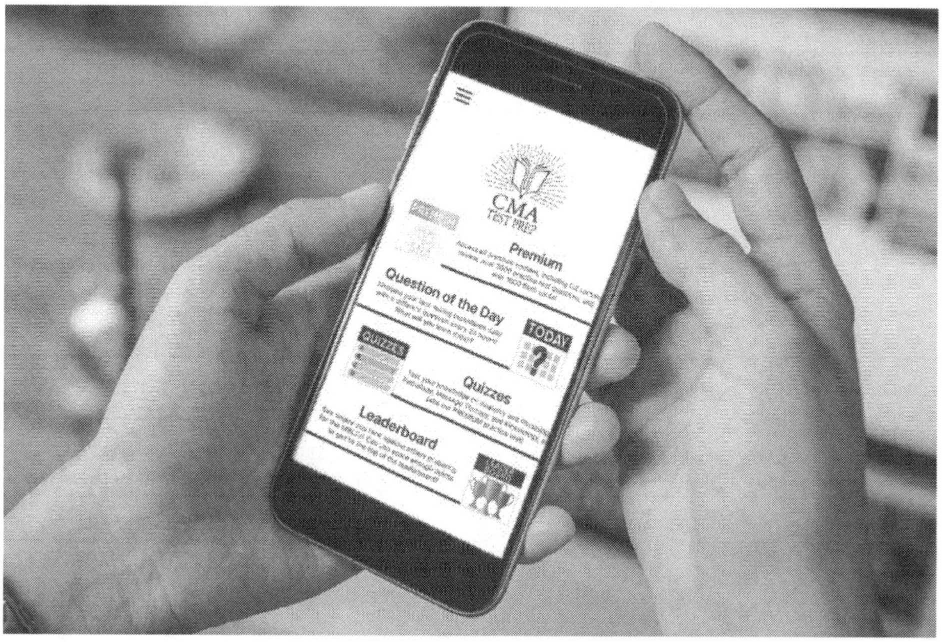

iPhone

Android

Presenting the brand new **CMA Test Prep App**! Available for iPhone and Android devices, the CMA Test Prep App features a full content review, 2200 practice test questions, a leaderboard so you can see how you stack up against other students taking practice tests, 1600 flash cards, and a fun matching assignment! Come learn on-the-go with the best CMA preparation app ever created! Free content includes 100+ practice test questions, and an updated Question of the Day every single day!

Just search for "**CMA Test Prep**" on the Apple App Store or Google Play Store, or scan the QR code for your device!

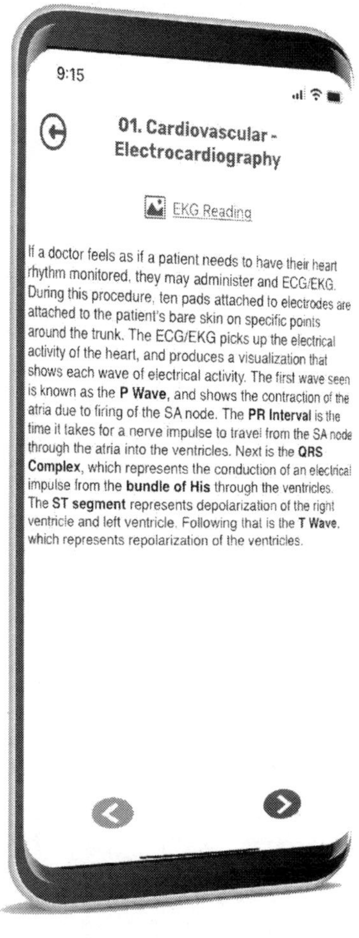

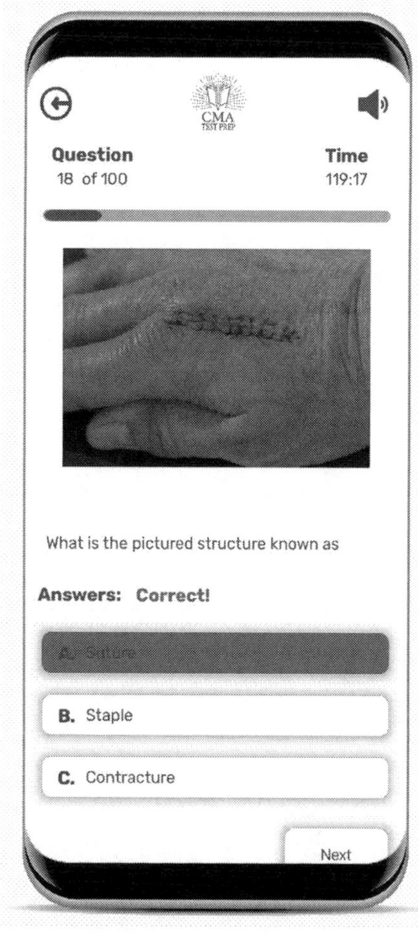

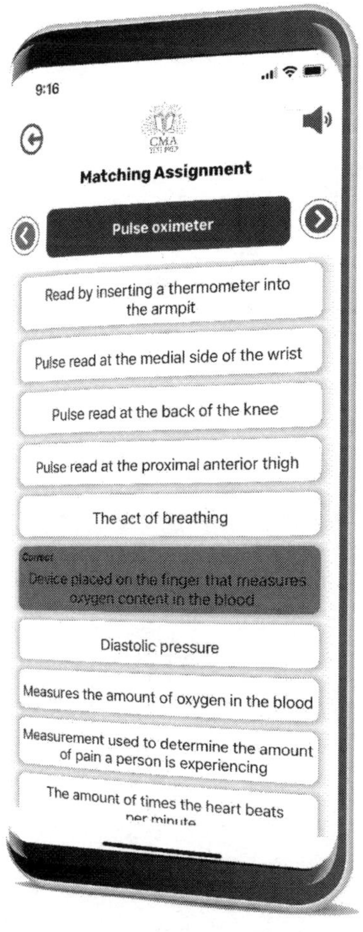

Made in the USA
Monee, IL
15 October 2026

65584646R10181